# ANNALS OF
# THE NEW YORK ACADEMY
# OF SCIENCES

Volume 944

EDITORIAL STAFF

*Executive Editor*
BARBARA M. GOLDMAN

*Managing Editor*
JUSTINE CULLINAN

*Associate Editor*
JOHN W. KENNEDY

The New York Academy of Sciences
2 East 63rd Street
New York, New York 10021

---

THE NEW YORK ACADEMY OF SCIENCES
(Founded in 1817)

BOARD OF GOVERNORS, September 2001–September 2002

TORSTEN N. WIESEL, *Chairman of the Board*
JOHN F. NIBLACK, *Vice Chairman of the Board*
BILL GREEN, *Past Chairman*
RODNEY W. NICHOLS, *President and CEO* [ex officio]

*Honorary Life Governors*
WILLIAM T. GOLDEN    JOSHUA LEDERBERG

JOHN T. MORGAN, *Treasurer*

*Governors*

| | | |
|---|---|---|
| ELEANOR BAUM | D. ALLAN BROMLEY | KAREN E. BURKE |
| LAWRENCE B. BUTTENWIESER | | PRAVEEN CHAUDHARI |
| JOHN H. GIBBONS | MICHAEL GOLDEN | RONALD L. GRAHAM |
| JACQUELINE LEO | WILLIAM J. McDONOUGH | SANDRA PANEM |
| RICHARD RAVITCH | RICHARD A. RIFKIND | JOHN J. ROCHE |
| SARA LEE SCHUPF | JAMES H. SIMONS | LEE VANCE |

HELENE L. KAPLAN, *Counsel* [ex officio]   NANCY B. EISENBERG, *Interim Secretary* [ex officio]

# BIOARTIFICIAL ORGANS III

## Tissue Sourcing, Immunoisolation, and Clinical Trials

ANNALS OF THE NEW YORK ACADEMY OF SCIENCES
Volume 944

# BIOARTIFICIAL ORGANS III

## Tissue Sourcing, Immunoisolation, and Clinical Trials

*Edited by*
*David Hunkeler, Alan Cherrington,*
*Aleš Prokop, and Ray Rajotte*

The New York Academy of Sciences
New York, New York
2001

*Copyright © 2001 by the New York Academy of Sciences. All rights reserved. Under the provisions of the United States Copyright Act of 1976, individual readers of the* Annals *are permitted to make fair use of the material in them for teaching and research. Permission is granted to quote from the* Annals *provided that the customary acknowledgment is made of the source. Material in the* Annals *may be republished only by permission of the Academy. Address inquiries to the Permissions Department (permissions@nyas.org) at the New York Academy of Sciences.*

Copying fees: *For each copy of an article made beyond the free copying permitted under Section 107 or 108 of the 1976 Copyright Act, a fee should be paid through the Copyright Clearance Center, Inc., 222 Rosewood Drive, Danvers, MA 01923 (www.copyright.com).*

∞ *The paper used in this publication meets the minimum requirements of American National Standard for Information Sciences—Permanence of Paper for Printed Library Materials. ANSI Z39.48-1984.*

## Library of Congress Cataloging-in-Publication Data

Bioartificial organs III : tissue sourcing, immunoisolation, and clinical trials / edited by David Hunkeler ... [et al.].
   p. ; cm. — (Annals of the New York Academy of Sciences, ISSN 0077-8923 ; v. 944)
   Includes bibliographical references and index.
   ISBN 1-57331-342-4 (cloth : alk. paper) — ISBN 1-57331-343-2 (pbk. : alk. paper)
   1. Artificial organs—Congresses. 2. Biomedical materials—Congresses. 3. Transplantation of organs, tissue, etc.—Congresses. 4. Pancreatic beta cells—Transplantation—Congresses. 5. Blood substitutes—Congresses. I. Title: Bioartificial organs 3. II. Title: Bioartificial organs three. III. Hunkeler, David. IV. Series.
   [DNLM: 1. Artificial Organs—Congresses. 2. Biocompatible Materials—Congresses. 3. Tissue Culture—Congresses. 4. Transplantation Tolerance—Congresses. WO 176 B61471 2001]
   Q11 .N5 vol. 944
   [RD130]
   500 s—dc21
   [617.9'5]

                                        2001044610
                                            CIP

K-M Research/CCP
*Printed in the United States of America*
**ISBN 1-57331-342-4** (cloth)
**ISBN 1-57331-343-2** (paper)
**ISSN 0077-8923**

ANNALS OF THE NEW YORK ACADEMY OF SCIENCES

Volume 944
November 2001

# BIOARTIFICIAL ORGANS III: TISSUE SOURCING, IMMUNOISOLATION, AND CLINICAL TRIALS[a]

*Editors*
DAVID HUNKELER, ALAN CHERRINGTON, ALEŠ PROKOP, AND RAY RAJOTTE

## CONTENTS

| | |
|---|---|
| Acknowledgments | xi |

### Part I. Introduction and Historical Perspective

| | |
|---|---|
| Allo Transplants Xeno: As Bioartificial Organs Move To The Clinic. Introduction. *By* DAVID HUNKELER | 1 |
| Bioartificial Organs: Glossary of Terms | 7 |
| Historical Perspectives of Hybrid Hepatic Assist Devices: Tissue Sourcing, Immunoisolation, and Clinical Trial. *By* YUKIHIKO NOSÉ | 18 |

### Part II. Tissue Sourcing

| | |
|---|---|
| Use of Small Animal Models for Screening Immunoisolation Approaches to Cellular Transplantation. *By* RONALD G. GILL | 35 |
| *In Vitro* Maturation of Neonatal Porcine Islets: A Novel Model for the Study of Islet Development and Xenotransplantation. *By* TANYA M. BINETTE, JANNETTE M. DUFOUR, AND GREGORY S. KORBUTT | 47 |

### Part III. Immunoisolation and Encapsulation

| | |
|---|---|
| Hydrogels for Biomedical Applications. *By* ALLAN S. HOFFMAN | 62 |
| Production of Alginate Beads by Emulsification/Internal Gelation. *By* D. PONCELET | 74 |
| Non-Invasive Monitoring of a Bioartificial Pancreas *in Vitro* and *in Vivo*. *By* IOANNIS CONSTANTINIDIS, ROBERT LONG, JR., COLIN WEBER, SUSAN SAFLEY, AND ATHANASSIOS SAMBANIS | 83 |

[a]This volume is the result of a conference entitled **Bioartifical Organs III: Tissue Sourcing, Immunoisolation, and Clinical Trials**, held on October 7–11, 2000, in Davos, Switzerland.

NMR Spectroscopy in β Cell Engineering and Islet Transplantation.
*By* KLEARCHOS K. PAPAS, CLARK K. COLTON, JOHN S. GOUNARIDES,
ERIC S. ROOS, MARY ANN C. JAREMA, MICHAEL J. SHAPIRO,
LEO L. CHENG, GARY W. CLINE, GERALD I. SHULMAN, HAIYAN WU,
SUSAN BONNER-WEIR, AND GORDON C. WEIR ....................... 96

Optimal Conditions of Transplantable Binary Polyelectrolyte Microcapsules.
*By* ARTUR BARTKOWIAK........................................... 120

Mass Production of Embryoid Bodies in Microbeads. *By* JOSEF P. MAGYAR,
MOHAMED NEMIR, ELISABETH EHLER, NICOLAI SUTER,
JEAN-CLAUDE PERRIARD, AND HANS M. EPPENBERGER................. 135

Soft, Porous Poly(D,L-lactide-co-glycotide) Microcarriers Designed for *ex Vivo*
Studies and for Transplantation of Adherent Cell Types Including
Progenitors. *By* ARRON S.L. XU AND LOLA M. REID ................ 144

Pectin-Based Microspheres: A Preformulatory Study. *By* ELISABETTA ESPOSITO,
RITA CORTESI, GIOVANNI LUCA, AND CLAUDIO NASTRUZZI ............ 160

Approaches to Development of Microencapsulated Form of the Live
Measles Vaccine. *By* E.A. NECHAEVA, N. VARAKSIN, T. RYABICHEVA,
M. SMOLINA, T. KOLOKOLTSOVA, A. VILESOV, N. AKSENOVA,
R. STANKEVICH, AND R. ISIDOROV................................ 180

## Part IV. Biomaterial Purification and Compatability

Purification of Polymeric Biomaterials. *By* CHRISTINE WANDREY AND
DIANELYS SAINZ VIDAL .......................................... 187

A Novel Class of Amitogenic Alginate Microcapsules for Long-Term
Immunoisolated Transplantation. *By* ULRICH ZIMMERMANN,
FRANK THÜRMER, ANETTE JORK, MEIKE WEBER, SASKIA MIMIETZ,
MARKUS HILLGÄRTNER, FRANK BRUNNENMEIER, HEIKO ZIMMERMANN,
INES WESTPHAL, GÜNTER FUHR, ULRIKE NÖTH, AXEL HAASE,
ANDRE STEINERT, AND CHRISTIAN HENDRICH ....................... 199

Transplantation of Alginate Microcapsules with Proliferating Cells in Mice:
Capsular Overgrowth and Survival of Encapsulated Cells of Mice and
Human Origin. *By* ANNE MARI ROKSTAD, BÅRD KULSENG,
BERIT L. STRAND, GUDMUND SKJÅK-BRÆK, AND TERJE ESPEVIK......... 216

## Part V. Islet and Bioartificial Pancreas

An Overview of the Immune System with Specific Reference to Membrane
Encapsulation and Islet Transplantation. *By* DEREK W.R. GRAY .......... 226

Cellular Support Systems for Alginate Microcapsules Containing Islets,
as Composite Bioartificial Pancreas. *By* RICCARDO CALAFIORE,
GIOVANNI LUCA, MARIO CALVITTI, LUCA M. NERI, GIUSEPPE BASTA,
SILVANO CAPITANI, ENNIO BECCHETTI, AND PAOLO BRUNETTI........... 240

Preclinical Development of the Islet Sheet. *By* RICHARD STORRS,
RANDY DORIAN, SCOTT R. KING, JONATHAN LAKEY, AND HORACIO RILO.. 252

Engineering Tolerance into Transplanted β Cell Lines. *By* BERNARD THORENS, PHILIPPE DUPRAZ, AND SANDRA COTTET............................ 267

*In Vitro* Test of New Biomaterials for the Development of a Bioartificial Pancreas. *By* N. LEMBERT, P. PETERSEN, J. WESCHE, P. ZSCHOCKE, A. ENDERLE, M. DOSER, H. PLANCK, H.D. BECKER, AND H.P.T. AMMON............. 271

Newly Developed Aminopropyl-Silicate Immunoisolation Membrane for a Microcapsule-Shaped Bioartificial Pancreas. *By* SHINJI SAKAI, TSUTOMU ONO, HIROYUKI IJIMA, AND KOEI KAWAKAMI................ 277

## Part VI. Bioartificial Kidney and Liver

The Role of a Bioengineered Artificial Kidney in Renal Failure. *By* WILLIAM H. FISSELL, JASON KIMBALL, SHERRILL M. MACKAY, ANGELA FUNKE, AND H. DAVID HUMES............................ 284

Derivation of Pharmacokinetics Equations for Quantitative Evaluation of Bioartificial Liver Functions. *By* Y.-G. PARK, H. IWATA, AND Y. IKADA ... 296

Development of a Hybrid Liver Support System. *By* I.M. SAUER, N. OBERMEYER, D. KARDASSIS, T. THERUVATH, AND J.C. GERLACH...... 308

Advances in Bioartificial Liver Assist Devices. *By* JOHN F. PATZER II........ 320

Effect of Flow Configuration and Membrane Characteristics on Membrane Fouling in a Novel Multicoaxial Hollow-Fiber Bioartificial Liver. *By* JEFFREY M. MACDONALD, STEPHEN P. WOLFE, INDRAJIT ROY-CHOWDHURY, HIROSHI KUBOTA, AND LOLA M. REID...... 334

Evaluating the Performance of a Hybrid Artificial Liver Support System With a Recoverable Hepatic Failure Rat Model. *By* HIROYUKI IJIMA, AYAKO NOGUCHI, TAKEYUKI KATSUNO, TSUTOMU ONO, KOHJI NAKAZAWA, KAZUMORI FUNATSU, AND KOEI KAWAKAMI......... 344

Development of a Coculture Model of Encapsulated Cells. *By* LAURENCE CANAPLE, NATHALIE NURDIN, NELA ANGELOVA, DAVID HUNKELER, AND BÉATRICE DESVERGNE...................... 350

## Part VII. Blood Substitutes and Endocrinology: Clinical Trials

Present Status of Modified Hemoglobin as Blood Substitutes and Oral Therapy for End Stage Renal Failure Using Artificial Cells Containing Genetically Engineered Cells. *By* THOMAS MING SWI CHANG..................... 362

β Cell Replacement for the Treatment of Diabetes. *By* JOSÉ OBERHOLZER, CHRISTIAN TOSO, FRÉDÉRIC RIS, PASCAL BUCHER, FRÉDÉRIC TRIPONEZ, ALP DEMIRAG, JINNING LOU, AND PHILIPPE MOREL................... 373

## Part VIII. Tissue Engineering

Standards and Guidelines for Biopolymers in Tissue-Engineered Medical Products: ASTM Alginate and Chitosan Standard Guides. *By* MICHAEL DORNISH, DAVID KAPLAN, AND ØYVIND SKAUGRUD........ 388

Hepatic Progenitors and Strategies for Liver Cell Therapies. *By* R. SUSICK, N. MOSS, H. KUBOTA, E. LECLUYSE, G. HAMILTON, T. LUNTZ, J. LUDLOW, J. FAIR, D. GERBER, K. BERGSTRAND, J. WHITE, A. BRUCE, O. DRURY, S. GUPTA, AND L.M. REID............................ 398

Formation of Sertoli Cell–Enriched Tissue Constructs Utilizing Simulated Microgravity Technology. *By* DON F. CAMERON, JOELLE J. HUSHEN, STANLEY J. NAZIAN, ALISON WILLING, SAM SAPORTA, AND PAUL R. SANBERG ............................ 420

The Influence of Extracellular Matrix on the Generation of Vascularized, Engineered, Transplantable Tissue. *By* OLIVER C.S. CASSELL, WAYNE A. MORRISON, AURORA MESSINA, ANTHONY J. PENINGTON, ERIK W. THOMPSON, GEOFFREY W. STEVENS, JILSKA M. PERERA, HYNDA K. KLEINMAN, JOHN V. HURLEY, ROSALIND ROMEO, AND KENNETH R. KNIGHT ............................................. 429

An Approach to Constructing Three-Dimensional Tissue. *By* IN KAP KO AND HIROO IWATA ................................. 443

## Part IX. Perspectives

Objectively Assessing Bioartificial Organs. *By* D. HUNKELER, A. REHOR, I. CEAUSOGLU, U. SCHULDT, L. CANAPLE, P. BERNARD, A. RENKEN, L. RINDISBACHER, AND N. ANGELOVA............................. 456

Bioartificial Organs in the Twenty-first Century: Nanobiological Devices. *By* ALEŠ PROKOP ............................................... 472

Index of Contributors ................................................ 491

**Financial assistance was received from:**
- BELLEVUE ASSET MANAGEMENT
- EUROPEAN COMMUNITY THROUGH THE COST 840 ENCAPSULATION NETWORK
- FONDS NATIONAL SUISSE
- INOTECH ENCAPSULATION AG
- JUVENILE DIABETES FOUNDATION INTERNATIONAL
- NATIONAL INSTITUTES OF HEALTH (USA)
- NATIONAL SCIENCE FOUNDATION (USA)
- NISCO ENGINEERING
- NOVARTIS PHARMACEUTICALS CANADA INC.
- PRONOVA BIOMEDICAL
- UNITED ENGINEERING FOUNDATION

The New York Academy of Sciences believes it has a responsibility to provide an open forum for discussion of scientific questions. The positions taken by the participants in the reported conferences are their own and not necessarily those of the Academy. The Academy has no intent to influence legislation by providing such forums.

# Acknowledgments

The organizing committee would like to thank Barbara Hickernell and her staff at the United Engineering Foundation for their efforts, over two years, to bring the third Bioartificial Organs conference to fruition. It was at their initiative that we moved the American-centered biannual event to Europe. The attendance, quality of presentations, and debate, as well as the new participants, are strong testaments to their vision. We would also like to thank the following organizations for financial support: Bellevue Asset Management, European Community through the COST 840 Encapsulation Network, Fonds National Suisse, Inotech Encapsulation AG, Juvenile Diabetes Foundation International, National Institutes of Health (USA), National Science Foundation (USA), Nisco Engineering, Novartis Pharmaceuticals Canada Inc., Pronova Biomedical, and the United Engineering Foundation.

The organizers acknowledge the fine work of Alan Cherrington on the awards committee and congratulate the lifetime recipient, Anthony Sun, of the University of Toronto. The outstanding Scientific Achievement award was presented to Ray Rajotte of the University of Alberta. The organizing committee and session chairs are also grateful for the technical advice provided prior to and during the conference by UEF Biotechnology Liaison, Allen Laskin. The organizer would like to thank the co-organizers for their support in writing the grants that funded the event and the postconference reports, as well as in selecting the topics, session chairs, and recommending invited speakers. The event, and the subsequent book, would not have been possible without their continued dedication, which has now spanned eight years and three events. The invaluable contributions and advice of the past Bioartificial Organs Chair, Aleš Prokop, are particularly noteworthy, as is the contribution of José Maria Hernandez Gil for providing the original design for the cover art and Klaus Eichler for his advice on the organization of large events.

The organizer is indebted to the assistance of Ingrid Margot. The majority of the speakers and authors benefited from her excellent organizational skills. Ingrid also participated in the logistics of Bioartificial Organs III, in Davos, as well as in the associated Biotechnology Market. Simply, had the organizer been left to himself, the event would not have taken place. Ingrid, thank you for so much. That you fulfilled your job description is evident to all, that you succeeded wonderfully is a trophy for yourself, and let me thank you on behalf of all the participants. As a note in closing, when one hires a partner, as a secretary to a conference surely is, one hopes that this person has both big dreams and feet firmly planted in reality. It is so very often difficult to identify such individuals *a priori*, but Ingrid Margot is just such a person. It should also be footnoted, hopefully without embarrassing her, that she also raised one-sixth of the funds for the Bioartificial Organs conference. For so very much of her help, this book is dedicated to Ingrid Margot.

DAVID HUNKELER
*Lausanne, Switzerland*
*March 15, 2001*

# Allo Transplants Xeno:
# As Bioartificial Organs Move To The Clinic

## Introduction

DAVID HUNKELER

*Laboratory of Polyelectrolytes and BioMacromolecules,*
*Swiss Federal Institute of Technology, Lausanne, Switzerland*

### BACKGROUND

The Bioartificial Organs conference series was initiated in 1993 by Aleš Prokop at Vanderbilt University. The first meeting, which attracted 75 attendees to Nashville, Tennessee, was held in July 1996. BIO+AO II was held in Canmore, Alberta, Canada in July 1998, involving 100 participants and, during October 7–12, 2000, the third conference in the series was held in Davos, Switzerland. BIO+AO cloisters groups that do not normally interact at meetings, including biotech and medtech executives, medical professionals, and biotech and medtech academics, all of whom are approximately equally represented. Interdisciplinary and international spin-offs are part of the deliverables from the conference, which could be more appropriately considered a retreat.

Bioartificial organs, as a discipline, addresses advances in cell transplantation that have recently included the remarkable successes in islet therapy for the treatment of diabetes. It also involves the development of novel materials, and their purification, as well as the interaction between science and regulation, as for example, with respect to the depyrogenation of natural and synthetic materials intended for human transplantation. The developments, since the Canmore meeting in 1998, include new start-up firms and not-for-profit foundations, the advancement in clinical trials, and consolidation in research and development, along with an increase in funding, both public and private.

Overall, bioartificial organs are forecast to be a multibillion-dollar industry by 2007 and they participate during the coming years' anticipated renaissance in the valuation of the biotech industry, and shareholder value in general. Commercially, bioartificial organs embed the principles of the old economy, including innovation, in-house development, and excess capacity.

Address for correspondence: David Hunkeler, Laboratory of Polyelectrolytes and BioMacromolecules, Swiss Federal Institute of Technology, Lausanne, Switzerland.
<david.hunkeler@epfl.ch>

# BIOARTIFICIAL ORGANS III: TISSUE SOURCING, IMMUNOISOLATION, AND CLINICAL TRIALS

The Davos meeting attracted 88 participants from five continents and 17 countries. It focused, as did the preceding two meetings,[1] on the interface between biotechnology, medicine and materials science, highlighting clinical advances in immunoisolated cell transplantation. Bioartificial organs include extracorporeal devices, such as the novel bioartificial kidney, as well as existing clinical therapies for hepatic failure, applied as a bridge to whole-organ transplantation. For the first time, the bioartificial heart was also presented. Specific advances, highlighted during Bioartificial Organs III, included an update on the Edmonton Protocol[2] involving allograft islet transplantation as a diabetes therapy, and a new understanding of the glucose cycle. Clinical trials on artificial blood substitutes and the control of pain were also summarized.

## *Diabetes Reversal and the Bioartificial Pancreas*

Ray Rajotte's Surgical Medical Research Institute (University of Alberta) has been able to stabilize the blood glucose levels for brittle diabetics, for more than one year. Rajotte believes the minute-to-minute control provided by islet "cell" therapy will reduce the end stage complications of diabetes. For example, 30% of the patients in the present study are expected to avoid death by kidney failure. In addition to his preliminary revelations in the *New England Journal of Medicine* disclosure, Rajotte reported in Davos, for the first time, that the thirteen patients who have been off insulin have exhibited no deterioration in C-peptide or hemoglobin levels. This 100% diabetes reversal should be weighed against historical data for islet transplantation (10% success for patients treated between 1990 and 1999). The 13 patients required an average of 11,000 islets per kilogram of body mass, with two transplants, carried out in the radiology department, as outpatients. All patients were at work the following day.

Rajotte noted that steroids are deleterious to islets and that minimizing the cold ischemia time is crucial. The elimination of xenoproteins and the isolation of islets immediately after receiving the tissue are also critical. Rajotte further commented that, in Alberta, the pancreas is the priority tissue, which certainly may account for the fact that this institute reports islets with higher stimulation, and better cryopreservability, than all others globally. In many centers the pancreas is removed only late in the cadaver process.

A JDF-funded multicenter trial involving six hospitals in the US, one in Canada, and three in Europe will attempt to repeat the diabetes reversal achieved with the Edmonton Protocol. In terms of the future, Rajotte believes that, as important as the new results are, a clinical therapy for diabetes requires a bioartificial pancreas. Therefore, he and Greg Korbutt, are encapsulating islets in calcium-alginate to enhance viability. The alginate microbeads reduce the number of islets required for diabetes reversal from 2,000 to 500 in mice models, due to the presence of an attachment matrix. The cotransplantation of islets in Sertoli cells, protecting islets from immune response, is also being investigated as alternative transplant sites for the bioartificial pancreas. Rajotte and others feel that drainage into the portal vein is necessary and, therefore, he targets bioartificial pancreas transplantation into a recoverable omental pouch.

## *New Advances in the Treatment of Diabetes*

Alan Cherrington of Nashville's Vanderbilt University Medical Center noted that the beta cell, in its natural conformation, responds exquisitely to minute changes in blood sugar. For example, when the blood sugar decreases from 105 to 100 mg/dl, the beta cell turns off completely, within minutes. Cherrington also reported that glucose is absorbed portally; one-third is taken up the liver, one-third by muscles, and one-third by the rest of the body. However, if glucose is delivered peripherally, only 10% of glucose enters the liver, with 56% in the muscle tissue, and 34% elsewhere. Insulin plays an important role in triggering glucose uptake by muscle and liver. When insulin is delivered peripherally it increases the role of muscle and diminishes the role of the liver. Therefore, one completely changes glucose bioavailability by delivering insulin peripherally, such as by injection. By choosing a peripheral site for insulin's delivery the glucose "fuel" can induce hyperglycemia and desensitization of the beta cells. Cherrington concluded that, "if we want a cure, we will have to deliver insulin portally."

Glucagon secretion is also extremely sensitive to glucose changes. For example, with a 20% decrease in the glucose concentration, glucagon secretion changes several fold. The flow of blood through the pancreas is from the beta-alpha in the cells. Therefore, the alpha cells watch what the beta cells do, implying that any bioartificial pancreas based on genetically modified beta cells will also have to include a modified alpha cell, secreting in the correct fashion. Neither are presently available. Genetic engineering may eventually provide a therapy for the two hundred million type I diabetics globally. However, it will likely require a generation before such therapy could be clinically tested, during which time Americans alone pay 120 billion dollars per year for treatment of the disease. For these reasons, and because it is unlikely that the human pancreatic tissue supply, estimated at up to 30,000 organs per year, will saturate, the allograft bioartificial pancreas is touted as the next therapy for diabetes, at least prior to 2020. According to Cherrington, the route to the bioartificial pancreas will likely be preceded by the replacement of whole-organ pancreas transplantation with naked islet transplantation.

## *Clinical Trials: Artificial Hemoglobin and Central Nervous System Applications*

Phase III clinical trials are under way, in the United Kingdom and Canada, for a third generation artificial hemoglobin. Thomas Chang (McGill University, Montreal) employs microencapsulated hemoglobin, enzymes, and microorganisms, coupled with absorbents and hormones. Bioartificial blood replaces macromolecular approaches wherein the first and second generation of polyHb involved crosslinking the Hb to increase the circulation half-life. Such "artificial cells" are also being investigated for end-stage renal failure. Patrick Aebischer (Cantonal Hospital, Lausanne) is applying differentiated murine C2C12 cells for ALS, following clinical trials with bovine chromaffin cells for pain control in terminally ill cancer patients. In the allo model, some C2C12 cells survived for one month. Total death was observed in xenotherapy (subcutaneous). These investigators looked at membranes of different cutoffs

(30, 70, and 280 kDa) with no advantage for xenotransplants. Aebischer concluded that it is not a complement/antibody problem that leads to rejection and that they would require both encapsulation and immunosuppression (possibly FK506).

### *Cellular Immunity to Immunoisolated Transplants*

Ron Gill, of the University of Colorado, seeks to use immunology's principles for cell and genetically engineered tissue transplants. He has observed two pathways involved in the failure of immunoisolated cells. The direct pathway, in which the donor cells sheds antigens and there is a CD-8 dependant recognition, dominates for allografts. In contrast the xenograft sheds the antigen but requires host-derived costimulants (indirect pathway). The xenograft response is, therefore, very dependent on the host CD4 cells. Specifically, the indirect response involving APCs (antigen presenting cells) stimulate the CD4 of the host and provokes a cytokine response. Gill says that, given that immunoisolation is based on molar mass cutoff, one can block the direct ingress of CD8 cells. However, it is uncertain what egress diffusion characteristics are needed to block the shed antigens, painting a skeptical future for immunoprotection with respect to xenotherapy.

Derek Gray, of Oxford University, noted that, for allografts, a slight MHC mismatch results in graft rejection. Therefore, the direct mechanism is the recognition of a T cell as a result of events in the MHC pathway. The indirect pathway involves a reaction of the recipient's dendritic cells in response to shed proteins or peptides. In allografts, islets transplanted into the portal vein, for example, will likely be surrounded by a blood clot, which will not hinder diffusion. For xenografts, xenoantibodies and extensive molecular incompatibility leads to activation of "all defense mechanisms" and the likelihood of hyperacute rejection. For the indirect pathway, the membrane will not block the shed proteins, unless they are too small to function. To address this, Gray noted that immunogenic peptides coming from the graft will likely be quite small, on the order of 8–15 amino acids.

Gray postulated that as one moves from allograft to concordant xenograft to discordant xenograft to primate xenograft, the complexity of the immune barrier must increase. In the first few months following transplantation there will be an adaptation, or "operational tolerance", which is most powerful for large organs, such as the liver and heart. Gray also reported that the acceptance of the graft has elements very similar to the acceptance of autoimmunity. In conclusion, we are aware of many mechanisms that turn on the autoimmune system, but are unaware of how to turn them off. Overall, Gray does not believe that one can immunoprotect xenotissue, though membranes may work for allotransplantation.

### *New Directions for Cell Therapy*

The main conference conclusion was that allotransplantation is a viable approach to cell transplantation. Furthermore, the supply of cadaveric human tissue, for example, for islets used in the treatment of diabetes, is not expected to saturate until approximately 2015. Given the risks—now demonstrated rather than perceived—involved in xenotransplantation, and the unlikeliness that immunoprotection can be developed with ingress and egress control at very different cutoffs, *publicly funded allotransplantation seems to have supplanted privately financed xenotherapies.*[3]

One author, Clark Colton of MIT, even noted that membrane-based therapies now seem insufficient for xenotransplantation. Overall, the advantage of xenotransplantation (onco-saftey, via suicide genes) seems grossly outweighed by its disadvantages, specifically biosafety and xenooses/PERV.

The use of genetically modified tissue, although perhaps having less risk, will be even more problematic than initially perceived. For example, although insulin-secreting beta cells have been cloned, complementary alpha and delta cells are also needed and the action must be in the proper sequence. Therefore, genetically modified cell-based research will need to orient itself toward reconstruction of the entire endocrine system, rather than the function of specific cells. The most optimistic predictions for the success of such research target the year 2020.

Bioartificial organ retrievability was agreed to as necessary, although the site of transplantation, for safe explantation, was debated, with the omental pouch (Rajotte, Edmonton), the liver (Morel, Geneva), and the subcutaneous sites (IsletSheet Medical, San Francisco) proposed. For all but the subcutaneous applications, microcapsules are the preferred "device" geometry with a critical diameter of 400 micrometers now agreed to by various experts, including Sun (Toronto), Colton (Cambridge), Calafiore (Perugia), and Hunkeler (Lausanne). Furthermore, immunoisolation devices for allotransplantation will have to differ from those for xenotransplantation. *This is a paradigm shift in development since, pre-Davos, it had been assumed that xenograft therapies in small-animal models could be used in clinical scale-up.* The conference also concluded that bioartificial organs will require coimmobilization to recreate an endocrine system. For example, a bioartificial pancreas will likely also benefit from the immune privilege provided by coencapsulated Sertoli cells. The effect of albumin on the regulation of the glucose metabolism also points the way to a joint bioartificial pancreas and liver, since hepatocytes and islets provide strong synergies when in close proximity.

Specific features of bioartifical organs that are both necessary and, in a post-Davos context, available include:

- *Calcium independence.*
- *Membrane-containing microcapsules:* membrane diameters approximately one-tenth of the device thickness (400 micrometers) will be needed. These are being tested for diabetes in an omental pouch (Edmonton) and the portal vein of the liver (Geneva).
- *Freeze-thaw stability:* microcapsules based on elastic thick-walled chemistry (alginate, cellulose sulfate, and synthetic oligocations, such as polymethylene-co-guanidine or polyvinyl amine) can be used for long-term (six-month) cell cryopreservation, with yields exceeding 85%.
- *Endotoxin reduction:* polysaccharides are available with endotoxin levels five to ten times below that regulated by the FDA, for alginate and cellulose sulfate, respectively.
- *Xenofree buffers:* the buffers employed should be xeno-protein free (Edmonton Protocol).
- *Appropriate metrics and monitoring:* the indicators employed to assess auto-, allo-, and xenograft function will require international standardization,[4] with watchdog agencies now created, for example by the OECD and WHO.[5]

Overall, this third bioartificial organs conference has set the stage for seven years of allotherapy-based development, anticipating a relatively widespread clinical bioartificial pancreas by 2007. Non-profit foundations and startups were announced at the conference, alongside a surprisingly large number of patents, as a means to saturate the clinic with microencapsulated human tissue, prior to moving on to considering the risks involved in genetically modified cells. The future for xenotransplantation was viewed as bleak.

## REFERENCES

1. HUNKELER, D. 1999. Bioartificial organs transplanted from research to reality. Nat. Biotech. **17:** 335.
2. SHAPIRO, A.M.J., J.R.T. LAKEY, E.A. RYAN, *et al.* 2000. Islet transplantation in seven patients with type 1 diabetes mellitus using a glucocorticoid-free immunosuppressive regimen. N. Engl. J. Med. **343**(4): 230–238.
3. BIRMINGHAM, K. 2000. Merger signals shift in xenotransplantation research. Nat. Med. **6:** 1195.
4. HUNKELER, D. 2000. Nature biotechnology, objectively assessing bioartificial organs. Nat. Biotech. **18:** 1021.
5. 2000. Plans drawn up for xenotransplantation watchdog. Nature **407:** 666.

# Bioartificial Organs: Glossary of Terms

*Acute Liver Failure.* The etiology of acute liver failure is of toxic origin and includes drugs and mushrooms, as well as infectious virus hepatitis. Acute liver failure causes progredient brain dysfunction, leading to death of the patient. This development occurs within 1–2 weeks. In parallel, the patient's organ may recover and regeneration has often been proven histologically. Treatment of acute liver failure conventionally involves intensive care, with survival rates of approximately 50%. In highly urgent cases, liver transplantation, with life-long immunosuppression, is performed. By temporarily replacing the liver function, a bridge to transplantation is possible in case of delay in procuring an organ.

*Alginate (Synonym: Salt of Alginic Acid).* A marine or bacterial polysaccharide with carboxylic functionality on the sugar backbone. Alginate complexes tenaciously with multivalent ions or oppositely charged polyelectrolytes. The microstructure consists of guluronic (G) and mannuronic (M) acid residues. The former produces hydrogels with good mechanical strength, whereas the latter provides elasticity and flexibility. Hydrogels formed with alginate are both selective (barium binds stronger than calcium) and cooperative with respect to the M blocks. Gels produced with calcium can shrink, or swell. The swelling is most severe for microbeads less than 0.3 mm in diameter.

*Allogenic.* Different genetic constitution within the same species.

*Allograft.* Organ or tissue involved in allotransplantation.

*Allotransplantation.* Transplantation between genetically non-identical individuals within the same species.

*Alpha Cells.* Pancreatic cells that secrete glucagon.

*ASTM.* Abbreviation for the American Society for Testing of Materials, who establish guidelines for tissue-engineered products and microcapsules.

*Anastomosis.* A traumatic or surgical opening between two or more normally distinct spaces or organs.

*Antigen-Specific Cells.* T and B lymphocytes bearing unique receptors capable of binding specific antigens expressed by transplanted cells.

*Artificial Red Blood Cells.* Synthetic or hybrid materials prepared in the laboratory to replace red blood cells for use in transfusion and other applications where red blood cells are normally required.

*Autograft.* Transfer of tissue within an individual.

*Autoimmune Disease.* Arising from, and directed at, an individual's own tissue.

*Autotransplantation.* Transplantation, generally of cells, derived from a whole organ explanted from the same donor. The transplantation of islets from patients having a pancreatectomy is an example.

*Autologous Cell Line.* Cultured cell lines derived from the same individual.

*Beta Cells.* Pancreatic cells that secrete insulin.

*Bioartificial Organ (Synonym: Hybrid Bioartificial Organ).* A *transplantable* device providing a mechanically stable *biocompatible,* non-*biodegradable* host to living cells. Examples include immunoisolated *macro-* and *microencapsulated* cells used for *immunoisolation,* such as the bioartificial pancreas (islets), liver (hepatocytes), and parathyroid (thyroid). Applications generally involve allo- and xenografts of *exocrine* tissues, as well as the treatment of neurological disorders and hormone-deficient diseases. Human tissue is derived from cadavers with the potential of immortalized cells lines based on pluripotent stem cell technology at the forefront of biomedical research and ethical debates. Bioartificial cartilage, skin, and bone belong to a second category of bioartificial organs in which cells are seeded to an, often biodegradable, substrate. The latter class of bioartificial organs can be considered to be part of the general area of tissue engineering. Overall, bioartificial organs comprise cells that are immunoisolated by elastic polymers or semipermeable membranes derived from synthetic and naturally occurring products such as *polysaccharides.*

*Biocompatibility.* The ability of a material to perform with an appropriate host response in a specific application.[1]

*Biodegradable.* From a biomaterial context, biodegradability refers to the decomposition of the implanted or transplanted device to molecules of lower molar mass. This occurs either through biological processes or the action of enzymes or bacteria.

*Biomimetic Material.* An artificial material that resembles the original, biologically produced precursor in micro- and macrostructure.

*Bioreactor.* A device for the culture of cells, or microorganisms, that enables the use of the cell performance as extracorporeal hybrid organ for temporary organ support (for example, hybrid liver support), or the products of the cells (for example, production of monoclonal antibodies for therapeutic use). Applications of bioreactors for the production of cells (for example, cell proliferation systems for blood stem cell tranplantation) are also under development. The first generation of medical bioreactors was adopted from dialysis/plasma separation hollow-fiber membranes or flat-sheet cartridges (two-compartment devices). The second generation of bioreactors incorporated oxygenation (three-compartment devices), with the third generation based on the incorporation of at least four evenly distributed compartments. Bioreactors enable decentralized oxygenation and controlled mass exchange with low gradients and, thus, high-density three-dimensional culturing of tissue.

*Bioresorbable.* From a biomaterial context, *bioresorbable* refers to the dissolution of the implanted or transplanted device to molecular fragments that are sufficiently low in molar mass to be metabolized and cleared through urine.

*BB Rat.* A spontaneously diabetic rat.

*C-Peptide.* The thirty amino-acid metabolically inactive peptide chain that connects the A and B strands of insulin in proinsulin. C-peptide can be detected in the blood as a marker of the insulin production by islets since it is removed in the conversion of proinsulin to insulin.

*Cardiomyocytes.* Heart muscle cells.

*Cell Transplantation (Synonym: Cell Therapy).* Treatment of normally an *autoimmune,* neurodegenerative or hormone-deficient disease through the transplantation of cells

# GLOSSARY OF TERMS

either to the same site as the cells in the existing organs, or to other sites where their efficacy can be optimized.

*Cellulose Sulfate.* An anionic polysaccharide used, alone or in combination with other *polyanions,* in the *symplex* formation with *polycations* to produce *permselective microcapsules.*

*Chitosan.* A cationic polysaccharide derived from the abundant natural polymer, chitin. Chitosan is often used as a biocompatible polymer coupled with various bioencapsulation techniques. Chemically, chitosan is a copolymer composed of 2-amino-2-deoxy-D-glucopyranose and 2-acetamido-2-deoxy-D-glucopryanose units.

*Cryopreservation.* Storage of tissue or tissue-material constructs at extremely low temperatures, usually employing liquid nitrogen, to preserve function and bank cells for future use.

*Coencapsulation. Immobilization* of more than one cell type, within a *microcapsule.* Generally this is used to enhance *in vivo* durability of a *transplant.* The most typical example includes the use of *Sertoli* cells to provide an *immunoprivilege* for *islets.*

*Confocal Laser Scanning Microscopy.* Unlike optical microscopy, only a spot of a minimum size in the specimen is illuminated in confocal microscopy. To enable an image to be formed from this, the specimen must be scanned. The image of the spot is directed through a pinhole stop in an intermediate image plane. As a result, only light from the focal plane can reach the detector (a photomultiplier). All other (out-of-focus) planes are blocked out. This results in an "optical section". The images are stored electronically and displayed on a monitor. A series of optical sections can be recorded by moving a motor a slight distance along the $z$-axis each time an image has been recorded, after which the next image is then also recorded. Such a $z$-series permits the electronic reconstruction of the three-dimensional structure using suitable computer programs. Visible light, ultraviolet or infrared laser lines can be used.

*Composite Bioartificial Pancreas.* Combination of islets with cells that offer immunoprotection (e.g., Sertoli cells) and "nursing" cells. The latter release growth factors and cytokines that are associated with neurotrophic effects. Astrocytes provide an example of a nursing cell.

*Concordant and Discordant Xenografts.* Concordant xenografts are from phylogenetically related species in which the recipient does not demonstrate naturally occurring antibodies reactive to donor species (e.g., primate to human). Discordant xenografts are from phlyogenetically divergent species in which the recipient does spontaneously demonstrate antibodies ("natural antibodies") reactive to the donor species (e.g., porcine to human).

*Cytokine.* Low molar mass hormone-like glycoprotein released by cells of the immune system and regulating the immune response. Examples include interferon and interleukin, the latter being an accepted nomenclature for a cytokine once its amino acid structure is known.

*Cytotoxicity.* Detrimental to cells and referring to the effect of an antibody on a specific antigen, frequently regulating the activity of complement.

*Dalton.* Unit of mass that equals the atomic weight of a hydrogen atom, or $1.657 \times 10^{-24}$ g. It is, more typically, expressed in kilodaltons (kDa), which signifies kilograms per mole.

*Depyrogenation.* Removal, or reduction, in the pyrogen (e.g., *endotoxin*) level. Precipitation, filtration, and chromatographic separation are common means, usually used in combination to depyrogenate biomaterials or medicaments.

*Dermagraft™.* A living, human, dermal replacement developed for the treatment of conditions in which the skin has been injured or destroyed. Dermagraft is produced by seeding neonatal foreskin fibroblasts onto a three-dimensional scaffold consisting of *bioresorbable* material. The cells grow and divide, producing ullagens, extracellular matrix proteins, and growth hormones found in normal, healthy human donors. Dermagraft also has an anti-inflammatory activity. The "bioartificial skin" is in clinical trials for partial thickness burns and cardiovascular applications.

*Diabetes Mellitus.* A metabolic disease manifesting a deficiency or absence of insulin secretion by the pancreas. It is characterized by hyperglycemia and an alternation of protein and fat metabolisms. Diabetes mellitus includes two categories of diseases: Type-I, insulin-dependant and Type-II, non-insulin-dependent. There may be a Type-III, gestational, form and a Type-IV, due to impaired glucose tolerance. The latter encompasses all other forms of diabetes, including those that are associated with pancreatic disease, hormonal changes, and genetic or other anomalies.

*Direct Pathway (Synonym: Donor Major Hisocompatability Complex-Restricted).* Antigen presentation in which T-cells engage native HGC molecules directly on the surface of donor-derived antigen-presenting cells. This is the dominant pathway for *allograft* rejection.

*EMEA.* Abbreviation for the European Agency for the Evaluation of Medicinal Products.

*Edmonton Protocol.* Islet allotransplantation involving xenoprotein-free buffers. Intrahepatic islet transplantation was carried out as soon as sufficient tissue mass was available, with patients given an IV antibiotic treatment with oral vitamin stimulation. A low-dose immunosuppression was applied immediately prior to transplantation. Pentamide was inhaled once per month to avoid infection.

*Electrostatic Droplet Generation.* Vibration of a needle, at frequencies in the thousands of hertz range, produces a uniform stream of submillimeter liquid droplets, generally in the absence of satellite peaks. Particle size distributions have stand ard deviations below 3%, but the technique is not applicable for high solution viscosities.

*Encapsulation.* One of a family of immobilization procedures that includes adsorption and entrapment. Encapsulation involves the use of natural or synthetic materials, including ceramics, metals, and polymers, although the latter are preferred for biomedical applications. This surrounds the material to be encapsulated, such as a drug or cell, providing a diffusive barrier that controls the ingress to and egress from the encapsulate. The prefix *micro* is related to the capsule size and is used for systems between one and one-thousand micrometers. Nanocapsules have also been developed. Encapsulation can also include non-permeable systems that are degradable, such as those used for vaccines.

*Endocrine Tissue.* Secretes hormones into the bloodstream.

*Endogenous.* Originating or produced within the organism or one of its parts.

*(Full) Endocrine Replacement Therapy (Synonym: Bioartificial Graft).* Concept of co-immobilization of cells that provide costimulatory factors. For example, the albumin released from hepatocytes will likely aid in the survival of microencapsulated islets, as will the immunoprotection offered by Sertoli or amniotic cells.

*Endotoxins.* Lipopolysaccharides, a component of a Gram-negative bacterial cell wall, induce fever in mammals. Endotoxins are anionic and have molar masses similar to that of many components of immobilization systems and tend to aggregate, rendering separation difficult.

*Exocrine Tissue.* Secretes outwards, into or through a duct. For example, the exocrine pancreas produces enzymes that are needed in internal digestion.

*Extracellular Matrix.* Region surrounding an animal cell's membrane. The three primary constituents include collagens, which provide strength, adhesive proteins, such as elastin, laminin, and fibronectin, and proteoglycan fillers. In some tissue, such as the liver, this space is insignificant, whereas in connective tissues and cartilage this is the most important part .

*FasL (Synonym: Fas Ligand).* A cell surface protein similar to a tumor necrosis factor. When T cells are activated, they express FasL, including apoptosis (cell death following a characteristic pattern: cell shrinkage, fragmentation, and destruction of the DNA). The failure of FasL interactions has been associated with autoimmune diseases.

*FDA.* Abbreviation for the Food and Drug Administration of the United States, Department of Health and Human Services.

*Fibroblast Cells.* A family of cells, present in all tissues, arising from three germ layers. These cells produce collagenous fibers and give rise to connective tissue.

*Fibrosis.* Formation of fibrotic tissue as a reparative or reactive process.

*Foreign Body.* Reaction response to a non-natural material usually involving macrophages.

*Gene Transfer (Ex Vivo).* Cells from a donor are explanted, propagated *in vitro*, genetically modified to express a desired gene product and than reimplanted to the same patient.

*Gene Transfer (In Vivo).* DNA is introduced, either in viral vectors or as a liposome-DNA complex, directly in to a patient's tissue where DNA uptake, followed by gene expression, occurs. This has been tested clinically for cystic fibrosis.

*Glucagon.* A polypeptide hormone that is produce in the alpha cells of the pancreas and released in response to decreases in blood glucose. Glucagon stimulates *de novo* synthesis of glucose. It is an insulin counter hormone.

*Guluronic Acid.* A C-5 epimer of *mannuronic acid.*

*Hepatocytes.* The major cellular component of the liver, representing 80% of the cell population, the hepatocyte is the primary metabolic and detoxification center of the body. Hepatocytes, parenchymal cells, are responsible for intermediate metabolism (gluconeogenesis, fatty acid, and amino acid), protein and macromolecule synthesis, immune and hormonal system modulation, biotransformation (e.g., urea synthesis, gluconuridation, and sulfation), oxidative detoxification (primarily through the cytochrome P450 enzyme system), and *exocrine* secretion of bile. Immortalized hepatocytes are under investigation for liver support systems.

*Hollow Fibers.* Tubular *semipermeable* polymeric device with an internal diameter, usually, on the order of one millimeter. This can be sealed and used to store cells, occasionally in an *alginate* matrix. They are often polysulfone- or polyacrylonitrile-based, although new chemistries based on polyisoprene have also been developed. They are typically applied, in a *bioartificial* organ context, for applications involving the *transplantation* of approximately one million cells (e.g., central nervous system), or where *subcutaneous* recovery is desirable.

*Homeostasis.* Equilibrium within the body environment with respect to temperature and fluid content.

*Hybrid Liver.* Liver support devices that replace the organ function outside the body. Extracorporeal blood perfusion/plasma separation enables temporary liver support. There are biological systems with organ perfusion methods and artificial systems with detoxification/adsorption methods. Hybrid liver support devices incorporate a bioreactor with artificial components and based on use of metabolically active liver cells, as the biologic component. The combination is called a hybrid system. Hybrid liver support circuits may also incorporate artificial detoxification cartridges, for example, with charcoal or resin.

*Hydrogel.* Water-swollen polymer networks that may contain upwards of approximately 15 wt% water to 99 wt% water. The polymer network may be held together by covalent linkages, physical interactions, such as ionic complexes, or hydrophobic domains, or molecular entanglements.

*Hyperacute Rejection.* Immediate, dramatic rejection of a transplant due to the pre-existing presence of donor-reactive antibodies in the host. This form of rejection is observed in response to *discordant xenografts,* in which the recipient spontaneously develops xenograft-reactive "natural" antibodies in the absence of intentional prior immunization with xenograft antigens. *Necrosis* is usually observed within three days.

*Hyperglycemic.* An abnormally elevated level of glucose in the circulating blood, seen in patients with diabetes mellitus.

*Hypoglycemia.* An abnormally low blood glucose concentration. In the context of *bioartificial organs,* this can be created, for example by transplanted $\beta$ *cells,* due to the lack of presence of the $\alpha$ *cell* and the *glucagon* hormone.

*Hypoxia.* Insufficient oxygen supply in tissues and blood, for example, due to lack of blood perfusion. *Anoxia* describes a situation with a total lack of oxygen in the tissue.

# GLOSSARY OF TERMS

*Immunoglobulins.* A group of glycoproteins present in the serum and tissue fluids that recognize and bind to antigens. There are five classes of immunoglobulins: IgM, IgG, IgA, IgD, and IgE (synonym: antibody).

*Immunoisolation.* Utilization of a, generally polymeric, barrier to protect the host from the graft, and vice versa. Immunoisolation "devices" include hollow fibers, microcapsules and flat sheets.

*Immunologically Privileged Sites.* Includes the brain, certain regions of the eye, the ovaries, placenta, testes, and the pregnant uterus. In these sites the antigens do not elicit immune responses under normal circumstances. Grafts placed into these sites are said to be "tolerated". The interaction between the privileged tissue and T cells are inhibited by blood–tissue barriers.

*Implantation.* Surgical insertion of a tissue-free material or device.

*Indirect Pathway (Synonym: Host MHC-restricted).* Antigen presentation in which donor-derived antigens are captured by recipient APC, degraded and represented in association with recipient MHC molecules, in contrast to the *direct pathway.* The indirect pathway is the major xenograft response and involves antigen-presenting cells stimulating the CD4 helper T cells of the host, which provoke cytokines.

*Insulinoma.* A type of islet cell adenoma that secretes insulin. These tumors of the pancreas cause excess secretion of insulin, thus lowering the blood glucose level to a point causing illness.

*Internal Gelation.* Method of preparing calcium alginate beads wherein the calcium source is internal to the alginate droplet, often in the form of calcium carbonate. This emulsion-based method provides a more homogeneous *hydrogel* than for beads gelled with calcium chloride, which is contained in an external solution and must first diffuse into the bead. Particle size distributions are broader than for individual droplet methods, such as those prepared electrostatically or with *air-stripping.*

*Ionotropic Gelation.* Formation of a hydrogel through the reaction of a multivalent electrolyte with a polyelectrolyte bearing oppositely charged groups. The most common example involves calcium chloride and sodium alginate.

*Islet of Langerhans.* Cluster of endocrine cells found in the pancreas (e.g., alpha, beta, and delta) producing hormones such as insulin.

*Islet Sheet.* Multilayered construction of alginate where *islets* are cast as a thin flat sheet, optionally with a reinforcing polymer, which is sandwiched on both sides by an acellular immunoprotective alginate layer. The construct is crosslinked throughout.

*Insulin.* A polypeptide hormone, secreted by *beta cells* in the islets of *Langerhans.*

*Intraperitoneal.* Within the abdominal cavity.

*JDFI.* Abbreviation for the Juvenile Diabetes Foundation International.

*Lipopolysaccharide (Synonym: Endotoxin).* Consists of three biologically, chemically, genetically and serologically different parts. These are non-polar lipid compounds, referred to as lipid A, the so-called core oligosaccharide, and a heteropolysaccharide representing the surface antigen. Lipopolysaccharides are an important component of the outer membrane of Gram-negative bacteria.

*Liposomal Enzyme Deficiency.* Group of more than 40 separate diseases manifesting a deficiency in the enzyme responsible for macromolecular catabolism. One such variant accumulates glycosaminoglycans, which can lead to cell and organ dysfunction.

*Macrophages.* Large mononuclear phagocytic amebic cells important in innate immunity, in the early adaptive phases of the host defense as antigen-presenting cells, and as effector cells in humoral and cell-mediated immunity.

*Mannuronic Acid.* A uronic acid derivative of mannose made by converting the primary alcohol group of mannose to a carboxyl group.

*Matrigel.* A synthetic material that closely resembles the basement membrane composition (types I-V collagens, glycoproteins, proteoglycans, hyaluronic acid, and lamilin). Matrigel is effective for the attachment and differentiation of both normal and transformed anchorage-dependent cell types, such as neurons and *hepatocytes.* The biological response of cells in Matrigel can be improved.

*Membrane.* Amorphous substance with a thickness significantly smaller than its surface dimensions. In general, *permeability* is restricted for molecules above a certain size, or for macromolecules of a given charge or conformation.

*Microbeads and Microcapsules.* Submillimeter hydrogels formed via either ionotropic gelation or polyelectrolyte complexation. A microbead has a uniform morphology, whereas a microcapsule contains an inner core that can be liquefied postformation, and a permselective membrane. The resulting membrane provides diffusional resistance against high molar mass materials, with a *molar mass cut-off* generally in the 50–100 kDa range, approximately half of that for *microbeads.* The cationic nature of microcapsule surface is expected to be responsible for cell overgrowth (*foreign body reaction*), which is often not observed in *alginate* microcapsules.

*Microgravity.* Existence of a gravitational force, as expressed by the product of the gravitational constant and the difference in the density of a suspended object in a fluid, one one-millionth of that encountered at sea level.

*Mitogenic.* Causing mitosis (reproduction of cells) or transformation.

*MMCO (Synonym: Molar Mass Cut-Off).* The molar mass cut-off (MMCO) is synonymously referred to as the molecular weight cut-off (MWCO). Generally, the MMCO is denoted by the minimum average molar mass of a solute that is 90% excluded by the capsule membrane. MMCO determines the upper limit for molecular transport across the membrane.

*Nanoparticles.* Submicron-sized colloids postulated to improve the speed of drug or hormone delivery via the high surface-to-volume ratio caused by miniaturization.

*Necrosis.* Localized death of a cell or organ due to a chemical or physical injury, as opposed to apoptosis, which is a biologically programmed form of cell death. As an example, necrosis can occur as the result of loss of nutrient supply, or, in bioartificial organs, due to oxygen diffusion limitations. *Necrotic* is referred to, or associated with, necrosis.

*NOD Mice.* Non-obese diabetic (NOD) mice that are characterized by the development of spontaneous, autoimmune diabetes.

*Non-Autologous Cell Lines.* Cell lines established from another individual of the same species (allogeneic cell lines) or from another species (xenogeneic cell lines).

*Normoglycemia (Synonym: Euglycemia).* Blood glucose levels in the range of 80–120 mg/dl, as observed in non-diabetics.

*Oligomer.* A macromolecule with, generally, less than one hundred repeat units. Physical parameters change with the number of monomeric units. The end group functionality usually influences behavior in contrast to polymers.

*Oligosaccharide.* A compound made up of the condensation of a small number of monosaccharide units.

*Omental Pouch.* Pocket created between peritoneal folds between the stomach and another abdominal organ. These pouches generally contain cells or *bioartificial organs*.

*PPARs.* Factors that can bind fatty acid ligands. All pathways in the fatty acid metabolism are governed by PPAR.

*Parathyroid Glands and Hormones.* In humans, there are four parathyroid glands localized in the thyroid. Parathyroid hormones, synthesized by the gland, are essential for life, since removal of the parathyroid glands is associated with a high mortality rate due to a lack of calcium in plasma. Hypersecretion of parathyroid hormones may occur and provokes hypercalcemia, hypophosphatemia leading to demineralization of bones, and the formation of kidney stones.

*Parkinson's Disease.* A group of syndromes described by James Parkinson, observed mainly in elderly individuals, and marked by tremor, muscle rigidity, and poverty of movement. It is due to the degenerescence (cell death) of dopaminergic neurons in specific brain areas, such as the thalamus, putamen, and the caudate nucleus.

*Permeability.* A metric used to describe mass transport of a solute $i$ within a membrane is the permeability coefficient, or permeability, $P_i$. The permeability is defined in various ways that are context dependent. Typically the permeability $P_i$ of solute $i$ in the matrix (cm$^2$/s) is the product of a transport property, the diffusion coefficient $D_i$ (cm$^2$/s) and a thermodynamic property, the partition coefficient $K_i$ (dimensionless): $P_i = D_i \cdot K_i$. This equation assumes concentration-independent diffusion and partition coefficients. The equation is valid for matrices in which the solute is transported by two ways: diffusion through pores and dissolution in the matrix. For a grossly porous membrane, containing a high amount of water, the latter mechanism (interaction between matrix and solute) can be neglected. Consequently, methods for the determination of permeability coefficient approaches, based on Fick's first law of diffusion, exist, in which the membrane thickness is usually considered in the equations. Gel permeability can involve steric, electrostatic and conformational factors.

*PERV (Abbreviation for Porcine-Derived Endothelial Retroviruses).* Viruses can be transmitted across species and, in particular, within the context of *xenotransplantation,* to humans. Suspicion of PERV was to a large extent the reason behind a call for a moratorium on xenotransplantation. Exposure of isolated islets to *in vitro* and *in vivo* blood has been shown to result in acute islet damage.[2] It has also been reported that pig islets can infect human cells in culture, providing the first evidence that PERV is transcriptionally active and infectious across species.[3]

*Polyanion (Synonym: Anionic Polyelectrolyte).* A negatively charged polyelectrolyte that can either be a polysaccharide, such as alginate, or a synthetic material, such as polyacrylic acid. Can form symplexes with polycations that are the membrane component of spherical microcapsules.

*Polycation (Synonym: Cationic Polyelectrolyte).* A positively charged polyelectrolyte, such as poly-L-lysine that complexes with a polyanion, such as alginate, to form a microcapsule.

*Polyelectrolyte.* Macromolecule with charges on the backbone or side chains. Materials with positive and negative charges, on separate monomer units on one polymer chain are referred to as polyampholytes. If the charges are on the same subunit then the nomenclature zwitterion (betaine) is employed.

*Polyelectrolyte Complex (Synonym: Symplex).* Reaction product between oppositely charged polyelectrolytes.

*PolyHemoglobin.* Covalent crosslink of a number of hemoglobin molecules together to form larger molecules, using bifunctional agents like glutaraladehyde. This has been successfully used in Phase III clinical trials as an *artificial red blood cell* substitute.

*Poly-L-lysine.* A *polycation,* generally with molar masses in the tens of *kilodaltons,* which is applied, with alginate, to microencapsulate cells for transplantation.

*Polylactic-co-Glycolic Acid (Synonym: PLGA).* Biodegradable copolymers where the rate of degradation can be altered between days and months by varying the ratio of lactic acid to glycolic acid monomeric units.

*Portal Vein.* A large vein conveying the blood flow from the abdominal organs to the liver. It ramifies in smaller branches within the liver.

*Proximal Tubule Cell.* A differentiated epithelial cell lining the first part of the renal tubule and receiving the ultrafiltrate formed in the kidney glomerular filtration apparatus.

*Quaternary Microcapsule.* Chemistry involving a blend of *polyanions* (*alginate* and *cellulose sulfate*) that are gelled in calcium chloride. The *polycation* polymethylene-co-guanidine reacts *in situ* or subsequently, to form the outer membrane.

*Renal Tubular Assist Device.* A bioreactor cartridge containing renal tubule cells to provide transport, metabolic, and endocrinologic activity in the treatment of kidney failure.

*Rotating Cell Culture System.* A bioreactor for three-dimensional cell aggregation under conditions of law shear force, high mass transfer, and *microgravity.* The system, originally developed by NASA, balances the sedimentation force, due to gravity, with centrifugal forces caused by rotation.

*Secretague.* An agent promoting secretion, mostly of hormones, for example, of insulin upon glucose or an amino acid stimulus.

*Sertoli Cells.* Cells that originally are located in the male testis, where they seem to help development of, and protect the germinal cells, through their maturation process, from autoimmune destruction. Molecular crosstalk between Sertoli, Leydig, and peritubular cells play a role in constituting the so called "blood–testicular barrier". The functional competence of Sertoli cells is mediated by sophisticated molecules, including several factors, that not only favor cell growth but also seem to contrast apoptosis (or programmed cell death) pathways. In an attempt to enhance islet graft longevity. Sertoli cells have been recently proposed for islet cotransplantation in *diabetic* animal models. Sertoli cells are expected to have a direct mitogenic effect on β cells and to release immunomodulatory molecules.

*Stem Cells.* Cells capable of both indefinite proliferation and differentiation into specialized cells. This serves as a continuous source of new cells for such tissues as blood and testes. Totipotent stem cells are capable of giving rise to an entire organism whereas pluripotent stem cells are capable of giving rise to different kinds of cells, but not an entire organism.

*Somatic Gene Therapy.* A "universal" recombinant cell line engineered to secrete desired gene products. These are often enclosed in a permselective membrane, generally polymeric, and transplanted to a given patient. In contrast to *ex vivo* and *in vivo* gene transfer, the cells can be transplanted into a variety of patients since the microcapsule can, in principle, prevent graft rejection without recourse to immunosuppressive drugs.

*(Air) Stripping.* Concentric flow of air or an inert gas around a syringe pulls liquid droplets that can have diameters below the internal diameter of the syringe. Particle size distributions have standard deviations of less than 5%. The technique is applicable to high viscosity fluids.

*Syngraft (Synonym: Isograft).* Tissue or organ transplanted between two genetically identical individuals.

*Thrombogenicity.* The tendency for a material to induce thrombus-formation (clotting) when in contact with blood.

*Tissue Engineering.* Distinguished from cellular transplantation by the presence of three-dimensional structures (scaffolds or templates).

*Transplantation.* Surgical introduction of a part, or the whole, of a tissue or organ taken from another individual or animal. Contrasts with implantation, in which non-living materials is introduced.

*Transcutaneous.* Delivery across the skin.

*Vascularization.* The presence of an irrigating vessel system within a tissue.

*Xenogenic.* Foreign substance/tissue introduced into an organism.

*Xenotransplantation.* Transplantation of tissues across a species barrier (see concordant and discordant grafts).

## REFERENCES

1. WILLIAMS, D.F. 1987. Definitions in Biomaterials (Progress in Biomaterials), Vol. 4. Elsevier.
2. BENNET, W., B. SUNDBERG, T. LUNDGREN, *et al.* 2000. Transplantation **69:** 711.
3. VAN DEER LAAN, L.J., C. LOCKEY, B.C. BRIFFETH, *et al.* 2000 Nature **407:** 90.

# Historical Perspectives of Hybrid Hepatic Assist Devices

## Tissue Sourcing, Immunoisolation, and Clinical Trial

YUKIHIKO NOSÉ

*Michael E. DeBakey Department of Surgery,*
*Baylor College of Medicine, Houston, Texas, USA*

ABSTRACT: A hybrid hepatic assist device using canine liver tissues was developed and clinically applied 38 years ago. However, for many years practical hybrid hepatic assist devices were not clinically introduced owing to the many difficulties encountered in employing cultured hepatocytes. These problems include: (1) maintenance of viable cultured cells, (2) maintenance of normal hepatocyte function with these cells, (3) elimination of toxic substances generated by non-viable cultured and/or stored cells, (4) elimination of immunological factors generated by cultured cells and by the patient, and (5) difficulties of the biocompatible immunological barrier for cells against the patient. Fortunately, recent progress in apheresis and biomaterial technologies enable us to isolate cultured cells immunologically and yet maintain effective metabolic functions for the patient. These technologies generate an immunological barrier of a hybrid hepatic assist device for the patients. Proper adsorption columns developed for apheresis procedures enable us to remove the toxic substances released by non-viable cells. Recent development of oxygen-carrying macromolecules enable us to provide sufficient oxygen supply to the cultured cells and to maintain their normal cellular function, not only during the cultured period of time, but also during their actual clinical application. Together with the advancement of cell culture technologies, including the proper cultured environments and cellular seeding environments, these technologies, primarily developed for therapeutic apheresis, should be able to provide more effective and safe hybrid artificial organs.

KEYWORDS: bioartificial organs; hybrid artificial organ; hybrid hepatic assist; immunological isolation; properly functioning cells; oxygen delivery; removal of toxic substance

## INTRODUCTION

Historically, the first bioartificial metabolic organ applied in patients was reported in 1963 by the present author.[1] Since that time and for many years, bioartificial organs were considered impractical. However, during the last decade substantial progress in tissue culture technologies have again focused on bioartificial organs for various types of clinical application.

Address for correspondence: Yukihiko Nosé, M.D., Ph.D., Professor of Surgery, Michael E. DeBakey Department of Surgery, Baylor College of Medicine, One Baylor Plaza, Houston, TX 77030 USA. Voice: 713-798-4434; fax: 713-798-3985.
ynose@bcm.tmc.edu

In this paper, historical attempts for a hybrid hepatic assist and lessons to be learned from historical bioartificial organs, primarily the hybrid metabolic assist device and non-hybrid metabolic and immunological assist devices, are discussed.

## THE FIRST HYBRID HEPATIC ASSIST

It was more than 40 years ago, in 1957, that an attempt to develop a hybrid hepatic assist device using canine hepatocytes was initiated by this author at the University of Hokkaido, School of Medicine, Sapporo, Japan (see FIGURE 1).

In order to develop a practical metabolic reactor, fresh canine liver tissues were initially employed (see FIGURE 2). It was believed that this was the first reported attempt to construct a hybrid metabolic artificial organ.[2] To provide minimal metabolic function for a patient, it was necessary to generate approximately 150 grams of 200-μ-thick slices of liver tissue. Initially, approximately 1–2 mm-thick slices were made. However, it was quickly realized the thickness should be less than 200 μ because effective oxygen penetration into the tissues was only possible to about 100 μ deep. It was a difficult challenge to maintain the viability of these liver slices during preparation. At that time, no practical tissue culture technologies had been developed. Thus, freshly harvested heterologous liver tissues were considered to offer the only possible source for achieving metabolic function for the hepatic assist. In addition, it was necessary to have these tissues readily available whenever the clinical need presented itself. Thus, freeze–thawed liver tissue applications were made from frozen liver slices.

These liver tissues were kept in an oxygenated medium in which essential amino acids, glucose, albumin, and vitamins were added. This medium was circulated through the artificial kidney unit, like a dialysate. The membrane used for this

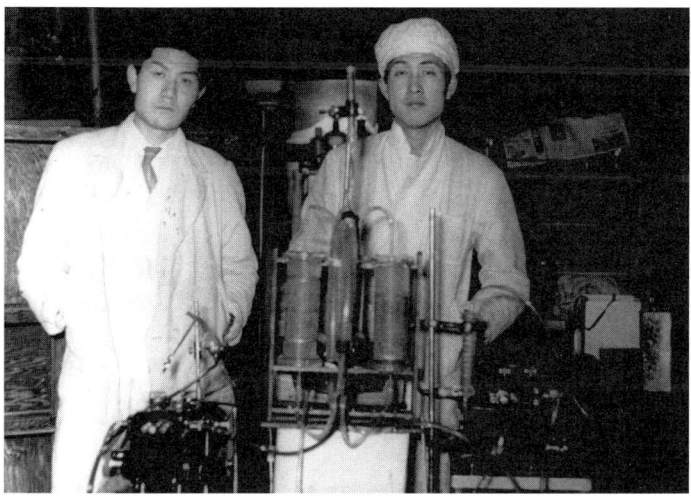

**FIGURE 1.** Yukihiko Nosé (*left*) behind the first hybrid hepatic assist device in 1959.

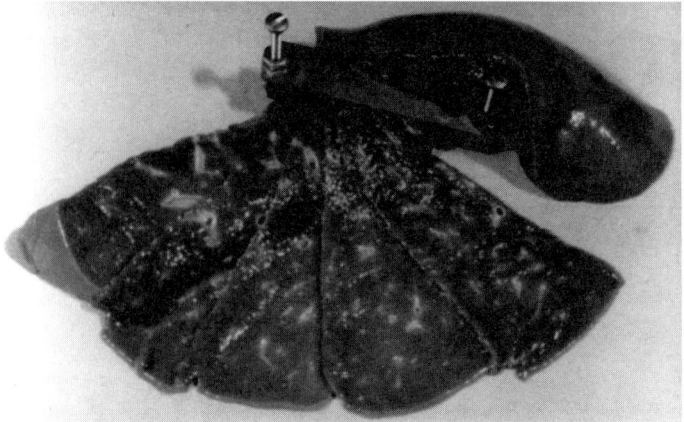

**FIGURE 2.** Freshly harvested canine liver slices.

application was a gel-type cellulose membrane with a molecular cut off in the range of 50,000 daltons, very similar to the high performance hemodialysis membrane available today (see FIGURE 3).

FIGURE 4 shows the original 1969 model of the extracorporeal metabolic reactor. Two cylinders are shown at the center of the figure, each containing approximately 100 grams of liver tissue. One chamber was exchanged every hour with fresh liver tissues. At the front of these liver tissue-containing columns, a foaming column can be seen. This is a bubble oxygenator, and the medium was fully oxygenated before being circulated through the liver tissue columns.

How to keep the hepatocyte function extracorporeally? By the supply of sufficient nutritions and sufficient oxygen. Nutritional supply to the cells was relatively simple.

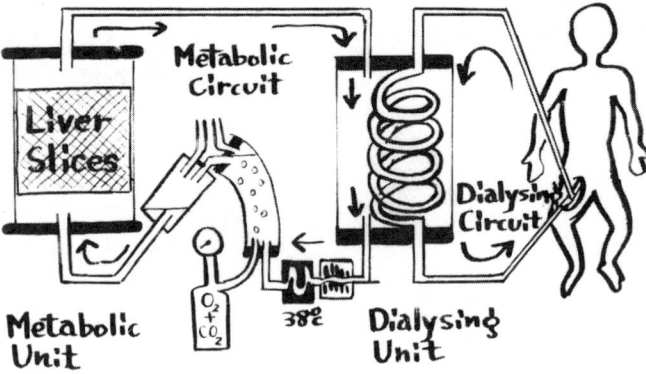

**FIGURE 3.** Schematic illustration of the first hybrid hepatic assist device using fresh and/or freeze-thawed liver slices (1959).

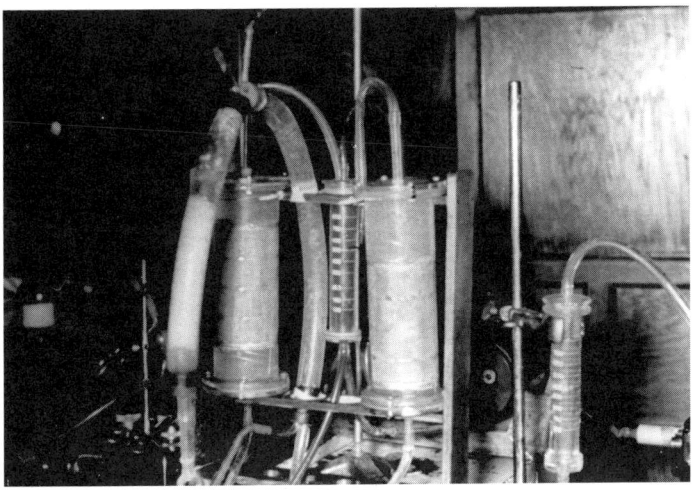

**FIGURE 4.** Actual hybrid hepatic assist device for experimental use (1959).

Unfortunately, the oxygen supply to cells without red cells or oxygen-carrying macromolecules was difficult. The reason for this difficulty is shown in FIGURE 5. The left side of FIGURE 5 shows the gas condition of the arterial blood, and the right side shows the gas condition of the venous blood.[3] Tissues use 5 cc of oxygen from 100 cc of blood (19 cc minus 14 cc). These are from red cells. Unfortunately, without red cells, only approximately 0.2 cc of oxygen from 100 cc of blood is available in plasma (0.3 cc minus 0.13 cc). This is the normal gas condition. Even though the plasma

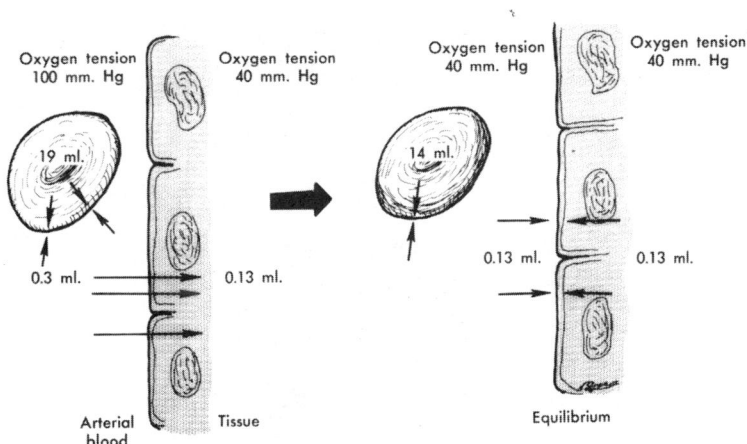

**FIGURE 5.** Oxygen content in arterial and venous blood. The $O_2$ content in red cells and in plasma are shown.

is oxygenated with 100% oxygen, it is very difficult to supply even 1 cc of oxygen to the tissue by perfusing it with a non-red cell–containing perfusate.

How to deliver oxygen properly to cells? It is necessary to add an oxygen-carrying agent to the perfusate. Typically, this is hemoglobin. Otherwise, we would have to use blood as the perfusate. In the event that a cellular mix up of red cells with hepatocytes is expected, a membrane or separator should be used between these two cells, similar to a membrane oxygenator. This is another problem. Unfortunately, stroma-free hemoglobin cannot be used because of its toxicity. Thus, it is necessary to consider the development of oxygen-carrying macromolecules. These should be immunologically inert and should not stimulate coagulation cascade, a complement, or other body defense system in the body.

A stabilized conjugated hemoglobin was developed to be able to meet most of these basic requirements for oxygen-carrying macromolecules.[4,5] FIGURE 6 shows such a macromolecule. This 10% crosslinked Hb conjugate is able to supply all the necessary oxygen, performing as an artificial blood. The molecular weight of the conjugate is 90,000 daltons, and its size is between that of albumin and $\gamma$ globulin.

Returning to 40 years previously, the freezing of the liver tissue should be discussed briefly. Freezing the tissue was accomplished three different ways: freezing in liquid air (–196°C), freezing in dry ice (–70°C), and freezing in a –5°C freezer. Rapid freezing was best; yet, surprisingly, the slowest freezing was also acceptable. For thawing, rapid thawing directly in a 37°C medium proved to be best. An explanation of these two acceptable freezing methods is as follows. Rapid freezing creates small ice crystals in the cell but does not damage the cellular structure. Slow freezing creates large ice crystals outside of the cell but also does not damage the cellular structure. So the rapid freezing method was employed and the tissue frozen by dropping it directly in liquid air.

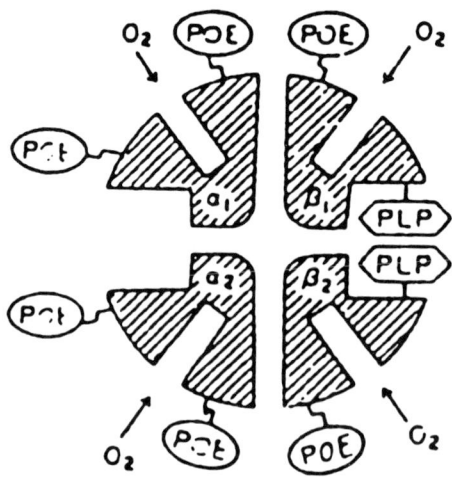

**FIGURE 6.** Schematic structure of conjugated hemoglobin.

The aim of this extracorporeal metabolic reactor was to use the enzymatic function of hepatocytes, regardless of the cells being "alive" or "dead." Thus, the frozen liver tissue was vacuum-dried and kept refrigerated in the vacuum container (see FIGURE 7). Fortunately, these freeze-dried liver granules demonstrated a reduced, yet acceptable, metabolic function of the hepatocytes. This was approximately 25% of fresh liver tissues. Since the supply of freeze-dried liver tissues was abundant and easily made, and these tissues were 2–4 times more available than fresh liver tissue, the freeze-dried liver granules were used in clinical studies. The freeze-dried liver granules, 200 μ in diameter, demonstrated urea synthesis, glyconeogenesis, and ammonia detoxification, even for up to two hours.

The performance of the clinically applicable hepatic assist device was simplified with the availability of freeze-dried liver granules. The freeze-dried liver granules were added to a medium in a big tank and bubbled with 95% oxygen and 5% $CO_2$. The patient's blood circuit with a gel-type cellulose membrane unit was immersed inside this tank. Gas bubbles were used to agitate the medium (see FIGURE 8).

By March of 1962, this device was employed for four acute liver insufficiency patients,[1] using approximately 100 g of dry liver granules. This is equivalent to approximately 500 g of fresh liver tissue. Fortunately, two out of four patients were salvaged from acute liver insufficiency followed by surgical intervention. A paper on this subject was presented at the 1963 ASAIO congress and elsewhere.[1] This was the same year Dr. Tom Starzl in Denver attempted the first liver transplantation.[6] Since our hybrid assist device was also reported in the same year, the author was honored to share symposia on liver transplantation versus hepatic assist with Dr. Starzl.

On one occasion, Dr. Starzl commented to the author, "Yuki, you're wrong! You are just trying to get the patient's abnormal metabolic status back to normal. Your method does not cure a patient's diseased liver condition. If your hepatic assist is

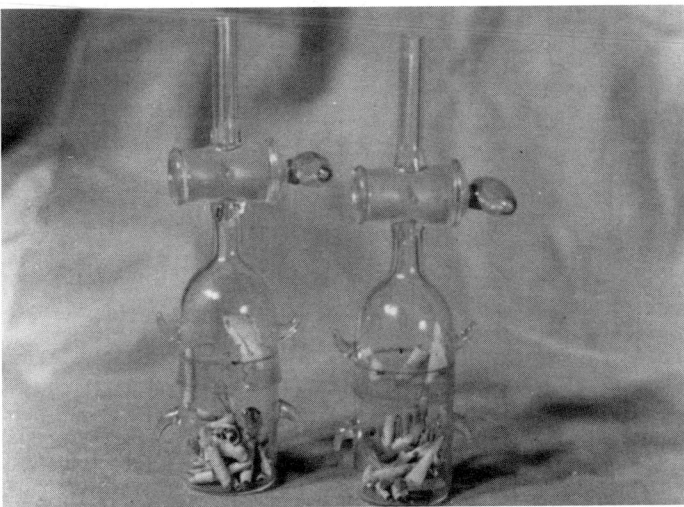

**FIGURE 7.** Freeze-dried liver slices in vacuum containers.

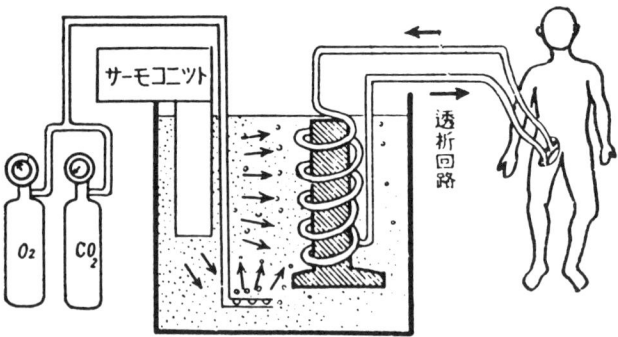

**FIGURE 8.** Schematic illustration of the hybrid hepatic assist device using freeze-dried liver granules (1961).

effective for improving patients' hepatocyte functions, then it would be better than a liver transplantation. However, normalizing all metabolic conditions of the patient cannot be termed an artificial liver." He said there were the two very important principles for treating acute liver insufficiency, and they were different from what this author had intended to achieve at that time. One was to improve the microcirculation within the liver tissues and stop the damage of hepatocytes. For almost 40 years, I had ignored the warning Dr. Starzl had given me and was pursuing the wrong treatment of patients with acute liver insufficiency aiming to normalize their hematological metabolic parameters.

## PROBLEMS ASSOCIATED WITH HYBRID HEPATIC ASSIST

In addition to heeding Dr. Starzl's warning, we should critically look at a hybrid hepatic assist strategy. Even though during the last 40 years, the author has strongly believed that the future of hepatic assist should be the hybrid hepatic assist, there are several difficult issues to solve before it can becomes a safe and effective hepatic assist device.

### *Storage of Viable Hepatocytes*

First, in order to use cultured hepatocytes for clinical application, these cells must be frozen in order to make them available whenever there is a clinical need for these hepatocytes. Since during the freeze–thawing process, we lose approximately 20% of hepatocytes, the toxic substances released from these dead cells should be removed before clinical application. Currently, an adsorption column to remove endotoxins is becoming available.[7] Such adsorption columns and various types of membrane separators[8] could be used for this application. A more detailed description of this issue is made in a later section. Very often we forget this very important preparation prior to clinical application. However, our future aim is to eliminate the freezing requirement for cultured hepatocytes. Sufficient supply of viable cultured hepatocytes is considered necessary.

TABLE 1. **Hepatocyte function during tissue culture**

>   Altered metabolic function
>   Due to culture
>   Due to freeze-thawing
>   Non or partially viable cells
>   Toxic substance release
>   Altered metabolic function
>   Cellular function changes at lower oxygen supply environment

## *Maintenance of Normal Hepatocyte Function*

Another important issue is that the hepatocytes change their function during the cultured period (see TABLE 1). These functional alterations should be critically examined. This is not a negative statement. It can be advantageous. It is possible to customize those cultured hepatocytes to our benefit. It may be possible to boost the desired hepatocyte functions for hepatic assist during the culture period. The most important factors to consider for these altered hepatocyte functions are that the cells still be alive but under altered metabolic function. Sometimes, and very often, these hepatocytes do not really function to assist the desired metabolic function and generate toxic substances. They would not be therapeutically advantageous to use as a metabolic reactor. As this author has already mentioned, properly cultured cells in an ideal metabolic environment with the proper gas condition should be maintained. Hepatocyte functional changes in a lower oxygen supply environment should be noted.

## *Elimination of Immunological Impact of Using Homologous or Heterologous Hepatocytes*

Another important factor to consider in hybrid hepatic assist, using foreign hepatocytes, is eliminating the immunological factors from hepatocytes, and eliminating the immunological insult to the patient. A biocompatible membrane separator could be effectively utilized to allow metabolism of molecules smaller than albumin but not allow any molecules larger than γ globulin.[8] Certainly a patient's leukocytes would not be exposed directly to cultured hepatocytes.

## METABOLIC AND IMMUNOLOGICAL ASSIST WITHOUT HEPATOCYTES

After the author came to the USA in 1962, he initiated metabolic assist using and expanding the hemodialysis technology. In other words, he made an attempt to develop a metabolic and immunological assist device without tissue materials. These technologies are primarily called membrane plasmapheresis technologies[8,9] and include plasma separators, plasma fractionators, and high performance hemodialyzers. These dialyzers should be used as hemodiafiltration apparatus primarily aimed at removing cytokines.

With these devices, it was possible to achieve plasma exchange, plasma perfusion, hemodiafiltration or hemodialysis (macromolecular changes up to the albumin level), plasma filtration, including double filtration, cryofiltration,[10] and thermofiltration.[11] Furthermore, through the introduction of various types of adsorption columns, plasma adsorption technologies were introduced.

## Plasma Exchange

FIGURE 9 shows the filters we developed, primarily with several Japanese companies, during the past 30 years. Plasma exchange means to separate the entire diseased plasma that has been removed from whole blood and to exchange it with healthy normal plasma (see FIGURE 10). Approximately 20% of the blood that passed through the filter was removed by the plasma separator at a transmembrane pressure of less than 50 mmHg (see FIGURE 11).

Initially, this author's group treated many patients suffering from liver failure with the plasma exchange method. Almost all patients recovered from coma; however, this procedure was not successful for more than 30% of the patients. At death, the patients' liver tissues were necrotic. It was finally realized that plasma exchange was not helping the recovery of liver function. Actually, this procedure was removing "hepatocyte growth factors" in the liver failure plasma of patients and donated "hepatocyte suppressor factors" that exist in a healthy individual. Because of the removal of the hepatocyte growth factors and the addition of hepatocyte suppressor factors, the procedure did not contribute to the recovery of the patients' liver functions.

## Plasma Adsorption

It was decided that only the toxic factors should be removed from liver failure patients by using adsorbents.[12] The plasma of the patients was separated by the

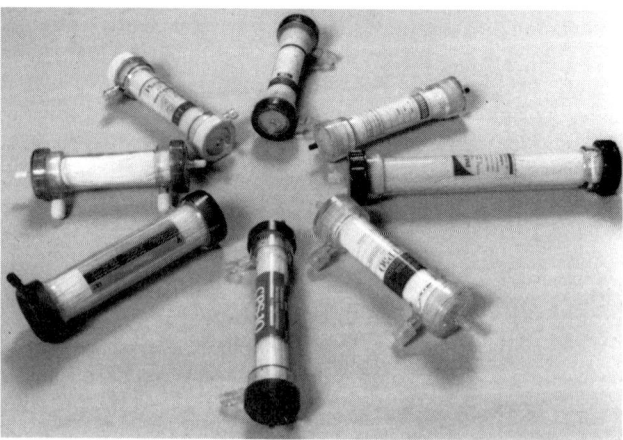

**FIGURE 9.** Various types of plasma separators and plasma fractionators.

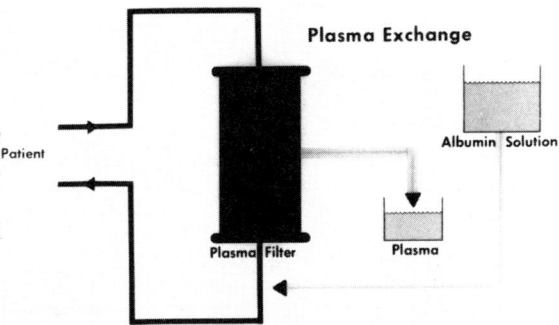

**FIGURE 10.** Schematic illustration of plasma exchange.

membrane plasma separator. The separated plasma was perfused over the adsorbent column of the liver toxins (see FIGURE 12).

FIGURE 13 shows the BR601 column used for one hyperbilirubinemia patient. For the second and third procedures, two columns were used. Even for the fourth procedure, the effective removal of bilirubin can be seen here. After seven sessions, this patient completely recovered from a comatose condition, her appetite became normal, and she was walking inside the hospital. Again, her bilirubin level increased after the plasma adsorption procedures were stopped (see FIGURE 14). Perhaps a liver transplant should have been performed on this patient. Unfortunately, in 1980, liver transplants were not always considered to be successful. In spite of an additional five plasma perfusions, this patient did not recover.

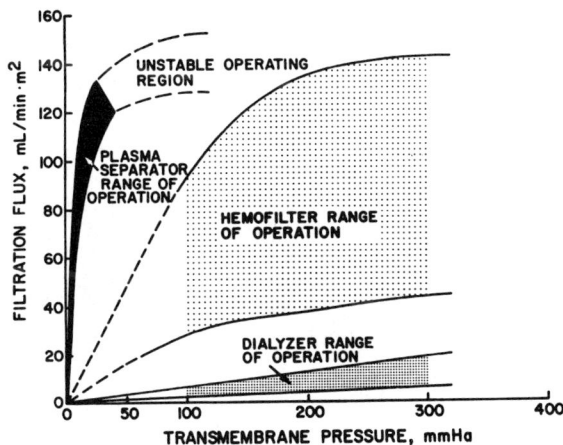

**FIGURE 11.** Filtration flux of plasma separator, hemofilter, and hemodialysis filters at various transmembrane pressures.

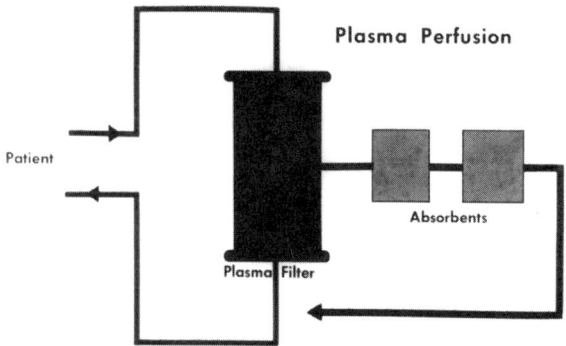

**FIGURE 12.** Schematic illustration of plasma adsorption.

It was clear that this method of hepatic assist was effective for symptomatic relief. If the patient had been treated more extensively, there would have been more symptomatic recovery but no improved chance for survival.

### Plasma Filtration

Therefore, consideration was given to the idea that there might be immunological factors involved, and subsequently double-filtration technologies were introduced. After plasma was separated, it was passed through the plasma fractionation filter. The removal of immunologically active macromolecules was performed by this secondary filter (see FIGURE 15).

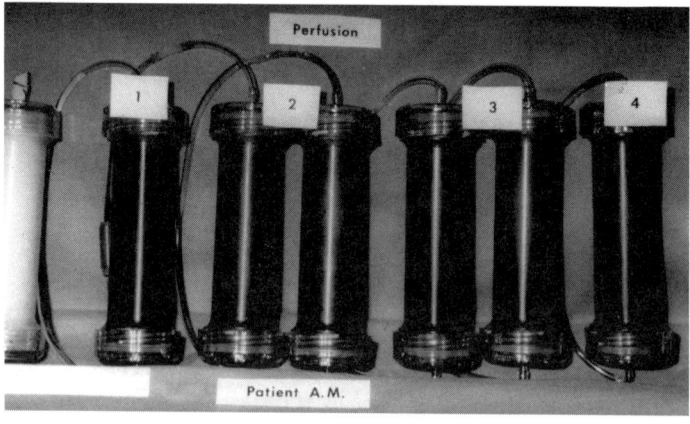

**FIGURE 13.** BR 601 columns used for patient AM, 50-year-old female (see FIG. 18) suffering from hyperbilirubinemia (initial four treatments).

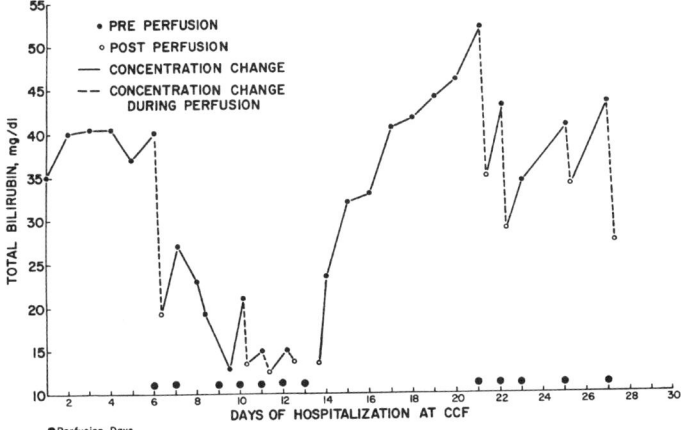

**FIGURE 14.** Total bilirubin levels of patient AM during the initial seven sessions and subsequent five sessions of plasma adsorption treatment.

The Kuraray 5A filter removed molecules larger than 100 KD, including λ globulin and immuno complexes. The Kuraray 2A filter removed any molecules larger than albumin molecules (see FIGURE 16). To the far right in FIGURE 16 the sieving characteristics of the plasma separator are shown, and on the far left those of hemodialyzers. When this plasma fractionation was performed at near zero temperature, a fibrinogen–fibronectin–heparin conjugate was formed and a more effective immunologically active macromolecule removal was established. It was called cryofiltration[10] (see FIGURE 17). When plasma fractionation was performed at near

## Plasma Filtration

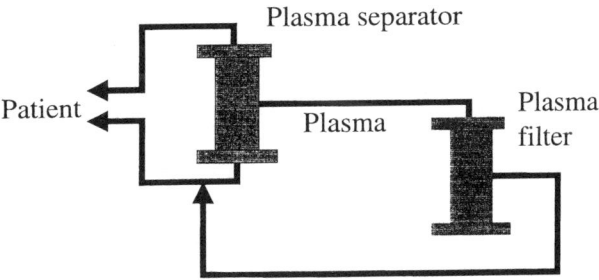

**FIGURE 15.** Schematic illustration of plasma filtration or plasma fractionation.

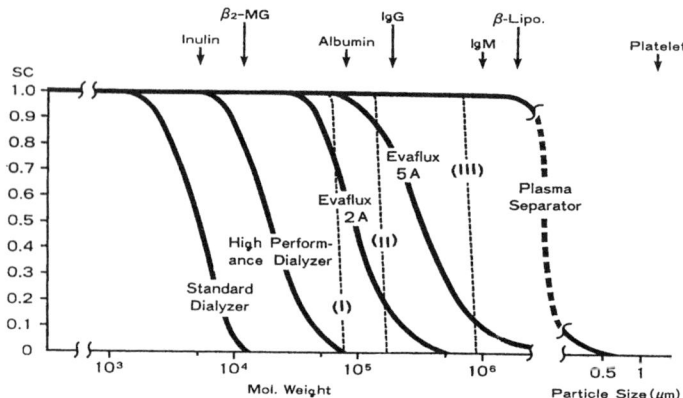

**FIGURE 16.** Sieving coefficients of Kuraray 5A and 2A plasma fractionators. The 5A fractionators separate IgG or larger macromolecules and the 2A fractionators separate albumin or larger macromolecules. Sieving coefficients of the plasma separator (*right*) and hemodialyzer (*left*) are also shown.

body temperature, a more effective removal of lipids was accomplished. This procedure was called thermofiltration.[11]

It was demonstrated that by using these various types of blood purification systems, it would be possible to maintain chronic liver failure patients for long term. One patient suffering from sclerosing cholangitis was kept alive for longer than five years with these various types of treatments. This patient was the longest surviving

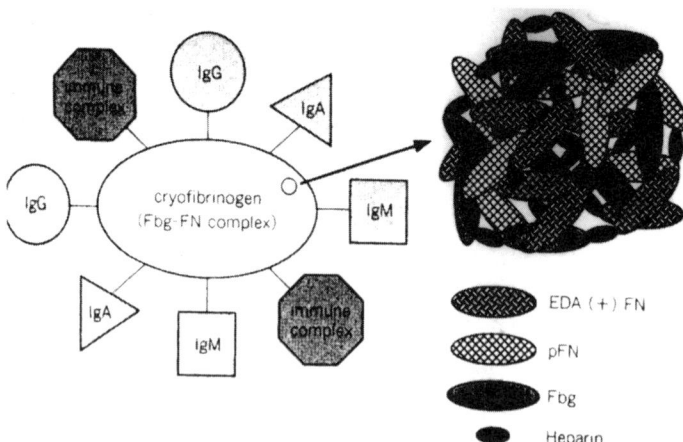

**FIGURE 17.** Schematic illustration of cryogel. The basic structures are fibrinogen–heparin–fibronectin complexes. Other macromolecules are also included in the cryogel.

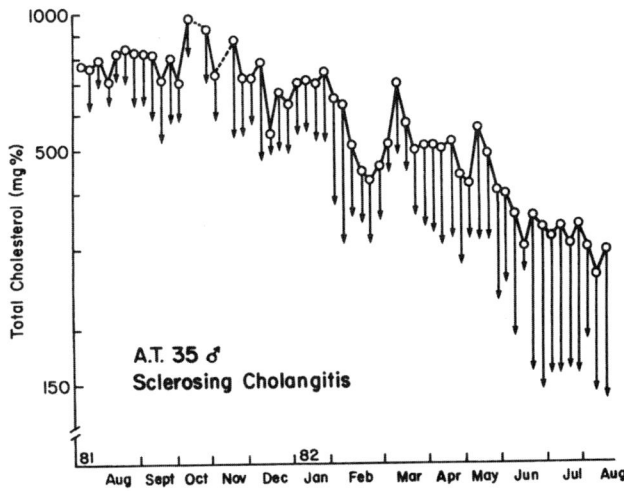

**FIGURE 18.** Total cholesterol levels of the patient AT (35 to 36 years old) suffering from sclerosing cholangitis during the first year of treatment.

patient[13] with these plasmapheresis procedures. The initial one-year total cholesterol levels of this patient are shown in FIGURE 18.

## METABOLIC ASSIST VERSUS HEPATIC ASSIST

In conclusion, none of our efforts to develop a hepatic assist device for normalizing the metabolic condition in blood helped to increase the survival rate of liver failure patients. The current method of applying a hepatic assist device provides only a bridge to transplantation. One should not forget about a hepatic assist device that helps to recover a patient's liver function, as Dr. Starzl warned this author 37 years ago.

What is the future of the artificial liver? This author believes it should not be metabolic assist but hepatic assist. The device should help and stimulate hepatocyte growth in the patient.

## HEPATIC ASSIST: CURRENT STATUS

The current and most effective means of treatment for fulminant hepatic failure are the combination therapies involving continuous hemodiafiltration (removal of small and low level molecules smaller than albumin, such as cytokines) and continuous plasma exchange (removal of entire plasma containing toxic substances caused by or resulting from the disease).[14] Symptomatically, almost all patients with acute liver insufficiency who received this type of non-hybrid hepatic assist recovered from hepatic coma. It is extremely important to attempt the treatment of hepatic-failure–causing diseases at the same time as treating liver failure syndromes. Treatment of acute hepatitis A, acute hepatitis B, and non-A, non-B hepatitis (now hepatitis C) caused by designated viruses should include antivirals and immunosuppresant therapies. Fulminant autoimmune and drug-induced hepatitis should be treated by immunosuppressant and other agents. Of course, it is also necessary to provide hepatocyte growth factors. The overall survival rate of fulminant hepatic failures in selected centers in Japan is almost at the same level as is transplantation in the U.S. For chronic liver diseases, it is possible to maintain a patient's metabolic parameters in physiologically acceptable ranges by repeated plasma exchanges and plasma perfusion over absorbents for as long as five years.[13]

## IMMUNOLOGICAL SEPARATION OF HEPATOCYTES FROM AND TO THE PATIENT

Hybrid artificial organs use heterologous or homologous tissues for their reactors. The naturally immunological issues between cultured cells and patients should be properly addressed. For hepatic assist, a reduced level in the patient's liver functions allows minimal immunological consideration. However, this immunological issue should be considered carefully.

As described in the previous section, immunologically active macromolecules that either originated from cultured cells or in patients can be removed effectively through the use of plasma fractionators and/or immunoadsorbents. Plasma fractionators effectively remove any molecules larger than IgG. Furthermore, albumin metabolism or metabolic activities smaller than albumin molecules are possible for cultured cells if Kuraray 2A filters are employed for separating the patient's blood from the cultured cells. With these apheresis technologies, immunological barriers can be established (see TABLE 2).

If this immunological barrier membrane is used, the proper delivery of $O_2$ within the cultured cell chamber should be considered, as already described. In addition, it is essential that biocompatibility issues of the immunological barrier membrane be considered (see TABLE 3).

In order to achieve this objective, we should provide hepatocyte growth factors to patients. We should find a method for improving microcirculation in liver tissues and we should find a method for increasing the oxygen supply to liver tissues.

The author believes in the recent progress of hybrid hepatic assist utilizing hepatocyte growth and maintenance. Technologies developed through a bioartificial liver will benefit many patients currently suffering from liver failure.

TABLE 2. Molecular cutoff of immunogically active macromolecules

| |
|---|
| Separation of IgG or higher molecules possible |
| Separation of albumin or lower molecules possible |
| Separation of whole plasma macromolecules possible |

TABLE 3. Biocompatibility of barrier material

| |
|---|
| Humoral compatibility |
|     Coagulation factors |
|     Complement activation |
| Cellular compatibilities |
|     Platelet adhesion and aggregation |
|     White thrombus |
| Erythrocyte compatibilities |
|     Red thrombus |
|     Hemolysis |

## CONCLUSIONS

To establish an effective hepatic assist system, it is expected that a hybrid artificial liver is the final goal in using cultured hepatocytes. Currently, there are several problems to overcome before such a hybrid system can be used as a clinically feasible device. They include the following:

- Use of hepatocytes harvested from normal human liver tissues or tumor cells.
- Hepatocytes harvested from heterologous origin or not.
- Maintenance of normal hepatocyte functions for cultured cells.
- Maintenance of viable hepatocyte function with an oxygen rich environment.
- Requirement to keep cultured hepatocyte frozen whenever clinical needs arise.
- Removal of dead cells or hypofunctioning cells and their non-desirable decomposed tissues and/or released toxic substances.

Hepatocyte suppressor factors exist in the plasma of healthy individuals whereas hepatocyte growth factors exist in the plasma of hepatic failure patients. Thus, exchanging a patient's plasma with that of a normal individual will eliminate the possible hepatocyte growth or regeneration of damaged hepatocytes. In addition, hepatocyte microcirculation could be improved to stimulate the growth of hepatocytes. This could be achieved by infusing oxygen-carrying macromolecules to the patient.

The hepatic assist device aimed at symptomatic relief through the removal of toxic substances from the patient's plasma does not contribute to the survival of hepatic failure patients.

## REFERENCES

1. NOSÉ, Y., J. MIKAMI, Y. KASAI, et al. 1963. An experimental artificial liver utilizing extracorporeal metabolism with sliced or granulated canine liver. Trans. Am. Soc. Artif. Int. Organs. **9**: 358–362.
2. MITO, M., A. NISHIMURA & Y. NOSÉ. 1959. Studies on extracorporeal circulation to an artificial liver. Sogoigaku (Japanese text). **16**(8): 761–762.

3. NOSÉ, Y. 1973. Manual on Artificial Organs. Volume II. The Oxygenator. 27 (Figure 2-2). The C.V. Mosby Co. St. Louis.
4. MATSUSHITA, M., A. YABUKI, M. NASU, et al. 1987. Oxygen transport by a pyridoxolated-hemoglobin-polyoxyethylene conjugate. Trans. Am. Soc. Artif. Intern. Organs **33:** 352–355.
5. HORI, M. & Y. NOSÉ. 1987. Proceedings of the International Symposium on Stabilized Hemoglobin. 1–95, Cleveland, Ohio. ISAO Press.
6. STARZL, T.E., T.L. MARCHIORO & K.N. VONKAULLA. 1963. Homotransplantation of the liver in humans. Surg. Gynecol. Obstet. **117:** 659–676.
7. KODAMA, M., H. AOKI, K. HANAZAKA & T. TANI. 1991. New development of hemoadsorption. Intensive Critical Care Med. **3**(2): 143–150.
8. NOSÉ, Y., P.S. MALCHESKY, J.W. SMITH & R.S. KRAKAUER. 1983. Plasmapheresis. Therapeutic Application and New Techniques. 436. Raven Press, New York.
9. NOSÉ, Y. & P.S. MALCHESKY. 1981. Technical aspects of membrane plasmapheresis. *In* Therapeutic Membrane Plasmapheresis (I). T. Oda, Ed.: 3–14. Proccedings of the First Symposium on Therapeutic Plasmaphereis held by Japanese Society for Therapeutic Plasmapheresis. June 20, 1981. FK Schattauer Verlag, Stuttgart and New York.
10. NOSÉ, Y., T. HORIUCHI, P.S. MALCHESKY, et al. 1982. Therapeutic cryogel removal in autoimmunodisease. What is cryogel? *In* Therapeutic Plasmapheresis (II). T. Oda, Ed.: 15–25. Proceedings of the Second Sympsium on Therapeutic Plamapheresis. FK Schattauer Verlag, Stuttgart and New York.
11. NOSÉ, Y., M. USAMI, P.S. MALCHESKY, et al. 1985. Clinical thermofiltration: intitial application. Artif. Organs **9:** 425–427.
12. ASAMURA, Y., P.S. MALCHESKY, I. ZAWICKI, et al. 1980. Clinical hepatic support by on-line plasma treatment with multiple sorbents—evaluation of system performance. Trans. Am. Soc. Artif. Intern. Ogans **26:** 400–404.
13. MALCHESKY, P.S., S. OMOKAWA & Y. NOSÉ. 1988. Chronic hepatic assist. Artif. Organs **12**(4): 300–304.
14. YOSHIBA, M., K. INOUE, K. SEKIYAMA & I. KOH. 1996. Favorable effect of new artificial liver support on survival of patients with fulminant hepatic failures. Artif. Organs **20:** 1169–1172.

# Use of Small Animal Models for Screening Immunoisolation Approaches to Cellular Transplantation

RONALD G. GILL

*Barbara Davis Center for Childhood Diabetes,*
*University of Colorado Health Sciences Center, Denver, Colorado, USA*

ABSTRACT: It has been recognized for many years that immunoisolation strategies form an attractive approach to preventing the rejection of cellular allografts and xenografts. Although immunoisolation has proven dramatically successful in some cases, the results have tended to be somewhat variable. Although many advances have been made in the development of biocompatible materials for separating host immune cells from the transplanted tissues, much of the experimentation in this area has been outcome driven. That is, the nature of host reactivity and/or biomaterial design resulting in the failure of some immunoisolation strategies has mostly been undefined. A first premise of this discussion is that immunoisolation is primarily cell isolation and not antigen isolation, *per se.* That is, although varied membrane barriers are designed to prevent cell–cell contact between host and donor cells, soluble antigens derived from the transplant are likely to gain access to the host immune system. A key question centers on the degree and consequence of this type of antigen presentation in the host to the immunoisolated transplant. To address this and related concerns, this overview presents a simple paradigm for using defined rodent (mouse) models for systematically screening the efficacy of immunoisolated cellular transplants. The proposition is made that understanding the basis of graft failure will aid in the design of future immunoisolation technologies.

KEYWORDS: small animal models; screening immunoisolation; cellular transplantation

## ADVANTAGES AND DISADVANTAGES OF DEFINED SMALL-ANIMAL (MOUSE) MODELS

The main proposition of this discussion is that defined transgenic or gene-targeted (knockout) mouse models can be used to assess the nature of immune recognition of immunoisolated transplants. Such models are especially useful for troubleshooting in those cases in which immunoisolated tissues fail to demonstrate durable function *in vivo.* There are clear advantages to using defined mouse models for assessing immunoisolation technologies. Relative to large-animal models, even the most complex mouse genetic knockout models are inexpensive and represent a reduced scale of

Address for correspondence: Ronald G. Gill, Ph.D., Barbara Davis Center for Childhood Diabetes, University of Colorado Health Sciences Center, 4200 East 9th Ave., Box B-140, Denver, CO 80262, USA. Voice: 303-315-6390; fax: 303-315-4124.
ron.g.gill@uchsc.edu

reagents and tissue required for testing the efficacy of immunoisolation. Perhaps more important are the vast array of transgenic and defined genetic knockout models uniquely available in mice. Such models allow for testing the impact of pathways involving either broad (e.g., humoral versus cellular) or precise (e.g., individual cytokines or effector molecules) immune components on the function of immunoisolated grafts. For example, such models can distinguish between responses ranging from humoral complement-dependent tissue injury to cellular T lymphocyte-dependent damage, results that can have great utility in directing immunoisolation design (see below).

However, as useful as such knockout models are in dissecting mechanisms of immune-mediated responses, there are also disadvantages to using small animal models. First, mouse models do not reflect the large scale of tissue preparation required for clinical transplantation. That is, transplanting relatively small amounts of immunoisolated tissues into rodents allows for the use of highly selected, uniformly treated tissues that may not be feasible in large-scale preparations required in a large animal or human. For example, we have been able to individually hand select completely coated microencapsulated pancreatic islets in sufficient numbers to transplant mice, an approach that is not applicable for large animal use. Other key disadvantages include the potential anatomical, metabolic, or immunologic differences between small and large animal models. For example, it is possible that some forms of innate immune responses, such as those generated by macrophage or complement activation, are more vigorous in large outbred animal models than those found in rodent models. Thus, some immune pathways relevant in large animal models may be under represented in rodent models. Taken together, it is important to consider both the positive and negative features of rodent models when evaluating the general utility of experimental results.

## DISTINGUISHING BIOCOMPATIBILITY FROM TRANSPLANTATION IMMUNITY

Although immunoisolation technology can have many disparate applications, there is general interest in grafting tissues either from the same species (allografts) or from differing species (xenografts). In order to embark on a systematic evaluation of immunoisolation technology *in vivo,* it is important to first define key endpoints of graft evaluation. Proposed in FIGURE 1 is a sample progression of checkpoints encountered towards the ultimate goal of achieving successful immunoisolation of discordant tissue xenografts. The initial rate-limiting property essential to the success of immunoisolation is that of biocompatibility. Any biomaterial considered for tissue transplantation must be suitable for durable graft function and be immunologically inert relative to the host. That is, the biomaterials used must be compatible both with the grafted cells or tissues and with the host itself. If either of these two forms of tissue compatibility is insufficient, then graft survival will be in jeopardy. On one hand, immunoisolated tissues can be subject to failure due to non-immunologic factors such as chronic nutritional or oxygen deprivation due to the site of implantation and/or to the barrier design.[1–3] This is especially relevant in that most immunoisolation strategies employ non-vascularized devices in which nutrient and

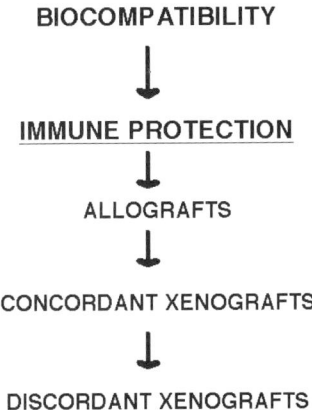

**FIGURE 1.** Sequential progression of assessing immunoisolation strategies.

oxygen delivery to the graft depend on diffusion, imparting biophysical limitations to any immunoisolation strategy suitable for durable graft survival and function. Conversely, the biomaterials used for immunoisolation must also be compatible with the host. It is commonly appreciated that some materials, such as impure alginate preparations used for microencapsulation, can trigger host inflammatory reactions to the immune barrier itself resulting in graft dysfunction.[4,5] Therefore, given these concerns, it is essential first to determine the biocompatibility of the immunoisolation strategy independently of transplantation immunity. This is best accomplished through isografting in which genetically identical or autologous tissues are transplanted to the host. This approach is outlined in FIGURE 2: tissues from an inbred mouse strain (BALB/c) are grafted into another BALB/c recipient. In this way, tissue dosing, site of implantation, and longevity of graft function can be monitored to optimize the inherent biocompatibility of the immunoisolation technology without the confounding variable of allograft or xenograft immunity. Adequately addressing this

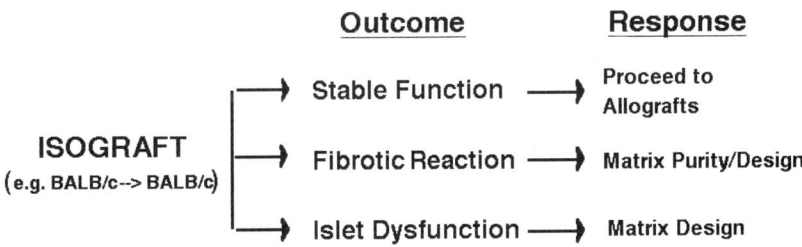

**FIGURE 2.** Assessing the biocompatibility of immunoisolation materials with pancreatic islet isografts.

paramount problem of biocompatibility is essential prior to evaluating the efficacy of immunoisolation strategies for immune protection of allografts or xenografts.

## IMMUNE PROTECTION FOR IMMUNOISOLATED TISSUES: DIRECT AND INDIRECT RESPONSES TO GRAFT ANTIGENS

Although solving issues of biocompatibility of immunoisolation materials with both the host and the donor tissue is essential, the primary goal of this field is to afford immune protection to the transplant. Immunoisolation was predicated on the rationale that preventing cell–cell contact between the host and the donor would attenuate the response. For example, for many years a major paradigm has been that cytotoxic T cells play a key role in graft rejection through a cognate interaction with the grafted cells. Supporting this view is evidence that cellular graft rejection can be highly cell-specific,[6,7] implicating a precise, cell–cell recognition in rejection consistent with the activity of cytotoxic T cells. However, it has become apparent that responses to both allografts and xenografts are more complex than previously appreciated. Therefore, the design of immunoisolation technology requires a consideration of the types of T cell responses that can occur in response to the graft. This initial focus on T lymphocytes as rate-limiting cells in tissue rejection is derived from numerous observations that most tissue allografts or xenografts are spontaneously accepted in T cell-deficient mice (e.g., athymic nude or scid mice) despite the presence of functional innate immune system components such as natural killer (NK) cells, myeloid lineage cells, and complement pathways.[8,9] Although these varied innate immune system elements greatly contribute to host reactivity, graft-destructive responses in mice appear to be fundamentally T cell-dependent. For example, our own laboratory routinely transplants allogeneic mouse, or xenogeneic rat, porcine, and human pancreatic islets into T cell-deficient mice without any discernible host response deleterious to the graft.

Given the T cell-dependent nature of graft rejection, it is essential to consider how T cells may contribute to the response against tissues sequestered within an immunoisolation barrier. T lymphocytes primarily recognize antigens as peptides presented in association with major histocompatibility complex (MHC) molecules. CD8 T cells recognize antigens presented in association with class I MHC molecules whereas CD4 T cells generally recognize antigens presented by class II MHC molecules.[10] However, *two* signals are required for T lymphocyte activation, engagement of the antigen-specific T cell receptor (signal 1) and a second non-antigen-specific inductive signals signal, or costimulator, provided by an antigen presenting cell (APC).[11] A variety of receptor–ligand interactions can provide costimulatory activity, such as CD28[12] expressed by T cells interacting with the CD80 and CD86[13] cell-surface molecules expressed by APC and activated B cells.[14] Germane to this discussion, two primary forms of graft antigen presentation can fulfill this two-signal requirement for T cell activation: (1) *Direct* (or donor MHC-restricted) antigen presentation, in which T cells engage native donor MHC–peptide complexes expressed on the surface of graft-derived APCs; and (2) *indirect* (or host MHC-restricted) antigen presentation, in which donor-derived antigens are captured by recipient APCs, degraded, and re-presented in association with recipient MHC molecules. Importantly, exogenous antigens are generally processed and presented by class II MHC molecules and thus invoke a predominantly CD4 T cell response,[15] although such captured antigens can also be presented by MHC class I-restricted cross-presentation.[16] The distinction between these two antigen presentation pathways is of great importance regarding immunoisolated tissues. T cells of *direct* specificity for MHC antigens on the surface of donor cells require a cell–cell, or cognate interaction with the graft APCs whereas T cells specific for donor-derived peptides presented by MHC molecules on the surface of host APCs do not. Thus, although tissue isolation strategies that prevent cell–cell contact between donor cells and host immune cells are expected to block the direct pathway as defined above (see FIGURE 3), the indirect pathway is expected to be more problematic. That is, whereas the direct pathway may be excluded by immunoisolation, there is still the potential for graft peptide antigens to traverse the isolating membrane and be presented by host-type APCs. The degree and consequence of this type of response to immunoisolated tissues is largely undefined, but has been observed in the response to immunoisolated tissues[17] and would explain the finding that CD4 T cells can participate in the response to encapsulated islets.[18,19]

In the case of pancreatic islet transplants, our own experience suggests that *direct* T cell reactivity predominates in allograft immunity whereas *indirect* reactivity predominates in xenograft immunity.[15] That is, although both donor APCs and MHC class I expression are required for islet allograft rejection, *host* CD4 T cells, APCs, and MHC class II expression are important for islet xenograft rejection.[15] This latter finding is consistent with a CD4-dependent *indirect* response in which donor antigens are presented by MHC class II antigens expressed on host-type APCs (FIG. 3). It is important to emphasize that these distinctions are not absolute; in many cases indirect reactivity occurs to allografts whereas direct reactivity occurs to xenografts. However, this general scheme implies that the direct pathway dominates alloreactivity whereas the indirect pathway dominates islet xenoreactivity. If this primary role for direct reactivity in alloimmunity is the case, then allogeneic tissues would be

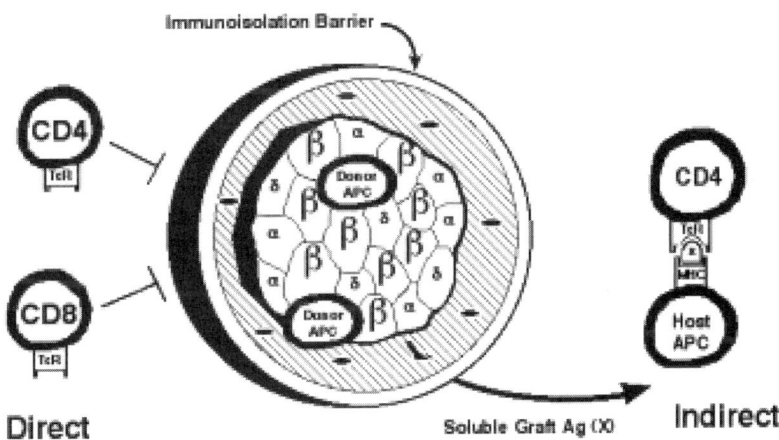

**FIGURE 3.** Contribution of *direct* (donor APC-dependent) and *indirect* (host APC-dependent) T cell reactivity to an immunoisolated islet transplant.

expected to have considerable benefit from strategies that exclude cell–cell contact with the graft. However, if indirect reactivity is primary for xenograft immunity, then the benefit of immunoisolation for xenograft survival is less certain (FIG. 3). As mentioned above, because nutrient, waste, and oxygen exchange within capsules or other devices depends on diffusion, there are limits on the thickness and porosity of the immunoisolation membrane that are conducive for tissue viability. This means that some degree of sensitization of the host is likely through the release of soluble antigens and subsequent presentation by the indirect pathway (FIG. 3). Antibody responses, which are a surrogate marker of the indirect pathway resulting from a CD4 T cell-B cell interaction,[15] have been observed in response to immunoisolated xenografts.[20] If the xenograft response is a result of this indirect pathway, then one might expect that immunoisolated xenogeneic tissues would be more vulnerable to recognition than would allogeneic tissues. This disparity between allograft and xenograft survival in immunoisolation devices has been reported.[19]

A major unanswered question centers on the extent of such indirect CD4 T cell reactivity to immunoisolated xenografts. There are dramatic examples whereby immunoisolation can facilitate xenograft survival[21–25] indicating that immunoisolation can be beneficial for the implantation of xenogeneic cells. However, other studies indicate that CD4-dependent immunity can result in the destruction of immunoisolated xenografts.[18,19] It is unclear what properties of biomaterials promote the survival of xenografts in some settings or permit destructive responses to occur in others. The remainder of this discussion focuses on the use of defined mouse models for screening the nature of immune protection provided by immunoisolation technology.

## TROUBLESHOOTING FOR IMMUNOISOLATED ALLOGRAFTS AND XENOGRAFTS

Once it is clear that an immunoisolation approach is biocompatible with both the graft and the host, it is essential to determine the degree of immune protection afforded by the barrier. As implied above, provided that an immunoisolation material maintains a structural barrier preventing cell–cell contact between the graft and the recipient, the primary T cell-dependent pathway of concern is the *indirect* pathway of antigen recognition. However, to confirm this concept, it is reasonable to ensure than an immune barrier affords suitable protection to cell or tissue allografts (see FIGURE 4). For example, the rejection of xenografts, but not allografts within a defined immunoisolation barrier supports the concept that rejection is a result of xenograft immunity and is not simply a structural or biocompatibility design flaw. This approach was used successfully in discerning the nature of xenograft failure in macroencapsulation devices.[19] That is, CD4 T cell-dependent reactivity was found to trigger xenograft but not allograft rejection in the same model system,[19] presumably via exaggerated *indirect* CD4 T cell recognition of the xenogeneic cells relative to the allogeneic graft.

Assuming that allografts can indeed survive within a defined immunoisolation system, a key issue will be troubleshooting the potential event that xenogeneic tissues

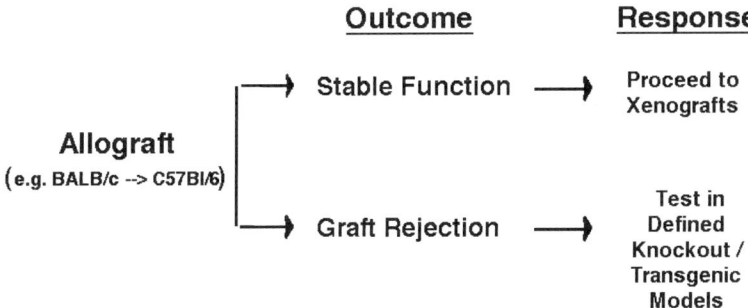

**FIGURE 4.** Assessing allograft function in immunoisolation barriers.

are rejected. Solving this problem would be most useful for determining the modifications in materials and/or adjunct therapies required for xenograft survival. Depicted in FIGURE 5 are only a handful of candidate mouse models currently available that can be applied to the study of immunoisolated xenografts. For example, an ongoing debate in the field centers on the nature of soluble effector molecules that may participate in the injury to immunoisolated tissues. Since only those molecules capable of traversing the isolation barrier have access to the graft, defining such effector molecules has great importance for future barrier modification. Humoral elements such as antibodies and complement components are potentially key participants in target injury. However, proinflammatory cytokines such IL-1, TNF, and IFN-γ are also well known for inflicting injury to tissues such as pancreatic islets.[26–29] Furthermore, IL-1 in some cases is capable of mediating islet injury to encapsulated islets *in vitro*,[30,31] implicating such cytokines as potential mediators of injury to immunoisolated tissues

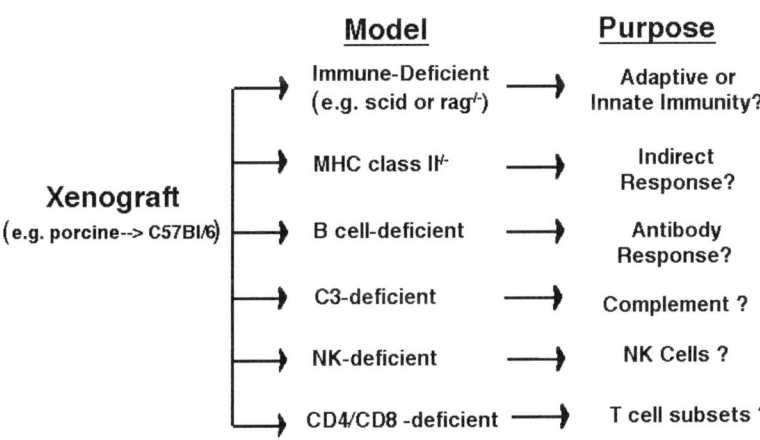

**FIGURE 5.** Assessing immunoisolated xenografts in defined genetic mouse knockout models.

during an inflammatory response. However, some forms of microencapsulation appear less sensitive to cytokine-mediated injury.[32] Since mice that are genetically deficient in these varied cytokines are available, the use of such animals as recipients could clarify the role of these candidate molecules in mediating tissue injury.

Despite this long standing implication of soluble molecules as mediators of tissue dysfunction within immunoisolation devices, there is actually little published data on the effector mechanisms involved *in vivo*. For example, although it is clear that xenografts elicit vigorous antibody responses, such antibodies surprisingly are not actually required for the acute cellular rejection of either concordant (rat) or discordant (porcine) non-immunoisolated xenografts in mice.[33,34] This result can also extend to the cellular rejection of immunoisolated xenografts, in which CD4 T cells, in the absence of B cells or antibodies, can result in graft rejection in some cases.[19] This issue of correlation versus causation greatly impacts the immunoisolation field. For example, finding the presence of xenoreactive antibodies may prompt the development of barrier membranes with reduced porosity that excludes such antibodies. However, this course of action may only result in reduced tissue viability without a clear indication that the antibody response is actually injurious to the immunoisolated tissues. A means of testing the potential pathogenic role for antibody and complement pathways in the response to encapsulated xenografts is to use B cell and/or complement-deficient models to establish a causal requirement of these pathways to tissue injury. In the latter case, complement component C3-knockout mice exist that are deficient in both classical and alternate pathways of complement activation. The use of these models can aid in either implicating or excluding a primary role for these key humoral pathways in inflicting damage to immunoisolated xenografts (FIG. 5).

Conversely, it is possible that T cell-dependent inflammation, independent of humoral immunity, contributes to the failure of immunoisolated xenografts. Confirmation that such graft failure is indeed a result of CD4 T cell-dependent *indirect* presentation can be accomplished through the use of knockout models that are either CD4- or MHC class II-deficient (FIG. 5). Macrophages, APCs that can be activated by CD4 T cells via indirect recognition, can clearly participate in the injury to immunoisolated tissues.[35,36] This type of inflammatory injury would most likely result from cytokines and other mediators, such as reactive oxygen species, with much lower molecular mass than represented by antibody and complement components. Fortunately, knockout models for most key inflammatory cytokines also exist, permitting a dissection of cytokine requirements for tissue injury if desired. Distinguishing the role of antibody/complement pathways, mentioned above, from smaller molecules such as cytokines in triggering tissue injury is most important for developing immunoisolation strategies. For example, if IL-1 were found to be a key mediator of tissue injury, then it would probably not be realistic to design barriers to exclude this molecule; IL-1 may be comparable in molecular mass to many therapeutic molecules (e.g., 5–30 kd) required from the immunoisolated cells. Furthermore, decreasing the porosity of barriers to exclude cytokines with an approximate molecular weight range of 10–30 kd may lead to an unacceptable sacrifice in tissue viability. Taken together, whether or not an isolation barrier can be used practically as a molecular sieve for soluble effector molecules depends greatly on the relative contribution and local concentrations of individual candidate molecules to tissue injury. Alternatively, it is possible that local inflammation does not actually lead to pathogenic concentrations of effector molecules within the immunoisolation device, *per se,* but rather leads to a consumption of oxygen and nutrients in the local microenvironment, essentially starving the graft.[37] If this were the case, reducing the molecular weight exclusion properties of the barrier membrane may only exacerbate the problem.

## SPECIAL CONSIDERATION FOR XENOGRAFTS: IMMUNOISOLATION FOR BIOCONTAINMENT OF ZOONOSES

The focus of this discussion has been on the use of immunoisolation materials for immune protection of allogeneic and xenogeneic cells. However, an important concern has been raised concerning the potential transfer of pathogens, or zoonoses, within xenogeneic tissues to the host. This issue has come to the forefront given the demonstration that porcine endogenous retroviruses (PERV) can result in cross-species infection *in vitro* and *in vivo*.[38,39] It is notable, however, that evidence to date has not indicated PERV transmission to either humans or primates transplanted with porcine cell or tissue xenografts.[40–43] Nevertheless, the potential exposure of xenograft recipients to defined or undefined zoonoses requires careful consideration. In this respect, immunoisolation technologies may play an additional benefit by forming a potential containment barrier to reduce the risk of such pathogen exposure, analogous to the use of macroencapsulation devices to contain neoplastic cells.[44] The potential use of immunoisolation for this adjunct purpose depends entirely on the requirements for graft survival described above. That is, for immunoisolation barriers to prevent the egress of zoonoses, the exclusion characteristics of the selective membrane must be sufficient to contain the defined pathogens (e.g., PERV). However, whether such membrane properties are compatible with the robust survival and function of the immunoisolated xenograft would need to be empirically determined. It is plausible that immunoisolation materials could serve simultaneous immune-protective and biosafety functions in the future.

## CONCLUSION

In summary, identifying rate-limiting immune mechanisms involved in the potential injury to immunoisolated tissues will greatly aid in the continuing development and application of this technology. A final speculation on this topic pertains to the original supposition that immunoisolation permits cellular but not antigen sequestration of the transplant. It is probably important to distinguish between these two issues. Although preventing cell–cell contact is currently feasible and realistic, preventing exposure of the host to potentially small molecular weight donor-derived antigens may not be readily feasible. Thus, attempts to greatly restrict the molecular mass of soluble molecules that can readily traverse a size-selective barrier may not be warranted without clear evidence that defined cellular pathways and candidate effector molecules indeed contribute to tissue injury *in vivo*. Otherwise, an unacceptable sacrifice in graft viability may be made without a corresponding benefit in immune protection.

## REFERENCES

1. COLTON, C.K. & E.S. AVGOUSTINIATOS. 1991. Bioengineering in development of the hybrid artificial pancreas. J. Biomech. Eng. **113:** 152–170.
2. SCHREZENMEIR, J., J. KIRCHGESSNER, L. GERO, *et al.* 1994. Effect of microencapsulation on oxygen distribution in islets organs. Transplantation **57:** 1308–1314.
3. DE VOS, P., J.F.M. VAN STRAATTEN, A.G. NIEUWENHUIZEN, *et al.* 1999. Why do nicroencapsulated islet grafts fail in the absence of fibrotic overgrowth? Diabetes **48:** 1381–1388.
4. VANDENBOSSCHE, G.M.R., M.E. BRACKE, C.A. CUVELIER, *et al.* 1993. Host reaction against empty alginate-polylysine microcapsules: influence of preparation procedure. J. Pharm. Pharmacol. **45:** 115.
5. DE VOS, P., B. DE HAAN & R. VAN SCHLIFGAARDE. 1997. Effect of the alginate composition on the biocompatibility of alginate-polylysine microcapsules. Biomaterials **18:** 273.
6. ROSENBERG, A.S. & A. SINGER. 1988. Evidence that the effector mechanism of skin allograft rejection is antigen-specific. Proc. Natl. Acad. Sci. USA **85:** 7739–7742.
7. SUTTON, R., D.W.R. GRAY, P. MCSHANE, *et al.* 1989. The specificity of rejection and the absence of susceptibility of pancreatic islet β cells to nonspecific immune destruction in mixed strain islets grafted beneath the renal capsule in the rat. J. Exp. Med. **170:** 751–762.
8. CZITROM, A.A., S. EDWARDS, R.A. PHILLIPS, *et al.* 1985. The function of antigen-presenting cells in mice with severe combined immunodeficiency. J. Immunol. **134:** 2276–2280.
9. LAUZON, R.J., K.A. SIMINOVITCH, G.M. FULOP, *et al.* 1986. An expanded population of natural killer cells in mice with severe combined immunodeficiency (SCID) lack rearrangement and expression of T cell receptor genes. J. Exp. Med. **164:** 1797–1802.
10. SWAIN, S.L. 1983. T cell subsets and the recognition of MHC class. Immunol. Rev. **74:** 129–142.
11. LAFFERTY, K.J., S.J. PROWSE & C.J. SIMEONOVIC. 1983. Immunobiology of tissue transplantation: a return to the passenger leukocyte concept. Annu. Rev. Immunol. **1:** 143–173.
12. JUNE, C.H., J.A. LEDBETTER, P.S. LINSLEY, *et al.* 1990. Role of the CD28 receptor in T-cell activation. Immunol. Today **11:** 211–216.
13. CHEN, C., A. GAULT, L. SHEN, *et al.* 1994. Molecular cloning and expression of early T cell costimulatory molecule-1 and its characterization as B7-2 molecule. J. Immunol. **152:** 4929–4936.
14. SCHWARTZ, R.H. 1992. Costimulation of T lymphocytes: The role of CD28, CTLA-4, and B7/BB1 in interleukin-2 production and immunotherapy. Cell **71:** 1065–1068.
15. GILL, R.G. 1998. Direct and indirect pathways of immunity to pancreatic islet transplants. Transplant. Rev. **12:** 85–95.
16. KURTS, C., W.R. HEATH, F.R. CARBONE, *et al.* 1996. Constitutive class I-restricted exogenous presentation of self antigens *in vivo*. J. Exp. Med. **184:** 923–930.
17. ZEKORN, T.D.C., U. ENDL, U. SEIBERS, *et al.* 1995. Evidence for an antigen-release induced cellular immune response against alginate-polylysine encapsulated islets. Xenotransplantation **2:** 116.
18. WEBER, C.J., S. ZABINSKI, T. KOSCHITZKY, *et al.* 1990. The role of $CD4^+$ helper T cells in the destruction of microencapsulated islet xenografts in NOD mice. Transplantation **49:** 396–404.
19. LOUDOVARIS, T., T.E. MANDEL & B. CHARLTON. 1996. $CD4^+$ T cell mediated destruction of xenografts within cell-impermeable membranes in the absence of $CD8^+$ T cells and B cells. Transplantation **61:** 1678–1684.
20. LANZA, R.P., A.M. BEYER & W.L. CHICK. 1994. Xenogeneic humoral responses to islets transplanted in biohybrid diffusion chambers. Transplantation **57:** 1371–1375.
21. LANZA, R.P., D.H. BUTLER, K.M. BORLAND, *et al.* 1991. Xenotransplantation of canine, bovine, and porcine islets in diabetic rats without immunosuppression. Proc. Natl. Acad. Sci. USA **88:** 11100–11104.

22. LANZA, R.P., A.M. BEYER, J.E. STARUK, et al. 1993. Biohybrid artificial pancreas: Long-term function of discordant islet xenografts in streptozotocin diabetic rats. Transplantation **56**: 1067–1072.
23. LANZA, R.P., W.M. KUHTREIBER, D. ECKER, et al. 1995. Xenotransplantation of porcine and bovine islets without immunosuppression using uncoated alginate microspheres. Transplantation **59**: 1377–1284.
24. SUN, Y., X. MA, D. ZHOU, et al. 1996. Normalization of diabetes in spontaneously diabetic cynomologus monkeys by xenografts of microencapsulated porcine islets without immunosuppression. J. Clin. Invest. **98**: 1417–1422.
25. HASSE, C., T. BOHRER, P. BARTH, et al. 2000. Parathyroid xenotransplantation without immunosuppression in experimental hypoparathyroidism: long-term in vivo function following microencapsulation with a clinically suitable alginate. World J. Surg. **24**: 1361–1366.
26. PUKEL, C., H. BAQUERIZO & A. RABINOVITCH. 1988. Destruction of rat islet cell monolayers by cytokines. Synergistic interactions of interferon-γ, tumor necrosis factor, lymphotoxin, and interleukin1. Diabetes **37**: 133–136.
27. MANDRUP-POULSEN, T., G.A. SPINAS, S.J. PROWSE, et al. 1987. Islet cytotoxicity of interleukin 1. Influence of culture conditions and islet donor characteristics. Diabetes **36**: 641–647.
28. RABINOVITCH, A., W. SUMOSKI, R.V. RAJOTTE, et al. 1990. Cytotoxic effects of cytokines on human pancreatic islet cells in monolayer culture. J. Clin. Endocrinol. Metab. **71**: 152–156.
29. BENDTZEN, K., T. MANDRUP-POULSEN, J. NERUP, et al. 1986. Cytotoxicity of human p I 7 interleukin-1 for pancreatic islets of Langerhans. Science **232**: 1545–1547.
30. COLE, D.R., M. WATERFALL, M. MCINTYRE, et al. 1992. Microencapsulated islet grafts in the BB/E rat: a possible role for cytokines in graft failure. Diabetologia **35**: 231.
31. KING, A., A. ANDERSEN & S. SANDLER. 2000. Cytokine-induced functional suppression of microencapsulated rat pancreatic islets in vitro. Transplantation **70**: 380–400.
32. TAI, I.T., I. VACEK & A. SUN. 1995. The alginate-poly-L-lysine-alginate membrane: evidence of a protective effect on microencapsulated islets of Langerhans following exposure to cytokines. Xenotransplantation **2**: 37.
33. GILL, R., L. WOLF, D. DANIEL, et al. 1994. CD4 T cells are both necessary and sufficient for islet xenograft rejection. Transplant. Proc. **26**: 1203.
34. BENDA, B., A. KARLSSON-PARRA, A. RIDDERSTAD, et al. 1996. Xenograft rejection of porcine islet-like cell clusters in immunoglobulin- or Fc-receptor γ-deficient mice. Transplantation **62**: 1207–1211.
35. WIEGAND, F., K.-D. KRONCKE & V. KOLB-BACHOFEN. 1993. Macrophage-generated nitric oxide as cytotoxic factor in destruction of alginate-encapsulated islets. Transplantation **56**: 1206–1212.
36. KESSLER, L., C. JESSER, Y. LOMBARD, et al. 1996. Cytotoxicity of peritoneal murine macrophages against encapsulated pancreatic rat islets: in vivo and in vitro studies. J. Leuk. Biol. **60**: 729–736.
37. BRAUKER, J., L.A. MARTINSON, S.K. YOUNG, et al. 1996. Local inflammatory response around diffusion chambers containing xenografts. Nonspecific destruction of tissues and decreased local vascularization. Transplantation **61**: 1671–1677.
38. VAN DER LAAN, L.J., C. LOCKEY, B.C. GRIFFETH, et al. 2000. Infection by porcine endogenous retrovirus after islet xenotransplantation in SCID mice. Nature **407**: 90–94.
39. MARTIN, U., M.E. WINKLER, M. ID, et al. 2000. Productive infection of primary human endothelial cells by pig endogenous retrovirus (PERV). Xenotransplantation **7**: 138–142.
40. MARTIN, U., G. STEINHOFF, V. KIESSIG, et al. 1998. Porcine endogenous retrovirus (PERV) was not transmitted from transplanted porcine endothelial cells to baboons in vivo. Transpl. Int. **11**: 247–251.
41. HENEINE, W., A. TIBELL, W.M. SWITZER, et al. 1998. No evidence of infection with porcine endogenous retrovirus in recipients of porcine islet-cell xenografts. Lancet **352**: 695–699.

42. PARADIS, K., G. LANGFORD, Z. LONG, *et al.* 1999. Search for cross-species transmission of porcine endogenous retrovirus in patients with living pig tissue. Science **285:** 1236–1241.
43. ELLIOTT, R.B., L. ESCOBAR, O. GARKAVENKO, *et al.* 2000. No evidence of infection with porcine endogenous retrovirus in recipients of encapsulated porcine islet xenografts. Cell Transplant. **9:** 895–901.
44. LOUDOVARIS, T., S. JACOBS, S. YOUNG, *et al.* 1999. Correction of diabetic NOD mice with insulinomas implanted within Baxter immunoisolation devices. J. Mol. Med. **77:** 219–222.

# *In Vitro* Maturation of Neonatal Porcine Islets

## A Novel Model for the Study of Islet Development and Xenotransplantation

TANYA M. BINETTE, JANNETTE M. DUFOUR, AND GREGORY S. KORBUTT

*Surgical-Medical Research Institute, Department of Surgery, University of Alberta, Edmonton, Alberta, Canada*

ABSTRACT: The mechanisms involved in islet neogenesis have remained largely unexplored due to lack of an appropriate model. Furthermore, with the recent advances in islet transplantation, the need for alternative islet tissue sources is greater than ever. Therefore, the authors have refined a neonatal porcine islet (NPI) maturation model that offers an ideal tool to gain insight into islet growth as well as an alternative source of transplantable tissue. Recent knowledge in islet growth has resulted in endocrine tissue being derived from human pancreatic precursor tissue *in vitro*. The potential for large scale production of endocrine tissue *in vitro* has been indicated, however, more investigation must be done on the various signals and pathways involved in pancreatic development to optimize this technique. The authors believe that their NPI *in vitro* maturation model provides an ideal tool to study islet growth and maturation. Transduction of the NPI to overexpress genes of interest (i.e., PDX-1) or exposure of the NPI to various culture conditions will allow us to determine the effects on islet maturation. An understanding of NPI development gained will not only allow us to mature this unlimited tissue source for optimal xenotransplantation, but also elude to how human pancreatic endocrine precursor cells may be used to solve the current islet tissue supply problem.

KEYWORDS: maturation; neonatal porcine islets; islet development; PDX-1; xenotransplantation

## INTRODUCTION

In insulin-dependent (type 1) diabetes mellitus (IDDM), an autoimmune attack on an individual's pancreas, causes their insulin producing β cells to be destroyed. The β cells are located in the islets of Langerhans,[1] which are scattered throughout the pancreas. Impaired insulin production results in inadequate glucose metabolism leaving the diabetic individual with very high blood glucose levels.[2] Pathogenesis of IDDM includes genetic predisposition and environmental factors (indicated by localized populations where incidence of diabetes is high). Diabetics require daily insulin injections as well as an exercise regime and balanced diet[3] and still encounter complications due to transient periods of hyperglycemia. Acute complications

Address for correspondence: Gregory S. Korbutt, Surgical-Medical Research Institute, 1074 Dentistry/Pharmacy Building, University of Alberta, Edmonton, Alberta, Canada T6G 2N8.

korbutt@ualberta.ca

include ketoacidosis (which in the most severe cases leads to coma), hypoglycemic episodes due to over treatment with exogenous insulin, and increased susceptibility to infections. Chronic complications such as kidney malfunction, nerve impairment, blindness, and cardiovascular disease[4] all contribute to the decreased lifespan of the diabetic individual, up to one-third shorter than the average non-diabetic.[3] These complications of diabetes lead to psychosocial consequences for the patient, from guilt for transmitting a genetic disorder, to adjusting to life without vision, to difficulties in obtaining life insurance and the high cost of treatment.[5]

## CLINICAL ISLET TRANSPLANTATION

Transplanting insulin-producing tissue may replace the need for daily insulin injections.[6] Although insulin therapy restores the regular lifestyle of the individual, the search for a more permanent and controlled physiological method of restoring glucose homeostasis is promising.[7] For more than 30 years pancreas transplants have been conducted[7] despite the complicated surgical procedure, significant morbidity and mortality, and chronic immunosuppression of the recipients. Therefore, the risks associated with pancreas transplantation are sometimes greater than the complications resulting from living with the disease. Isolated islet transplantation offers a potentially lower risk, since islets can be tested for donor compatibility and, perhaps, manipulated *in vitro* to avoid rejection.[6] Although human islet transplants have been a reality since 1987,[8] only within the past two years have they become an effective treatment for a population of diabetics.[9] Along with advances in islet purification, a novel steroid-free immunosuppressive regime (Daclizumab, Sirolimus, and low dose Tacrolimus) has increased the success (measured by insulin independence for one year) of islet transplantation from 8% to 100%, the longest term of insulin independence being 24 months posttransplant.[9] However, even after improvements in the islet isolation procedure, in order to achieve insulin independence patients must receive more than 9,000 islet equivalents per kilogram body weight, which requires a minimum of two donor pancreases for each patient.

Presently, in the United States, the number of newly diagnosed IDDM patients is ten times the number of consenting organ donors every year.[10] The goal of transplanting pancreatic endocrine tissue is to prevent complications associated with periodic hyperglycemia normally experienced by type I diabetics using daily insulin treatment. Insulin independence early in the course of the disease would curb the subsequent complications, although until an ample, transplantable, insulin-producing source is found this goal will not be achieved. Several sources of insulin-producing tissue are being considered to solve the "islet supply" problem. Porcine[11–15] and bovine[16] islets, fish-Brockman bodies,[17] genetically engineered insulin-secreting cell lines,[18–20] and *in vitro* production of human fetal[21] or adult[22] β cells are the major candidates.[23]

## WHY NEONATAL PORCINE ISLETS?

Xenotransplantation involves cross species tissue exchange. Pigs are most likely to provide a solution to the organ supply problem. Pigs breed rapidly, have large litter sizes, can be housed in a pathogen-free environment, are inexpensive, ethically acceptable, and have many morphological and physiological similarities to humans. Porcine insulin has also been used safely in the treatment of type 1 diabetics and is structurally similar to human insulin.[24]

Adult pigs are not considered a good source of islet tissue sinces age, breed, and quality of the organs result in varying success in regard to islet yield and viability.[23] Although adult porcine islets produce insulin, they are fragile, which makes them very hard to maintain in tissue culture. This becomes a problem if the islets are exposed to culturing procedures to reduce graft immunogenicity or to temperature variations (low temperatures used to store islets, or to combine islets from several donors). Collagenase digestion of fetal porcine pancreas, however, results in an abundant yield of viable islet-like cell clusters that can restore normoglycemia in diabetic nude mice two months posttransplantation.[11] However, fetal pancreatic $\beta$ cells taken from rat, pig, and human respond poorly to glucose.[25] A more promising solution appears to be neonatal porcine pancreatic islet tissue. Viable NPI cells are successfully isolated in large numbers by culturing collagenase digested pancreas for nine days.[25] It has been shown that the poor response of fetal $\beta$ cells to glucose is rapidly converted to an adult-like pattern after birth.[26] This leads to the obvious conclusion that neonatal islets, having growth potential and being not as fragile as adult islets, are a possible solution for xenotransplantation tissue to treat hyperglycemia in type 1 diabetics. Not only are NPI successfully maintained in tissue culture, they also respond well to a glucose challenge *in vitro* secreting significant amounts of insulin.[25]

Transplantation of 2,000 NPI was able to restore diabetic (alloxan induced) nude mice to a normoglycemic state within 6–8 weeks posttransplantation. Normoglycemia was maintained for upwards of 11 months posttransplantation. On removal of the grafted tissue a state of hyperglycemia returned. Examination of the cellular insulin contents of the harvested grafted kidneys showed an increase in insulin content 5–20 times that of what it was on the day of transplant.[6]

## WHY NEONATAL PORCINE ISLETS AS A MODEL FOR ISLET NEOGENESIS?

Knowing that *in vitro* cultured NPI response to glucose exceeds that of fetal islets *in vitro*,[25] and assuming that this is due to more functionally mature $\beta$ cells, it may be concluded that NPI have undergone $\beta$ cell growth and maturation. Furthermore we have also seen, using our *in vitro* model of micoencapsulating and culturing NPI in autologous serum, an increased proportion of insulin- and glucagon-positive cells in conjunction with increased numbers of NPI cells. Taken together, this culture system causes the expansion of islet endocrine cells and in particular an increased mass of $\beta$ and $\alpha$ cells. Associated with this *in vitro* cell expansion is an elevated expression of the homeodomain transcription factor PDX-1 as well as proinsulin mRNA. We believe that the alginate microcapsule provides an extracellular support matrix whereas the autologous serum is a source of species-specific growth/mitogenic factors and in combination they induce differentiation and/or proliferation of NPI cells *in vitro*.

This *in vitro* expansion of β and α cells may involve two distinct pathways: (1) differentiation of ductal epithelium into β and α cells (neogenesis), and (2) proliferation of preexisting differentiated β and α cells. Our current data in part support this concept since:

  (a) Cytokeratins (CK) have been shown to be markers of islet ductal cell differentiation,[27] and during our culture system the proportion of CK-7 positive NPI ductal cells decreases by 28% to less than 5%. This corresponds to an increased proportion of endocrine cells; suggesting differentiation of ductal cells into endocrine cells and thus a subsequent loss of CK-7 expression.
  (b) CK-7 reactivity in β and α cells has been suggested to provide evidence for the differentiation of duct cells into islet endocrine cells since these double positive cells are believed to be transitional cytodifferentiated cellular phenotypes.[27]
  (c) It has been suggested that during regeneration of pancreatic endocrine cells, PDX-1 is upregulated in newly dividing ductal cells as well as islets.[28] In our model we see a progressive increase in PDX-1 expression and we also frequently observe ductal cyst formation "budding" from the NPI cell aggregates and that these ductal cells stain intensely for PDX-1.

This system not only provides us with an unlimited supply of islet tissue, it also is an excellent model of islet development that should theoretically mimic human pancreatic islet development and can thus be used as a model for studying human islet proliferation and neogenesis.

## ISLET β CELL DEVELOPMENT

All pancreatic cells differentiate from the ductal epithelium and evidence shows that both exocrine and endocrine cells are derived from the same population of precursor cells. It has been observed during development, that some endocrine cells stain double-positive for two hormones and progressively each cell is restricted to express only one.[26] However, Herrara[29] recently designed experiments that clearly indicate that β cells do not activate the glucagon promoter at all during development and α cells similarly do not turn on the insulin promoter. He suggests, as does Jensen,[30] that insulin/glucagon double-positive cells may appear later in islets, but dual hormone expression is not involved in islet cell development. Early in development, all pancreatic precursor cells express pancreatic and duodenal homeobox gene-1 (PDX-1). Exocrine cells lose the PDX-1 phenotype and begin to express p48 and finally amylase whereas endocrine cells maintain PDX-1 expression, adopting a neurogenin 3 (Ngn3)-positive phenotype followed by expression of NeuroD/Beta2.[30] A review of pancreatic development by Slack[31] warns us that at this point it is difficult to make conclusions about development due to genes being turned on and off by various cells at various stages of development. However, the consensus seems to be that both β and α cells begin to express Pax 6, shortly after which α cells begin to produce glucagon and subsequently stop expressing PDX-1. β cells maintain PDX-1 and Pax 6 expression while also expressing Pax 4 and finally producing insulin. Somatostatin-producing δ cells also express PDX-1 during development and throughout maturity. Other key genes that are activated/inactivated during islet cell development include Brain 4, Nkx 6.1, Nkx 2.2, and Isl 1.[30]

It appears that there are two separate mechanisms by which islet β cells develop: replication of preexisting β cells (proliferation) or differentiation of β cells from ductal cells (neogenesis).[26] In adult β cells the rate of mitosis is low and, despite the presence of ductal epithelium, there is a terminal nature of β cell differentiation, indicating that the entire repertoire of β cells is established during the neonatal period.[32] Only due to extreme stimulus will precursor cells in the adult pancreatic ducts differentiate to replenish the islet population. Some experimental examples of extreme stimulus include partial pancreactomy, cellophane wrapping of the head of the pancreas, or clinically, shortly after onset of IDDM or severe liver disease.[26] In humans it has been observed that during neonatal development there is a progressive dominance of terminally differentiated endocrine cells that are derived from a polymorphic endocrine subpopulation of islet cells.[33] During this development, the β cells develop their main function, to respond to physiological levels of blood glucose. There are likely three stages involved in development: (1) proliferation of the ductal epithelium (cells budding off), (2) differentiation of budding cells into new islet (endocrine) cells, and (3) amplification of the preexisting β cells. Toward the end of the neonatal period, there is a rapid decrease in proliferation of islet cells. From transplantation experiments, it has been demonstrated that a critical β cell mass must be achieved (via growth and/or differentiation) before normoglycemia is achieved.

We believe that porcine pancreatic development may be directly extrapolated to predict human pancreatic development. The NPI maturation system allows us to closely examine postnatal development of the endocrine pancreas—a period during which very few mature β cells are present and the population is largely composed of ductal precursor cells.[25] Using confocal laser scanning microscopy to observe the morphology of islets stained for insulin and CK7 (ductal cell marker), some cells stain yellow indicating they are double positive for CK7 (red) and insulin (green). A large percentage of the cell population is CK7 positive precursor cells, indicating the growth potential of NPI. Following tissue culture as described by Korbutt,[25] NPI are composed of 24% insulin-containing cells and a total of 35% fully differentiated endocrine cells. The remaining 57% of the islet cells are nongranulated epithelial cells with a subpopulation of ductal endocrine precursor cells identified by expression of CK7.[23] Rayat (personal communication) has shown that after transplantation, NPI CK7 positive ductal cells decrease in number, presumably being replaced by insulin-positive β cells that can be seen budding off ducts. This supports the concept that in neonates, β cells differentiate from ductal precursor (CK7-positive) cells. The presence of such a high percentage of CK7-positive cells in the neonatal islet supports the theory that endocrine cells differentiate from ductal cells and that this idea is indeed very plausible and worthy of further investigation. In order to overcome the lag time before normoglycermia is achieved in transplants using NPI, the growth factors and signals involved in the differentiation of ductal cells into endocrine cells must first be understood. Understanding of the mechanisms involved in β cell development will ultimately provide insight into alternative sources of human tissue for islet transplantation.

## PANCREATIC AND DUODENAL HOMEOBOX GENE-1 (PDX-1)

A homeobox is a short (180 base pair) conserved DNA sequence encoding a DNA-binding motif that is known for its presence in genes involved in the development and cell differentiation of many organisms.[34] As indicated by the name, PDX-1 is selectively produced in the pancreas and duodenum. It appears to function both in the regionalization of the gut endoderm (to form the beginnings of the pancreas) and in β cell maturation. A mouse that is homozygous pdx-1$^{-/-}$ is born without a pancreas and does not survive.[35–38] A study reported by Stoffers et al.[35] described the case of a female born without a pancreas. As was expected, a (frame shift) mutation was located in the pdx-1 gene resulting in the production of a much shorter protein (16 kD instead of 42–43 kD), which may interfere with normal PDX-1 function. It is speculated that a less severe pdx-1 mutation may impair PDX-1 functions and result in downregulation of insulin gene transcription. Prolonged high glucose levels (hyperglycemia) impair insulin production and also appear to reduce insulin transcription by down regulation of PDX-1.[39,40]

Along with its role in pancreatic development, PDX-1 is expressed in the developing pancreatic duct and is associated with insulin, glucagon, and amylase expression during morphogenesis and differentiation.[41] Later in development, PDX-1 becomes phenotypically specific, expressed mainly in β cells, δ cells, and pancreatic ductal cells.[41] A few days after being partially pancreatectomized, rats demonstrated elevated expression of PDX-1 mRNA and protein in pancreatic ducts (β cell precursors).[42] This experiment mimics ontogeny as the pancreas is undergoing regeneration and indicates, along with the observation that PDX-1 is expressed in β cells at a higher rate than in other endocrine cells, that PDX-1 is (in part) responsible for β cell neogenesis. PDX-1 expression declines during development and is restricted to β and δ cells in adult islets (in the nuclei of 91% of β cells and in 15% of δ cells) suggesting that it is a regulator of the insulin gene.[43–46]

Exploration of the role of PDX-1 in β cell proliferation and differentiation is of interest due to its potential applications in pre-transplant culturing of NPI to achieve a higher β cell mass, thereby shortening the lag period between transplantation and normoglycemia in islet transplant recipients. These studies are also relevant to exploring other sources for development of transplantable human islet tissue.

Due to the critical role of PDX-1 in β cell neogenesis and islet development it is important to understand the regulation of PDX-1 transcription and translation as well as the factors involved in the activation of PDX-1 protein (i.e., phosphorylation, nuclear localization, DNA binding, and transactivation). A better understanding of the mechanisms of PDX-1 activation may lead to improved *in vitro* and *in vivo* techniques to increase β cell mass. Factors involved in the regulation of PDX-1 include the transcription factor, upstream stimulatory factor (USF), and hepatocyte nuclear factor 3 (HNF3), the insulinotropic hormone glucagon-like peptide 1 (GLP-1), and a GLP-1 analog exendin-4 as well as glucose, insulin, transforming growth factor beta (TGFβ) and PDX-1 itself.

Regulation of PDX-1 occurs on several levels. First the mRNA must be transcribed from the pdx-1 gene and then the mRNA translated into protein. Next the protein must be modified (by posttranslational modification, shuttling to the nucleus, binding DNA, and transactivation) to allow PDX-1 to be fully functional. Transcriptional regulation occurs by several transcription factors that bind specific sites in the regions upstream (5′) to the pdx-1 gene, which then leads to increased levels of PDX-1 mRNA. These factors (described below) are also known to be important in the β cell specific transcription of PDX-1 mRNA. In addition, hormones are also able to regulate the production of PDX-1 mRNA and protein.

To identify factors involved in the β cell specific transcription of PDX-1, the 5′ flanking region of the endogenous pdx-1 promoter was studied. Regions in the promoter between bp −2809 and −1958 as well as an E box element located at bp −107 to −102 were shown to be involved in controlling β cell specific expression of PDX-1.[47–50] Mutational and functional analysis of HNF3 like sites within area I (−2694 to −2561 bp) and II (−2139 to −1958 bp) demonstrated that HNF3 (a regulator of endodermal cell lineage development) binds to these sites and is involved in the β cell specific expression of PDX-1 that is controlled by these sites.[47,48] Moreover, PDX-1 mRNA levels were downregulated in HNF3 homozygous null β cells.[48] Another group has shown that HNF3 can bind to and transactivate two regions in the PDX-1 promoter between bp −2809 to −2655 and −2233 to −2097, both of which have been shown to confer β cell-specific activation. The region from bp −2809 to −2655 was also shown to bind PDX-1 and it was demonstrated that PDX-1 acts cooperatively with HNF3 to regulate its own transcription at this site.[49] Together these results indicate that HNF3 has an essential role in cell-type–specific PDX-1 transcription and that PDX-1 may autoregulate itself. In addition, upstream stimulatory factor (USF) binds to the PDX-1 gene promoter at an E box and functionally regulates the expression of PDX-1 gene in differentiated pancreatic β cells.[50]

Other factors able to upregulate PDX-1 mRNA and protein production, GLP-1 and exendin-4, are interesting because they have been shown to stimulate β cell proliferation and neogenesis.[51–54] Exendin-4 treatment of diabetic mice was able to increase the pancreatic expression of PDX-1 as well as enhance β cell neogenesis and islet size.[54] Exendin-4 was also able to stimulate the replication of β cells and differentiation of β cells from ductal tissue.[53] These results imply that upregulation of PDX-1 leads to increased β cell mass and underline the importance to further study factors involved in regulation of PDX-1 expression.

PDX-1 protein is regulated at several levels including phosphorylation, transactivation, DNA binding, and nuclear translocation. Translation of the PDX-1 mRNA produces a 284-amino acid protein (see FIGURE 1) with a calculated molecular mass of 31 kDa and an observed molecular mass of 46 kDa. This change in molecular mass is believed to be due to protein phosphorylation and PDX-1 is known to have nine putative phosorylation sites at $Ser^{61}$, $Ser^{66}$, $Ser^{125}$, $Thr^{152}$, $Thr^{187}$, $Ser^{211}$, $Ser^{212}$, $Thr^{231}$, and $Ser^{232}$.[55] Moreover, high glucose has been shown to stimulate conversion from the inactive 31 kDa form of PDX-1 found in the cytoplasm to the active 46 kDa phosphorylated form localized predominantly in the nucleus.[56] This translocation was shown to be activated through phosphatidylinositol 3-kinase (PI3K).[56,57] Protein phosphorylation is known to regulate the activity of many proteins and can do so at all levels of protein regulation. In the case of PDX-1,

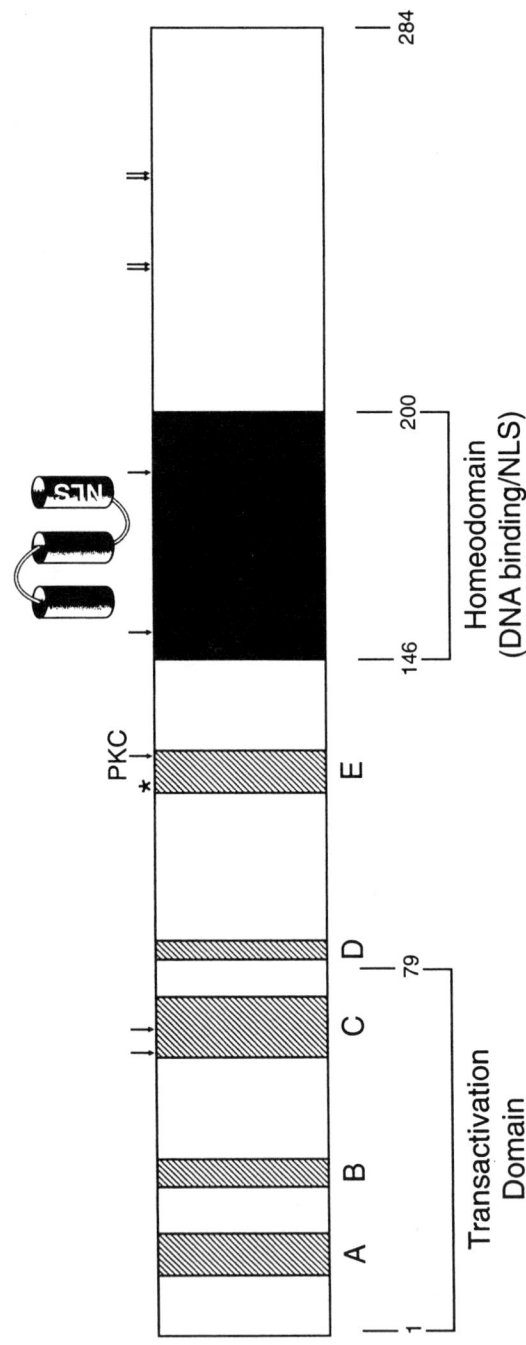

**FIGURE 1.** Schematic representation of PDX-1 protein indicating potential phosphorylation sites (↓). *, PBX-1 interaction site; NLS, nuclear localization signal; PKC, potential protein kinase C phosphorylation site.

phosphorylation is involved in translocation of the protein from the cytoplasm to the nucleus, and has been shown to increase the ability of PDX-1 to bind DNA and to upregulate transcription (transactivational activity).[56–59]

The transactivation domain is located in the N-terminus within the first 79 amino acids (FIG. 1) and is stimulated by glucose.[60–62] This domain contains the necessary regions for PDX-1 to regulate the glucose stimulated expression of the insulin gene that is most likely controlled through specific protein interactions between the transactivation domain of PDX-1 and other transcription factors that regulate insulin transcription. Three evolutionarily conserved subdomains within this region, subdomain A (amino acids 13–22) subdomain B (amino acids 32–38) and subdomain C (amino acids 60–73) are important for transactivation (FIG. 1).[60] Subdomains A, B, and C are required for interactions between PDX-1 and basic helix-loop-helix proteins (i.e., E2/5, E12, E47, etc.) that bind as a heterodimeric complex to the E2 element of the insulin promoter. However, so far a direct PDX-1–E2A protein complex has not been demonstrated.[60] Subdomain D (amino acids 81–85) has little or no effect on regulation of the insulin gene. Deletion of subdomain E (amino acids 117–126) had no effect on activation of the insulin promoter even though this deletes the region containing a potential PKC phosphorylation site and the region known to interact with PBX-1 (a homolog of extradenticle that binds cooperatively with homeodomain proteins in *Drosophila melanogaster*).[62,63] PBX-1 interaction having no effect on the insulin promoter is not surprising because this interaction is required for somatostatin expression in δ cells, but not insulin expression in β cells.[63]

The DNA binding domain and nuclear translocation signal are both found in the homeodomain that consists of three helices and is located between amino acids 146 and 206 (FIG. 1). The homeodomain encodes a 61 amino acid motif that forms a helix–turn–helix structure that is highly conserved.[64] The homeodomain binds DNA at A-T rich regions and regulates the insulin promoter by binding to the A box at a core consensus sequence of TAAT.[64] One nuclear localization signal (NLS) located in helix three of the homeodomain is present in PDX-1. The NLS is 16 amino acids long (**RH** IKIWFQN **RR** MKW **KK**) with three pairs of basic residues (shown in bold) essential for nuclear targeting.[55,65]

Factors known to regulate PDX-1 protein activation are TGFβ, glucose, GLP-1, exendin-4, and insulin, of which glucose is the best studied. TGFβ has been shown to increase PDX-1 DNA binding activity, transactivational activity, and nuclear localization whereas glucose, GLP-1, and insulin have been shown to increase PDX-1 DNA binding and transactivational activity.[58,59,61,66–70] Treatment of INS-1 cells with TGFβ leads to an increase in PDX-1 protein levels in nuclear extracts, increased DNA binding to the PDX-1 responsive A3 site of the insulin promoter, and increased activity of the insulin promoter.[66] The TGFβ stimulation of the insulin promoter was found to be due to activation through the A3 site.[66]

The stimulated DNA binding and transactivational activity may be due to protein phosphorylation since GLP-1, insulin, and glucose are all able to increase IP3K activity.[67,68,70] Moreover, glucose has been shown to increase PDX-1 DNA binding activity, and transactivation in a phosphorylation dependent manner.[58,59] These studies of PDX-1 protein regulation have for the most part been studied in the context of insulin gene production in cell lines, therefore further studies are needed to determine the role PDX-1 protein regulation has in primary β cell development.

Although much is known about the regulation of PDX-1, there is still much to learn about the mechanisms of PDX-1 regulation. Moreover, it is clear that PDX-1 has an important role in the differentiation and proliferation of β cells in the pancreas and in the β cell specific expression of the insulin gene. However, the precise role of PDX-1 and the factors involved in PDX-1 regulation in β cell neogenesis and proliferation need to be elucidated. In addition, further understanding the mechanisms of PDX-1 activation is important in the design of culture conditions that will enhance the expansion of NPI from ductal and endocrine tissues for the treatment of diabetics.

## DEDIFFERENTIATION AND TRANSDIFFERATION OF ACINAR AND DUCTAL TISSUE

Although islet isolation techniques have been modified to increase the yield of purified islets, even if the resulting yield exceeds the current 60% of pancreatic islets allowing the donor to transplant ratio to be 1:1, there will still never be enough organ donors to satisfy the tissue demand. Recent literature has described the ability of acinar cells to dedifferentiate and subsequently (re) adopt a ductal cell phenotype.[71–73] Taken together with Bonner-Weir's technique of large scale production of endocrine tissue from human ductal tissue acquired postislet isolation,[74] there is much promise of an alternative source of large amounts of human islet tissue that may be modified *in vitro* to be transplanted to a larger population of diabetics.

During human islet isolation, typically 20 ml of tissue is discarded once the islets are purified. This tissue contains mostly exocrine cells, however a small proportion of unpurified islets and a significant amount of ductal tissue remain. Pancreatic tumors in humans primarily contain CK19-positive cells, indicating they are of ductal origin.[71] However, observations of transgenic animals designed to develop pancreatic tumors indicate that these ductal cell tumors may be the result of acinar cell transdifferentiation.[75] Hall *et al.* hypothesized that the acinar tissue dedifferentiates to a ductal precursor phenotype, and this ductal tissue has the capacity to expand *in vivo*, indicating that *in vitro* manipulation of acinar tissue may expand ductal (pancreatic precursor) tissue.[71] *In vitro*, culturing human acinar tissue in media containing 10% fetal calf serum results in transdifferentiation to a ductal (CK19-positive) phenotype. This has been repeated in rat[72] using CK20 as a ductal cell marker where 60% of the transdifferentiated cells are binuclear, indicating they are of an acinar origin. In both rat and human, once acinar tissue has transdifferentiated, some of this ductal tissue has been shown to express PDX-1 protein and message, indicating these cells have the potential to be pancreatic precursor cells.[72,73] It has been shown in both the NOD mouse[76] and human[74] that ductal tissue may differentiate and become functional islet/endocrine tissue *in vitro*. The authors believe that their *in vitro* NPI maturation model provides the necessary tools to elucidate the mechanisms involved in ductal cell differentiation. Freshly isolated NPI include exocrine and ductal tissue that, in the appropriate culture conditions, may expand the endocrine cell mass by transdifferentiating. These recent advances in islet cell development indicate potential for a human tissue source that will make allotransplantation of islets an available treatment for type 1 and 2 diabetics.

## CONCLUSION

Our model of NPI maturation was developed with the belief that this would be the most abundant, practical source of insulin-producing tissue. There are still obstacles to overcome, such as xenoantigens expressed on all porcine tissue that trigger hyperacute rejection in humans and the fear of incorporation of porcine endogenous retrovirus (PERV) into human DNA. Since pig cloning has become a reality,[77] it is only a matter of time before transgenic pigs, which do not express xenoantigens, will be developed.

In the meantime we have seen, in neonatal porcine tissue, evidence of ductal tissue differentiating into endocrine tissue. Recently there have been reports of human exocrine tissue dedifferentiating and expressing a ductal (precursor) phenotype under specific culture conditions[71] as well as human pancreatic ductal tissue differentiating into PDX-1 positive tissue *in vitro*[74] indicating the possibility of differentiation into endocrine cells. Taken together, this indicates potential for *in vitro* expansion of human cadaveric, autologous, or fetal tissue. As we gain knowledge about PDX-1 and other factors involved in islet growth and maturation, we should be able to perfect the expansion of β cells from ductal precursor cells.

Expansion of human islet tissue *in vitro* presents many exciting options for islet cell transplantation. Perhaps, instead of requiring two or more cadaveric pancreata to normalize a patient, one pancreas could supply enough tissue (once expanded) to transplant into several patients. Autografts would be an appealing way to avoid immunosuppression since tissue from a portion of the patient's own pancreas could be used to expand and differentiate into islet tissue that could be transplanted. Both of these methods are especially practical when dealing with type 2 diabetes since there is no autoimmune destruction of β cells, such as occurs in type 1 diabetes.

## REFERENCES

1. GEPTS, W. 1965. Pathological anatomy of the pancreas in juvenile diabetes mellitus. Diabetes **14:** 619–633.
2. NATHAN, D.M. 1992. The rationale for glucose control in diabetes mellitus. Endocrinol. Metabol. Clin. North Am. **21:** 221–235.
3. VOET, D. & J.G. VOET. 1990. Energy metabolism: integration and organ specialization. Biochemistry **25:** 737–738.
4. NATHAN, D.M. 1993. Long-term complications of diabetes mellitus. N. Engl. J. Med. **23:** 1676–1685.
5. RYAN, E., E.L. TOTH & A. RABINOVICH. 1999. Diabetes mellitus and hypoglycemia. *In* Endocrinology and Metabolism, Med 423 Course. 279–305.
6. KORBUTT, G.S., G.L.WARNOCK & R.V. RAJOTTE. 1997. Islet transplantation. *In* Physiology and Pathophysiology of the Islets of Langerhans. Ch. **53:** 397–410.
7. KELLY, W.D., R.C. LILLEHEI, F.K. MERKEL, *et al.* 1967. Allotransplantation of the pancreas and duodenum along with the kidney in diabetic nephropathy. Surgery **61:** 827–837.
8. BRENDAL, M.D. 1997. Clinical islet transplantation: registry report. Report #7.
9. SHAPIRO, A.M.J., J.R.T LAKEY, E.A. RYAN, *et al.* 2000. Islet transplantation in seven patients with type 1 diabetes mellitus using a glucocorticoid-free immunosuppressive regimen. New Engl. J. Med. **343**(4): 230.
10. SMITH, R.M. & T.E. MANDEL. 1998. Transplantation treatment for diabetes. Immunol. Today **19**(10): 444–447.

11. KORSGREN, O., L. JANSSON, D. EIZIRIK & A. ANDERSSON. 1991. Functional and morphological differentiation of fetal porcine islet-like clusters after transplantation into nude mice. Diabetologia **34:** 379–386.
12. GROTH, C.G., O. KORSGREN, A. TIBELL, *et al.* 1994. Transplantation of porcine fetal pancreas to diabetic patients. Lancet **344:** 1402–1404.
13. LUI, X., K.F. FEDERLIN, R.G. BRETZEL, *et al.* 1991. Persistent reversal of diabetes by transplantation of fetal pig proislets into nude mice. Diabetes **40:** 858–866.
14. DAVALLI, A.M., Y. OGAWA, L. SCALIA, *et al.* 1995. Function, mass and replication of porcine and rat islets transplnated into diabetic nude mice. Diabetes **44:** 104–111.
15. RICORDI, C., C. SOCCI, C. DAVALLI, *et al.* 1989. Isolation of the elusive pig islet. Surgery **107:** 688–694.
16. MARCHETTI, P., R. GIANNARELLI, S. COSIMI, *et al.* 1995. Massive isolation, morphological and functional characterization, and xenotransplantation of bovine pancreatic islets. Diabetes **44:** 375–381.
17. WRIGHT, J.R., S. POLVI & H. MACLEAN. 1992. Experimental transplantation with principal islets of teleost fish (Brockman bodies). Long-term function of tilapia islet tissue in diabetic nude mice. Diabetes **41:** 1528–1532.
18. FERBER, S., H. BELTRANDELRIO, J.H. JOHNSON, *et al.* 1994. GLUT-2 gene transfer into insulinoma cells confers both low and high affinity glucose-stimulated insulin release. J. Biol. Chem. **269:** 11523–11529.
19. KNAACK, D., D.M. FIORE, M. SURANA, *et al.* 1994. Clonal insulinoma cell line that stably maintains correct glucose responsiveness. Diabetes **43:** 1413–1417.
20. EFRAT, S., D. FUSCO-DEMANE, H. LEMBERG, *et al.* 1995. Conditional transformation of a pancreatic beta-cell line derived from transgenic mice expressing a tetracycline-regulated oncogene. Proc. Natl. Acad. Sci. USA **92:** 3576–3580.
21. KOVER, K. & W.V. MOORE. 1989. Development of a method for isolation of islets from human fetal pancreas. Diabetes **38:** 917–924.
22. HAYEK, A., G.M. BEATTIE, V. CIRULLI, *et al.* 1995. Growth factor/matrix-induced proliferation of human adult beta-cells. Diabetes **44:** 1458–1460.
23. KORBUTT, G.S., Z. AO, M. FLASHNER & R.V. RAJOTTE. 1997. Neonatal porcine islets as a possible source of tissue for humans and microencapsulation improves the metabolic response of islet graft posttrasplantation. Ann. N.Y. Acad. Sci. **831:** 294–303.
24. SOCCI, C., C. RICORDI, A.M. DAVALLI, *et al.* 1989. Selection of donors significantly improves pig islet isolation yield. Horm. Metab. Res. **25**(Suppl. 1): 32–35.
25. KORBUTT, G.S., J.F. ELLIOTT, Z. AO, *et al.* 1996. Large scale isloation, growth, and function of porcine neonatal islet cells. J. Clin. Invest. **97:** 2119.
26. BONNER-WEIR, S. & F.E. SMITH. 1994. Islet cell growth and the growth factors involved. Trends Endocrinol. Metab. **5:** 60–64.
27. BOUWENS, L., R.N. WANG, DE BLAY EMMY, *et al.* 1994. Cytokeratins as markers of ductal cell differentiation and islet neogenesis in the neonatal rat pancreas. Diabetes **43:** 1279.
28. SHARMA, A., D.H. ZANGEN, P. REITZ, *et al.* 1999. The homeodomain protein IDX-1 increases after an early burst of proliferation during pancreatic regeneration. Diabetes **48:** 507.
29. HERRERA, P.L. 2000. Adult insulin- and glucagon-producing cells differentiate from two independent cell lineages. Development **127**(11): 2317–22.
30. JENSEN, J., R.S. HELLER, T. FUNDER-NIELSEN, *et al.* 2000. Independent development of pancreatic alpha- and beta-cells from neurogenin3-expressing precursors: a role for the notch pathway in repression of premature differentiation. Diabetes **49:** 163.
31. SLACK, J.M.W. 1995. Developmental biology of the pancreas. Development **121:** 1569–1580.
32. VINIK, A., G. PITTENGER, R. RAFAELOFF & L. ROSENBERG. 1992. Factors controlling pancreatic islet neogenesis. Tumor Biology **14:** 184–200.
33. ROSSELIN, G. & S. EMAMI. 1997. Growth and differentiation of the islet cells in neonates. *In* Pancreatic Growth and Regeneration. Karger Landes Systems. Basel. **3:** 44–95.

34. PESHAVARIA, M. & R. STEIN. 1997. PDX-1: an activator of genes involved in pancreatic development and islet gene expression. *In* Pancreatic Growth and Regeneration. Karger Landes Systems. Basel. **4:** 96–107.
35. STOFFERS, D.A., N.T. ZINKIN, V. STANOJEVIC, *et al.* 1997. Pancreatic agenesis attributable to a single nucleotide deletion in the human *IPF1* gene coding sequence. Nature Genetics **15:** 106–110.
36. JONSSON, J., L. CARLSSON, T. EDLUND & H. EDLUND. 1994. Insulin-promoter-factor 1 is required for pancreas development in mice. Nature **371:** 606–609.
37. OFFIELD, M.F., T.L. JETTON, P.A. LABOSKY, *et al.* 1996. PDX-1 is required for pancreatic outgrowth and differentiation of the rostral duodenum. Development **122:** 983–995.
38. AHLGREN, U., J. JONSSON & H. EDLUND. 1996. The morphogenesis of the pancreatic mesenchyme is uncoupled from that of the pancreatic epithelium in IPF1/PDX1-deficient mice. Development **122:** 1409–1416.
39. SEUFERT, J., G.C. WEIR & J.F. HABENER. 1998. Differential expression of the insulin gene transcriptional repressor CCAAT/enhancer-binding protein β and transactivator islet duodenum homeobox-1 in rat pancreatic β cells during the development of diabetes mellitus. J. Clin. Invest. **101**(11): 2528–2539.
40. JONAS, J, A. SHARMA, W. HASENKAMP, *et al.* 1999. Chronic hyperglycemia triggers loss of pancreatic β cell differentiation in an animal model of diabetes. J. Biol. Chem. **274**(20): 14112–14121.
41. STOFFERS, D.A., M.K. THOMAS & J. F. HABENER. 1997. Homeodomain protein IDX-1: a master regulation of pancreas development and insulin gene expression. Trends Endocrinol. Metab. **8**(4): 145–151.
42. ZANGEN, D.H., S. BONNER-WEIR, C.H. LEE, *et al.* 1997. Reduced insulin, GLUT2 and IDX-1 in beta cells after partial pancreatectomy. Diabetes **46:** 258–264.
43. PESHAVARIA, M., L. GAMER, E. HENDERSON, *et al.* 1994. X1Hbox 8, an endoderm-specific Xenopus homeodomain protein, is closely related to a mammalian insulin gene transcription factor. Mol. Endocrinol. **8:** 806–816.
44. PEERS, B., J. LEONARD, S. SHARMA, *et al.* 1995. Insulin expression in pancreatic islet cells relies on cooperative interactions between the helix loop helix factor E47 and the homeobox factor STF-1. Mol. Endocrinol. **8:** 1798–1806.
45. SERUP, S., H.V. PETERSEN, E.E. PENDERSEN, *et al.* 1995. The homeodomain protein IPF-1/STF-1 is expressed in a subset of islet cells and promotes rat insulin 1 gene expression dependent on an intact E1 helix-loop-helix factor binding site. Biochem. J. **310:** 997–1003.
46. GUZ, Y., M.R. MONTMINY, R. STEIN, *et al.* 1995. Expression of murine STF-1, a putative insulin gene transcription factor, in β cells of pancreas, duodenal epithelium and pancreatic exocrine and endocrine progenitors during ontogeny. Development **121:** 11–18.
47. WU, K.L., M. GANNON, M. PESHAVARIA, *et al.* 1997. Hepatocyte nuclear factor 3beta is involved in pancreatic beta-cell-specific transcription of pdx-1 gene. Mol. Cell Biol. **17:** 6002–6013.
48. GERRISH, K., M. GANNON, D. SHIH, *et al.* 2000. Pancreatic beta cell-specific transcription of pdx-1 gene. The role of conserved upstream control regions and their hepatocyte nuclear factor 3beta sites. J. Biol. Chem. **275:** 3485–3492.
49. MARSHAK, S., E. BENSHUSHAN, M. SHOSHKES, *et al.* 2000. Functional conservation of regulatory elements in the pdx-1 gene: PDX-1 and hepatocyte nuclear factor 3beta transcription factors mediate beta-cell-specific expression. Mol. Cell Biol. **20:** 7583–7590.
50. QIAN, J., E.N. KAYTOR, H.C. TOWLE & L.K. OLSON. 1999. Upstream stimulatory factor regulates Pdx-1 gene expression in differentiated pancreatic beta cells. Biochem. J. **341:** 315–322.
51. WANG, X., C.M. CAHILL, M.A. PINEYRO, *et al.* 1999. Glucagon-like peptide-1 regulates the beta cell transcription factor, PDX-1, in insulinoma cells. Endocrinology **140:** 4904–4907.

52. PERFETTI, R., J. ZHOU, M.E DOYLE & J.M. EGAN. 2000. Glucagon-like peptide-1 induces cell proliferation and pancreatic-duodenum homeobox-1 expression and increases endocrine cell mass in the pancreas of old, glucose-intolerant rats. Endocrinology **141**(12): 4600-4605.
53. XU, G., D.A. STOFFERS, J.F. HABENER & S. BONNER-WEIR. 1999. Exendin-4 stimulates both β-cell replication and neogenesis, resulting in increased β-cell mass and improved glucose tolerance in diabetic rats. Diabetes **48**: 2270–2276.
54. STOFFERS, D.A., T.J. KIEFFER, M.A. HUSSAIN, et al. 2000. Insulinotropic glucagon-like peptide 1 agonists stimulate expression of homeodomain protein IDX-1 and increase islet size in mouse pancreas. Diabetes **49**: 741–748.
55. MOEDE, T., B. LEIBIGER, H.G. POUR, et al. 1999. Identification of a nuclear localization signal, RRMKWKK, in the homeodomain transcription factor PDX-1. FEBS Lett. **461**: 229–234.
56. MACFARLANE, W.M., C.M. MCKINNON, Z.A. FELTON-EDKINS, et al. 1999. Glucose stimulates translocation of the homeodomain transcription factor PDX1 from the cytoplasm to the nucleus in pancreatic β-cells. J. Biol. Chem. **274**: 1011–1016.
57. RAFIQ, I., G. DA SILVA XAVIER, S. HOOPER & G.A. RUTTER. 2000. Glucose-stimulated preproinsulin gene expression and nuclear trans-location of pancreatic duodenum homeobox-1 require activation of phosphatidylinositol 3-kinase but not p38 MAPK/SAPK2. J. Biol. Chem. **275**: 15977–15984.
58. FURUKAWA, N., T. SHIROTANI, E. ARAKI, et al. 1999. Possible involvement of atypical protein kinase C (PKC) in glucose-sensitive expression of the human insulin gene: DNA-binding activity and transcriptional activity of pancreatic and duodenal homeobox gene-1 (PDX-1) are enhanced via calphostin C-sensitive but phorbol 12-myristate 13-acetate (PMA) and Go 6976-insensitive pathway. Endocr. J. **46**: 43–58.
59. MACFARLANE, W.M., M.L. READ, M. GILLIGAN, et al. 1994. Glucose modulates the binding activity of the β-cell transcription factor IUF1 in a phosphorylation-dependent manner. Biochem. J. **303**: 625–631.
60. PERSHAVARIA, M., E. HENDERSON, A. SHARMA, et al. 1997. Functional characterization of the transactivation properties of the PDX-1 homeodomain protein. Mol. Cell Biol. **17**: 3987–3996.
61. PETERSEN, H.V., M. PESHAVARIA, A.A. PEDERSEN, et al. 1998. Glucose stimulates the activation domain of the PDX-1 homeodomain transcription factor. FEBS Lett. **431**: 362–366.
62. PERSHAVARIA, M., M.A. CISSELL, E. HENDERSON, et al. 2000. The PDX-1 activation domain provides specific functions necessary for transcriptional stimulation in pancreatic beta-cells. Mol. Endocrinol. **14**: 1907–1917.
63. PEERS, B., S. SHARMA, T. JOHNSON, et al. 1995. The pancreatic factor STF-1 binds cooperatively with Pbx to a regulatory element in the somatostatin promoter: importance of the FPWMK motif and of the homeodomain. Mol. Cell Biol. **15**: 7091–7097.
64. SANDERS, M. & M.S. GERMAN. 1997. The β cell transcription factors and development of the pancreas. J. Mol. Med. **75**: 327–340.
65. HESSABI, B., P. ZIEGLER, I. SCHMIDT, et al. 1999. The nuclear localization signal (NLS) of PDX-1 is part of the homeodomain and represents a novel type of NLS. Eur. J. Biochem. **263**: 170–177.
66. SAYO, Y., H. HOSOKAWA, H. IMACHI, et al. 2000. Transforming growth factor beta induction of insulin gene expression is mediated by pancreatic duodemal homeobox gene-1 in rat insulinoma cells. Eur. J. Biochem. **267**: 971–978.
67. MACFARLANE, W.M., S.B. SMITH, R.F.L. JAMES, et al. 1997. The p38/reactivating kinase mitogen-activated protein kinase cascade mediates the activation of the transcription factor insulin upstream factor 1 and insulin gene transcription by high glucose in pancreatic β-cells. J. Biol. Chem. **272**: 20936–20944.
68. BUTEAU, J., R. RODUIT, S. SUSINI & M. PRENTKI. 1999. Glucagon-like peptide-1 promotes DNA sysnthesis, activates phosphatidylinositol 3-kinase and increases transcription factor pancreatic and duodenum homeobox gene 1 (PDX-1) DNA binding activity in beta (INS-1) cells. Diabetologia **42**: 856–864.

69. HUSSAIN, M.A. & J.F. HABENER. 2000. Glucagon-like peptide 1 increases glucose-dependent activity of the homeoprotein IDX-1 transactivating domain in pancreatic beta-cells. Biochem. Biophys. Res. Commun. **274:** 616–619.
70. WU, H., W.M. MACFARLANE, M. TADAYYON, *et al.* 1999. Insulin stimulates pancreatic-duodenal homeobox factor-1 (PDX1) DNA-binding activity and insulin promoter activity in pancreatic β cells. Biochem. J. **344:** 813–818.
71. HALL P.A. & N.R. LEMOINE. 1992. Rapid acinar to ductal transdifferentiation in cultured human exocrine pancreas. J. Pathol. **166:** 97.
72. ROOMAN, I., Y. HEREMANS, H. HEIMBERG & L. BOUWENS. 2000. Modulation of rat pancreatic acinoductal transdifferentiation and expression of PDX-1 *in vitro*. Diabetologia **43:** 907–914.
73. GMYR, V., J. KERR-CONTE, S. BELAICH, *et al.* 2000. Adult human cytokeratin 19-positive cells reexpress insulin promoter factor 1 *in vitro*: further evidence for pluripotent pancreatic stem cells in human. Diabetes **49:** 1671–1680.
74. BONNER-WEIR, S., M. TENEJA, G.C. WEIR, *et al.* 2000. *In vitro* cultivation of human islets from expanded ductal tissue. Proc. Natl. Acad. Sci. USA **97:** 7999–8004.
75. SANDGREN, E.P., C.J. QUAIFE, A.G. PAULOVICH & R.D. PALMITER. 1991. Pancreatic tumor pathogenesis reflects the causative genetic lesion. Proc. Natl. Acad. Sci. USA **88:** 93–97.
76. RAMIYA, V.K., M. MARAIST, K.E. ARFORS, *et al.* 2000. Reversal of insulin-dependent diabetes using islets generated *in vitro* from pancreatic stem cells. Nature Medicine **6:** 278–282.
77. ONISHI, A., M. IWAMOTO, T. AKITA, *et al.* 2000. Cloning by microinjection of fetal fibroblast nuclei. Science **289:** 1188–1190.

# Hydrogels for Biomedical Applications

ALLAN S. HOFFMAN

*Bioengineering Department, University of Washington, Seattle, Washington, USA*

ABSTRACT: This paper reviews the composition and synthesis of hydrogels, the character of their absorbed water, and permeation of solutes within their swollen matrices. The most important properties of hydrogels relevant to their biomedical applications are also identified, in particular for use of hydrogels as drug and cell carriers, and as tissue engineering matrices.

KEYWORDS: hydrogels; tissue engineering; matrices; scaffolds

## INTRODUCTION

Because of their hydrophilic character and potential for biocompatibility, hydrogels (HGs) have been of great interest to biomaterial scientists for many years.[1–8] Early work in the 1980s by Yannas and coworkers[9] demonstrated the successful application of natural polymer hydrogels as artificial burn dressings. More recently, hydrogels have become especially attractive to tissue engineers as matrices for regenerating a wide variety of tissues and organs.[10,11] Hydrogels are hydrophilic polymer networks that may absorb from 10–20% (an arbitrary lower limit) up to thousands of times their dry weight in water.[2] Hydrogels may be chemically stable or they may degrade and eventually disintegrate and dissolve. They are called *reversible*, or *physical* gels when the networks are held together by molecular entanglements, and/or secondary forces including ionic, H-bonding or hydrophobic forces. Sometimes physical gels can form from biospecific recognitions, such as concanavalin A with a polymeric sugar, or streptavidin with a polymeric biotin. All of these interactions are reversible and can be disrupted by changes in physical conditions such as ionic strength, pH, temperature, application of stress, or addition of specific solutes. Physical hydrogels are not homogeneous, since clusters of molecular entanglements, or hydrophobically or ionically associated domains can create inhomogeneities. Free chain ends or loops also represent transient network defects in physical gels.

When a polyelectrolyte is combined with a multivalent ion of the opposite charge, it may form a physical hydrogel known as an *ionotropic* hydrogel. The pioneering work of Lim and Sun[12] demonstrated the successful application of calcium alginate microcapsules for cell encapsulation. Furthermore, when polyelectrolytes of opposite charges are mixed, they may gel or precipitate depending on their concentration, the ionic strength, and pH of the solution. The products of such ion-crosslinked systems are known as complex coacervates, or polyion complexes. Indeed, the calcium alginate capsules of Lim and Sun were coated with a complex coacervate of alginate-

Address for correspondence: Allan S. Hoffman, Sc.D., Bioengineering Department, Box 352255, University of Washington, Seattle, WA 98195, USA.
hoffman@u.washington.edu

PLL in order to stabilize the capsule. More recently, complex coacervates and polyion complex hydrogels have become especially attractive as tissue engineering matrices.[13–18]

Hydrogels are called *permanent* or *chemical* gels when they are covalently-crosslinked networks. Wichterle and Lim[19] pioneered in synthetic hydrogels for biomedical uses with the development of hydrogels based on PHEMA crosslinked with EGDMA, and these hydrogels have been very successful as soft contact lenses. In the crosslinked state they reach an equilibrium swelling level in aqueous solutions that depends mainly on the crosslink density (estimated by the MW between crosslinks, $M_c$). Like physical hydrogels, chemical hydrogels are not homogeneous. They usually contain regions of low water swelling and high crosslink density, called "clusters", that are dispersed within regions of high swelling, and low crosslink density. This may be due to hydrophobic aggregation of crosslinking agents, leading to high crosslink density clusters.[20] In some cases, depending on the solvent composition, temperature, and solids concentration during gel formation, phase separation can occur, and water-filled *voids* or *macropores* can form. In chemical gels, free chain ends represent gel network "defects" that do not contribute to the elasticity of

TABLE 1A. Natural polymers used to synthesize hydrogels

| | |
|---|---|
| Anionic polymers | hyaluronic acid, alginic acid, carrageenan, chondroitin sulfate, dextran sulfate, pectin |
| Cationic polymers | chitosan, polylysine |
| Amphipathic polymers | collagen (gelatin), carboxymethyl chitin, fibrin |
| Neutral polymers | dextran, agarose, pullulan |

TABLE 1B. Synthetic polymers used to synthesize hydrogels[a]

| | |
|---|---|
| Polyesters | PEG-PLA-PEG, PLA-PEG-PLA, PLGA-PEG-PLGA, PHB, P(PF-co-EG), P(PEG/PBO terephthalate) |
| Other polymers | P(MMA-co-HEMA), PEG-bis-(PLA-acrylate), PEG-g-P(AAm-co-Vamine), PEG +/− CDs, PAAm, P(NIPAAm-co-AAc), P(NIPAAm-co-EMA), PVAc/PVA, PNVP, P(biscarboxy-phenoxy-phosphazene) P(AN-co-allyl sulfonate), P(GEMA-sulfate) |

[a]See GLOSSARY for definitions of terms.

TABLE 1C. Combinations of natural and synthetic polymers used in hydrogels[a]

| |
|---|
| P(PEG-co-peptides), alginate-g-(PEO-PPO-PEO), chitosan-g-(PEO-PPO-PEO), P(PLGA-co-serine), P(HPMA-g-peptide), P(HEMA/Matrigel®), HA-g-NIPAAm, collagen-acrylate, alginate-acrylate |

[a]See GLOSSARY for definitions of terms.

the network. Other network defects are chain "loops" and entanglements, which also do not contribute to the permanent network elasticity.

There are many different macromolecular structures that are possible for physical and chemical hydrogels. They include the following: crosslinked or entangled networks of linear homopolymers, linear copolymers, and block or graft copolymers; polyion-multivalent ion, polyion–polyion or H-bonded complexes; hydrophilic networks stabilized by hydrophobic domains; and IPNs or physical blends. Hydrogels may also have many different physical forms, including (1) solid molded forms (e.g., soft contact lenses), (2) pressed powder matrices (e.g., pills or capsules for oral ingestion), (3) microparticles (e.g., as bioadhesive carriers or wound treatments), (4) coatings (e.g., on implants or catheters; on pills or capsules; or coatings on the inside capillary wall in capillary electrophoresis), (5) membranes or sheets (e.g., as a reservoir in a transdermal drug delivery patch; or for two-dimensional

TABLE 2A. Methods for synthesizing physical hydrogels[a]

| |
|---|
| Warm a polymer solution to form a gel (e.g., PEO-PPO-PEO block copolymers in $H_2O$) |
| Derivatize a hydrophilic polymer with hydrophobic groups that form domains. |
| Cool a polymer solution to form a gel (e.g., agarose or gelatin in $H_2O$) |
| Crosslink a polymer in aqueous solution, using freeze–thaw cycles to form polymer microcrystals (e.g., freeze–thaw PVA in aqueous solution) |
| Lower pH to form an H-bonded gel between two different polymers in the same aqueous solution (e.g., PEO and PAAc) |
| Mix solutions of a polyanion and a polycation to form a complex coacervate gel (e.g., sodium alginate plus polylysine) |
| Gel a polyelectrolyte solution with a multivalent ion of opposite charge (e.g., $Na^+alginate^- + Ca^{++} + 2Cl^-$) |

[a]See GLOSSARY for definitions of terms.

TABLE 2B. Methods for synthesizing chemical hydrogels[a]

| |
|---|
| Crosslink polymer solids or solutions with: |
|     radiation (e.g., irradiate PEO in H2O) |
|     chemical crosslinkers (e.g., treat collagen with glutaraldehyde or a bis-epoxide) |
|     multi-functional reactive compounds (e.g., PEG + diisocyanate = PU hydrogel) |
| Copolymerize monomer + crosslinker (e.g., HEMA + EGDMA) |
| Copolymerize monomer + multifunctional macromer (e.g., bis-methacrylate terminated PLA-PEO-PLA + photosensitizer + visible light radiation) |
| Polymerize a monomer within a different solid polymer to form an IPN hydrogel (e.g., AN + starch) |
| Chemically convert a hydrophobic polymer to a hydrogel (e.g., partially hydrolyze PVAc to PVA; or PAN to PAN/PAAm/PAAc) |

[a]See GLOSSARY for definitions of terms.

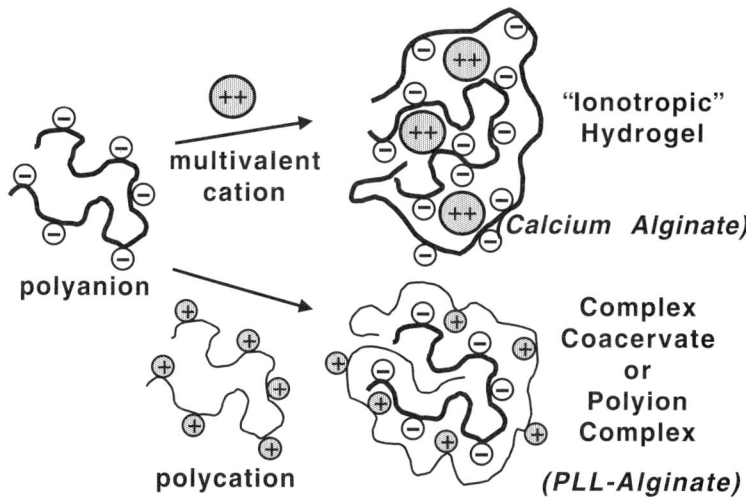

**FIGURE 1.** Synthesis of ionic hydrogels showing, as an example, the calcium-alginate/poly(L-lysine) system.

electrophoresis gels), (6) encapsulated solids (e.g., in osmotic pumps), and (7) liquids (e.g., that form gels on heating or cooling).

A wide and diverse range of polymer compositions have been used to fabricate hydrogels; TABLE 1 summarizes the many varied compositions. The compositions can be classified into natural polymer hydrogels,[21–30] synthetic polymer hydrogels,[31–38] and combinations of the two classes.[39–44] Many different routes have been

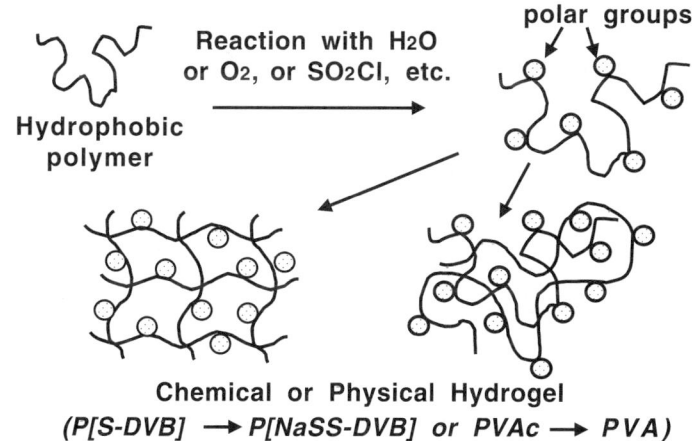

**FIGURE 2.** Synthesis of hydrogels by chemical modification of polymers.

used to synthesize hydrogels. These routes are summarized in TABLE 2 and shown schematically in FIGURES 1 to 5.

## WATER IN HYDROGELS

The character of the water in a hydrogel can determine the overall permeation of nutrients into and cellular products out of the gel. When a dry hydrogel begins to absorb water, the first water molecules entering the matrix will hydrate the most polar, hydrophilic groups, leading to *primary bound water*. As the polar groups are hydrated, the network swells, and exposes hydrophobic groups, which also interact with water molecules, leading to hydrophobically-bound water, or *secondary bound water*. Primary and secondary bound water are often combined and simply called the *total bound water*. After the polar and hydrophobic sites have interacted with and bound water molecules, the network imbibes additional water, due to the osmotic

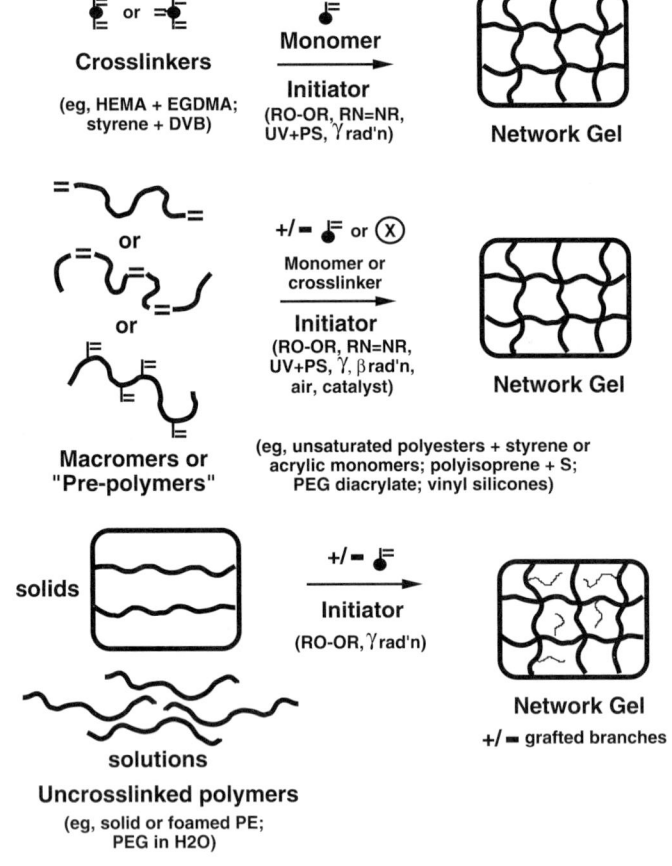

**FIGURE 3.** Free radical syntheses of network gels.

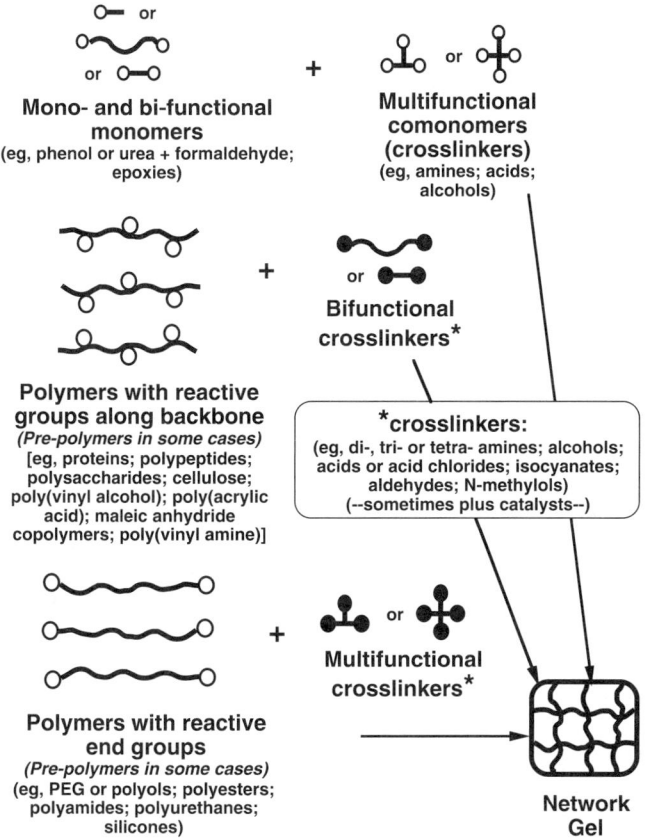

**FIGURE 4.** Condensation syntheses of network hydrogels.

driving force of the network chains towards infinite dilution. This additional swelling is opposed by the covalent or physical crosslinks, leading to an elastic network retraction force. Thus, the hydrogel reaches an equilibrium swelling level. The additional swelling water that is imbibed beyond the total bound water is called *free water* or *bulk water,* and is assumed to fill the space between the network chains, and/or the center of larger pores, macropores, or voids. As the network swells, if the network chains or crosslinks are degradable, the gel begins to disintegrate and dissolve, at a rate depending on its composition. It should be noted that a gel used as a tissue engineering matrix may never be dried, but the total water in the gel is still comprised of *bound* and *free* water.

There are a number of methods used by researchers to estimate the relative amounts of free and bound water, as fractions of the total water content. The two major methods used to characterize water in hydrogels are based on the use of small molecular probes and DSC. When probe molecules are used, the labeled probe solution is equilibrated with the hydrogel, and the concentration of the probe molecule

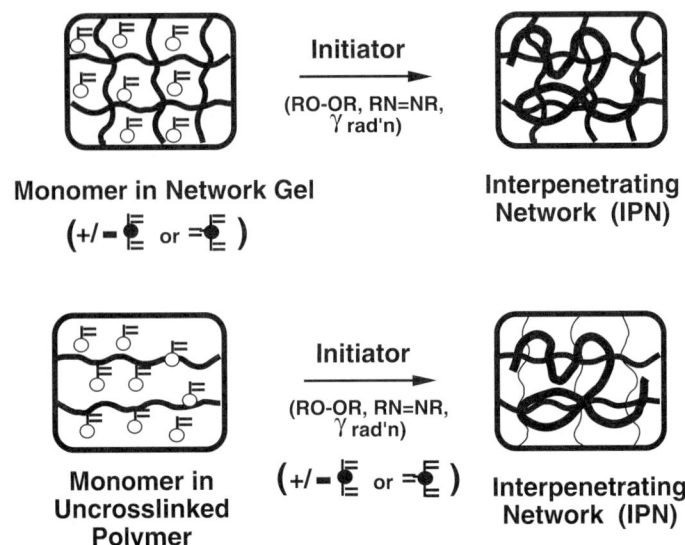

**FIGURE 5.** Free radical syntheses of inter-penetrating networks (IPNs).

in the gel at equilibrium is measured. Assuming that only the free water in the gel can dissolve the probe solute, one can calculate the free water content from the amount of the imbibed probe molecule and the known (measured) probe molecule concentration in the external solution. The bound water is then obtained by difference of the measured total water content of the hydrogel and the calculated free water content. Additional assumptions for use of this technique are that: (1) the solute does not affect the free and bound water distribution in the gel, (2) all of the free water in the gel is accessible to the solute, (3) the solute concentration in the free water of the hydrogel is equal to the solute concentration in the external solution, and (4) the solute does not interact with the gel matrix chains.

The use of DSC is based on the assumption that only the free water may be frozen, thus it is assumed that the endotherm measured when warming the frozen gel represents the melting of the free water, and that value will yield the amount of free water in the hydrogel sample being tested. The bound water is then obtained by difference of the measured total water content of the hydrogel test specimen and the calculated free water content, similar to the above.

## PORES AND PERMEATION IN HYDROGELS

The amount of water in a hydrogel, that is, the volume fraction of water, and its free versus bound water character determines the absorption (or partitioning) and diffusion of solutes through the hydrogel. Pores may be formed in hydrogels by phase separation during synthesis, or they may exist as smaller pores within the network.[44] The average pore size, the pore size distribution, and the pore interconnections are important factors of a hydrogel matrix that are often difficult to quantify, and are usually included together in the parameter called "tortuosity". The effective diffusion path length across a hydrogel film barrier is estimated by the film thickness times the ratio of the pore volume fraction divided by the tortuosity. These factors, in turn, are most influenced by the composition and crosslink density of the hydrogel polymer network.

Labeled molecular probes of a range of molecular weights (MWs) or molecular sizes are used to probe pore sizes in hydrogels. Fluorescein-labeled dextrans are usually used. The same assumptions and restrictions apply to these probes as those for small molecular probes used to characterize free and bound water in a hydrogel.

Probe solute permeation is a useful method for characterizing pores and their interconnections in hydrogels. The probe solute size and shape, its relative hydrophilic and hydrophobic character, and the availability of *free* water molecules to

TABLE 3A. Important properties of hydrogels relevant to their use as tissue engineering matrices

| Type of hydrogels | physical gel |
| --- | --- |
| | chemical gel |
| Molecular structures | linear polymers |
| | block copolymers |
| | graft copolymers |
| | interpenetrating networks (IPNs) |
| | polyblends |
| Composition of the hydrogel | natural polymers and their derivatives |
| | synthetic polymers |
| | combinations of natural and synthetic polymers |

TABLE 3B. Important properties or added functions of hydrogels relevant to their use as tissue engineering matrices

| Degradable or non-degradable |
| --- |
| Injectable or prefabricated solid |
| Mechanical strength |
| Ease of handling |
| Shape and surface/volume ratio |
| Closed versus open pores |
| Water content and character |
| Chemical modification (e.g., cell adhesion ligands) |
| Added bioactive components (cells, drugs) |
| Sterilizability |

hydrate and dissolve the solute molecules and pore interconnections, are important factors governing solute permeation through any particular hydrogel. The permeation coefficient, $P$, is the product of the partition coefficient, $K$, and the apparent diffusion coefficient, $D_{app}$.

The partition coefficient, $K$, and uniformity of a protein/peptide drug loaded within a hydrogel depends on the protein/peptide size, shape, and net charge; the ionic, polar, apolar groups of the polymer, total available *free* water within the hydrogel; the addition of partition enhancers, such as PEG, to the solution; temperature, pH, and ionic strength, and the drying method, if the hydrogel has been dried, since that often leaves a higher concentration of the drug at the outer regions of the hydrogel. If a protein drug is being loaded into a hydrogel and if the protein has a net charge opposite to that of the hydrogel, then it may plug the pores at the surface during loading into the gel. On the other hand, if it has a net charge that is the same as that of the gel, then it may be excluded from the gel by Donnan exclusion. When loading a protein into a gel, the ionic strength, pH and buffer used in the protein solution may individually or together control the amount and distribution of the protein loaded into the gel.

The "effective" or "apparent" diffusion coefficient of the probe molecule, $D_{app}$, is equal to $D_o$ times the ratio of the pore volume fraction divided by the tortuosity, where $D_o$ is the diffusion coefficient in free water and the ratio of the pore volume fraction divided by the tortuosity is always less than 1.

There is always a portion of the imbibed water in a hydrogel that is not available for drug permeation due to pore "dead ends", small pores that are less than the diameter of the drug molecule, H-bonded or hydrophobically *bound* water, and drug–matrix polymer interactions.

## HYDROGELS AS TISSUE ENGINEERING MATRICES

Hydrogels are increasingly studied as matrices for tissue engineering. TABLES 3A and 3B listing the important parameters and properties of hydrogels for this application. TABLE 4 identifies the important advantages and disadvantages of hydrogels as

TABLE 4. **Hydrogels as tissue engineering matrices**

| | |
|---|---|
| Advantages | Aqueous environment can protect cells and fragile drugs such as peptides, proteins, oligonucleotides, DNA. |
| | Good transport of nutrient to cells and products from cells. |
| | May be easily modified with cell adhesion ligands. |
| | Can be injected *in vivo* as a liquid that gels at body temperature. |
| | Should be biocompatible. |
| Disadvantages | Can be hard to handle. |
| | Usually mechanically weak. |
| | Difficult to load with drugs and cells and then crosslink *in vitro* as a prefabricated matrix. |
| | May be difficult to sterilize. |

matrices for tissue engineering. One significant advantage is the ease with which one may covalently incorporate cell membrane receptor peptide ligands, in order to stimulate adhesion, spreading, and growth of cells within the hydrogel matrix.[10,39,46] It is clear that there are both significant advantages and disadvantages to the use of hydrogels in tissue engineering and the latter will need to be overcome before hydrogels can be more widely applied.

## GLOSSARY OF TERMS

CD, cyclodextrin
DVB, divinyl benzene
DX, p-dioxanone
EG, ethylene glycol
EGDMA, ethylene glycol dimethacrylate
HA, hyaluronic acid
HG, hydrogel
IPN, inter-penetrating network
MBAAm, methylene-bis-acrylamide
P(…), poly(….)
PAAc, poly(acrylic acid)
PAAm, polyacrylamide
PAGE, polyacrylamide gel electrophoresis
PAN, polyacrylonitrile
PBO, poly(butylene oxide)
PCL, polycaprolactone
PEG, poly(ethylene glycol)
PEI, poly(ethylene imine)
PEO, poly(ethylene oxide)
PEMA, poly(ethyl methacrylate)
PF, propylene fumarate
PGEMA, poly(glucosylethyl methacrylate)
PHB, poly(hydroxy butyrate)
PHEMA, poly(hydroxyethyl methacrylate)
PHPMA, poly(hydroxypropyl methacrylamide)
PLA, poly(lactic acid)
PLGA, poly(lactic-co-glycolic acid)
PMMA, poly(methyl methacrylate)
PNIPAAm, poly(N-isopropyl acrylamide)
PNVP, poly(N-vinyl pyrrolidone)
PPO, poly(propylene oxide)
PS, polystyrene
PVA: poly(vinyl alcohol)
PVAc, poly(vinyl acetate)
PVamine, poly(vinyl amine)

## REFERENCES

1. PARK, K., W.S.W. SHALABY & H. PARK, Eds. 1993. Biodegradable Hydrogels for Drug Delivery. Technomic Publishing Company.
2. HARLAND, R.S. & R.K. PRUD'HOMME, Eds. 1992. Polyelectrolyte Gels: Properties, Preparation, and Applications. American Chemical Society, Washington D.C.
3. SHALABY, S.W., C.L. MCCORMICK & G.B. BUTLER, Eds. 1991. Water-soluble Polymers: Synthesis, Solution Properties, and Applications. American Chemical Society, Washington D.C.
4. PEPPAS, N.A., Ed. 1987. Hydrogels in Medicine and Pharmacy, Vols I–III. CRC Press, Inc., Boca Raton.
5. ULBRICH., K., V. SUBR, P. PODPEROVÁ & M. BURESOVÁ. 1995. Synthesis of novel hydrolytically degradable hydrogels for controlled drug release. J. Contr. Rel. **34:** 155–165.
6. HOFFMAN, A.S. 1997. Intelligent polymers. In Controlled Drug Delivery. K. Park, Ed. ACS Publications, ACS, Washington D.C.
7. HARRIS, J.M. & S. ZALIPSKY, Eds. 1997. Poly(ethylene glycol) Chemistry and Biological Applications. ACS Symposium Series, ACS, Washington D.C.
8. CRESCENZI, V., M. DENTINI & A.E.J. DE NOOY. 2000. Novel synthetic routes to hydrogels. ACS Polymer Preprints **41**(1): 718.
9. YANNAS, I.V., E. LEE, D.P. ORGILL, et al. 1989. Synthesis and characterization of a model extracellular matrix that induces partial regeneration of adult mammalian skin. PNAS **86:** 933–937.
10. HUBBELL, J.A. 1998. Synthetic biodegradable polymers for tissue engineering and drug delivery. Curr. Opin. Sol. State Mater. Sci. **3:** 246–251.
11. KIM, B.S., J. NIKOLOVSKI, J. BONADIO & D.J. MOONEY. 1999. Cyclic mechanical strain regulates the development of engineered smooth muscle tissue. Nature Biotech. **17:** 979–983.
12. LIM, F. & A.M. SUN. 1980. Microencapsulated islets as bioartificial pancreas. Science **210:** 908–910.
13. MATTHEW, H.W., S.O.SALLEY, W.D. PETERSON & M.D. KLEIN. 1993. Complex coacervate microcapsules for mammalian cell culture and artificial organ development. Biotechnol. Prog. **9:** 510–519.
14. DE CHALAIN, T., J.H. PHILLIPS & A. HINEK. 1999. Bioengineering of elastic cartilage with aggregated porcine and human auricular chondrocytes and hydrogels containing alginate, collagen, and kappa-elastin. J. Biomed. Mater. Res. **44:** 280–288.
15. KUO, C.K. & P.X. MA. 2000. Diffusivity of three-dimensional ionically-crosslinked alginate hydrogels. ACS Polymer Preprints **41**(2): 1661.
16. HSU, F.Y., S.W. TSAI, F.F. WANG & Y.J. WANG. 2000. The collagen-containing alginate/poly(L-lysine)/alginate microcapsules. Art. Cells Blood Subs. Immob. Biotech. **28:** 147–154.
17. DILLON, J.P., X.J. YU, A. SRIDHARAN, et al. 1998. The influence of physical structure and charge on neurite extension in a 3D hydrogel scaffold. J. Biomater. Sci. Pol. Edn. **9:** 1049–1069.
18. SECHRIEST, V.F., Y.J. MIAO, C. NIYIBIZI, et al. 1999. GAG-augmented polysaccharide hydrogel: a novel biocompatible and biodegradable material to support chondrogenesis. J. Biomed. Mater. Res. **49:** 534–541.
19. WICHTERLE, O. & D. LIM. 1960. Hydrophilic gels in biologic use. Nature **185:** 117.
20. DRUMHELLER, P. & J.A. HUBBELL. 1995. Densely crosslinked polymer networks of PEG in trimethylolpropane triacrylate for cell adhesion-resistant surfaces. J. Biomed. Mater. Res. **29:** 201–215.
21. KIM, H.D., D.A. D'AUGUSTA & R.H. LI. 2000. Formulation of hyaluronic acid ester-based injectable carriers for the delivery of rhBMP-2. Trans. Soc. Biomtls. 626.
22. HUNTER, C.J., A.C. SHIEH, R.M. NEREM & M.E. LEVENSTON. 2000. Effects of collagens I and II and chitosan on chondrocyte behavior in fibrin gel cultures. Trans. Soc. Biomtls. 306.
23. CHENITE, A., D. WANG & C. CHAPUT. 2000. Novel in situ autogelling chitosan solutions for injectable implants. Trans. Soc. Biomtls. 549.

24. ATKINSON, B.L., J.P. ELTON, M.A. RENAUD, et al. 2000. A comparative analysis of unique, injectable gels for BMP delivery. Trans. Soc. Biomtls. 492.
25. CLAPPER, D.L., M.J. BURKSTRAND, S.J. CHUDZIK & J.J. BENEDICT. 2000. A photocrosslinked collagen/BMP matrix promotes bone formation in vivo. Trans. Soc. Biomtls. 115.
26. CHOW, K.S. & E. KHOR. 2000. Novel fabrication of open-pore chitin matrices. Biomacromol. **1:** 61–67.
27. MARLER, J.J., A. GUHA, J. ROWLEY, et al. 2000. Soft tissue augmentation with injectable alginate and syngeneic fibroblasts. Plast. Reconstr. Surg. **105:** 2049–2058.
28. YAMAMOTO, M., Y. TABATA & Y. IKADA. 1999. Growth factor release from gelatin hydrogel for tissue engineering. J. Bioact. Biocompat. Pols. **14:** 474–489.
29. CAMPOCCIA, D., P. DOHERTY, M. RADICE, et al. 1998. Semisynthetic resorbable materials from hyaluronan esterification. Biomater. **19:** 2101–2127.
30. PRESTWICH, G.D., D.M. MARECAK, J.F. MARECAK, et al. 1998. Controlled chemical modification of hyaluronic acid. J. Contr. Rel. **53:** 93–103.
31. JEONG, B., Y.H. BAE & S.W. KIM. 2000. Biodegradable thermosensitive hydrogels for injectable drug delivery systems. Trans. Soc. Biomtls. 1491.
32. ICHI, T., J. WATANABE, T. OOYA & N. YUI. 2000. Design of hydrogels crosslinked by biodegradable polyrotaxanes. Trans. Soc. Biomtls. 1438.
33. MARCOLONGO, M., K. TSANG, J. THOMAS, et al. 2000. Novel hydrogel copolymers for intervertebral disc replacement. Trans. Soc. Biomtls. 191.
34. STILE, R.A., W.R. BURGHARDT & K.E. HEALY. 1999. Synthesis and characterization of injectable PNIPAAm-based hydrogels that support tissue formation in vitro. Macromol. **32:** 7370–7379.
35. SEFTON, M.V., M.H. MAY, S. LAHOOTI & J.E. BABENSEE. 2000. Making microencapsulation work: conformal coating immobilization gels and in vivo performance. J. Contr. Rel. **65:** 173–186.
36. TAGUCHI, T., A. KISHIDA, N. SAKAMOTO & M. AKASHI. 1998. Preparation of a novel functional hydrogel consisting of a sulfated glucoside-bearing polymer. J. Biomed. Mater. Res. **41:** 386–391.
37. SUGGS, L.J. & A.G. MIKOS. 1999. Development of poly(propylene fumarate-co-ethylene glycol) as an injectable carrier for endothelial cells. Cell Transplant. **8:** 345–350.
38. CRUISE, G.M., O.D. HEGRE, F.V. LAMBERTI, et al. 1999. In vitro and in vivo performance of porcine islets encapsulated in interfacially photopolymerized PEG diacrylate membranes. Cell Transpln. **8:** 293–306.
39. LUTOLF, M., A.B. PRATT, B. VERNON, et al. 2000. Collagenase-sensitive PEG hydrogels for controlled tissue regeneration. Trans. Soc. Biomtls. 651.
40. OHYA, S., Y. NAKAYAMA & T. MATSUDA. 2000. Molecular design of artificial extracellular matrix: preparation of thermoresponsive hyaluronic acid. Trans. Soc. Biomtls. 1297.
41. GIN, H., B. DUPUY, A. BAQUEY, et al. 1990. Lack of responsiveness to glucose of microencapsulated islets of langerhans after three weeks implantation in the rat—influence of complement. J. Microencap. **7:** 341–346.
42. CAO, Y.L., A. RODRIGUEZ, M. VACANTI, et al. 1998. Comparative study of the use of PGA, calcium alginate and pluronics in the engineering of autologous porcine cartilage. J. Biomater. Sci. Pol. Edn. **9:** 475–487.
43. ELISSEEFF, J., K. ANSETH, D. SIMS, et al. 1999. Transdermal photopolymerization for minimally invasive implantation. PNAS **96:** 3104–3107.
44. GRIFFITH, L.G. 2000. Polymeric biomaterials. Acta Materialia **48:** 263–277.
45. WOERLY, S. 1997. Porous hydrogels for neural tissue engineering. Porous Mater. Tiss. Eng. **250:** 53–68.
46. BORKENHAGEN, M., J.F. CLEMENCE, H. SIGRIST & P. AEBISCHER. 1998. Three-dimensional extracellular matrix engineering in the nervous system. J. Biomed. Mater. Res. **40:** 392–400.

# Production of Alginate Beads by Emulsification/Internal Gelation

D. PONCELET

*École Nationale d'Ingénieurs des Techniques des Industries Agricoles et Alimentaires (Enitiaa), BP 82225, 44322 Nantes, France*

> ABSTRACT: Alginate microspheres were produced by emulsification/internal gelation of an alginate sol dispersed within vegetable oil, followed by a reduction in pH to release calcium from an insoluble salt. Microspheres with mean diameters ranging from 50 to 1,000 μm were obtained with standard deviations ranging from 35 to 45% of their mean value. Smooth, spherical beads were obtained with the narrowest size dispersion when using low guluronic and low viscosity alginate and a carbonate complex as calcium vector. The calcium salt must also be included within the alginate sol as a very fine powder to promote homogeneous gelation. Internal gelation was also tested with the dropping method. Observation of the beads produced revealed that the structure of the beads is more homogeneous than observed with external gelation. Shrinking is more important, although the diffusion of large molecules is faster with internal versus external gelation.
>
> KEYWORDS: alginate bead production, emulsification, internal gelation, microspheres

## INTRODUCTION

Encapsulation in hydrogel beads remains one of the most usual methods of cell immobilization. Dropping an alginate solution into a calcium-gelifying bath permits one to produce relatively large quantity of beads although the productivity is inversely proportional to the bead volume.[1] Therefore, producing small beads in large quantity remains a challenge particularly under sterile conditions.

An emulsification/internal gelation method is proposed for producing small diameter alginate beads in large quantity. The difficulty in using dispersion/external gelation techniques with ionic polysaccharide is that the calcium source ($CaCl_2$) is insoluble in the oil phase. As an alternative, internal gelation of the dispersed alginate droplets may be initiated by releasing $Ca^{2+}$ from an insoluble complex (calcium salt) through pH reduction.[2] By controlling the conditions under which the water-in-oil dispersion is produced, the bead size can be controlled from a few microns to millimeters in diameter. The purpose of this paper is to report latest developments in obtaining the narrowest size distribution.

Address for correspondence: D. Poncelet, Enitiaa, BP 82225, 44322 Nantes cedex 3, France. Voice: 33 2 51 78 54 25; fax; 33 2 51 78 54 67.
poncelet@enitiaa-nantes.fr

## MATERIALS AND METHODS

### Reagents

Grinsted and SKW alginates were obtained, respectively, from Grinsted Products, Brabrand, Denmark, and SKW Bio Industries, Paris, France and used as received. Canola oil was provided by Canada Packers, Montreal, Canada. Calcium carbonate (Setacarb) was obtained from Omya Paris. Other products, Span 80, calcium citrate, calcium chloride, sodium bicarbonate and acetic acid were purchased from Sigma.

### Preparation of Alginate Solution

Sodium alginate (1 to 4% w/v) was dissolved by mixing in a Waring blender or other high-shear device for two minutes. Solutions stood for at least one hour to allow deaeration, and acid (or base) was generally added to adjust the pH to the desired value (typically 7.5).

### Bead Production

Alginate (20 ml) was mixed with 1 ml of a suspension of insoluble calcium salt (500 mM $Ca^{2+}$ equivalent). The carbonate, citrate, monohydrogenophosphate, oxalate, and tartrate salts of calcium were tested. The alginate–calcium salt mixture (21 ml) was dispersed in 100 ml canola oil in a turbine reactor by stirring at 200 to 500 rpm for 15 minutes. With continued agitation, 20 ml of canola oil containing 80 µl glacial acetic acid were then added to the emulsion, liberating divalent calcium for gelation of the alginate polyanions. After five minutes, the oil–bead suspension was added with gentle mixing to 150 ml of a 50 mM calcium chloride solution. After complete partitioning of beads to the aqueous phase, the oil was discarded, and the beads filtered on a 30 µm sieve and washed with 1% Tween solution.

While testing the internal gelation with extrusion techniques, the solution mentioned above was dropped in an acidic bath at different pH. Beads were left to stand for 10 min and then washed with water and kept in saline solution.

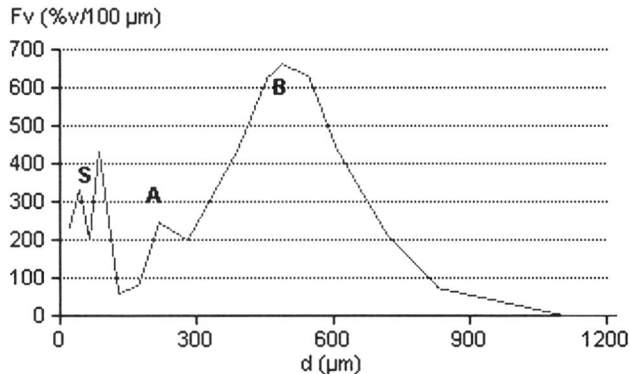

**FIGURE 1.** Typical size distribution of alginate bead batch.

### Microbead Characterization

The volume distributions of beads were estimated using a Malvern 2605-Lc particle size analyzer. A typical size distribution (see FIGURE 1) was composed of two main peaks (A and B) and several small satellite peaks (S). The main peak (A or B) was characterized by its mean diameter and standard deviation values. The mean diameter of the main peak was evaluated by the mode (maximum frequency) and the standard deviation was obtained from the peak width at half height (FIG. 1). Reproducibility tests for the mean and standard deviation were evaluated to 15 and 8% of the mode, respectively. Mechanical resistance was evaluated qualitatively by viewing the rupture of beads under pressure microscopically.

### Blue Dextran Release

Beads were suspended in a blue dextran solution (Sigma) for two hours and then transferred into distilled water. The blue dextran concentration was estimated by optical density. The ratio of the concentration in the solution, at a given time, to the concentration observed at complete release, was taken as the metric.

## RESULTS

The size distribution of alginate beads prepared by emulsification/internal gelation (FIG. 1) was polymodal with two main peaks (A and B) and several small peaks (S). The distribution of the main peaks is a function of the type of alginate and calcium vector (see TABLE 1). Calcium oxalate, tartrate, phosphate, carbonate, and citrate were evaluated. In the working pH range (greater than pH 5), only citrate and carbonate salts permit spherical bead formation with moderate size polydispersities. More complex size distribution is formed with calcium citrate, whereas calcium carbonate often results in a single main peak. Beads prepared with calcium carbonate were more spherical than those prepared with calcium citrate. The lack of sphericity was attributed to some incomplete coalescence of the drops during the gelation period.

A combination of low guluronic and low or medium viscosity alginate and calcium carbonate gave the narrowest size distribution, whereas combining high guluronic and high viscosity alginate with calcium citrate provided the most complex multimodal distribution. Under optimum conditions, peak A was eliminated except for very high viscosity alginate. In summary, the use of calcium carbonate in place of citrate strongly increases peak B to the detriment of peak A. The use of an alginate with a high guluronic content favors dominance of peak A.

The amount of calcium introduced into the alginate sol required to ensure complete gelation was 100 mM. However, a number of insoluble calcium complex grains were apparent in the resulting beads. The calcium concentration was then reduced to 25 mM without observing any change in bead size, shape, or mechanical strength.

The initial pH of the alginate sol was set to 8 but was later reduced to 7.5 when using calcium carbonate. The final pH was varied by changing the amount of acetic acid introduced to the dispersion system and/or by use of carbonate buffer. For final pH values lower than or equal to 6.5, strong and spherical beads were obtained with calcium carbonate complex. Beads were stronger and more spherical when using

TABLE 1. Effect of calcium vector and alginate type on size distribution

| Calcium Vector (50 mM $Ca^{2+}$) | Alginate Viscosity (cp at 1%) | Guluronic Content[a] | Mode (μm) | Standard Deviation (%) | Peak A (%) | Peak B (%) | Peak S (%) |
|---|---|---|---|---|---|---|---|
| Citrate | 100 | low | 720 | 34 | 78 | 16 | 6 |
|  | 158 | low | 660 | 35 | 78 | 18 | 4 |
|  | 480 | low | 690 | 35 | 78 | 20 | 2 |
|  | 1,300 | low | 720 | 36 | 84 | 10 | 6 |
|  | 1,464 | high | 610 | 34 | 85 | 5 | 10 |
|  | 1,694 | high | 620 | 34 | 87 | 4 | 9 |
|  | >2,000 | low | 670 | 29 | 77 | 16 | 7 |
| $CaCO_3$ | 100 | low | 423 | 36 | — | 88 | 12 |
|  | 158 | low | 346 | 41 | — | 76 | 14 |
|  | 480 | low | 423 | 36 | — | 88 | 12 |
|  | 1,300 | low | 308 | 53 | — | 87 | 13 |
|  | 1,464 | high | 390 | 56 | 35 | 58 | 7 |
|  | 1,694 | high | 385 | 51 | 37 | 51 | 18 |
|  | >2,000 | low | 318 | 65 | 17 | 73 | 10 |

[a]Low, about 40% to high, about 70%, from providers sources.

larger amounts of acetic acid while limiting the pH reduction by enhancing the buffer capacity of the alginate solution.

Commercial calcium citrate or carbonate powders consist of grains with diameters of 30 μm. For small microbead formulation (50 to 300 μm), the calcium salt particle size was reduced to ensure a more homogeneous dispersion within the alginate. Prior to use, the calcium carbonate suspension was thus sonicated with an ultrasonic homogenizer, or the dry powder was ground with a mortar and pestle to disrupt the aggregates (from 30 μm to 2.5 μm). Microbeads obtained with ground or sonicated calcium powder resulted in gels with a higher mechanical resistance, improved sphericity, and the absence of residual calcium grains.

The gelation time was estimated, qualitatively, by measuring the stickiness or adhesion of alginate sol after mixing with the calcium salt (see FIGURE 2). At pH 8, gelation occurred within a few minutes using citrate, whereas the alginate–calcium carbonate mixture was still in a liquid state after 48 hours. Following acidification to pH 6.5, gelation occurred within a few seconds, was quasi instantaneous with calcium carbonate, and within 20 sec for the calcium citrate.

### *Modeling Internal Gelation*

The release of calcium may be written as follows

$$Ca_xA_z \Leftrightarrow Ca^{2+} + zA^{(2x/z)-}$$

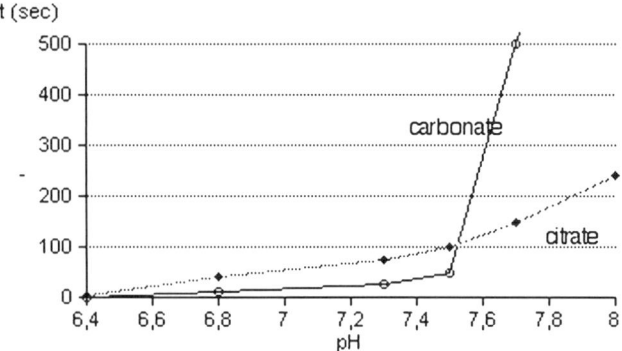

**FIGURE 2.** Gelification time of alginate solutions containing calcium vector at various pH values.

where A represents the anion. The free calcium concentration, [Ca$^{2+}$], and the total free anion concentration, $C_A$ (sum of the basic and acid forms), are related, at equilibrium, by

$$\frac{C_A}{z} = \frac{[Ca^{2+}]}{x}. \tag{1}$$

The free basic anion concentration, [A], is given by

$$[A] = \varphi_0 C_A, \tag{2}$$

where $\varphi_0$ is the partition coefficient calculated from the acidity constants of the chemical species A and the pH.[3] Finally the solubility product may be written as follows

$$L = [Ca^{2+}]^x[A]^z. \tag{3}$$

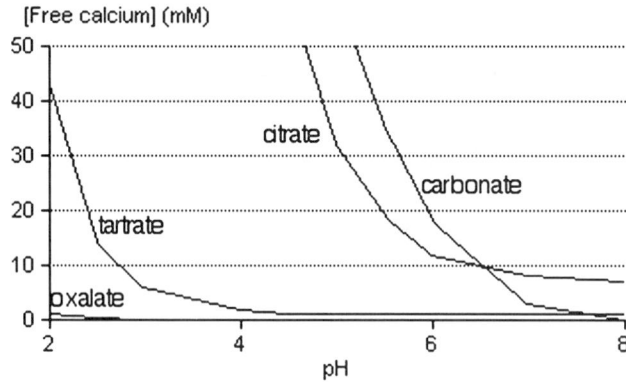

**FIGURE 3.** Free calcium concentration function of the calcium vector and pH.

Combining Equations (**1**) to (**3**) leads to:

$$[Ca^{2+}] = x + z\sqrt{L\left(\frac{x}{\varphi_0}\right)^z}. \qquad (4)$$

FIGURE 3 gives the free calcium concentration as a function of the pH for various calcium vectors. Calcium is not released from oxalate or tartrate complex in the pH range of interest (pH > 5). The release of calcium occurs over a narrower pH range with calcium carbonate than with calcium citrate. At pH 7–8, the calcium concentration with calcium citrate remains higher than 8 mM, and initiate gelation of the alginate.

## Physicochemical Parameter Influences

The Alginate viscosity had little influence on the size distribution (TABLE 1). Increasing the viscosity by a factor of 100 reduces the peak mode by less than 10%. However, the size dispersion is smallest for low viscosity alginate. In contrast, increasing the surfactant concentration decreased the mean bead size asymptotically as the surfactant concentration approached 1%.

## Extrusion-based Technology

Internal gelation could be applied to an extrusion-based technology. The alginate/calcium carbonate suspension was dropped in an acidic solution at different pH. TABLE 2 shows the influence of the bath pH on the droplet size and the shrinking factor (defined as the fraction of volume reduction during gelation). Correct beads could only be obtained in the gelation bath at a pH of six or below. The beads produced by internal gelation have lower mean sizes, and higher shrinking than those produced by external gelation. The shrinking factor increases with a reduction of the pH. Under optical microscopy, the internal gelation based beads shown a more homogenous structure (see TABLE 3). Large molecules (blue dextran at 2,000,000 daltons) escape faster from the internal gelation based beads than external gelation based beads (TABLE 3), indicating a higher egress permeability.

TABLE 2. Effect of the gelifying bath composition and pH on size and shrinking factor of beads done by extrusion

| Bath | pH | $d$ (mm) | Shrinking (%) |
|---|---|---|---|
| CaCl$_2$ 40mM | 6.6 | 3 | 0.6 |
| HAc/NaAc 3% | 3.0 | 2 | 0.92 |
| | 4.0 | 2.2 | 0.88 |
| | 5.0 | 2.4 | 0.86 |
| | 6.0 | 2.8 | 0.8 |
| | 6.5 | 2.9 (?) | 0.7 |
| | 7.0 | no gelation | — |

TABLE 3. Effect of the gelifying bath composition and pH on size and shrinking factor of beads done by extrusion

| Bath | pH | Time | Release | Pore Structure[a] |
|---|---|---|---|---|
| $CaCl_2$ | 6.6 | 15 days | 11% | inhomogeneous[b] |
| HAc/NaAc | 5 | 15 days | 60% | homogeneous |

[a] Optical observation under a microscope.
[b] Inhomogeneity refers to the presence of pores, channels, and so forth, not to an alginate concentration profile.

## DISCUSSION

The physicochemical conditions of alginate bead formation via internal gelation with a calcium vector primarily influences of the size distribution of the resulting microbeads. Physicochemical factors include the type and form of the calcium vector, its concentration, the initial and final pH values, and the selection of alginate composition and structure.

Alginate solutions at 2%w correspond to 103 mM of guluronic or manuronic monomers. The alginate was crosslinked with 25 mM divalent calcium (50 mM positive charge). Only the guluronic groups link sufficiently to calcium to produce strong gels even though all of the monomeric units have not been cross-linked. A calcium/alginate monomer ratio of 1/4 (25mM/100mM) seems to be sufficient to ensure strong bead formation. Higher ratios lead to residual insoluble calcium in the beads.

Calcium availability within the alginate gel is assured by achieving a homogeneous distribution within the alginate sol and from droplet to droplet. This assumes that the number of calcium vector grains is rather larger than the alginate droplets. If this is not the case, it will result in aggregation of the beads. However, spherical beads smaller than 50 μm may be formed using a higher calcium concentration and/or a smaller grain size.

Neutral pH values are appropriate for live cell immobilization. Acid tolerant cultures such as lactic acid bacteria may be immobilized at a lower pH range (7 initial to 5 final). The selection of a suitable calcium vector for internal gelation is, therefore, quite important. Over the pH range of interest, the concentration of free calcium must be very low initially with rapid release of calcium while reducing pH. A pKa value of the anions in the working range (6.5 to 7.5) is optimal for cell immobilization. Oxalate and tartrate were unacceptable, since they did not released calcium within a suitable pH range. Calcium phosphate was also rejected because of the large grain size, resulting in poor gelation.

A citrate complex resulted in large beads with a high variability in the size distribution. At pH 8, gelation was completed within four minutes whereas at a lower pH (6 to 6.5) gelation was not particularly fast (20 sec), although more rapid than under basic conditions. In contrast, calcium carbonate–alginate sol remained stable for more than 48 hours at pH 7.5. By reducing the pH to 6 or 6.5, essentially instantaneous gelation resulted. The beads were smaller and spherical and the size distribution was typically unimodal. The difference in behavior between the citrate and carbonate complexes relates to the stoichiometry that defines the slope of the calcium release as a function of pH. A molecular calcium to anion ratio of 1 into the calcium vector ensures the maximum slope, permitting work within a smaller pH range.

The alginate composition is also an important parameter in alginate bead formulation. A high guluronic content and homopolymer blocks lead to higher interaction alginate/calcium and hence stronger gels. Moreover, in the emulsification method, premature gelation occurs faster with high guluronic alginate.

### *Microbead Size Distribution*

The droplet size distributions in emulsions and resulting bead diameter distributions are determined by the relation between the dispersive forces and either the surface tension or the viscosity of the discontinuous phase. With citrate complex as the calcium vector, the alginate bead size distribution was independent of the surfactant concentration and the alginate viscosity. It was expected that the pregelation of the alginate was masking the other effects. When using carbonate complex, the alginate viscosity had no effect on the mean size but the bead diameter was dependent on the surfactant concentration and, thus, the interfacial tension. Pregelation is, therefore, no longer a dominant factor in determining the size distribution.

In summary, the narrowest size distribution alginate bead produced by emulsification and internal gelation was obtained by using low guluronic and low viscosity alginate, small and dispersed grains of calcium carbonate complex, within the pH range of 7.5 (initial) to 6.5 (final). The distribution was characterized by one main peak with a standard deviation of 36% representing 90% of the total bead volume. Emulsification/internal gelation appears promising for large-scale immobilization within alginate gels.

Effect of pH To obtain good quality beads by extrusion/internal gelation, the gelifying bath must have a pH lower than 6. This does not imply that one decrease the pH in the beads since the release of calcium from calcium carbonate releases carbonate ions that act as a base. However, the need for low pH in the bath may be necessary to insure fast reaction at the droplet interface. In the case of external gelation method, the reaction between alginate and calcium at the droplet interface is very fast and a skin is formed very quickly, preventing the alginate from diffusing in the aqueous phase. This is a typical phenomenon in a symmetric membrane formation. Such fast reaction at the interface is most probably necessary in the case of the internal gelation.

### *Thermodynamic of Shrinking and Swelling*

A larger shrinking of the beads formed by internal gelation is most probably due to the fact that the reaction takes place simultaneously throughout the volume of the beads. In the case of external gelation, when the gelled external layer becomes sufficiently rigid, gelation does not provoke additional shrinking. However, the external layer of beads formed by external gelation may be more compact than internally gelled core. This external layer then plays a role similar to a membrane. This is why the diffusion of large molecules is faster with beads formed by internal gelation, where gelation does not lead to such skin but most probably to large free space between compact alginate zones.

## CONCLUSION

Internal gelation seems to be a very promising method to form beads in a large scale, under sterile conditions with a relatively low mean size. However, it is difficult to expect size dispersion (standard deviation) lower than 30% of the mean size. Using internal gelation in combination with dropping techniques may also offer interesting alternatives, reducing the polydispersity to a 5–10% range. Additional work is, however, required to optimize the methods and to define the final properties of the beads and then the scope of applications.

## REFERENCES

1. PONCELET, D., B. PONCELET DE SMET, C. BEAULIEU & R.J. NEUFELD. 1992. Scale-up of gel bead and microcapsule production in cell immobilization. *In* Fundamentals of Animal Cell Encapsulation and Immobilization. M.F.A. Goosen, Ed.: 113–142. CRC Press, Boca Raton.
2. LENCKI, R.W.J., R.J. NEUFELD & T. SPINNEY. 1989. Microspheres and Method of Producing Same. U.S. Patent 4.822.534:Apr. 18, 1989.
3. PONCELET, D., A. PAUSS, H. NAVEAU, *et al.* 1985. Computation of physicochemical parameters, i.a. pH, in complex (bio)chemical system. Anal. Biochem. **150:** 421–428.

# Non-Invasive Monitoring of a Bioartificial Pancreas *in Vitro* and *in Vivo*

IOANNIS CONSTANTINIDIS,[a,b] ROBERT LONG, JR.,[a,b] COLIN WEBER,[c] SUSAN SAFLEY,[d] AND ATHANASSIOS SAMBANIS,[b,e]

[a]*Department of Radiology, Emory University, Atlanta, Georgia, USA*

[b]*Georgia Tech/Emory Center for the Engineering of Living Tissues, Atlanta, Georgia, USA*

[c]*Department of Surgery, Emory University, Atlanta, Georgia, USA*

[d]*Department of Ophthalmology, Emory University, Atlanta, Georgia, USA*

[e]*School of Chemical Engineering, Georgia Institute of Technology, Atlanta, Georgia, USA*

ABSTRACT: Monitoring biochemical processes relevant to the function, survival, and longevity of tissue-engineered pancreatic constructs is important for the development of an optimum construct design as well as patient care management after implantation. In this report we demonstrate the ability of nuclear magnetic resonance (NMR) techniques to monitor aspects of intracellular metabolism, overall morphology, and distribution of a microencapsulation based bioartificial pancreas *in vitro* and *in vivo*.

KEYWORDS: non-invasive monitoring; bioartificial pancreas; islets; BTC3 cells; alginate

## INTRODUCTION

It is estimated that 16 million people in the United States are currently diagnosed with diabetes, of which 10% are Type-1 diabetics.[1] The current treatment of multiple (4–5) daily insulin injections can afford these patients a near normal life. However, the stepwise blood glucose regulation granted by bolus injections of insulin is responsible for various detrimental complications manifested at later stages of life. Treatments that can yield physiologic glucose regulation, such as pancreas and islet transplantation, have recently shown significant promise[2] although the limited availability of donor organs and the lifelong requirement of immunosuppressive medication remain significant unsolved problems in islet tissue replacement.[3,4]

The bioartificial pancreas has the potential to be an efficacious clinical treatment that can provide physiologic blood glucose regulation without immunosuppressive medication, that is administered with relative ease, and that is readily available.[5–9] The design most commonly used to generate these tissue-engineered constructs is based on the microencapsulation of insulin-secreting cells in a biocompatible matrix

---

Address for correspondence: Ioannis Constantinidis, Department of Radiology, Emory University, Atlanta, GA 30322, USA.
iconsta@emory.edu

that provides mechanical support and, at least, partial immunoprotection.[5,6] Selecting the appropriate cell source for insulin secretion has been the subject of intense research.[10–12] The choices involve either mammalian islets or transformed β-cells. The principal advantage of using islets is physiologic control of blood glucose concentration. Their main disadvantages are the difficulty of isolation and their limited supply. An alternative choice is the use of cell lines that have been genetically modified to possess physiologic glucose-stimulated insulin secretion. The principal advantage of using such cell lines is the ease by which they can be propagated *in vitro* to large homogeneous populations. The disadvantages include subphysiological glucose responsiveness during prolonged cultivation,[11,13–17] and continuous growth within the capsule.[18] In terms of encapsulation biomaterials, several have been tested for effectiveness as the extracellular matrix; however, the most frequently used is the alginate/poly-L-lysine/alginate (APA) bead. Developing non-invasive imaging techniques that can monitor the viability and function of encapsulated cells as well as the integrity of the matrix is critical to understanding the function of these tissue-engineered constructs *in vitro* and *in vivo*.

NMR is an analytical tool that has been used by physicists and chemists to study the structure and dynamics of molecules since 1946.[19,20] NMR has the ability to simultaneously and non-invasively provide biochemical and structural information both *in vivo* and *in vitro*. In the field of tissue engineering, and particularly in the context of the bioartificial pancreas, application of NMR has been limited.[21–31] At present, our only means of assessing the efficacy for an implanted bioartificial pancreas is to measure blood glucose levels. It is obvious that recipient patients could be better managed by developing NMR-based methodology to monitor *in vivo* the viability, metabolic activity, and structural integrity of implanted bioartificial pancreatic constructs. This study represents the first step towards establishing a non-invasive *in vivo* monitoring method that uses existing magnetic resonance technologies that permit the evaluation of both intracellular metabolism and morphology of a microencapsulation-based bioartificial pancreas. The model constructs employed consist of porcine islets and insulin-secreting βTC3 murine insulinoma cells encapsulated in APA beads.

## MATERIALS AND METHODS

### Cell Culture and APA Encapsulation

βTC3 cells were obtained from the laboratory of Dr. Shimon Efrat (Department of Molecular Pharmacology, Albert Einstein College of Medicine, New York, NY). The cells were propagated as monolayers in T-flasks, and cultured in Dulbecco's modified eagles medium (DMEM) (D-5648, Sigma Chemical Co., St. Louis, MO) supplemented with L-glutamine to a final concentration of 6 mM, 15% heat-inactivated horse serum, 2.5% fetal bovine serum, and 1% penicillin/streptomycin solution as described elsewhere.[26] Only cells between passages 32 and 47 were employed for these experiments.

Adult porcine islets were provided by Dr. Bernard Hering (Department of Surgery, University of Minnesota). The islets were isolated, cultured overnight, and sent the following day by overnight mail to our institution. Islets were encapsulated within one hour of their arrival. Neonatal pig islets were isolated, cultured for nine days, and encapsulated as described by Weber, et al.[32]

Encapsulation of βTC3 cells and islets in APA beads was based on the initial protocol of Lim and Sun.[5] Adult porcine islets or freshly trypsinized βTC3 cells were suspended in a 2% alginate solution—Kelco LV for islets and Pronova biomedical type LVM for the βTC3 cells—and via an electrostatic bead generator droplets were allowed to fall in a 1.1% $CaCl_2$ solution producing calcium alginate beads. Both of these alginates have a high mannuronic acid content (greater than 60%) and have been shown to facilitate the proliferation of βTC3 cells.[25,33] The beads were subsequently treated with poly-L-lysine (MW 20,000–30,000, Sigma Chemical Co. St Louis, MO), and coated with alginate to form APA beads. Beads were 800 μm in diameter and contained initially $3.5 \times 10^7$ βTC3 cells/ml alginate or 20,000 islet equivalents per ml of alginate. The viability of encapsulated βTC3 cells, 24 and 48 hours after completion of this procedure, has been reported by our group to range between 60% and 85%.[26,34]

## *NMR Spectroscopy and Imaging*

All $^1H$ NMR data were acquired with a 4.7 T horizontal bore VARIAN 200/33 *INOVA* spectrometer. Freshly encapsulated βTC3 cells and islets were placed in a 1.3 mm inner diameter Teflon™ tube that allowed the beads to be stacked one on top of another. The NMR signal was detected with a home built solenoidal coil that surrounded the tube and was single tuned to the $^1H$ frequency. $T_2$ and diffusion weighted images were acquired within 24–48 hours after encapsulation. Typical acquisition parameters used for the diffusion weighted $^1H$ NMR images were: duration of dephasing/phasing gradients, 4 ms; echo time, 60–70 ms; repetition time, 2.5 s; the strength of dephasing gradient varied between 0–8 G/cm; the separation time of gradients varied between 10–40 ms. $T_2$ and diffusion weighted images were acquired using a standard spin–echo pulse sequence.

$^1H$ NMR spectra were acquired from both islets and βTC3 cells. Acquisition of $^1H$ NMR spectra in an aqueous environment demands the use of efficient water suppression techniques. Use of a spin–echo sequence that employs modified BIR-4 adiabatic pulses[35,36] enabled us to acquire spectra from both islets and βTC3 cells in the absence and presence of continuous perfusion. Suppression was accomplished by introducing a free precession period within the pulses to create minimum excitation at the water frequency and maximum excitation half way between the choline and lactate resonance. The length of the excitation pulse was 2.86 msec and that of the refocussing pulse was 3.32 msec. The repetition time was 2.39 sec and the echo time, TE/2, was 128 msec. The excitation bandwidth maximum was centered at 540 Hz or 2.70 ppm upfield of the water resonance. Use of this sequence resulted in the generation of an echo that contains optimum signal for the metabolites of interest and minimum signal for water.[31] The digitized full-echo signal was filtered, Fourier transformed, and fit in the frequency domain by Lorentzian model functions for each resonance in the frequency domain by routines supplied with the Sisco/Varian software.

## RESULTS AND DISCUSSION

### In vitro $^1H$ NMR Experiments

Neonatal porcine islets, packed in a Teflon™ tube, were imaged prior to encapsulation to establish the sensitivity of the NMR imaging techniques at 4.7 T to differentiate between the culture medium and the islet clusters. The tube was sealed at both ends and placed through a solenoidal coil. The islets were not perfused to avoid motion-related artifacts in the MR images due to medium flow. FIGURE 1 illustrates a $T_2$ (Panel A) and a diffusion (Panel B) weighted image of the neonatal porcine islets settled within the tube. Both images represent the same slice and were acquired sequentially within the same file. The echo time ($T_E$) was 70 msec and repetition time ($T_R$) was 4.0 sec. The strength of the dephasing gradient was 0–8 G/cm and the

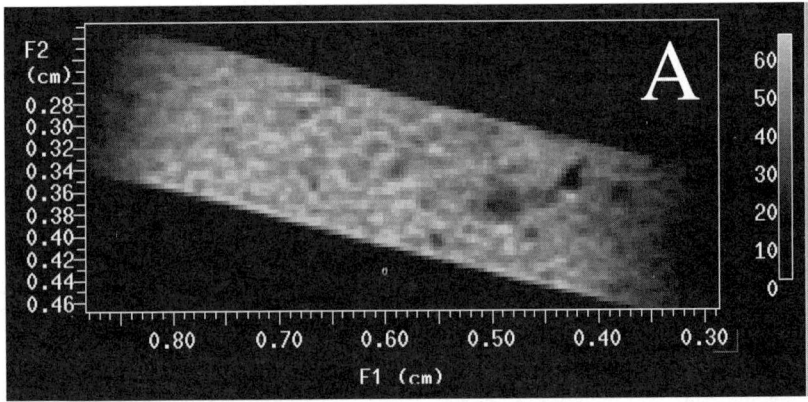

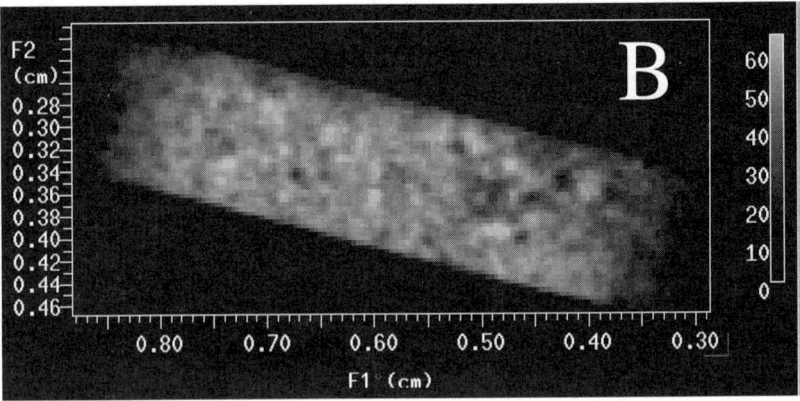

**FIGURE 1. A.** $T_2$ weighted image of unencapsulated neonatal porcine islets. **B.** Diffusion weighted image of the same slice as in **A**. Both images have a 40 × 40 μm in-plane pixel resolution and a 300 μm slice thickness

separation time between gradients was 40 ms. The images represent a 256 × 256 matrix and they are the average of four transients. With a 1 × 1 cm² field of view the resulting nominal spatial resolution is 40 × 40 μm in-plane and a slice thickness of 300 μm. The total acquisition time was 68 min. In the $T_2$ image the gray amorphous shapes represent the islets and the bright pockets between the islets represent the media. Based on this observation we can deduce that the $T_2$ of the islets is shorter than the surrounding medium. In the diffusion weighted image several regions of bright intensity are observed. It is postulated that the packing of islets at these

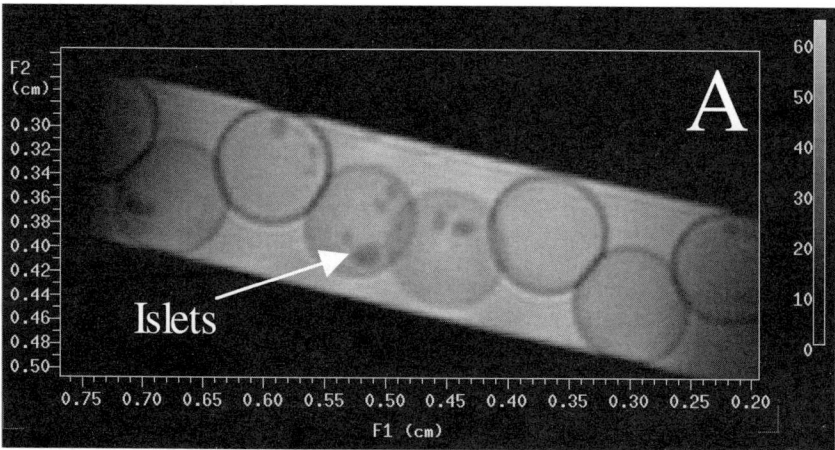

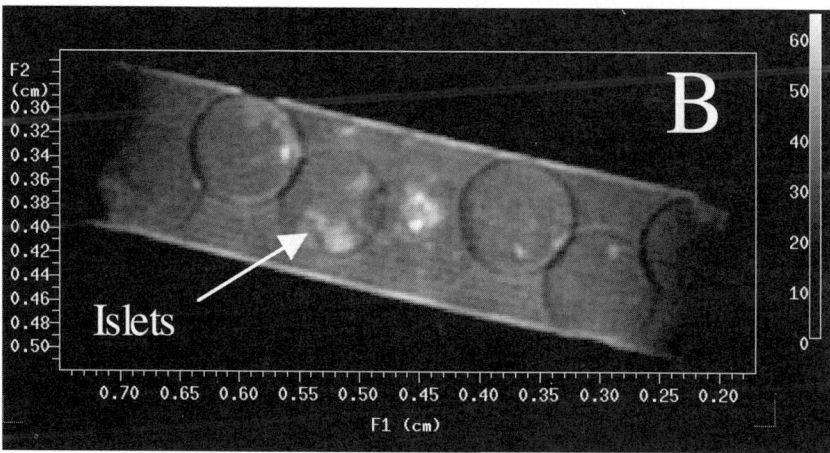

**FIGURE 2. A.** $T_2$ weighted image of APA encapsulated adult porcine islets. **B.** Diffusion weighted image of the same slice as in **A**. Both images have a 40 × 40 μm in-plane pixel resolution and a 400 μm slice thickness. The location of encapsulated islets can be clearly detected.

locations is tighter, thus decreasing water diffusion and increasing diffusion weighted contrast.

Once we established that unencapsulated islets were indeed visible by NMR imaging, we tried to determine if islets are also detectable in the encapsulating environment of an alginate matrix. For these experiments adult porcine islets were entrapped in APA beads. Upon completion of this protocol the beads were exposed to 50 mM citrate to resolubilize the internal alginate matrix; a common practice in the encapsulation of islets. APA capsules containing islets were stacked in a similar 1.3 mm inner diameter Teflon™ tube and filled with a medium designed to maintain the islets. FIGURE 2 illustrates a $T_2$ weighted (Panel A) and a diffusion weighted (Panel B) NMR image of several APA beads containing adult porcine islets. The acquisition parameters and pixel resolution for these images were similar ($T_R$ = 2.5 s, $T_E$ = 60 ms, 32 averages, strength of the dephasing gradient was 0–8 G/cm) to those discussed above in FIGURE 1. In both types of images the spherical contours of the APA beads are clearly demarcated. In the $T_2$ weighted image the islets appear darker than the liquefied alginate or the solution around them. Thus, the $T_2$ relaxation time of islets is shorter than both the culture medium and the alginate solution. In the diffusion weighted image the islets appear significantly brighter than the APA beads or the medium. In addition, we observe that bright areas are not restricted to the islets but they are observed in the vicinity of the islets as well. The reasons for this observation are not fully understood. However, we postulate that islets might secrete an extracellular matrix creating an added diffusion barrier. Based on these images it is apparent that both $T_2$ and diffusion weighted MR images can clearly identify the location of the encapsulated islets within a bioartificial pancreatic construct.

Given that an implantable bioartificial pancreas might consist of transformed β-cells we extended the NMR imaging experiments to include encapsulated βTC3 cells. Whereas in the islet preparations the APA beads were treated with citrate at the completion of encapsulation, APA beads containing βTC3 cells were not treated with citrate and, consequently, the beads remained gelled. We have determined that gelled APA beads are preferred for the encapsulation of βTC3 cells because they reduce the rate of cell proliferation and provide mechanical support to prolong the longevity of the cultures.[18] Like the islet experiments, APA beads containing βTC3 cells were stacked in a Teflon™ tube and sealed. FIGURE 3 illustrates MR images of 20 days old APA beads containing βTC3 cells. Panel A shows a $T_2$ weighted image whereas Panel B is the corresponding diffusion weighted image. In addition, a representative cross-section of an APA bead stained with hematoxylin/eosin is shown in Panel C. These images were acquired using the same acquisition parameters as were the images in FIGURE 2. In the $T_2$ weighted image APA beads are clearly detected against the culture medium whereas darker βTC3 cell aggregates at the periphery of the beads can also be seen. Based on these observations we deduced that the $T_2$ relaxation time of gelled alginate is shorter than the liquefied alginate solution (FIG. 2), thus the contrast between the alginate gel and the βTC3 cell clusters appears less obvious. In the diffusion weighted image, the cell aggregates at the periphery of the beads appear very bright, leading to the conclusion that βTC3 cells form tight aggregates, thus restricting the diffusion of water and possibly other nutrients and metabolites. This pattern of growth by βTC3 cells and the presence of a restrictive

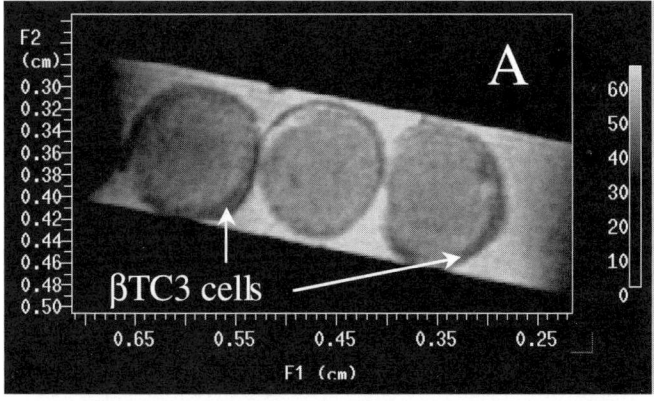

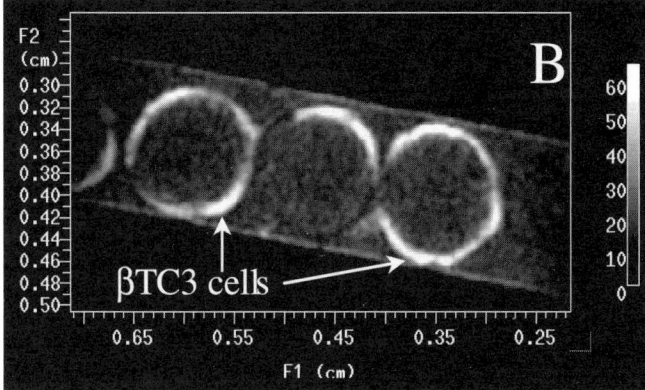

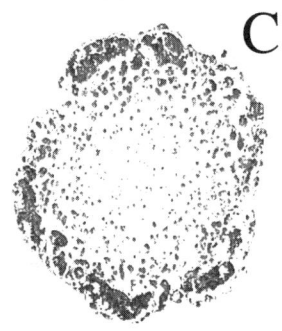

**FIGURE 3. A.** $T_2$ weighted image of APA encapsulated βTC3 cells. **B.** Diffusion weighted image of the same slice as in **A**. Both images have a 40 × 40 μm in-plane pixel resolution and a 400 μm slice thickness. **C.** Representative cross-section of an APA bead stained with hematoxylin/eosin.

environment at the periphery are supported by the histology cross-section showing large aggregates at the periphery and dead cells in the center of the beads (Panel C).

To measure changes in intracellular metabolites we performed a series of experiments in which $^1$H NMR spectra were acquired from both islets and βTC3 cells. FIGURE 4 shows representative $^1$H NMR spectra of unencapsulated neonatal porcine islets (Panel A) and βTC3 cells encapsulated in APA beads (Panel B). Both spectra were acquired using the same acquisition parameters. The islet spectrum (NT = 512, TR = 2.0, NP = 2048) was based on the sample of unencapsulated islets shown in FIGURE 1 and was, thus, collected in the absence of active perfusion. The total acquisition time for this spectrum was 20 min. The spectrum from encapsulated βTC3 cells was acquired from a larger volume of APA beads (about 4 ml) under constant perfusion with DMEM containing 16 mM glucose and the acquisition time was 2 min. The resonance assignments displayed in the figure are based on extract spectra and on published values of known chemical shifts. The similarities between the two spectra are remarkable. The resonance at 3.20 ppm labeled as total choline is known to be composed of the $-N^+(CH_3)_3$ groups of choline, phosphorylcholine, and glycerolphosphorylcholine. For the βTC3 cell line and culture conditions used in this study, extract spectra of monolayer cultures acquired at 400 MHz show that phosphorylcholine represents the major contributor to this signal (63.6 ± 4.0%) followed by glycerolphosphorylcholine (33.4 ± 4.0%), and choline (3.0 ± 0.4%).[31] The composition of this resonance for the adult porcine islets is not known. Upfield of the total choline resonance, the two broad resonances ranging between 2.35 and 2.07 ppm represent a mix of the β and γ protons of glutamate and glutamine (Glx), whereas the large resonance at 1.27 ppm is assigned to the $CH_3$ group of lactate. The shoulder downfield of the lactate peak at 1.43 ppm is assigned to alanine and the peak upfield of the lactate resonance at 0.94 ppm is assigned to the methyl resonances of several amino acids. Based on the composition of DMEM and the chemical shifts of the different amino acids, the compounds most likely contributing to this resonance are isoleucine, leucine, and valine.

## In vivo $^1$H NMR Experiments

Two BALB/c mice were implanted with 0.5 ml of APA beads by an intraperitoneal injection and the mice were imaged immediately after implantation (within two hours) and then one and three days later. The implanted beads measured 800 μm in diameter and contained βTC3 cells at a density of $7 \times 10^7$ cells/ml of alginate. Since this was a fresh preparation, βTC3 cells are distributed uniformly throughout the bead as single cells without the presence of large cell aggregates. Consequently, contrast from within the beads in the diffusion-weighted images is not expected and, therefore, not observed. FIGURE 5 contains two sagittal MR images of a mouse abdomen. Panel A shows a $T_2$ weighted MR image acquired three days after injection of the beads. Panel B shows a diffusion weighted MR image from the same slice as Panel A but zoomed at the region of the abdomen outlined by the dashed rectangle in Panel A. In this image the dark APA beads are clearly seen surrounded in a bright background. The dark signal intensity of the APA beads under diffusion weighting was anticipated since there are no cell aggregates to provide the contrast seen in FIGURE 3. The NMR parameters used to acquire these images were similar to those used for the *in vitro* images in FIGURES 1–3 with a larger field of view. These images

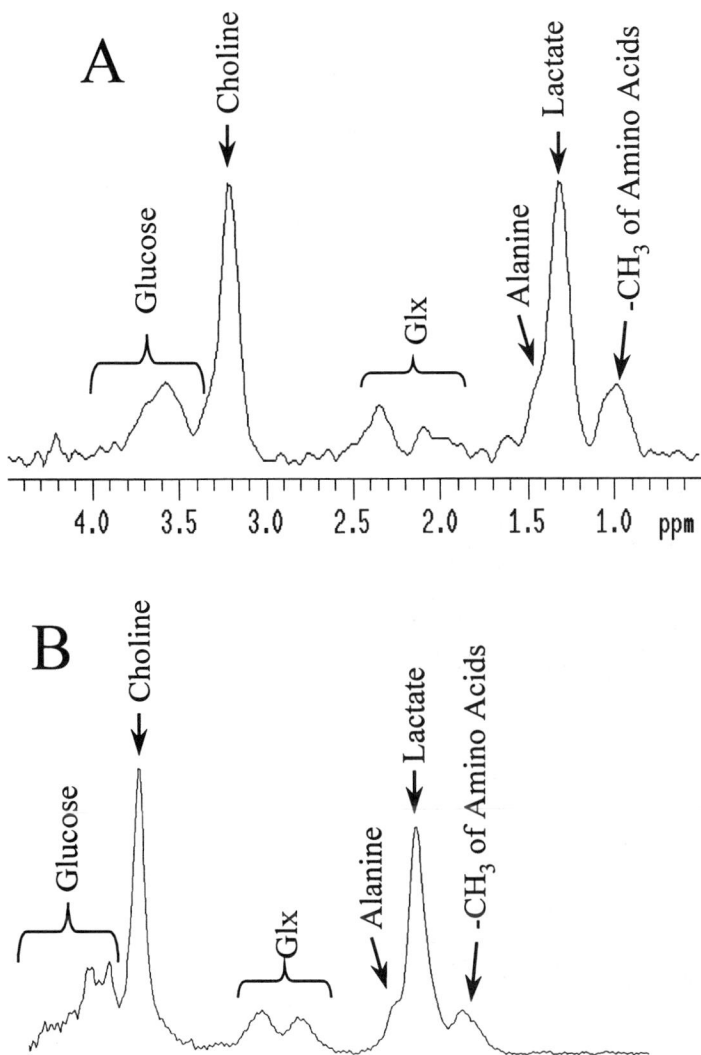

**FIGURE 4.** Water suppressed $^1$H NMR spectrum of neonatal porcine islets (**A**) and APA encapsulated βTC3 cells (**B**). Both spectra were acquired in the presence of DMEM medium (5 mM glucose for islets and 16 mM glucose for βTC3 cells).

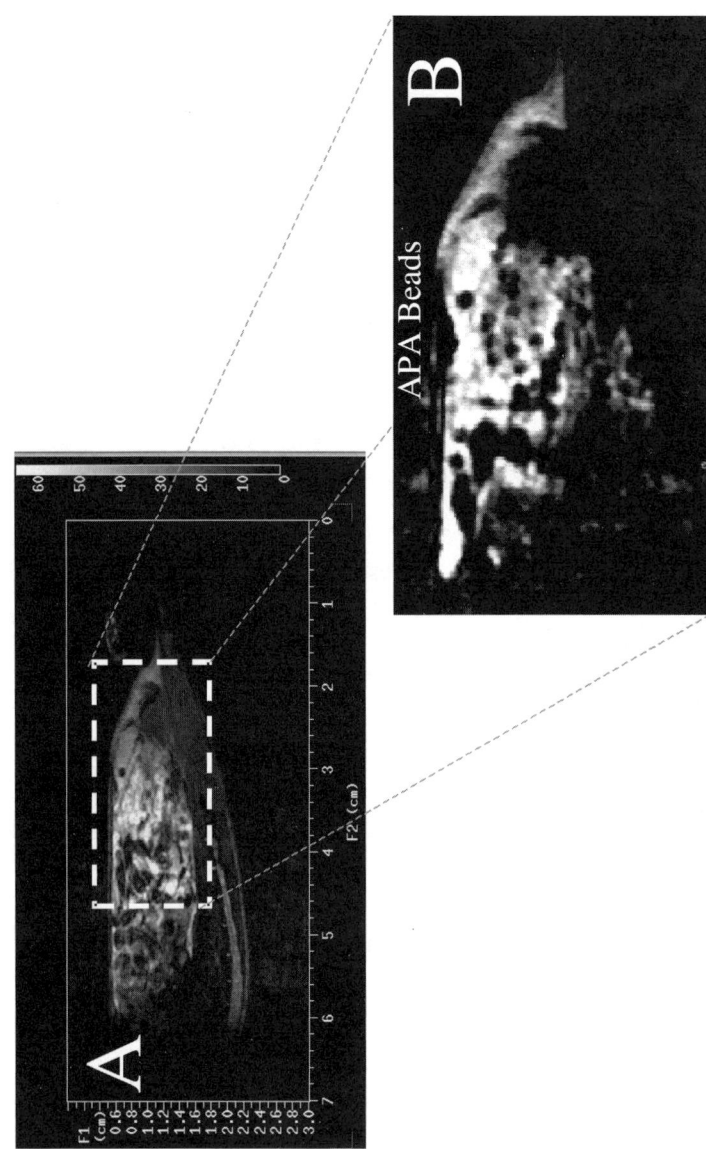

**FIGURE 5. A.** $T_2$ weighted MR image of the abdomen of a live BALB/c mouse three days after implantation of 0.5 ml APA beads. **B.** An expansion of the diffusion weighted image acquired from the same slice as in **A**. The dashed rectangle in **A** illustrates the region of interest displayed in **B**. A cluster of implanted APA beads is clearly seen as dark circles in bright background.

were acquired using a 3.8 cm diameter quadrature "birdcage" design RF coil. The spatial resolution of these images was 60 × 150 µm in-plane with a 1 mm slice thickness.

## CONCLUSIONS

Overall, we have demonstrated *in vitro* that $^1$H NMR imaging can be used to visualize islets or βTC3 cells within their encapsulated environment. Similarly, $^1$H NMR spectra of porcine islets and βTC3 cells are remarkably similar. With reference to matrix effects, the $T_2$ relaxation time of gelled alginate is shorter than the liquefied solution. Finally, we have shown that localizing implanted APA beads *in vivo* is feasible with the use of diffusion weighted imaging.

## ACKNOWLEDGMENTS

This work was supported by grants from the ERC Program of the National Science Foundation under Award Number EEC-9731643, and the NIH (DK47858, and RR13003). This financial support is greatly appreciated.

## REFERENCES

1. SERVICES USDoHaH. 1999. Conquering Diabetes. A strategic plan for the 21st century. A report of the congressionally-established Diabetes Research Working Group. Washington, D.C. Report No.: NIH Publication No. 99-4398.
2. SHAPIRO, A.M., J.R.T. LAKEY, E. RYAN, *et al.* 2000. Islet transplantation in seven patients with type I diabetes mellitus using a glucocorticoid-free immunosuppressive regimen. N. Engl. J. Med. **343:** 230–238.
3. ROBERTSON, R.P. 1992. Pancreatic and islet transplantation for diabetes-cures or curiosities. N. Engl. J. Med. **327:** 1861–1868.
4. SUTHERLAND, D.E.R. 1996. Pancreas and islet cell transplantation: now and then. Transplant. Proc. **28:** 2131–2133.
5. LIM, F. & A.M. SUN. 1980. Microencapsulated islets as bioartificial endocrine pancreas. Science **210:** 908–910.
6. SUN, A.M., W. PARISIUS, H. MACMORINE, *et al.* 1980. An artificial pancreas containing cultured islets of Langerhans. Artif. Organs **4:** 275–278.
7. REACH, G. 1993. Bioartificial pancreas. Diabet. Med. **10:** 105–109.
8. SOON-SHIONG, P. 1995. Encapsulated human islet transplant trials in type 1 diabetes patients. *In* Fetal Islet Transplantation. C.M. Peterson, L. Jovanovic-Peterson & B. Formby, Eds.: 137–149. Plenum Press, New York.
9. LANZA, R.P. & W.L. CHICK. 1997. Transplantation of encapsulated cells and tissues. Surgery **121:** 1–9.
10. HUGHES, S.D., J.H. JOHNSON, C. QUAADE & C.B. NEWGARD. 1992. Engineering of glucose-stimulated insulin secretion and biosynthesis in non-islet cells. Proc. Natl. Acad. Sci. USA **89:** 688–692.
11. EFRAT, S., D. FUSCO-DEMANE, H. LEMBERG, *et al.* 1995. Conditional transformation of a pancreatic beta-cell line derived from transgenic mice expressing a tetracycline-regulated oncogene. Proc. Natl. Acad. Sci. USA **92:** 3576–3580.
12. CLARK, S.A., C. QUAADE, H. CONSTANDY, *et al.* 1997. Novel insulinoma cell lines produced by iterative engineering of GLUT2, glucokinase, and human insulin expression. Diabetes **46:** 958–967.

13. RADVANYI, F., S. CHRISTGAU, S. BAEKKESKOV, *et al.* 1993. Pancreatic β-cells cultured from individual preneoplastic foci in a multistage tumorigenesis pathway: a potentially general technique for isolating physiologically representative cell lines. Mol. Cell. Biol. **13:** 4223–4232.
14. NEWGARD, C.B. & H. BELTRAN DEL RIO. 1995. Engineering a glucose responsive insulin secreting cell line. J. Cell. Biochem. Suppl. **21B:** 4.
15. KNAACK, D., M. FIORE, M. SURANA, *et al.* 1994. Clonal insulinoma cell line that stably maintains correct glucose responsiveness. Diabetes **43:** 1413–1417.
16. ISHIHARA, H., T. ASANO, K. TSUKUDA, *et al.* 1993. Pancreatic β-cell line Min6 exhibits characteristics of glucose metabolism and glucose-stimulated insulin secretion similar to those of normal islets. Diabetologia **36:** 1139–1145.
17. EFRAT, S., M. LEISER, M. SURANA, *et al.* 1993. Murine insulinoma cell line with normal glucose regulated insulin secretion. Diabetes **42:** 901–907.
18. CONSTANTINIDIS, I., I. RASK, R.C. LONG, JR. & A. SAMBANIS. 1999. Effects of alginate composition on the metabolic, secretory, and growth characteristics of entrapped βTC3 mouse insulinoma cells. Biomaterials **20:** 1969–1975.
19. BLOCH, F. & W.W. HANSEN. 1946. M. P. Nuclear induction experiment. Phys. Rev. **69:** 127.
20. PURCELL, E.M., H.C. TORREY & R.V. POUND. 1946. Resonance absorption by nuclear magnetic moments in solids. Physiol. Rev. **69:** 37–38.
21. SAMBANIS, A., K.K. PAPAS, P.C. FLANDERS, *et al.* 1994. Towards the development of a bioartificial pancreas: immunoisolation and NMR monitoring of mouse insulinomas. Cytotechnology **15:** 351–363.
22. KRIAT, M., J. FANTINI, J. VIOM-DURY, *et al.* 1992. Energetic metabolism of glucose, mannose and galactose in glucose starved rat insulinoma cells anchored on microcarrier beads. A phosphorous-31 NMR study. Biochimie **74:** 949–955.
23. MATSCHINSKY, F.M. 1996. A lesson in metabolic regulation inspired by the glucokinase glucose sensor paradigm. Diabetes **45:** 223–241.
24. CONSTANTINIDIS, I. & A. SAMBANIS. 1995. Towards the development of artificial endocrine tissues: 31P NMR spectroscopic studies of immunoisolated, insulin-secreting AtT-20 cells. Biotechnol. Bioeng. **47:** 431–443.
25. CONSTANTINIDIS, I., N.E. MUKUNDAN, M. GAMCSIK & A. SAMBANIS. 1997. Towards the development of a bioartificial pancreas: a $^{13}$C NMR study on the effect of alginate/poly-L-lysine/alginate entrapment on glucose metabolism by βTC3 mouse insulinoma cells. Cell. Mol. Biol. **43:** 721–729.
26. PAPAS, K.K., R.C. LONG, JR., I. CONSTANTINIDIS & A. SAMBANIS. 1997. Role of ATP and $P_i$ on the mechanism of insulin secretion in the mouse insulinoma βTC3 cell line. Biochem. J. **326:** 807–814.
27. CONSTANTINIDIS, I. & A. SAMBANIS. 1998. Non-invasive monitoring of tissue engineered constructs by nuclear magnetic resonance methodologies. Tissue Engin. **4:** 9–17.
28. PAPAS, K.K., R.C. LONG, JR., I. CONSTANTINIDIS & A. SAMBANIS. 1999. Towards the development of a bioartificial pancreas: I. Long-term propagation and basal and induced secretion from entrapped βTC3 cell cultures. Biotechnol. Bioeng. **66:** 219–230.
29. PAPAS, K.K., R.C. LONG, JR., I. CONSTANTINIDIS & A. SAMBANIS. 1999. Towards the development of a bioartificial pancreas: II. Effects of oxygen on long-term entrapped βTC3 cell cultures. Biotechnol. Bioeng. **66:** 231–237.
30. PAPAS, K.K., R.C. LONG, JR., A. SAMBANIS & I. CONSTANTINIDIS. 2001. Effects of short-term hypoxia on a bioartificial pancreatic construct. Cell Transpl. **9:** 415–422.
31. LONG, JR., R.C., K.K. PAPAS, A. SAMBANIS & I. CONSTANTINIDIS. 2000. *In vitro* monitoring of total choline levels in a bioartificial pancreas: $^1$H NMR spectroscopic studies of the effects of oxygen level. J. Magn. Reson. **146:** 49–57.
32. WEBER, C.J., M.K. HAGLER, J.T. CHRYSSOCHOOS, *et al.* 1997. CTLA4-Ig prolongs survival of microencapsulated neonatal porcine islet xenografts in diabetic NOD mice. Cell Transplantation **6:** 505–508.
33. STABLER, C., K. WILKS, A. SAMBANIS & I. CONSTANTINIDIS. 2001. The effects of alginate composition on encapsulated βTC3 cells. Biomaterials **22:** 1301–1310.

34. BENSON, J.P., K.K. PAPAS, I. CONSTANTINIDIS & A. SAMBANIS. 1997. Towards the development of a bioartificial pancreas: effects of poly-L-lysine on alginate beads with βTC3 cells. Cell Transplantation **6:** 395–402.
35. GARWOOD, M. & Y. KE. 1991. Symmetric pulses to induce arbitrary flip angles with compensation for RF inhomogeneity and resonance offsets. J. Magn. Reson. **94:** 511–525.
36. ROSS, B.D., H. MERKLE, K. HENDRICH, et al. 1992. Spatially localized in vivo $^1$H magnetic resonance spectroscopy of an intracerebral rat glioma. Magn. Reson. Med. **23:** 96–108.

# NMR Spectroscopy in β Cell Engineering and Islet Transplantation

KLEARCHOS K. PAPAS,[a] CLARK K. COLTON,[a] JOHN S. GOUNARIDES,[b]
ERIC S. ROOS,[b] MARY ANN C. JAREMA,[b] MICHAEL J. SHAPIRO,[b]
LEO L. CHENG,[c] GARY W. CLINE,[d] GERALD I. SHULMAN,[d]
HAIYAN WU,[a] SUSAN BONNER-WEIR,[e] AND GORDON C. WEIR[e]

[a]*Department of Chemical Engineering, Massachusetts Institute of Technology, Cambridge, Massachusetts, USA*

[b]*Novartis Pharmaceuticals, Analytics and BioNMR, Summit, New Jersey, USA*

[c]*Department of Pathology, Massachusetts General Hospital, Charlestown, Massachusetts, USA*

[d]*Yale University Medical School, New Haven, Connecticut, USA*

[e]*Joslin Diabetes Center, Harvard Medical School, Boston, Massachusetts, USA*

ABSTRACT: Islet transplantation is a promising method for restoring normoglycemia and alleviating the long term complications of diabetes. Widespread application of islet transplantation is hindered by the limited supply of human islets and requires a large increase in the availability of suitable insulin secreting tissue as well as robust quality assessment methodologies that can ensure safety and *in vivo* efficacy. We explore the application of nuclear magnetic resonance (NMR) spectroscopy in two areas relevant to β cell engineering and islet transplantation: (1) the effect of genetic alterations on glucose metabolism, and (2) quality assessment of islet preparations prior to transplantation. Results obtained utilizing a variety of NMR techniques demonstrate the following: (1) Transfection of Rat1 cells with the *c-myc* oncogene (which may be involved in cell proliferation and cell cycle regulation) and overexpression of *Bcl-2* (which may protect cells from stresses such as hypoxia and exposure to cytokines) introduce a wide array of alterations in cellular biochemistry, including changes in anaerobic and oxidative glucose metabolism, as assessed by $^{13}$C and $^{31}$P NMR spectroscopy. (2) Overnight incubation of islets and β cells in the bottom of centrifuge tubes filled with medium at room temperature, as is sometimes done in islet transportation, exposes them to severe oxygen limitations that may cause cell damage. Such exposure, leading to reversible or irreversible damage, can be observed with NMR-detectable markers using conventional $^{13}$C and $^{31}$P NMR spectroscopy of extracts. In addition, markers of irreversible damage (as well as markers of hypoxia) can be detected and quantified without cell extraction using high-resolution magic angle spinning $^1$H NMR spectroscopy. Finally, acute ischemia in a bed of perfused β cells leads to completely reversible changes that can be followed in real time with $^{31}$P NMR spectroscopy.

KEYWORDS: NMR; islet; β cell; transportation; transplantation; culture; quality; assessment; *c-myc*; *Bcl-2*; LDH; hypoxia; oxygen; lactate; phosphocholine; lipids; apoptosis

Address for correspondence: Klearchos K. Papas, Room 66-457, Department of Chemical Engineering, Massachusetts Institute of Technology, 77 Massachusetts Avenue, Cambridge, MA 02139-4307, USA. Voice: 617-252-1109; fax: 617-252-1651.
kpapas@mit.edu

## INTRODUCTION

Nuclear magnetic resonance (NMR) spectroscopy and imaging have been successfully applied to address a variety of questions related to cellular biochemistry, diabetes metabolism, brain function, organ transplantation, tumor biology, cancer treatment, apoptosis, gene therapy, and tissue engineering.[1-11] Advantages of NMR spectroscopy over conventional methods include the ability to identify and quantify multiple intracellular metabolites from a single NMR spectrum without separation to individual components, and when used non-invasively the ability to follow the progression and reversibility of the effects of metabolic stimuli or insults on intact cells or tissues. In this paper, we illustrate the use of NMR to investigate problems related to the development of improved insulin replacement therapies for the treatment of diabetes.

Type 1 diabetes is caused by autoimmune destruction of insulin-secreting β cells within islets of Langerhans in the pancreas. β cells secrete insulin in response to changes in blood glucose concentration in a highly regulated fashion and are responsible for achieving minute-to-minute regulation within physiological levels. Insulin deficiency results in prolonged hyperglycemia with serious long-term complications. Current treatments (e.g., insulin injections) do not provide tight regulation of blood glucose levels and, thus, do not alleviate the long-term complications of diabetes.[12] Both naked and encapsulated islet transplantation are being explored as alternative treatments that can provide more physiological blood glucose level control.[12-15] Recent dramatic improvement in the success rate of naked islet transplantation in humans[13] has prompted interest for more widespread application of this methodology, which requires a large increase in availability of suitable insulin secreting tissue[12,16-19] as well as methods for culture and transportation and, most importantly, robust quality assessment techniques that will ensure safety and *in vivo* efficacy. We explore the application of NMR to two major relevant areas: (1) effect of genetic alterations on glucose metabolism in β-cells, and (2) quality assessment of islet preparations prior to transplantation.

### *Effect of Genetic Alterations on Glucose Metabolism*

Genetic alterations may occur naturally, for example, associated with cell cycle progression and proliferation, or may be introduced artificially, for example, with the overexpression of anti-apoptotic genes by transfection with viral vectors. In order to explore the impact of genetic alterations on glucose metabolism, we studied Rat1 fibroblast cells transfected with two genes. These genes were *c-myc,* a gene associated with cell proliferation and cell cycle progression,[20-23] and *Bcl-2,* a gene associated with protection from proapoptotic stimuli.[24-28] Because *c-myc* is associated with upregulation of the cytosolic enzyme LDH[23,24] and *Bcl-2* is targeted on the mitochondria, we hypothesized that their expression at high levels may induce changes in the relative rates of oxidative and anaerobic glucose metabolism. We used $^{13}C$ NMR to investigate changes in glucose metabolism and $^{31}P$ NMR to investigate any other changes that may be related to cellular proliferation status. Changes in glucose metabolism may be particularly important for β cells and islets because glucose metabolism is believed to be tightly linked to β cell stimulus-secretion coupling.[29-47]

β-cells are thought to act as unique fuel sensors that translate changes in blood glucose concentration into changes in insulin secretion rate via a series of metabolic and electrophysiological events.[29–36] In the "fuel hypothesis", the increase in oxidative metabolism following glucose stimulation leads to an increase in intracellular [ATP] and in the [ATP]/[ADP] ratio, which initiates the cascade of events that leads to accelerated insulin exocytosis (see FIGURE 1).

The preferential stimulation of oxidative glucose metabolism, considered crucial for proper β-cell glucose sensing, is achieved by the combination of low levels of lactate dehydrogenase (LDH) and high levels of pyruvate carboxylase and mitochondrial glycerol phosphate dehydrogenase.[31–36] Several reports[34,38–43] demonstrate that alterations in the balance between oxidative and anaerobic glucose metabolism, which can be introduced by changes in the expression levels of enzymes such as

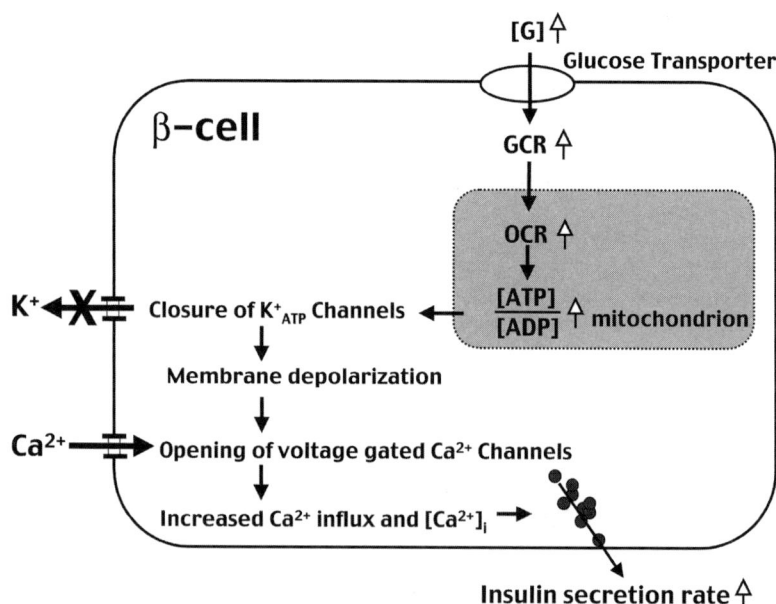

**FIGURE 1.** The "fuel hypothesis" for glucose-stimulated insulin secretion (GSIS) provides a link between metabolic and electrophysiological events. An increase in extracellular glucose concentration [G] results in an increase in the rate of glucose consumption (GCR), which, in turn, increases the oxygen consumption rate (OCR) as a result of the preferential entrance of glycolytically derived pyruvate into the TCA cycle, thereby stimulating mitochondrial oxidative metabolism. The resulting increase in the rate of ATP synthesis leads to an increase in intracellular [ATP] and in the [ATP]/[ADP] ratio, which are thought to cause closure of the ATP-sensitive $K^+$ channels, resulting in the depolarization of the cell membrane and opening of the voltage-gated $Ca^{2+}$ channels. This allows the influx of $Ca^{2+}$ ions into the cell, thus establishing a net increase in the intracellular $Ca^{2+}$ concentration. The elevated intracellular $Ca^{2+}$ concentration is thought to be the ultimate messenger for the increased rate of insulin exocytosis.

glucokinase, hexokinase, or LDH, or by defects in β cell mitochondria, impair glucose-stimulated insulin secretion (GSIS).

The limited human islet supply hinders large-scale application of islet transplantation.[12,17–19] Generation of large volumes of glucose-responsive, insulin-secreting tissue for transplantation by stimulating proliferation of preexisting adult islets, by inducing differentiation of dividing precursor cells, or by engineering glucose-responsive β cell lines is proposed as an alternative solution.[16–19,44–48] These approaches remain a challenge. Furthermore, rapidly proliferating β cells lose proper regulation of GSIS by a mechanism not fully understood, although changes in expression levels of key enzymes such as glucokinase and hexokinase, as well as *c-myc* and LDH, have been implicated.[46–51]

Rapidly proliferating cells express genes and enzymes such as *c-myc* and LDH, that are believed to facilitate efficient division.[52] Increased *c-myc* expression upregulates LDH in Rat1 fibroblasts[23,24] and in islets removed from pancreatectomized rats.[49–51] Because LDH overexpression alters the relative rates of anaerobic and oxidative glucose metabolism in β cells and islets, and because such alterations are believed to interfere with GSIS,[41,42] it is conceivable that actively proliferating β cells with elevated levels of *c-myc* and LDH may have impaired function.

The inherent susceptibility of β cells and islets to oxidative damage (presumably due to low expression of antioxidant enzyme genes) prompted the use of genetic modifications to improve β cell and islet defense mechanisms.[53,54] Examples include overexpression of antiapoptotic genes such as *Bcl-2* and *Bcl-$X_L$* that protect cells from a variety of proapoptotic stimuli, including hypoxia and cytokines.[25–28] Because these antiapoptotic genes are expressed primarily on the mitochondrial matrix, their overexpression may alter the relative rates of anaerobic and oxidative glucose metabolism[55] and impair GSIS.

Methods used to generate large numbers of β cells or islets must allow them to retain the biochemical features that render them glucose-responsive. Tools that will enable monitoring and characterization of changes in cellular bioenergetics and metabolism will be valuable in β cell and islet engineering and transplantation.

The ability of $^{31}$P, $^{13}$C, and $^1$H NMR spectroscopy to monitor cellular bioenergetics, metabolism, and oxygenation status has been demonstrated with extracts and with perfusion bioreactors using a variety of cell types, and more recently β cells.[2,3,6,8–10,56–59] $^{13}$C NMR is particularly suited for metabolic studies as it enables the identification and quantification of multiple metabolites from a single spectrum, as well as, the estimation of fluxes through different enzymatic pathways.[4,7,58–60] The levels, rates of incorporation, and the position of the $^{13}$C label in the carbon backbone of a metabolite can be used to determine absolute and relative fluxes through various enzymatic pathways.[4,7,58–60] FIGURE 2 depicts a highly simplified scheme of how $^{13}$C NMR can be used to identify and quantify changes in the relative rates of anaerobic and oxidative glucose metabolism that we use for the interpretation of results presented in this paper.

We used three cell lines, parental Rat1 fibroblast cells (R), R cells transfected with the *c-myc* oncogene (RM), and RM cells overexpressing the antiapoptotic gene *Bcl-2* (RMB) as models in exploring effects of genetic alteration on glucose metabolism. We demonstrate that $^{31}$P and $^{13}$C NMR reveal a wide array of cellular

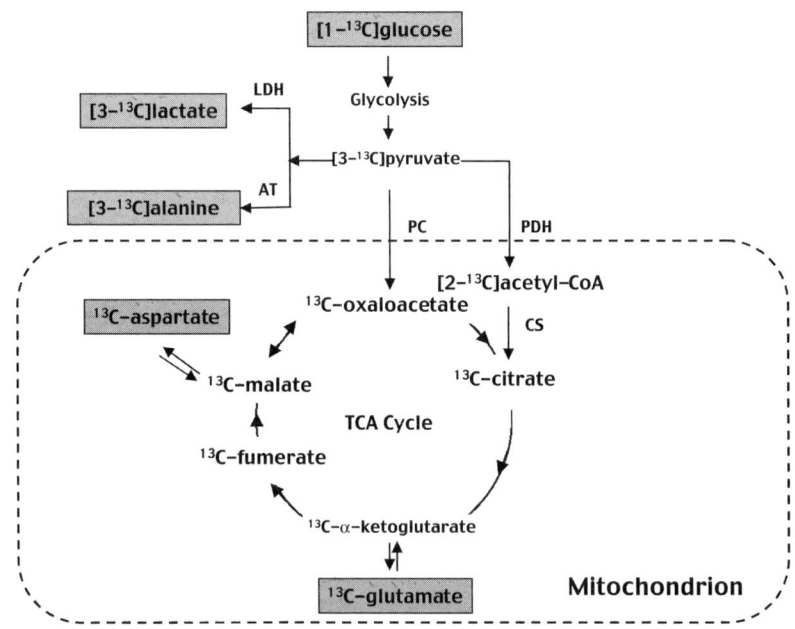

**FIGURE 2.** A simplified view of how NMR spectroscopy can be used to follow the fate of the $^{13}C$ label that originates in [1-$^{13}C$]glucose and undergoes reaction through anærobic and oxidative metabolism. The first digit in the bracket indicates the position of the label on the carbon backbone. Metabolites in *rectangles* ([3-$^{13}C$]lactate, [3-$^{13}C$]alanine, [$^{13}C$]aspartate, and [$^{13}C$]glutamate) are those that are found at the highest intracellular concentrations and thus give dominant signals in the $^{13}C$ NMR spectrum. Resonances detected include those of [2-$^{13}C$]glutamate, [3-$^{13}C$]glutamate, [4-$^{13}C$]glutamate, [2-$^{13}C$]aspartate, and [3-$^{13}C$]aspartate (see FIGURE 6), collectively denoted for simplicity in this figure as [$^{13}C$]glutamate and [$^{13}C$]aspartate, respectively. Catabolism of [1-$^{13}C$]glucose through glycolysis produces [3-$^{13}C$]pyruvate. [3-$^{13}C$]pyruvate can be converted to [3-$^{13}C$]lactate in a reaction catalyzed by lactate dehydrogenase (LDH) or to [3-$^{13}C$]alanine in a reaction catalyzed by alanine aminotransferase (AT). Under non-oxygen limiting conditions, oxidative metabolism dominates, and pyruvate enters the tricarboxylic acid (TCA) cycle through the action of the enzymes pyruvate dehydrogenase (PDH) and pyruvate carboxylase (PC). The [$^{13}C$]-α-ketogluterate and [$^{13}C$]-malate generated by the TCA cycle are in equilibrium with the [$^{13}C$]-glutamate and [$^{13}C$]-aspatrate pool, respectively. Consequently, TCA cycle activity can be monitored by NMR spectroscopy based on the rate of $^{13}C$ label incorporation into glutamate and aspartate. Under oxygen limiting conditions or when mitochondrial inhibitors are used, the incorporation of $^{13}C$ label into TCA cycle intermediates declines, resulting in an observed decline in their resonance intensity in the $^{13}C$ NMR spectrum. In this situation, anaerobic metabolism dominates, pyruvate is converted into lactate, and there is a substantial accumulation of the $^{13}C$ label in this metabolite. Thus changes in the ratios of [$^{13}C$]-glutamate/[$^{13}C$]-lactate, and [$^{13}C$]-aspartate/[$^{13}C$]-lactate are good indicators of changes in the relative rates of oxidative and anaerobic glucose metabolism.

alterations including changes in the relative rates of anaerobic and oxidative glucose metabolism introduced by *c-myc* expression as well as *Bcl-2* overexpression.

### Quality Assessment

Large scale islet or β cell transplantation requires efficient and effective quality assessment methods. Insufficient islet volume or excessive islet damage may lead to a failure of the transplant. There is a need for reliable methods for evaluation of viable islet volume and identification of the presence of damaged tissue so as to ensure that an islet graft does not fail because of inadequate viable islet volume or poor islet quality.

Treatment of a single diabetic patient by islet transplantation requires 300,000–1,000,000 islet equivalents (IEQ). Delivery of this therapy requires handling large numbers of islets. Oxygenation of large numbers of islets in culture is thought to be a challenge. Poor oxygenation severely impairs GSIS and results in loss of viability both *in vitro* as well as *in vivo* following transplantation.[14,61–64] Islets are highly vascularized *in vivo* where they are exposed to arterial $pO_2$ levels. When removed from the pancreas, their intraislet capillary space collapses, and oxygen supply is dependent on diffusion from the surrounding medium. Central necrosis, resulting from oxygen limitations has been repeatedly observed in cultured islets.

In addition, transportation methods currently used (e.g., islets packed in the bottom of a centrifuge tube filled with liquid medium and shipped overnight at room temperature) may expose islets to severe oxygen limitations as well as other stresses (e.g., additional nutrient limitations, toxic metabolite accumulation, pH changes). Such exposures may cause reversible as well as irreversible damage. Strategies that minimize damage during culture, storage, and transportation are needed. Furthermore, methods that can provide markers with which to identify adverse conditions are of importance.

We examined markers of damage with a variety of methods. We conducted studies with conventional $^{13}C$ NMR measurements with extracts of RINm5F cells and porcine islets to identify markers of hypoxia. We extended these studies with intact βTC3 cells using high-resolution magic angle spinning proton NMR (HRMAS $^1H$ NMR) spectroscopy and identified similar markers of hypoxia as well as peaks related to mobile lipids (not detectable in aqueous phase extracts) that have been associated with apoptosis.[2,3] We also conducted studies with perfused RINm5F and βTC3 cells exposed to stresses expected to result in reversible as well as irreversible damage. Exposure to Procide (a commercially available fungicide) resulted in the permanent loss of all $^{31}P$ NMR detectable signals originating from RINm5F cells. On the other hand, a one-hour exposure of βTC3 cells to ischemia resulted in a reversible decline in the ATP/Pi ratio, which recovered to pre-exposure levels after removal of the stress.

## MATERIALS AND METHODS

### Cell Lines, Islets, and Culture Conditions

RINm5F cells were obtained from ATCC (CRL 11605), and confluent monolayer cells of passages between 20–35 were used. Mouse insulinoma βTC3 cells were obtained from Dr. Shimon Efrat (Albert Einstein College of Medicine, Bronx, NY). Cells of passages between 27–42 were used. Parental Rat1 fibroblast cells, Rat1 cells transfected with the *c-myc* oncogene, as well as Rat1-*myc* cells overexpressing *Bcl-2* were obtained from Dr. Carlo Nalin (Novartis Pharma, Summit, NJ). Cells of passage number 10–30 were used. Culture medium was replaced daily, and cell cultures were split 1:50 every four days and replated. Cell lines were cultivated at 37°C in a humidified incubator with 95% air/ 5% $CO_2$ and were passaged in either T-150 $cm^2$ or T-175$cm^2$ flasks. Cells were fed (unless indicated otherwise) every other day with fresh Dulbecco's modified eagle's medium (DMEM), supplemented with 16 mM glucose, 10% (v/v) fetal bovine serum, and 1% (v/v) penicillin streptomycin (Sigma, P-0781). Adult porcine islets were obtained from the Islet Core Facility at the Joslin Diabetes Center one day after isolation and overnight culture at room temperature.

### Glucose, Lactate, and Total Protein Measurements

Glucose and lactate concentrations were measured in media aliquots using an Ektachem DT60II Analyzer. Total protein was measured with a commercially available kit using albumin standards (Pierce).

### Extraction Procedure and Sample Preparation

Following aspiration of the culture media, the cells were gently washed with Ringer's balanced saline solution (3 × 35 ml), and 5 ml of 4% (w/v) perchloric acid (PCA) was placed over the monolayer surface. The cells were then flash frozen with liquid nitrogen. The T-flasks were opened with a TC Flask Thermocutter, the cells were collected in a 50 ml centrifuge tube (Falcon), and 4 ml of 4% PCA was used to collect any residual material in the flask. This mixture was allowed to sit for one hour over ice, after which time the material was homogenized with a tissue-tearing homogenizer (Biospec Products Inc. Model No. 985-370). The cell mixture was centrifuged (1,840$g$ for 12 min), the supernatant was removed, and the cell debris was saved for protein analysis. The supernatant was neutralized to pH 6.3–6.8 using 2 M $K_2CO_3$. The mixture was again centrifuged (1840 $g$ for 12 min), and the supernatant was removed and lyophilized overnight. Lyophilized samples were dissolved in 1 ml of $D_2O$ containing 1.5 mg/ml 3-(trimethylsilyl)propionic-2,2,3,3-d4 acid, sodium salt (TMSPA), added as a chemical shift and quantification standard for both $^{13}C$ and $^1H$ NMR experiments, and 0.05mg/ml trisodium trimetaphosphate (TTP), added as a chemical shift and quantification standard for $^{31}P$ NMR experiments. 10 μl of 0.1M ethylenediamine tetraacetic acid in $D_2O$ (EDTA, pD (deuterium) 7.4) was added to chelate any residual paramagnetic species, which may adversely affect the NMR spectrum. The samples were adjusted to a pD of 7.2–7.4 using deuterochloric acid (DCl) and sodium deuteroxide (NaOD). A similar procedure was used for islet extracts with the omission of surface detachment by trypsinization, since islets were not attached to any surface.

### NMR Spectroscopy of Extracts

$^{31}$P and proton decoupled $^{13}$C NMR spectra were acquired at 161.98 MHz and 100.61 MHz, respectively on a Bruker DMX-400 wide-bore spectrometer (400 MHz $^1$H). Proton decoupled $^{13}$C NMR spectra were acquired with 25,000 transients, a spectral width of 21,186.44 Hz, 64 K complex data points, and a relaxation delay of 3.0 sec. For $^{31}$P NMR spectra, 15,000 transients were collected with 16 K complex points, a spectral width of 5,841.12 Hz, and relaxation delay of 3.0 sec. All spectra were recorded at 300 K. Spectra were processed using the UXNMR software package (Bruker). Prior to Fourier transformation an exponential line-broadening multiplication was applied to each data set. The line broadening factors applied were 0.8 Hz for $^{13}$C spectra, and 1.0 Hz for $^{31}$P spectra. Because all data for each nucleus were collected and processed under identical conditions, corrections for relaxation effects were not employed. The $^{13}$C chemical shifts were referenced relative to the TMSPA signal, which was set to −2.46 ppm. $^{31}$P chemical shifts were referenced relative to the phosphocreatine resonance at 0.00 ppm.

### NMR Studies with Perfused Cells

For the studies involving perfused cells, $^{31}$P spectra were acquired in 64 acquisition blocks in a perfusion bioreactor modified to fit a vertical wide-bore DMX-400 spectrometer and a perfusion system.[9,57] This process was repeated until sufficient signal to noise was achieved. $^{31}$P were recorded with 8,192 complex points and a relaxation delay of 3 sec. The spectral widths for $^{31}$P and $^{13}$C spectra were 5,841.12 Hz and 22,123.89 Hz, respectively. $^{31}$P chemical shifts were referenced to the phosphocreatine resonance at 0.00 ppm.

### HRMAS $^1$H NMR Spectroscopy

Cell samples were washed twice in PBS, frozen, and stored in liquid nitrogen until analyzed. Frozen cell samples were placed in the HRMAS sample rotor, weighed, and transferred into the NMR probe precooled at 3°C. Measurements were performed at 3°C on an MSL400 NMR spectrometer (proton frequency at 400.13 MHz) with a BDMAS probe (Bruker Instruments, Inc. Billerica, MA) custom modified for HRMAS analysis. Data were collected and analyzed as described elsewhere.[65,66]

## RESULTS AND DISCUSSION

### Effect of Genetic Alterations on Glucose Metabolism

We used $^{13}$C and $^{31}$P NMR spectroscopy to examine the effect of genetic alterations on glucose metabolism in three cell lines: Parental Rat1 (R) cells, Rat1 cells transfected with the *c-myc* oncogene (RM), and RM cells overexpressing the antiapoptotic gene *Bcl-2* (RMB). $^{13}$C NMR spectra from extracts of the three cell lines incubated under identical conditions revealed many changes in the incorporation

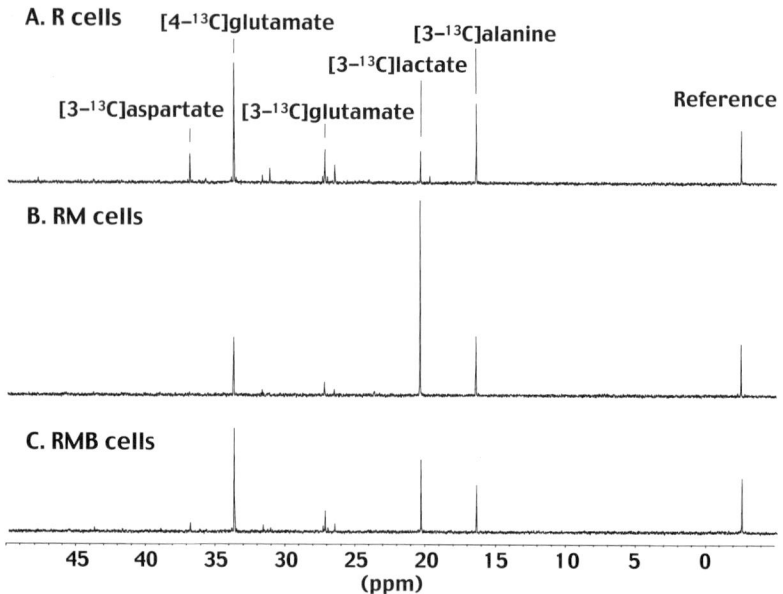

**FIGURE 3.** Typical $^{13}$C nmr spectra of extracts of monolayers of cell lines. Cells were incubated in DMEM with 20 mM [1-$^{13}$C]glucose for four hours prior to extraction. (**A**) Parental Rat1 Cells (R); (**B**) Rat1 cells transfected with the *c-myc* oncogene (RM); and (**C**) Rat1-*myc* cells overexpressing the antiapoptotic gene *Bcl-2* (RMB). Peak intensities reflect intracellular concentrations of the depicted metabolites.

of $^{13}$C label into markers of oxidative and anærobic glucose metabolism (see FIGURE 3). [4-$^{13}$C]glutamate and [3-$^{13}$C]aspartate were lower and [3-$^{13}$C]lactate was higher in RM when compared to R cells. The decrease in [4-$^{13}$C]glutamate and [3-$^{13}$C]aspartate in *c-myc*–transfected cells reflects a reduction in the rate of

**TABLE 1.** Effects of *c-myc* expression and *Bcl-2* overexpression on glucose metabolism of Rat1 cells

|  | R | RM | RMB |
| --- | --- | --- | --- |
| GCR | 456 ± 42 | 1161 ± 165 | 524 ± 14 |
| LPR | 452 ± 17 | 1681 ± 99 | 667 ± 19 |
| $Y_{L/G}$ | 1.0 ± 0.1 | 1.5 ± 0.1 | 1.3 ± 0.1 |

NOTE: Abbreviations for cell lines are the same as in caption to FIGURE 3. Glucose consumption rate (GCR) and lactate production rate (LPR) are expressed in nmol/hr·mg protein. The lactate yield on glucose, $Y_{L/G}$, defined as moles of lactate produced per mole of glucose consumed, is also equal to the ratio LPR/GCR. GCR and LPR were measured from the differences of the concentrations of glucose and lactate at the beginning and at the end of a four-hour time interval and the measured total protein per flask. Values represent mean ± SD; $n = 4$ for all measurements. All values for RM and RMB were significantly different from comparable values for R ($p < 0.05$).

oxidative glucose metabolism, and the increase in [3-$^{13}$C]lactate reflects an increase in the rate of anaerobic glucose metabolism. These observations are consistent with the higher glucose consumption rate (GCR), lactate production rate (LPR), and lactate yield in glucose ($Y_{L/G}$), as summarized in TABLE 1, as well as the lower ratios of [4-$^{13}$C]glutamate/[3-$^{13}$C]lactate, and [3-$^{13}$C]aspartate/[3-$^{13}$C]lactate measured in RM when compared to R cells (see FIGURE 4). RMB cells contained substantially higher levels of [4-$^{13}$C]glutamate and [3-$^{13}$C]aspartate and substantially lower levels of lactate than RM cells, thereby suggesting that overexpression of *Bcl-2* in RM cells increased the rate of oxidative and decreased the rate of anaerobic glucose metabolism. These observations are consistent with the lower GCR, LPR and $Y_{L/G}$ (TABLE 1), and with the higher ratios of [4-$^{13}$C]glutamate/[3-$^{13}$C]lactate, and [3-$^{13}$C]aspartate/[3-$^{13}$C]lactate measured in RMB when compared to RM cells (FIG. 4).

Expression of *c-myc* in Rat1 cells also introduced significant changes in the $^{31}$P NMR spectra (see FIGURE 5). The intracellular concentrations of phosphoethanolamine (PE) and phosphocreatine (PCr) were substantially reduced, whereas *c-myc* transfection had little effect on the levels of phosphocholine (PC) and nucleotide triphosphates (NTP), primarily ATP. As a consequence, the peak intensity ratios

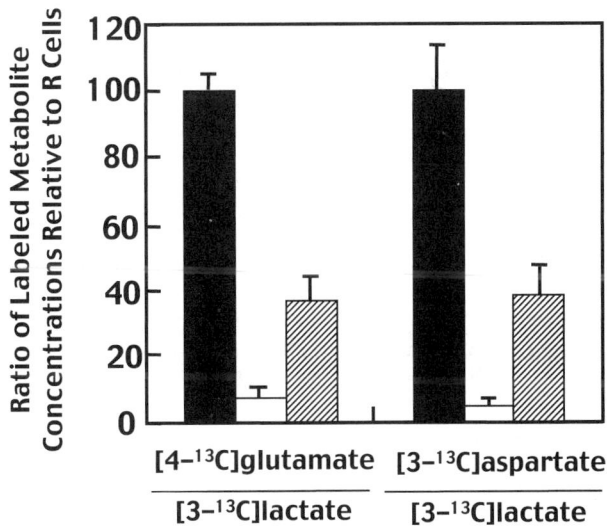

**FIGURE 4.** Ratios of $^{13}$C labeled metabolite concentrations for R, RM, and RMB cells that demonstrate *c-myc*- and *Bcl-2*-induced changes in relative ratios of oxidative and anærobic glucose metabolism in Rat1 cells. The graph summarizes the results obtained from quadruplicate flasks for each cell line. Concentrations were taken to be proportional to peak intensities of the respective metabolites in the $^{13}$C NMR spectrum, as indicated in FIGURE 3. *Error bars* represent standard deviations. The ratios of [4-$^{13}$C]glutamate to [3-$^{13}$C]lactate and [3-$^{13}$C]aspartate to [3-$^{13}$C]lactate are indicators of relative rates of oxidative and anaerobic metabolism, and they are substantially different between the three cell lines examined. ■, R; □, RM; ▨, RMB.

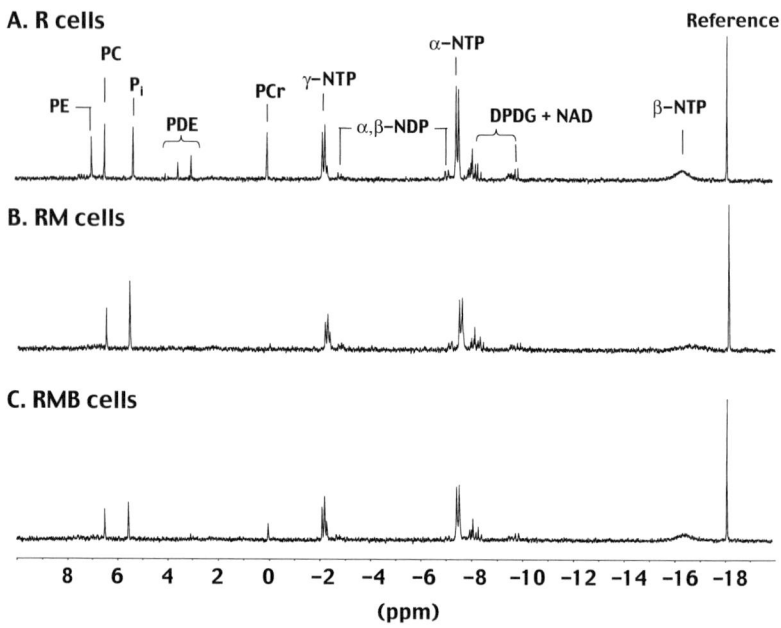

**FIGURE 5.** Typical $^{31}P$ nmr spectra of extracts of monolayers of (**A**) parental Rat1 cells (R); (**B**) Rat1 cells transfected with the *c-myc* oncogene (RM); and (**C**) Rat1-*myc* cells overexpressing the antiapoptotic gene *Bcl-2* (RMB). All cell lines were incubated as indicated in FIGURE 3. Large differences are observed in the resonances of phosphocreatine (PCr), phosphoethamolomine (PE), and phosphodiesters (PDE).

PC/PE and NTP/PCr were substantially higher in RM when compared to R cells. The phosphodiesters (PDE) glycerolphosphocholine (GPC) and glycerolphoethanolamine (GPE) were undetectable in RM cells (FIG. 5). Intracellular levels of PCr were higher in RMB when compared to RM cells but were still much lower than those in R cells. The levels of all other intracellular metabolites measured with $^{31}P$ NMR were not significantly different between RM and RMB cells.

These results demonstrate a strong effect of *c-myc* transfection on glucose metabolism in Rat1 cells. The increased $Y_{L/G}$ results from preferential conversion of pyruvate to lactate in RM cells and is consistent with *c-myc*–induced upregulation of LDH.[23,24] The observed increase of GCR in RM cells is expected in fast growing tumor cells. High rates of anærobic glucose metabolism may be necessary to support the energy requirements of rapidly proliferating tumor cells and to minimize oxidative stress[52] during phases of the cell cycle when maximal biosynthesis and cell division occur, and it may explain the high LPR exhibited by rapidly proliferating tumor cells. We suggest that actively proliferating β-cells or islets with elevated levels of *c-myc* and LDH may have alterations in the relative rates of anærobic and oxidative glucose metabolism and, therefore, impaired GSIS. Conversely, maturation and differentiation of β cells and lower rates of proliferation might lead to lower levels of *c-myc* and LDH and thus to normal glucose metabolism and GSIS.

Overexpression of *Bcl-2* in RM cells reduced the rate of anaerobic and increased that of oxidative glucose metabolism, introducing changes opposing those of *c-myc*. This shift may result from the physical presence of large amounts of *Bcl-2* on the mitochondria, which may affect their behavior and function. Alternatively, *Bcl-2* overexpression may alter expression and/or activity of cytosolic enzymes such as LDH. Some reports demonstrated that *Bcl-2* overexpression in β cells did not affect GSIS and protected from certain proapoptotic stimuli, including hypoxia.[25–26] Detailed information on effects of *Bcl-2* on β cell metabolism was not reported in these studies. In another study, overexpression of *Bcl-$X_L$* (an antiapoptotic gene from the same family) in islets caused an impairment of GSIS that resulted from a *Bcl-$X_L$* induced decline in β cell mitochondrial (oxidative) metabolism.[55] These differences in behavior may be the result of differences in the nature and expression levels of these genes or to differences in the nature of the cells transfected.

*C-myc* expression is implicated in the regulation of cell cycle and growth.[20–24] Elevated levels of phosphomonoesters (PC, PE, and the PC/PE ratio) and phosphodiesters (GPC, GPE) have been associated with increased cell growth and degradation in human tumors, malignant animal tumor models, and cell lines.[67–70] In a recent report, PE gradually increased as the stationary growth phase was approached, whereas PC decreased during log growth, the net effect being a substantially lower PC/PE ratio in stationary cultures compared to actively proliferating ones.[69] Our data demonstrate that *c-myc* expression substantially increases the ratio of PC/PE by decreasing the levels of intracellular PE. We also find that *c-myc* transfection reduces PCr to very low, and GPE and GPC to undetectable levels, though the precise role of these changes is not clear.

Our results demonstrate that NMR spectroscopy can be a potent tool for studying the effect of genetic alterations on cellular metabolism, particularly the absolute and relative rates of anærobic and oxidative glucose metabolism. Investigation of the metabolism of progenitor cells during culture and at various stages of treatment with agents that are believed to promote differentiation and maturation may provide insight on the underlying mechanisms as well as metabolite markers associated with this process. Furthermore, drastic alterations in cellular proliferation may result in changes in NMR-detectable markers such as phosphomonoesters and phosphodiesters that may be useful tools in islet and β cell engineering. NMR-detectable markers, which would help identify mature, well differentiated β cells with low proliferation rate may also be important for quality assessment prior to and possibly after islet transplantation.

## *β Cell and Islet Quality Assessment: Effects of Culture Conditions, Storage, and Transportation*

The large-scale application of islet transplantation to the treatment of diabetes will require the handling of hundreds of thousands of islets per patient. Central necrosis, believed to be the result of oxygen limitations, has been repeatedly observed in cultured islets.[14,15,61] In addition, transportation modes currently used may expose islets to severe oxygen limitations as well as other stresses. Such exposures during transportation may result in both reversible as well as irreversible damage. The results presented in the sections that follow are first steps in developing methods to assess such damage.

### Effects of Anoxia on RINm5F Cells and Porcine Islets Assessed with NMR-Detectable Markers

In order to search for NMR-detectable markers, we conducted preliminary experiments with cultured insulin-secreting RINm5F cells exposed to humidified gas phases of either 95%air/5%$CO_2$ (normoxia), or 95%$N_2$/5%$CO_2$ (anoxia). Intracellular levels of water-soluble metabolites in PCA-extracted cells were measured at the end of the 24-h incubation. $^{13}$C NMR (see FIGURE 6) revealed that anoxia inhibited $^{13}$C label incorporation into glutamate and aspartate (markers of oxidative glucose metabolism) with a concurrent increase in label incorporation into lactate (marker of anaerobic glucose metabolism). Anoxia resulted in a 12-fold increase in [3-$^{13}$C]lactate/[3-$^{13}$C]alanine, a 10-fold increase in [3-$^{13}$C]lactate]/[3-$^{13}$C]aspartate, and an 18-fold increase [3-$^{13}$C]lactate/[4-$^{13}$C] glutamate. In addition, $^{31}$P NMR of the same samples revealed that anoxia caused a 63% reduction in the intracellular levels of phosphocholine (PC) and a 37% reduction in the ATP/ADP ratio (see FIGURE 7). It is suspected that maintenance of appreciable ATP levels under anoxia is the result of an increase in the rate of anærobic glucose metabolism by RINm5F cells. This is consistent with the 2.2-fold increase in GCR and 3.4-fold increase in LPR measured

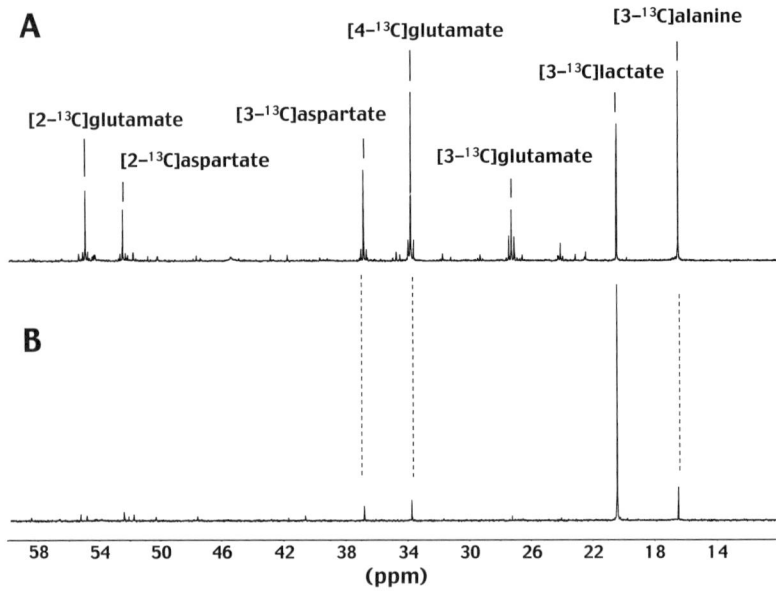

**FIGURE 6.** Typical $^{13}$C nmr spectra of extracts of RINm5F cells incubated in DMEM containing 20 mM [1-$^{13}$C]glucose for 24 h under either humidified atmosphere of (**A**) 95%Air/5%$CO_2$ (normoxia), or (**B**) 95%$N_2$/5% $CO_2$ (anoxia). Anoxia caused significant inhibition of incorporation of $^{13}$C lablel (originating from glucose) into glutamate and aspartate (markers of oxidative glucose metabolism) with a concurrent increase in the lactate signal (marker of anærobic glucose metabolism).

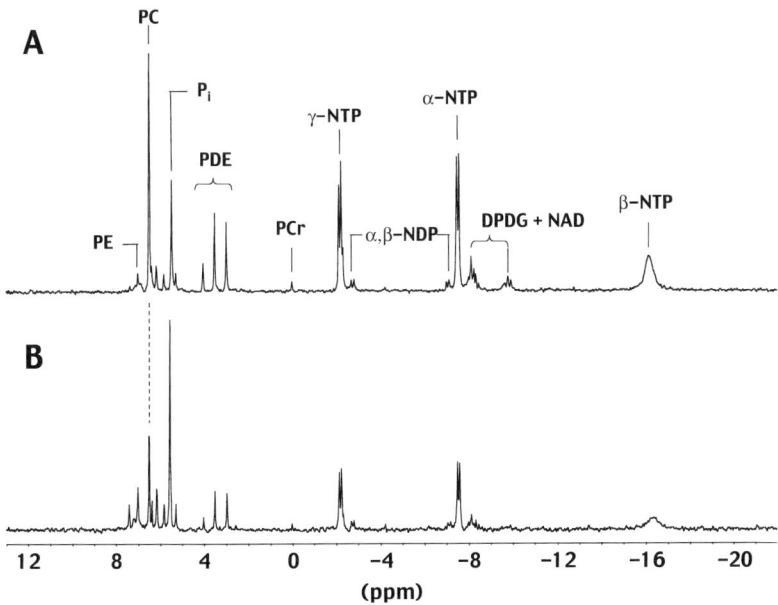

**FIGURE 7:** $^{31}$P NMR spectra of extracts of RINm5F cells incubated as indicated in FIGURE 6. Detected resonances include those of phosphocholine (PC), phosphoethanolamine (PE), phosphocreatine (PCr), inorganic phosphate (Pi), adenosine triphosphate (ATP), and adenosine diphosphate (ADP). Anoxia resulted in a decline in the resonance intensity of PC, an increase in Pi, and a decline in the ratio ATP/ADP. The maintenance of significant ATP levels under complete anoxia is attributed to the high levels of LDH present in these cells, which allows the continuation of anærobic glycolysis for energy generation.

in these cells under anoxic conditions and by the increase in $Y_{L/G}$ from 1.4 under normoxia to 2.0 under anoxia.

To investigate potential damaging effects of culture and transportation, we exposed porcine islets to typical culture and shipment conditions and obtained $^{13}$C NMR spectra of their extracts. Islets were cultured at the bottom of petri dishes at 37 or 24°C at a density of 333 IEQ/cm$^2$ or pelletized in the bottom of a tube filled with medium and stored at 24°C. The islets were incubated in glucose-free DMEM supplemented with 10mM [1-$^{13}$C]glucose and equilibrated with a 95% air, 5% CO$_2$.

As measured by relative peak heights in the $^{13}$C NMR spectra, concentrations of $^{13}$C labeled lactate were higher than those of TCA cycle intermediates (which were only detected at 37°C). The ratios of [3-$^{13}$C]lactate to [1-$^{13}$C]glucose were increased by 35% and 976% in islets cultured in the dish at 37°C and in the bottom of the tube at 24°C, respectively, when compared to those cultured at 24°C in the dish. The ratios of [3-$^{13}$C]lactate to [3-$^{13}$C]alanine were increased by 24% and 467% in islets cultured in the dish at 37°C and in the bottom of the tube at 24°C, respectively, when compared to those cultured at 24°C. The data suggest the islets were exposed to varying degrees of hypoxia that depended on the culture condition, most severely when cultured pelletized in the bottom of the tube at room temperature, and to a lesser extent when cultured in the petri dish at 37°C.

It is believed by some that any lactate generated from islets is contributed by non-β-cells within them or by contaminating exocrine tissue. Irrespective of the source of lactate, its presence at higher levels is indicative of hypoxia, a condition that all cells within the population are exposed to whether they secrete lactate or not. Furthermore, prolonged exposure of β cells within islets to hypoxia may upregulate LDH and thus may enable them to utilize glucose anærobically. Such changes in the β cell enzymatic machinery may be detrimental to islet function. Therefore lactate, as well its ratio to alanine, appear to be good markers of islet quality and oxygenation status.

## HRMAS $^1H$ NMR of βTC3 cells

HRMAS $^1H$ NMR offers advantages relative to conventional NMR techniques because lengthy extraction procedures are not needed and measurements require relatively low cell volumes. In addition, intracellular lipids, which are not water soluble and not detected in PCA extracts, can be observed with HRMAS $^1H$ NMR. Changes in such NMR observable cellular lipids have been associated with apoptosis,[2,3] and they can potentially serve as markers of cell damage both *in vitro* as well as *in vivo*.

The damaging and stressful nature of the transportation conditions that islets may experience in the bottom of 50 ml centrifuge tubes was further investigated with HRMAS $^1H$ NMR, employing insulin-secreting mouse insulinoma βTC3 cells as a model system. βTC3 cells are expected to be less sensitive to hypoxia than islets, since they express high levels of LDH and have the ability to generate energy via anærobic glycolysis.[8,10,64] Therefore, damage of these cells would be expected to be less than that of islets. Conditions were designed to induce varying degrees of damage and to simulate conditions that may be encountered during islet culture and transportation, including cells cultured overnight (1) as monolayers in T-flasks in a humidified incubator at 37°C (standard laboratory practice), (2) at the bottom of a 50-ml tube at room temperature (24°C) (common for transportation), (3) at the bottom of 50-ml tube at 37°C (more severe because of increased metabolism and oxygen supply limitations), and (4) at the bottom of a 50-ml tube at 5°C. In order to assess whether NMR detectable markers correlated with cell viability, samples of cells exposed to these conditions were collected and subjected to HRMAS $^1H$ NMR measurements and examination with trypan blue (TB) staining.

The HRMAS $^1H$ NMR spectra revealed differences in phosphocholine (PC), lactate (Lac), and alanine (Ala) peaks, and mobile lipid (ML) peaks representing $CH_2$ and $CH_3$ groups (see FIGURE 8). In the cells cultured as monolayers, Lac and the ratio Lac/Ala were at their lowest value, PC and the ratio PC/Lac were at their highest, and mobile lipids ($CH_2$) were barely detectable. Viability estimated by TB was highest in monolayer cells and lowest in pelletized cells incubated at 37°C.

As shown in TABLE 2, FIGURE 8, and by the trends in the ratios of the peak heights shown in FIGURE 9, the absolute levels and/or the ratios of Lac, Ala, PC, and the two ML peaks may be useful, sensitive markers of oxygenation status, as well as of reversible and/ or irreversible damage. The correlation between the intracellular levels of Lac as well as PC and oxygenation status is consistent with previously published $^{31}P$ and $^1H$ NMR studies on alginate-entrapped perfused βTC3 cells.[8,10,56]

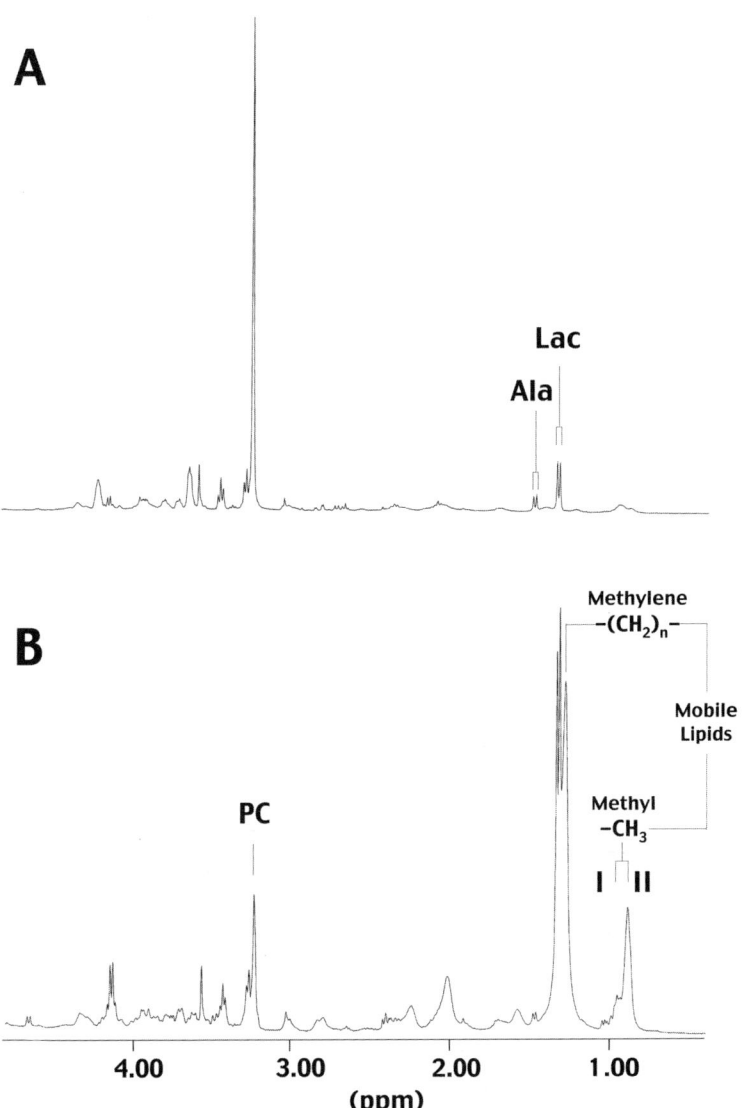

**FIGURE 8:** HRMAS $^1$H NMR spectra of βTC3 cells incubated overnight at 37°C in DMEM equilibrated with incubator air in flasks as monolayers (**A**) or palletized in the bottom of a 50-ml tube (**B**). Clearly resolved peaks include those originating from lactate (Lac), alanine (Ala), phosphocholine (PC), and the methylene (CH$_2$) and methyl (CH$_3$-I and CH$_3$-II) of mobile lipids (ML). Spectrum **B** shows substantial increases in Lac and the mobile lipids and a decline in PC. The changes in the PC/Ala, PC/Lac, and Lac/Ala ratios are consistent with exposure to hypoxic conditions, and the increase in the ratio CH$_2$/CH$_3$-I of mobile lipids is consistent with irreversible damage accompanying apoptosis.[2,3]

TABLE 2. HRMAS $^1$H NMR of βTC3 cells cultured for 24 hours

| | | | Ratio of spectrum peaks | |
|---|---|---|---|---|
| Cell condition | Temperature (°C) | Gas | Lac/PC | Lac/Ala |
| A. Monolayer | 37 | Air | 0.2 | 1.7 |
| B. Pelletized | 5 | Air | 0.6 | 7.2 |
| C. Pelletized | 24 | Air | 3.9 | 10.5 |
| D. Pelletized | 37 | Air | 5.7 | 15.5 |

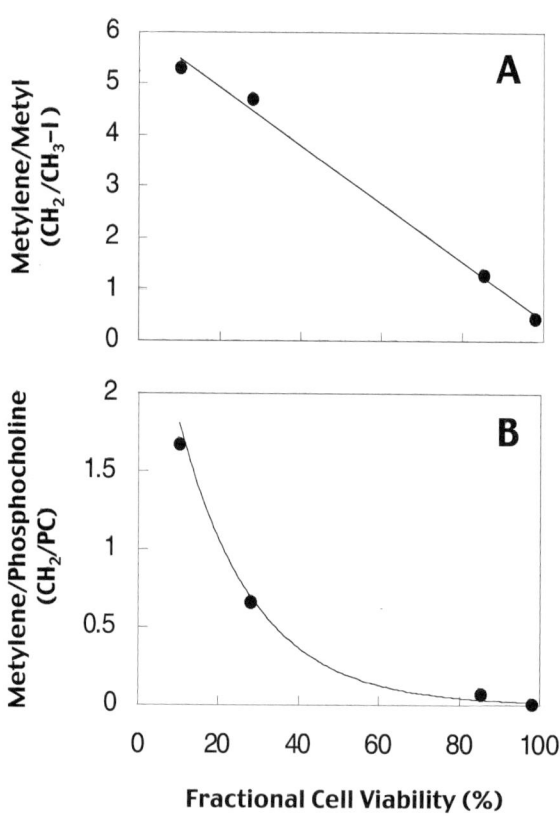

**FIGURE 9.** Relationship between HRMAS $^1$H NMR-detectable markers and fractional viability. βTC3 cells were cultured for 24 h under conditions inducing varying degrees of damage. Peak intensities of the relevant metabolites were obtained from spectra as depicted in FIGURE 8. Fractional viability was determined by trypan blue (TB) staining at the termination of each experiment for each condition. As indicated in panel **B**, for the conditions examined, the ratio of the methylene ($CH_2$) to the methyl ($CH_3$-I) of mobile lipids correlates especially well with fractional viability (measured with TB) in βTC3 cells.

The correlation between oxygenation status and the ratio Lac/Ala is also consistent with data from PCA extracts of RINm5F cells exposed to anoxia and the $^{13}$C NMR spectra of porcine islets. The observation of the ML (CH$_2$) resonance with HRMAS $^1$H NMR is particularly important because its appearance in the spectra is thought to reflect irreversible damage accompanying apoptosis.[2,3]

### Non-invasive NMR Measurements of Intact Perfused Cells

Information obtained using NMR coupled with cell perfusion allows non-invasive monitoring under well defined conditions for investigation of the time course and reversibility of the effects of exposures to stimuli and adverse conditions (such as hypoxia or ischemia) from the same sample, which serves as its own control.[8–10,56,57] An example is non-invasive, non-destructive assessment of viable

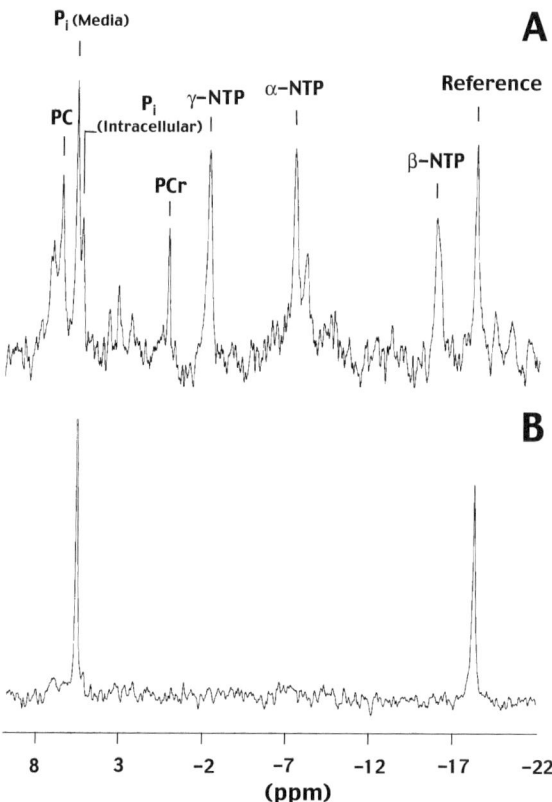

**FIGURE 10.** Effects of exposure to Procide (a commercially available fungicide) on $^{31}$P NMR spectra of RINm5F cells in a perfusion bioreactor: (**A**) spectrum prior to exposure to Procide; (**B**) spectrum two hours after a 30-min exposure to Procide. Purging the perfusion system of Procide for several hours did not result in recovery of ATP or other $^{31}$P containing metabolites, thereby demonstrating irreversible damage.

tissue volume of a fraction or an entire islet preparation at various steps during handling (e.g., immediately prior to after shipment and immediately prior to transplantation). *In vitro* monitoring of quality has been studied with βTC3 cells and can be easily extended to investigations with large numbers of islets.[8–10,56,57] Information on viable tissue volume can be obtained by simultaneous measurements of the cellular bioenergetic status as well as ATP generation rates utilizing $^{31}$P NMR spectroscopy because dead cells do not contain detectable levels of ATP (see FIGURE 10). For well-oxygenated cells at 37°C, intracellular pH, absolute levels of ATP, the ratio ATP/Pi, and ATP generation rates, which can be simultaneously measured with $^{31}$P NMR, provide reliable estimates of viable tissue volume. Combination with $^{1}$H

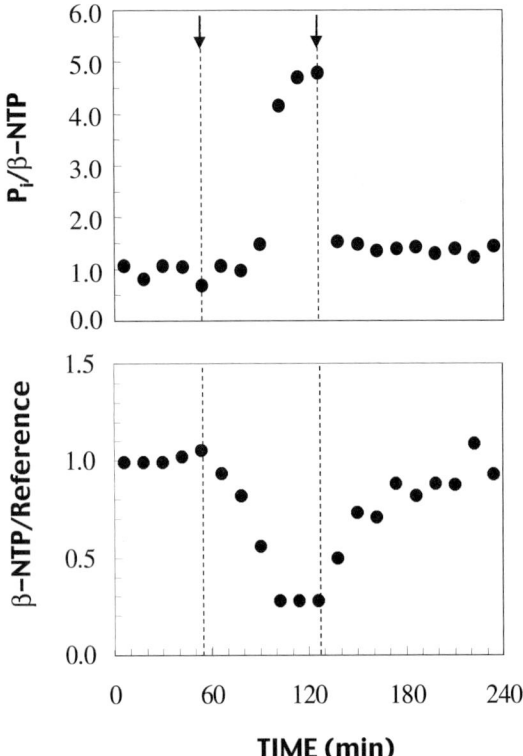

**FIGURE 11.** Effects of ischemia on $^{31}$P NMR spectra of βTC3 cells. Experiments were conducted in a perfusion system similar to that described in detail elsewhere,[9] and adapted for a vertical bore magnet. Ischemia was established by stopping the flow in the perfusion loop (*first arrow*) for one hour, and recovery was simulated by reinitiating the flow (*second arrow*). The transient decay of ATP and the Pi/ATP ratio, and their complete recovery after initiation of flow, indicates that exposure to the stressful conditions inflicted during this one-hour period is not sufficient to induce irreversible damage. This may not be true for islets, which may not be as capable as βTC3 cells in generating energy anærobically because of low levels of LDH in islets

NMR spectroscopy would provide additional information based on $^1$H NMR- detectable markers of oxygenation status as well as the presence or absence of damaged tissue.[2,3,8,9] With the large numbers of islets and β cells required for human transplantation, measurements of ATP as well as ATP generation rate can be conducted within minutes, conceivably within a bioreactor specifically designed for optimal culture, storage, and transportation and NMR compatibility so that repeated measurements can be conducted without breaking sterility.

NMR in conjunction with cell perfusion may be useful for monitoring growth and growth suppression, cell differentiation and maturation, and reversibility of damage imposed by exposures to stressful conditions and proapoptotic stimuli. As indicated in FIGURE 11, exposure of βTC3 cells to ischemia for one hour causes reversible changes but no apparent irreversible damage. Similar information for islets would be important because islets are often repeatedly packed in centrifuge tubes during handling as well as in syringes prior to transplantation. Identifying the time required to inflict irreversible damage is particularly important, as are questions related to differences between single and repeated exposures to such stresses, stress duration, and recovery time on the extent of irreversible damage and the time required before it is observable. These can be easily investigated by taking advantage of the non-invasive nature of NMR spectroscopy coupled with perfusion technology.

## CONCLUDING REMARKS

Recent improvements in treatment of type I diabetes with human islet transplantation highlight the need for alternative tissue sources for widespread application of this methodology, which will require innovations in islet and β cell engineering, expansion, or generation from precursor cells and methods for banking, culture, transportation, and quality assessment to ensure *in vivo* efficacy and safety. Our results suggest that exposure of islets to typical culture and shipment conditions for prolonged periods of time may result in damage because of severe oxygen and other nutrient limitations, as well as waste metabolite accumulation. Insufficient islet volume, impaired GSIS, or excessive islet damage may lead to a failure of an islet transplant. There is a need for reliable methods for the evaluation of viable and functional islet volume and for the identification of the presence of damaged tissue. Our results show that NMR spectroscopy is a powerful tool that can provide useful information on these issues and that its application in these areas in combination with currently existing or other new tools is promising.

## ACKNOWLEDGMENTS

This work was supported in part by a grant from the Juvenile Diabetes Foundation International Center for Islet Transplantation at Harvard Medical School.

## REFERENCES

1. BECKMANN, N., R.P. HOF & M. RUDIN. 2000. The role of magnetic resonance imaging and spectroscopy in transplantation: from animal models to man. NMR Biomed. **13:** 329–348.
2. BHAKOO, K.K. & J.D. BELL. 1997. The application of NMR spectroscopy to the study of apoptosis. Cell Mol. Biol. **43:** 621–629.
3. BLANKENBERG, F.G., P.D. KATSIKIS, R.W. STORRS, et al. 1997. Quantitative analysis of apoptotic cell death using proton nuclear magnetic resonance spectroscopy. Blood **89:** 3778–3786.
4. CLINE, G.W., I. MAGNUSSON, D.L. ROTHMAN, et al. 1997. Mechanism of impaired insulin-stimulated muscle glucose metabolism in subjects with insulin-dependent diabetes mellitus. J. Clin. Invest. **99:** 2219–2224.
5. EVANOCHKO, W.T., T.C. NG & J.D. GLICKSON. 1984. Application of in vivo NMR spectroscopy to cancer. Magn. Reson. Med. **1:** 508–534.
6. EVELHOCH, J.L., R.J. GILLIES, G.S. KARCZMAR, et al. 2000. Applications of magnetic resonance in model systems: cancer therapeutics. Neoplasia **2**(1–2): 152–165.
7. JEFFREY, F.M., A. RAJAGOPAL, C.R. MALLOY & A.D. SHERRY. 1991. $^{13}$C-NMR: a simple yet comprehensive method for analysis of intermediary metabolism. Trends Biochem. Sci. **16:** 5–10.
8. LONG, JR., R.C., K.K. PAPAS, I. CONSTANTINIDIS & A. SAMBANIS. 2000. In vitro monitoring of total choline levels in a bioartificial pancreas: $^1$H NMR studies of the effects of oxygen level. J. Mag. Resonance **146:** 49–57.
9. PAPAS, K.K., R.C. LONG, JR., I. CONSTANTINIDIS & A. SAMBANIS. 1997. Role of ATP and $P_i$ on the mechanism of insulin secretion in the mouse insulinoma βTC3 cell line. Biochem. J. **326:** 807–814.
10. PAPAS, K.K., R.C. LONG, JR., A. SAMBANIS & I. CONSTANTINIDIS. 1999. Towards the development of a bioartificial pancreas: II. Effects of oxygen on long-term entrapped βTC3 cell cultures. Biotech. Bioeng. **66:** 231–237.
11. SAUTER, A. & M. RUDIN. 1993. Determination of creatine kinase kinetic parameters in rat brain by NMR magnetization transfer. Correlation with brain function. J. Biol. Chem. **268:** 13166–13171.
12. MATHIEU, C. 2001. Current limitations of islet transplantation. Transplant. Proc. **33**(1–2): 1707–1708.
13. SHAPIRO, A.M., J.R. LAKEY, E.A. RYAN, et al. 2000. Islet transplantation in seven patients with type 1 diabetes mellitus using a glucocorticoid-free immunosuppressive regimen. N. Engl. J. Med. **343:** 230–238.
14. COLTON, C.K. 1995. Implantable biohybrid artificial organs. Cell Transplant. **4:** 415–436.
15. AVGOUSTINIATOS, E.S. & C.K. COLTON. 1997. Effect of external oxygen mass transfer resistances on viability of immunoisolated tissue. Ann. N.Y. Acad. Sci. **831:** 145–167.
16. RAMIYA, V.K., M. MARAIST, K.E. ARFORS, et al. 2000. Reversal of insulin-dependent diabetes using islets generated in vitro from pancreatic stem cells. Nat. Med. **6:** 278–282.
17. SACHS, D.H. & S. BONNER-WEIR. 2000. New islets from old. Nat. Med. **6:** 250–251.
18. BONNER-WEIR, S., M. TANEJA, G.C. WEIR, et al. 2000. In vitro cultivation of human islets from expanded ductal tissue. Proc. Natl. Acad. Sci. USA **97:** 7999–8004.
19. SORIA, B., E. ANDREU, G. BERNA, et al. 2000. Engineering pancreatic islets. Pflugers Arch. **440:** 1–18.
20. DANG, C.V. 1999. c-Myc target genes involved in cell growth, apoptosis, and metabolism. Mol. Cell. Biol. **19**(1): 1–11.
21. NASI, S., R. CIARAPICA, R. JUCKER, et al. 2001. Making decisions through Myc. FEBS Lett. **490**(3): 153–162.
22. PELENGARIS, S., B. RUDOLPH & T. LITTLEWOOD. 2000. Action of Myc in vivo proliferation and apoptosis. Curr. Opin. Genet. Dev. **10:** 100–105.
23. SHIM, H., C. DOLDE, C. BRIAN, et al. 1997. c-*Myc* transactivation of LDH-A: implications for tumor metabolism and growth. Proc. Natl. Acad. Sci. USA **94:** 6658–6663.

24. SHIM, H., Y.S. CHUN, B.C. LEWIS & C.V. DANG. 1998. A unique glucose-dependent apoptotic pathway induced by c-*Myc*. Proc. Natl. Acad. Sci. USA **95**: 1511–1516.
25. DUPRAZ, P., C. RINSCH, W.F. PRALONG, *et al.* 1999. Lentivirus-mediated Bcl-2 expression in betaTC-tet cells improves resistance to hypoxia and cytokine-induced apoptosis while preserving *in vitro* and *in vivo* control of insulin secretion. Gene Ther. **6**: 1160–1169.
26. IWAHASHI, H., T. HANAFUSA, Y. EGUCHI, *et al.* 1999. Cytokine-induced apoptotic cell death in a mouse pancreatic beta-cell line: inhibition by Bcl-2. Diabetologia **39**: 530–536.
27. JACOBSON, M.D. & M.C. RAFF. 1995. Programmed cell death and Bcl-2 protection in very low oxygen. Nature **374**: 814–816.
28. PAPAS, K.K., L. SUN, E.S. ROOS, *et al.* 1999. Change in lactate production in Myc-transfected cells precedes apoptosis and can be inhibited by Bcl-2 overexression. FEBS Lett. **446**: 338–342.
29. HELLERSTROM, C. 1967. Effects of carbohydrates on the oxygen consumption of isolated pancreatic islets of mice. Endocrinology **81**: 105–112.
30. HUTTON, J.C. & W.J. MALAISSE. 1980. Dynamics of $O_2$ consumption in rat pancreatic islets. Diabetologia **18**: 395–405.
31. SCHUIT, F., K. MOENS, H. HEIMBERG & D. PIPELEERS. 1999. Cellular origin of hexokinase in pancreatic islets. J. Biol. Chem. **274**: 32803–32809.
32. SCHUIT, F., A. DE VOS, S. FARFARI, *et al.* 1997. Metabolic fate of glucose in purified islet cells. Glucose-regulated anaplerosis in beta cells. J. Biol. Chem. **272**: 18572–18579.
33. JIJAKLI, H., J. RASSCHAERT, A.B. NADI, *et al.* 1996. Relevance of lactate dehydrogenase activity to the control of oxidative glycolysis in pancreatic islet β-cells. Arch. Biochem. Biophys. **327**: 260–264.
34. WOLLHEIM, C.B. 2000. Beta-cell mitochondria in the regulation of insulin secretion: a new culprit in type II diabetes. Diabetologia **43**: 265–277.
35. MATSCHINSKY, F.M. 1996. A lesson in metabolic regulation inspired by the glucokinase glucose sensor paradigm. Diabetes **45**: 223–241.
36. SCHUIT, F.C., P. HUYPENS, H. HEIMBERG & D.G. PIPELEERS. 2001. Glucose sensing in pancreatic β-cells: a model for the study of other glucose-regulated cells in gut, pancreas, and hypothalamus. Diabetes **50**: 1–11.
37. CIVELEK, V.N., J.T. DEENEY, K. KUBIK, *et al.* 1996. Temporal sequence of metabolic and ionic events in glucose-stimulated clonal pancreatic β-cells (HIT). Biochem. J. **315**(3): 1015–1019.
38. FREINKEL, N., N.J. LEWIS, R. JOHNSON, *et al.* 1984. Differential effects of age versus glycemic stimulation on the maturation of insulin stimulus-secretion coupling during culture of fetal rat islets. Diabetes **33**: 1028–1038.
39. PORTHA, B., M.H. GIROIX, P. SERRADAS, *et al.* 1988. Insulin production and glucose metabolism in isolated pancreatic islets of rats with NIDDM. Diabetes **37**: 1226–1233.
40. TANIGUCHI, S., K. TANIGAWA & I. MIWA. 2000. Immaturity of glucose-induced insulin secretion in fetal rat islets is due to low glucokinase activity. Horm. Metab. Res. **32**: 97–102.
41. AINSCOW, E.K., C. ZHAO & G.A. RUTTER. 2000. Acute overexpression of lactate dehydrogenase-A perturbs beta-cell mitochondrial metabolism and insulin secretion Diabetes **49**: 1149–1155.
42. ALCAZAR, O., M. TIEDGE & S. LENZEN. 2000. Importance of lactate dehydrogenase for the regulation of glycolytic flux and insulin secretion in insulin-producing cells. Biochem. J. **352**: 373–380.
43. ISHIHARA, H., H. WANG, L.R. DREWES & C.B. WOLLHEIM. 1999. Overexpression of monocarboxylate transporter and lactate dehydrogenase alters insulin secretory responses to pyruvate and lactate in beta cells. J. Clin. Invest. **104**: 1621–1629.
44. NEWGARD, C.B. 1994. Cellular engineering and gene therapy strategies for insulin replacement in diabetes. Diabetes **43**: 341–350.

45. TIEDGE, M., M. ELSNER, N.H. MCCLENAGHAN, et al. 2000. Engineering of a glucose-responsive surrogate cell for insulin replacement therapy of experimental insulin-dependent diabetes. Hum. Gene. Ther. **11:** 403–414.
46. KNAACK, D., D.M. FIORE, M. SURANA, et al. 1994. Clonal insulinoma cell line that stably maintains correct glucose responsiveness. Diabetes **43**(12): 1413–1417.
47. EFRAT, S., D. FUSCO-DEMANE, H. LEMBERG, et al. 1995. Conditional transformation of a pancreatic beta-cell line derived from transgenic mice expressing a tetracycline-regulated oncogene. Proc. Natl. Acad. Sci. USA **92:** 3576–3580.
48. ANTINOZZI, P.A., H.K. BERMAN, R.M. O'DOHERTY & C.B. NEWGARD. 1999. Metabolic engineering with recombinant adenoviruses. Annu. Rev. Nutr. **19:** 511–544.
49. JONAS, J.C., A. SHARMA, W. HASENKAMP, et al. 1999. Chronic hyperglycemia triggers loss of pancreatic beta cell differentiation in an animal model of diabetes. J. Biol. Chem. **274:** 14112–14121.
50. WEIR, G.C., D.R. LAYBUTT, H. KANETO, et al. 2001. Beta-cell adaptation and decompensation during the progression of diabetes. Diabetes **50**(Suppl. 1): S154–S159.
51. JONAS, J.C., R. LAYBUTT, G.M. STEIL, et al. 2001. Potential role of the early response gene c-myc in beta-cell adaptation to changes in glucose concentration. Diabetes **50**(Suppl. 1): S137.
52. BRAND, K. 1997. Aerobic glycolysis by proliferating cells: protection against oxidative stress at the expense of energy yield. J. Bioenerg. Biomembr. **29:** 355–364.
53. TIEDGE, M., S. LORTZ, J. DRINKGERN & S. LENZEN. 1997. Relation between antioxidant enzyme gene expression and antioxidative defense status of insulin-producing cells. Diabetes **46:** 1733–1742.
54. LENZEN, S., J. DRINKGERN & M. TIEDGE. 1996. Low antioxidant enzyme gene expression in pancreatic islets compared with various other mouse tissues. Free Radic. Biol. Med. **20:** 463–466.
55. ZHOU, Y.P., J.C. PENA, M.W. ROE, et al. 2000. Overexpression of Bcl-x(L) in beta-cells prevents cell death but impairs mitochondrial signal for insulin secretion. Am. J. Physiol. Endocrinol. Metab. **278:** E340–E351.
56. PAPAS, K.K., R.C. LONG, JR., I. CONSTANTINIDIS & A. SAMBANIS. 2000. Effects of short-term hypoxia on the bioenergetics and insulin secretion of alginate-entrapped mouse insulinoma βTC3 Cells. Cell Transplant. **9:** 415–422.
57. PAPAS, K.K., R.C. LONG, JR., A. SAMBANIS & I. CONSTANTINIDIS. 1999. Towards the development of a bioartificial pancreas: I. Effects of glucose on long-term entrapped βTC3 cell cultures. Biotech. Bioengin. **66:** 219–230.
58. CONSTANTINIDIS, I., N.E. MUKUNDAN, M.P. GAMCSIK & A. SAMBANIS. 1997. Towards the development of a bioartificial pancreas: a $^{13}$C NMR study on the effects of alginate/poly-L-lysine/alginate entrapment on glucose metabolism by βTC3 mouse insulinoma cells. Cell Mol. Biol. **43:** 721–729.
59. LEIBFRITZ, D. 1996. An introduction to the potential of $^1$H-, $^{31}$P- and $^{13}$C-NMR-spectroscopy. Anticancer Res. **16:** 1317–1324.
60. SHULMAN, R. & D. ROTHMAN. 2001. $^{13}$C-nmr of intermediary metabolism: implications for systemic physiology. Annu. Rev. Physiol. **63:** 15–48.
61. DIONNE, K.E., C.K. COLTON & M.L. YARMUSH. 1993. Effect of hypoxia on insulin secretion by isolated rat and canine islets of Langerhans. Diabetes **42:** 12–21.
62. SCHREZENMEIR, J., L. GERO, C. LAUE, et al. 1992. The role of oxygen supply in islet transplantation. Transplant. Proc. **24:** 2925–2929.
63. COLTON, C.K. & E.S. AVGOUSTINIATOS. 1991. Bioengineering in development of the hybrid artificial pancreas. J. Biomech. Eng. (Trans ASME) **113:** 152–170.
64. PAPAS, K.K., R.C. LONG, JR., I. CONSTANTINIDIS & A. SAMBANIS. 1996. Effects of oxygen on the metabolic and secretory activities of βTC3 cells. Biochim. Biophys. Acta **1291:** 163–166.
65. CHENG, L.L., I.W. CHANG, B.L. SMITH & R.G. GONZALEZ. 1998. Evaluating human breast ductal carcinomas with high-resolution magic-angle spinning proton magnetic resonance spectroscopy. J. Mag. Resonance **135:** 194–202.
66. CHENG, L.L., C.L. WU, M.R. SMITH & G.R. GONZALEZ. 2001. Non-destructive quantitation of spermine in human prostate tissue samples using HRMAS $^1$H NMR spectroscopy at 9.4 T. FEBS Lett. **494:** 112–116.

67. RUIZ-CABELLO, J. & J.S. COHEN. 1992. Phospholipid metabolites as indicators of cancer cell function. NMR Biomed. **5:** 226–233.
68. AIKEN, N.R. & R.J. GILLIES. 1996. Phosphomonoester metabolism as a function of cell proliferative status and exogenous precursors. Anticancer Res. **16:** 1393–1397.
69. TING, Y.T., T. SHERR & H. DEGANI. 1996. Variations in energy and phospholypid metabolism in normal and cancer human mammary epithelial cells. Anticancer Res. **16:** 1381–1388.
70. BHAKOO, K.K., S.R. WILLIAMS, C.L. FLORIAN, *et al.* 1996. Immortalization and transformation are associated with specific alterations in choline metabolism. Cancer Res. **56:** 4630–4635.

# Optimal Conditions of Transplantable Binary Polyelectrolyte Microcapsules

ARTUR BARTKOWIAK

*Polymer Institute, Technical University of Szczecin, Szczecin, Poland*

ABSTRACT: Binary polyanion/oligocation microcapsules, prepared in a one-step process, are proposed as an alternative to the common alginate/poly-L-lysine system used in bioencapsulation technology. The model system is based on natural polysaccharides and involves the anionic sodium alginate, or iota-carrageenan, complexed with cationic oligochitosan. This system has been characterized with respect to capsule formation, mechanical strength, and permeability. This paper provides a general description of the influence of the most pronounced parameters that can be used as a tool to modulate the properties of binary microcapsules. These parameters have been separated into two categories. The first, which includes molar mass of polyanion, pH, ionic strength, and concentration of both polyelectrolytes, can be used to simultaneously control capsule mechanical and structural properties. The second set, molar mass of polyanion and reaction time, influences only mechanical resistance without altering membrane permeability. Additional issues related to mechanical stability and the possible change of capsule properties following transplantation are discussed.

KEYWORDS: binary polyelectrolyte microcapsules; optimal conditions; mechanical resistance; permeability

## INTRODUCTION

The encapsulation of materials in polymeric microcapsules having permeable or semipermeable membranes surrounding a liquid core is well known in the art.[1] A wide variety of different approaches, based on numerous polymer chemistries, various processes of membrane formation and several encapsulation technologies have been described in the literature.[2] Encapsulation is currently employed in the food, agriculture, biotechnology, and biomedical industries. One of the important application of this technique is an encapsulation of biologically active species. In general, such therapies have the potential for the treatment of diseases requiring enzyme or endocrine replacement as well as in nutrient delivery via the encapsulation of enzymes, bacteria or cells. Examples of these medical applications are the encapsulation of islets of Langerhans for the treatment of diabetes mellitus, the use of encapsulated bioartificial organs targeted at treating neurodegenerative disorders, such as Parkinson's disease, Alzheimer's disease, and Huntington's chorea, and in the control of chronic pain and the administration of human growth factors.[3]

Address for correspondence: Artur Bartkowiak, Polymer Institute, Technical University of Szczecin, Pulaskiego 10, 70-322 Szczecin, Poland. Voice: +4891-4494088; fax: +4891-4494685.
barart@mailbox.tuniv.szczecin.pl

During the past two decades, due to the possibility of unique formation under physiological conditions and potential applications as microcapsules for medical implants, a variety of approaches based on polyelectrolyte complexes (PECs) have been studied. Several systems based on various polymer chemistries, processes of membrane formation, and encapsulation technologies have been evaluated.[4] At present one can distinguish two major groups of these systems in relation to a number of polyelectrolytic components (see FIGURE 1). In binary systems only two major components participate in complex formation. These complexes can be formed by polyanion/polyvalent metal cation or by polyanion/polycation interactions.

In multicomponent systems three or more components participate in complex formation. The most popular binary systems are based on the PEC of alginate and various polyvalent metal cations. However, the majority of these are not thermodynamically stable in physiological solution; the polyvalent cations within the complex are gradually replaced by monovalent ions. This leads to a continuous decrease of the capsule mechanical resistance, an increase of their porosity, and ultimately, disintegration of the system. Therefore, numerous groups all over the world have been looking for the best way to improve the mechanical stability of alginate/polyvalent metal capsules.

In the case of encapsulation of mammalian cells during the last two decades the overwhelming majority of researches restricted their studies to the alginate/$Ca^{2+}$/poly-L-lysine system (FIG. 1C), which was initially proposed twenty years ago by Lim and Sun.[5] Solid alginate/calcium beads are coated with a solution of oppositely charged poly-L-lysine and subsequently converted into a permeable capsule by liquefying the ionotropically gelled anionic polysaccharide. In practice such a multistep process is very difficult to control and requires complex technological solutions to be able to encapsulate living cells and perform the process under sterile conditions. Further disadvantages of this system that have been reported by some groups include limited mechanical properties and low biocompatibility.[6]

A very promising, single-step approach for forming capsules is based on complex formation between oppositely charged, high molecular weight polymers. In this method, a solution of a first polymer including the material to be encapsulated is preformed in droplets 0.2–5.0 mm in diameter and contacted with a second, oppositely

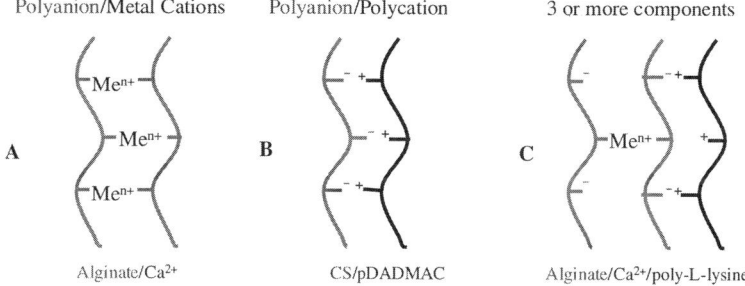

**FIGURE 1.** A schematic representation of PEC systems used in microencapsulation: (**A**) binary polyanion/metal cation; (**B**) binary polyanion/polycation; and (**C**) multicomponent.

charged, polymer.[7] Typically, droplets of the first polymer and the material to be encapsulated are generated using a capillary or spraying device and contacted with the second polymer, for example, by falling into a precipitation bath. The PEC reaction between the polymers at the surface of the droplet forms a membrane around a liquid core including the encapsulated material. In biotechnology if one is looking to optimize a process one attempts to minimize the number of variables. Therefore, binary systems, in which there are only two reactive components, seems to be promising. During the past decade few systematic studies related to binary capsules based on polyanion/polycation complexes have been reported.[4,8] This paper elucidates the general trends in modulation of the binary polyelectrolyte capsule properties as well as the optimal conditions for their formation.

## EXPERIMENTAL

### Alginate

Sodium alginate—Keltone HV (lot. 54650A) (Kelco/NutraSweet, San Diego, CA, USA) with intrinsic viscosity [η] of 880 mL/g in 0.1 M NaCl at 20°C was used for capsule preparations. This corresponds to a molar mass (MM) of 440,000. The preparation of sodium alginate samples of different MM have been described elsewhere.[9]

### Chitosan

Samples with varying molar masses of 1–4 kiloDaltons (kDa) were prepared by controlled radical degradation via continuous addition of hydrogen peroxide to 2.5% chitosan solution of pH 3.5–4.0 at 80°C. Chitosan with a MM of 50 kDa and a degree of deacetylation greater than 97% was used as the starting material (Hutchinson/McNeil Int., Philadelphia, USA, product E-055). All samples, after degradation as chloride salts, had similar polydispersities in MM (1.5–1.8) and high degrees of deacetylation (exceeding 95%). The degradation, characterization of polysaccharides, and preparation of solutions have comprehensively been described elsewhere.[10]

### Microcapsule Preparation and Characterization

Microcapsule preparation, conversion of chitosan, and permeability measurements, as well as mechanical testing and microscopic observation procedure are described elsewhere.[9,10] The detailed explanation of newly developed examination method of PEC alginate/oligochitosan membrane formation by applying the analytical ultracentrifugation synthetic boundary technique coupled with the twin scanning UV/VIS and Rayleigh interference optics has recently been reported.[11]

## RESULTS AND DISCUSSION

Recently, a new generation of binary microcapsules that can be prepared by using a PEC reaction between anionic polysaccharides and oligochitosan has been proposed.[12] This is unique relative to most polyelectrolyte complex systems in that it is based on natural polysaccharides and it involves a single step process to generate the membrane of microcapsule, avoiding the formation of a bead as a precursor.[13] TABLE 1 categorizes the influences on capsule properties into three groups related to polyelectrolyte structure, solution properties, and process of capsule formation. Because such complex system are often difficult to optimize via full or factorial experimental designs, general trends in modulation of binary polyelectrolyte capsule properties are highlighted in TABLE 1. To evaluate effects of selected parameters on the microcapsule properties two major metrics were used, the capsule mechanical resistance and the membrane porosity.

## Effect of Chitosan Molar Mass and Concentration

It was found that mechanical properties of the alginate/chitosan capsules are strongly dependent on the chitosan chain length, where the highest mechanical resistance is observed for low MM oligomers.[12] For the alginate/oligochitosan system, the molar mass of the chitosan is a key parameter in the formation of stable, elastic capsules with high modulus. Specifically, chitosan oligomers with molar masses between 2 and 20 kDa are favored.[13] For the chitosan of MM above 20,000 the membrane is very thin and has weak mechanical properties.[12] In this case the chitosan macromolecules are too large to penetrate the interface of the alginate solution and they create only a thin monolayer at the surface of the polyanion droplet.

By decreasing the chitosan MM below 20 kDa, the creation of capsules with increasing membrane thickness and mechanical properties is observed with a maximum strength at chitosan molar mass of 2–4 kDa. Below approximately 1 kDa a mechanical unstable PEC precipitate is formed due to too short oligocation chains that can not effectively crosslink the alginate macromolecules. In addition, increasing the oligochitosan concentration changes the kinetics of membrane formation, engendering a significant increase in mechanical stability and decrease of membrane cutoff. Moreover, since there is a significant correlation between the solubility of polysaccharides, such as chitosan and molecular weight, the use of an oligomeric polymer can both improve the solubility of the polymer at physiologically relevant pH and provide capsules having good mechanical properties.

TABLE 1. Parameters that exclusively control the properties of polyelectrolyte microcapsules

| Polyelectrolyte Structure | Solution Properties | Capsule Formation |
|---|---|---|
| *molar mass* | *polymer concentration* | *reaction time* |
| type of charge group | *ionic strength* | capsule diameter |
| *charge density* | *pH (around the pKa)* | method of formation |
| chain architecture | temperature | |
| hydrophobicity of backbone | | |

NOTE: Italicized text indicates parameters specifically discussed in this paper.

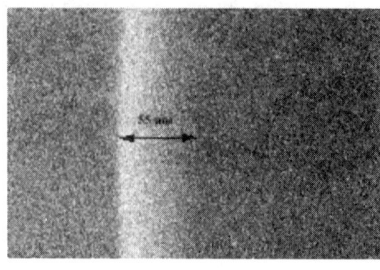 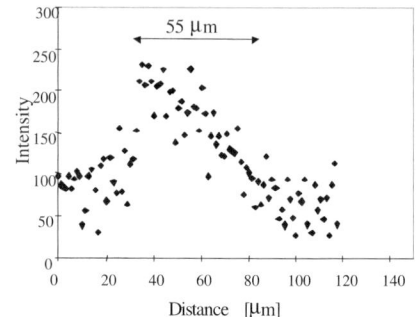

**FIGURE 2.** Photomicrograph of alginate/oligochitosan capsule membrane prepared in 0.01% eosin under fluorescence confocal microscope (*left*); and the intensity of the light in horizontal direction of the same picture analyzed using the Scion Image software (*right*).

### Structure of the PEC Membrane and an Effect of Reaction Time

Examination of microcapsules with a diameter in the range 2–2.5 mm under the optical microscope revealed the membrane thickness of 10 to 200 μm depending on the experimental conditions. From fluorescence intensity one can observe that capsules have asymmetric membrane structures with higher concentrations of chitosan close to the surface, gradually decreasing towards capsule center (see FIGURE 2). This agrees with a previous description of asymmetric capsule membrane formation between two oppositely charged polyelectrolytes as a two-step process.[14] Such membrane formation begins with the spontaneous creation of a semisolid complex "skin" at the droplet surface as a result of the phase separation process. After this initial step, a macroporous and heterogeneous membrane is build up, a process that is controlled by diffusion of the oligochitosan macromolecules. One could expect that the structural heterogeneity effects capsules properties where the capsule skin controls the membrane cutoff and the inner-membrane controls the mechanical resistance. This has been proven by measuring the capsule properties obtained after different reaction times (see TABLE 2). Generally, the mechanical strength of the

**TABLE 2. Properties of alginate/oligochitosam microcapsules as a function of reaction time**[a]

| Reaction Time | Membrane Thickness | Permeability (after 3 h) (%) | | Bursting Force |
|---|---|---|---|---|
| (min) | (μm) | 40 kDa | 110 kDa | (mN) |
| 5 | 40 | 33 | 24 | 50 ± 30 |
| 10 | 60 | 33 | 23 | 110 ± 60 |
| 15 | 80 | 32 | 23 | 200 ± 70 |
| 20 | 95 | 33 | 22 | 370 ± 150 |

[a]Capsules (2.5 mm in diameter) were obtained through a reaction between a 1% sodium alginate (Keltone HV) solution and a 1% chitosan $M_n$ = 2.8 kDa (pH 7.0, 0.9% NaCl).

capsules increases with reaction time due to the increase of the capsule wall thickness. However, no significant differences in the capsule permeability and the cutoff were measured. This indicates that the process of skin formation during the first minutes of reaction controls the cutoff of the membrane. However, the subsequent diffusion that controls building-up of the inner membrane is responsible for the mechanical resistance of the capsule.

For more detailed structure observation and to study the kinetics of binary membrane formation the analytical ultracentrifugation technique was applied.[11] In the experiment a special two-channel centerpiece was used in which the alginate solution was overlaid with the chitosan solution and scanned in the vertical direction using a special UV-light absorbance optical system. Based on obtained absorbance graphs one could follow the kinetics of the membrane formation. These results confirm the aforementioned heterogeneity of such a binary membrane (see FIGURE 3). Moreover, the broadening of the AUC-scans with time in the direction of chitosan solution that is observed after initial process of the skin formation indicates that the membrane also grows slowly with time in the direction of chitosan solution. This indicates that the large pores (greater than 18 nm) of the membrane, which correspond to the molar mass of dextran 150 kDa, permit the egress some of alginate macromolecules. On a macroscale this could be observed at high magnification of the capsule membrane as a "shaggy" type character of the surface (see FIGURE 4A). In the case of capsules obtained using similar principles, however, based on iota-carrageenan in the presence of gelling sodium cations that disable a diffusion of polyanion chains, one could see the highly smooth surface (FIG. 4B).[15]

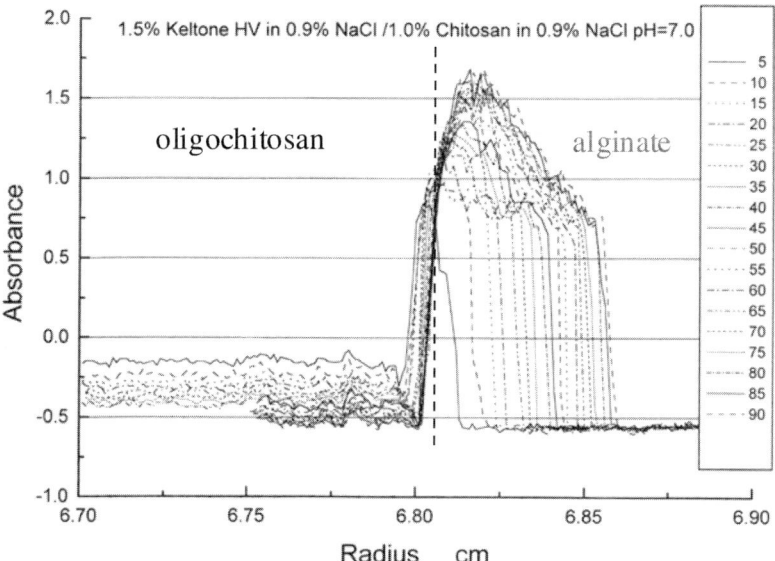

**FIGURE 3.** AUC absorption scans during layering and development of standard alginate/oligochitosan membrane (5,000 rpm, 370 nm, 20°C, scan time in min).[11]

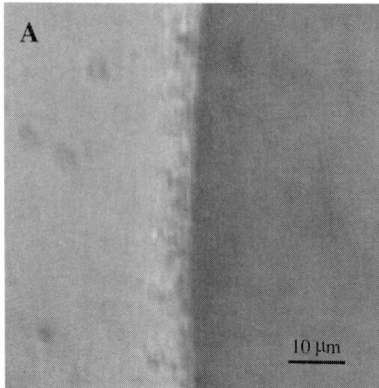 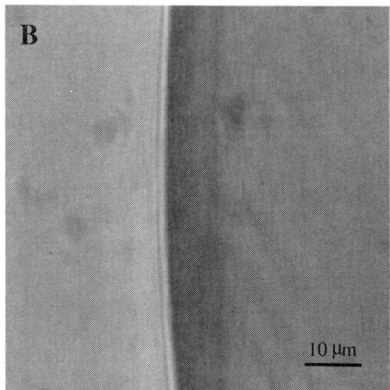

**FIGURE 4.** Photomicrographs of capsule membranes under a standard light microscope: (**A**) alginate/oligochitosan; (**B**) iota-carrageenan/Na$^+$/oligochitosan.

### pH and Ionic Strength

Chitosan, as a weak polybase, has limited solubility in the higher pH region where precipitation occurs when less than 30% of amino groups are in a protonated state. Therefore, one of the major disadvantages of using chitosan as polycation in bioencapsulation was the necessity of applying it at pH below 6.5. However for low MM chitosans (less than 6 kDa), which are preferable for mechanical stable binary capsule formation, precipitation occurs at higher pH values due to a shift in pKa toward higher values where it is possible to form capsule at neutral or even slightly basic solutions. The capsules obtained at different pH values between 6 to 7, in water or saline, varied in their surface roughness, membrane thickness, and morphology.[12] In general capsules prepared in water had smooth surfaces and their membrane thickness increased as a function of pH leading to a capsule of higher mechanical resistance. These differences can be explained by changes in chitosan protonation degree from 65% to 35% and this, in consequence, leads to a less crosslinked and more porous membrane where permeability is increasing with increasing of pH during capsule formation.

The presence of the low molecular salt accelerates the diffusion of the oligocations and leads to thicker and more resistant capsule walls, although with lower crosslinking density. With increasing sodium chloride concentration, a significant decrease in mechanical resistance and an increase in membrane porosity was found. Pronounced changes in both properties were observed in the same low ionic strength region up to 0.03 M salt concentration. Recently, based on the theoretical electrostatic interaction approach, a correlation between capsule properties and the Debye screening length $\lambda_D$ of polyanion chains has been shown.[16] This relation can be used as a tool to predict and modulate the binary capsule properties.

### Molar Mass and Concentration of Alginate

Two other parameters that influence the properties of binary capsules are the polyanion molar mass and concentration. The predominant factor that controls capsule mechanical strength is the MM of the polyanion; capsules prepared from alginate of 440 kDa have more than five times higher mechanical resistance than capsules of alginate 270 kDa.[5] The mechanical resistance also increases with concentration of alginate; however, increase of polyanion concentration by factor of two only doubles their mechanical resistance. The alginate concentration exerts a significant influence on capsule membrane porosity; with a decrease in concentration one can expect a decline of the charge density at the surface of the polyanion droplet, which leads to a less dense and more permeable membrane. Furthermore, since change in the alginate molar mass without changing its concentration does not affect the charge density at the surface of the droplet, no significant influence of the polyanion MM on capsule porosity was noticed. Similar relations were observed when alginate was replaced by iota-carrageenan in the same system.[15]

## Effect of Temperature

The temperature influences the viscosity of the polymer solutions, which in consequence may affect the capsule properties in a manner similar to that observed in the case of changing polyanion concentration. Furthermore, it is of a great importance for the rheological behavior of polyelectrolytes having thermoreversible gelation characteristics, where by changing the temperature during capsule formation, around their sol–gel transition point, one can modulate the properties of capsules, such as their permeability and mechanical resistance. For example for the iota-carrageenan/oligochitosan system the capsule membrane grows slower during incubation at lower temperature leading to higher relative crosslinking density and resulting in a lower permeability (see TABLE 3).[15] Moreover, the kinetics of diffusion of different molecules through the iota-carrageenan capsule wall can be controlled by variation of temperature. Therefore, such a system could find an additional application as a temperature-controlled delivery system.

## Selectivity of Chitosan Complexation

One interesting phenomenon that was found during the binary capsule formation is a selectivity of reaction with respect to length of oligochitosan chains. These results are based on GPC evaluation of chitosan chains that exclusively participate in capsule formation.[10] In all experiments the number average molar mass of chitosan was 2.6 kDa (see TABLE 4) in the starting solution. With an increase in pH, a significant

TABLE 3. Properties of capsules prepared at various temperatures[a]

| Temperature (°C) | Membrane Thickness (μm) | Chitosan Conversion (%) | Crosslinking Density[b] $-NH_3^+/-SO_3^-$ (mol/mol) | Permeability to Dextran 110 kDa (%) | Bursting Force (N) |
|---|---|---|---|---|---|
| 4 | 80 | 6.31 | 4.99 | 13 | 5.1 |
| 22 | 363 | 7.19 | 1.94 | 29 | 9.8 |
| 37 | 500 | 8.84 | 2.05 | 30 | 9.2 |

[a]Capsules were obtained through a reaction between a 1.2% iota-carrageenan (Fluka AG) in 3.67% HEPES buffer and a 1% chitosan $M_n$ = 2.7 kDa in 0.9% NaCl (pH 7.0, reaction 20 min).
[b]Chitosan/carrageenan charge group ratio in the capsule membrane.

TABLE 4. Molar masses of chitosan bonded during capsule formation[a]

| Solvent | pH | Chitosan Degree of Protonation (%) | $M_n$ of Chitosan (kDa)[b] |
|---|---|---|---|
| Water | 6.0 | 65 | 1.80 |
| | 6.5 | 50 | 1.85 |
| | 7.0 | 35 | 2.85 |
| 0.9% NaCl | 6.0 | 65 | 2.80 |
| | 6.5 | 50 | 3.40 |
| | 7.0 | 35 | 4.10 |

[a] Capsules (2.5 mm in diameter) were obtained through a reaction between a 1% sodium alginate (Keltone HV) solution and a 1% chitosan $M_n$ = 2.6 kDa (20 min reaction time).
[b] The $M_n$ of chitosan in the starting solution was 2.60 kDa.

shift of the complexed chitosan MM towards higher values was observed, both in salt-free and saline solutions. This is due to the decrease in chitosan degree of protonation at higher pHs where, to create stable membranes with similar number of crosslinking points, the higher MMs are preferentially involved in membrane formation (see FIGURE 5A). Furthermore, one can observe that the higher MM portion of chitosan is involved in membrane formation at greater ionic strength. The screening effect and the change of the polyanion coil conformation from an elongated into a more compact form leads to a larger distance between them and, as a result, preferentially longer chains of oligocation participate in the complex formation (FIG. 5B). Such selectivity was not exclusively found in the case of varying pH and the ionic strength during capsule formation. It was observed in the case of changing other parameters, such as reaction time, concentration, and MM of polyelectrolytes.[9,10] Therefore, one could expect that the aforementioned phenomenon is one of the main mechanisms responsible for the variation in capsule properties obtained under different reaction conditions.

### *Summary of Parameter Influences*

Summarizing the results presented one can distinguished six major groups of parameters that influence the binary capsule properties (see TABLE 5). Four variables simultaneously control capsule mechanical resistance and membrane cutoff. Specifically, the MM of the polycation and its charge density cause changes of properties in the same direction whereas the polyelectrolyte concentration and ionic strength produce contrary modifications. The last two groups (reaction time and polyanion concentration) influence only capsule mechanical resistance without changing the membrane cutoff, leading to a decoupling of the capsule mechanical resistance from their porosity. Furthermore, in most cases, one can observe a good correlation between mechanical resistance and membrane thickness, as well as between membrane porosity and crosslinking density.

The optimal conditions for binary polyelectrolyte capsule formation can be defined as those under which the mechanical stable capsule with required membrane porosity are formed (see TABLE 6). The first group of conditions is related to the polyanion solution, where a polyelectrolyte should be of relatively high molar mass,

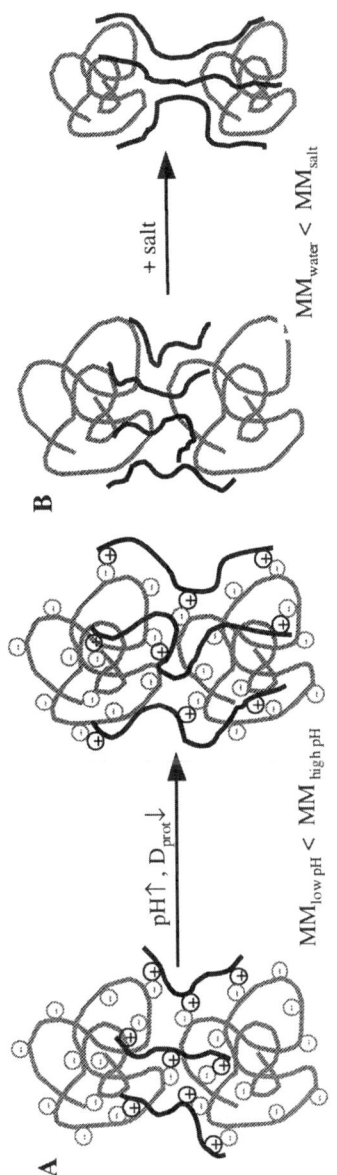

**FIGURE 5.** A schematic representation of a polyanion/oligocation PEC complexes as a function of (**A**) pH and (**B**) ionic strength.

TABLE 5. Effects of reaction parameters on binary polyelectrolyte capsule properties

| Variable | Membrane Thickness | Bursting Force | Crosslinking Density | Membrane Cutoff |
|---|---|---|---|---|
| ↑ Molar Mass of Polycation (outer) | ↓ | ↓ | ↑ | ↓ |
| ↑ pH (charge density ↓) | ↑ | ↑ | ↓ | ↑ |
| ↑ Ionic Strength | ↓ | ↓ | ↓ | ↑ |
| ↑ Polyanion/Oligocation Concentration | ↓ | ↑ | ↑ | ↓ |
| ↑ Reaction Time | ↑ | ↑ | ↓ | const. |
| ↑ Molar Mass of Polyanion (inner) | const. | ↑ | const. | const. |

preferentially higher than expected cutoff of the capsule to avoid the egress of the macromolecules from the capsules. The concentration should be 1 to 3% and the viscosity of the solution should in the range from 60 to 5,000 cPas, since below the lower limit the droplets cannot resist impact during the contact with the polycation solution and the upper value limits the preparation of homogenous polyanion solutions as well as the formation of the uniform spherical droplets during the atomization process. In the receiving bath the polycation macromolecules should be of the relative low MM (lower than 10,000). The concentration of polycation should be between 1–5% and the viscosity and the surface tension should be low enough to not disturb the entrance of the polyanion droplets into the receiving bath solution. Finally, both polyelectrolytes employed should be permanently charged with the charge density difference of between 2 and 4.

## *Encapsulation of Living Cells*

Transplantation of encapsulated cells may be helpful for many diseases in which a specific hormone or other substances secreted by cells are insufficient or lacking. Immunoprotection of transplanted cells is a promising way to avoid immune rejection. The encapsulation of living cells for biomedical applications to form bioartificial organs, such as a bioartifical pancreas, in which the capsule membrane acts as immunobarrier, is a multidisciplinary problem where many questions related to chemistry, biology, and technology remain.[17] Moreover, there are many technical obstacles that need to be identified. Therefore, during the formation and the optimization of microcapsules containing living cells one should consider additional variables related to the

TABLE 6. Optimal conditions of binary polyanion/oligocation capsule formation

| Polyanion Solution | Polycation Solution | Charge of Polyelectrolytes |
|---|---|---|
| high molar mass (higher than "cutoff") concentration 1–3% viscosity 60–5,000 cPas | low molar mass (2,000–10,000) concentration 1–5% low viscosity low surface tension | both should be "strong" polyelectrolytes (permanent charged) polyanion/polycation charge density difference (2–4 times) |

new components of the culture media, changes of the hydrodynamic behavior of the polyelectrolyte solution, polymer cytotoxicity, membrane biocompatibility, technological problems related to the capsule size, maximizing the rate of packing, and centering the cells within the capsules.

In every bioencapsulation system, the polymers that contact the cells must be non-cytotoxic, and the PEC membrane contacting the physiological fluid should be biocompatible. It is well known that high molar mass natural polysaccharides, such as sodium alginate and carrageenans, are non-cytotoxic.[2] These ionic polysaccharides are used in every country of the world as a food additive and are recognized by all regulatory agencies as safe and functional food ingredients. Chitosan is well known for its unusual antimicrobial activity against different groups of microorganisms, such as bacteria, yeast, and fungi.[18] Furthermore, binding of chitosan with DNA and inhibition of mRNA synthesis occurs via chitosan penetrating the nuclei of the microorganisms and interfering with the synthesis of mRNA and proteins.[19] Nevertheless, the capsule preparations proposed here do not involve a step in which the oligochitosan solution directly contacts immobilized cells; the short oligochains that create capsule membrane through a diffusion process could be in the contact with cells. Recently, it has been shown that low molar mass chitosan, obtained in radical degradation and purified by precipitation, is noncytotoxic against islets of Langerhans and genetically modified CHO cells.[20]

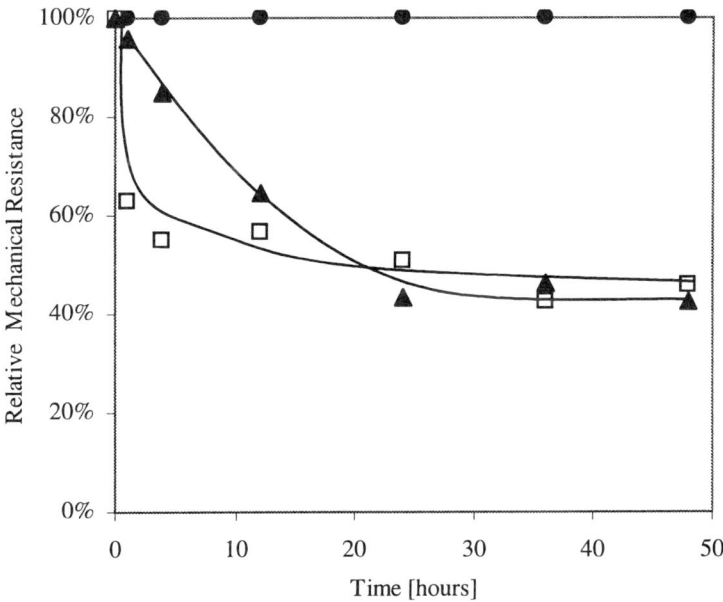

**FIGURE 6.** Changes of the capsule mechanical resistance stored in various salt solutions (●, 0.9% NaCl; □, MOPS; and ▲, PBS; a molarity of the HEPES and PBS solution corresponds to 0.9% NaCl).

Due to the relatively "weak" type of chemical bonds between charge groups within the PECs, the resulting microcapsules are sensitive to environmental conditions and, therefore, tend to change their properties during the change of storage conditions. The effect of new components on the properties of binary polyelectrolyte microcapsules can be visualized using alginate/oligochitosan microcapsules, prepared in saline and that, after formation, have been stored in three different solutions (see FIGURE 6). For capsules after 20 hours of seasoning, either in HEPES buffer or PBS solution, one can observe a significant reduction of mechanical resistance down to 50% of the initial value, whereas no change was observed for capsules kept in standard saline solution.

Another very important problem related to capsule stability is a possible change in capsule properties after transplantation. The mechanical resistance after transplantation should remain constant. However, in the case of the polyelectrolyte complexes, there will be always some decrease in mechanical resistance due to structure reorganization and egress of weak bonded oligocations or even polyanion molecules (see FIGURE 7A). The cutoff of the membrane, which should be strictly defined,

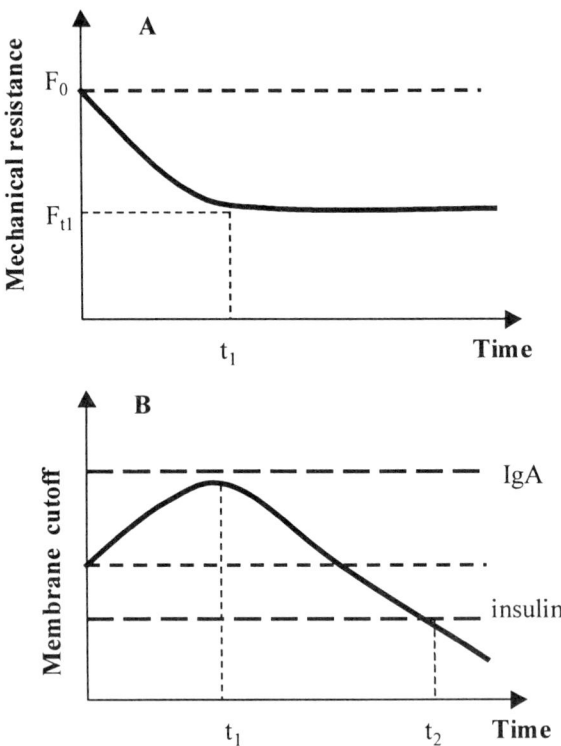

**FIGURE 7.** A schematic representation of the theoretical changes of PEC capsule properties following transplantation: (**A**) mechanical resistance; (**B**) membrane cutoff.

for example, in the case of the bioartificial pancreas, between the molar masses of insulin and antibodies, will initially increase due to the polyelectrolyte complex reorganization mentioned previously. Following this, one can observe a decrease in the cutoff caused by protein adsorption on the surface of the capsule, where un-compensated charges are present (FIG. 7B). Finally one could expect that, due to this process after some time $t_2$, the porosity will be lower than the size of hormone or nutrient molecules, leading first to lost of the functional properties and finally to necrosis of the cells.[17] All these complex issues—rate of the nutrients and oxygen transport as well as adsorption and denaturation of proteins in contact with PEC membrane—may impact the immunoprotection and metabolism of the encapsulated cells. Therefore, prior to applying any PEC system as bioartificial organs one should obtain the answers to the following questions:

1. What will be the mechanical resistance of the capsules after $t_1$ and is it high enough to resist all mechanical stresses in the body?;
2. What will be the capsule membrane cutoff at time $t_1$ and what is the life time of the device indicated by time $t_2$?

Only based on these answers can one correctly define the applicability and the life time of the system for the particular type of the bioencapsulation.

## CONCLUSIONS

A system based on the PEC between high molar mass alginate or iota-carrageenan and oligochitosan has been used as a model for description of optimal conditions of binary microcapsule formation. One can distinguish six major groups of parameters that influence binary capsule properties. Four of these simultaneously control capsule mechanical resistance and membrane cutoff and the last two groups influence only capsule mechanical resistance without changing membrane cutoff. These two categories of parameters may permit controlled manipulation during capsule formation to adjust the mechanical and structural properties. However, if one would like to optimize any selected system for the particular bioencapsulation application, the long term *in vitro* and *in vivo* stability of the microcapsule needs to be tested.

## ACKNOWLEDGMENT

I would like to thank Professor David Hunkeler from the Laboratory of Polyelectrolytes and BioMacromolecules (Swiss Federal Institute of Technology, Lausanne) for critical and helpful discussions, and for all his support during my stay in his group.

## REFERENCES

1. WILLAERT, R.G. & G.V. BARON. 1996. Gel entrapment and micro-encapsulation. Chem. Eng. Rev. **12**(1–2): 1–205.
2. RENKEN, A. & D. HUNKELER. 1998. Microencapsulation: a review of polymers and technologies with a focus on bioartificial organs. Polimery **43**(9): 530–537.

3. CHANG, T.M.S. 1997. Artificial cells and bioencapsulation in bioartificial organs. Ann. N.Y. Acad. Sci. **831:** 249–259.
4. PROKOP, A., D. HUNKELER, S. DIMARI, et al. 1998. Water soluble polymers for immunoisolation I: complex coacervation and cytotoxicity. Adv. Polymer Science **136:** 1–51.
5. LIM, F. & A.M. SUN. 1980. Microencapsulated islets as bioartificial endocrine pancreas, Science **210:** 908–909.
6. DE VOS, P., et al. 1997. Effect of alginate composition on the biocompatibility of alginate-polylisine microcapsules. Biomaterials **18:** 273–278.
7. DAUTZENBERG, H., W. JAEGER, J. KÖYZ, et al. 1994. Polyelectrolytes: Formation, Characterization and Application. Hanser, Munich, Vienna, New York.
8. DAUTZENBERG, H., et al. 1999. Development of cellulose sulfate-based polyelectrolyte complex microcapsules for medical applications. Ann. N.Y. Acad. Sci. **875:** 46–63.
9. BARTKOWIAK, A. & D. HUNKELER. 2000. Alginate-oligochitosan microcapsules: II. Control of mechanical resistance and permeability of the membrane. Chem. Mater. **12**(1): 206–212.
10. BARTKOWIAK, A. & D. HUNKELER. 1999. Alginate-oligochitosan microcapsules: a mechanistic study relating membrane and capsule properties to reaction conditions. Chem. Mater. **11**(9): 2486–2492.
11. WANDREY, C. & A. BARTKOWIAK. 2001. Membrane formation at interfaces examined by analytical ultracentrifugation techniques. J. Colloid. Surfaces A. **180**(1–2): 141–153.
12. BARTKOWIAK, A. & D. HUNKELER. 1999. New microcapsules based on oligoelectrolyte complexation. Ann. N.Y. Acad. Sci. **875:** 36–45.
13. BARTKOWIAK, A. & D. HUNKELER. 1998. Federal Institute of Technology, Lausanne, (assignee). UK Patent Application No. 2 135 954.
14. DAUTZENBERG, H., et al. 1996. Immobilisation of biological matter by polyelectrolyte complex formation. Ber. Bunsenges. Phys. Chem. **100:** 1045–1053.
15. BARTKOWIAK, A. & D. HUNKELER. 2001. Carrageenan-oligochitosan microcapsules: optimization of the formation process. J. Colloid. Surfaces B. **21:** 285–298.
16. BARTKOWIAK, A. 2001. Effect of the ionic strength on properties of binary alginate/oligochitosan microcapsules. J. Colloid Surfaces A. In press.
17. COLTON, C.K. 1995. Imptantable biohybrid artificial organs. Cell Transplant. **4**(4): 415–436.
18. YALPANI, M., F. JOHNSON & L.E. ROBINSON. 1992. Advances in Chitin and Chitosan. 543–555. Elsevier Applied Science, Amsterdam.
19. SUNDHARSHAN, N.R., D.G. HOOVER & D. KNOOR. 1992. Food Biotechnol. **5:** 45–57.
20. BARTKOWIAK, A. 2001. Binary Polyelctrolyte Microcapsules Based on Polysaccharides. Habilitation Thesis, Technical University of Szczecin (566), Polymer Institute (3).

# Mass Production of Embryoid Bodies in Microbeads

JOSEF P. MAGYAR,[a] MOHAMED NEMIR,[a] ELISABETH EHLER,[a] NICOLAI SUTER,[b] JEAN-CLAUDE PERRIARD,[a] AND HANS M. EPPENBERGER[a]

[a]Institute of Cell Biology, Swiss Federal Institute of Technology, ETH-Hönggerberg, CH-8008 Zurich, Switzerland

[b]Nisco Engineering Incorporated, Dufourstrasse 110, CH-8008 Zurich, Switzerland

ABSTRACT: Embryonic stem cells (ESC) are totipotent cells that can differentiate into a large number of different cell types. Stem cell-derived, differentiated cells are of increasing importance as a potential source for non-proliferating cells (e.g., cardiomyocytes or neurons) for future tissue engineering applications. Differentiation of ESC is initiated by the formation of embryoid bodies (EB). Current protocols for the generation of EB are either of limited productivity or deliver EB with a large variation in size and differentiation state. To establish an efficient and robust EB production process, we encapsulated mouse ESC into alginate microbeads using various microencapsulation technologies. Microencapsulation and culturing of ESC in 1.1% alginate microbeads gives rise to discoid colonies, which further differentiate within the beads to cystic EB and later to EB containing spontaneously beating areas. However, if ESC are encapsulated into 1.6% alginate microbeads, differentiation is inhibited at the morula-like stage, so that no cystic EB can be formed within the beads. ESC colonies, which are released from 1.6% alginate microbeads, can further differentiate to cystic EB with beating cardiomyocytes. Extended supplementation of the growth medium with retinoic acid promotes differentiation to smooth muscle cells.

KEYWORDS: embryonic stem cells; embryoid bodies; microbeads

## INTRODUCTION

Organ transplantation, as today's standard surgical treatment of organ failure, is mainly limited by the availability of donor organs. In recent years tissue-engineered artificial organs, generated from autogeneic or allogeneic cells, have been shown to provide a true alternative to organ transplantation. Living tissue equivalents are available for skin,[1] cartilage,[2] and bone,[3,4] and many more equivalents are in development.[5] This approach is successful for cell types that are capable of proliferation, for example, in vitro cultures provide a controlled and renewable reservoir for these cells. In case of non-dividing cells, however, other ways and sources need to be found. There are two principal ways: either a temporal release of postmitotic cells

Address for correspondence: Josef P. Magyar, Institute of Cell Biology, Swiss Federal Institute of Technology, ETH-Hönggerberg, CH-8008 Zurich, Switzerland. Voice: +41/1/633 33 54; fax: +41/1/633 10 69.

magyar@cell.biol.ethz.ch

from quiescence or the isolation of the stem cells of the cell type of interest. In the case of cardiomyocytes, neither of these possibilities were successful until now.[6]

Embryonic stem cells (ESC) are totipotent cells, originating from the inner cell mass of blastulas. They are able to differentiate to virtually all cell and tissue types *in vivo* as well as *in vitro*.[7,8] Therefore, ESC could serve as a source for the *in vitro* generation of postmitotic cells like cardiomyocytes. The full differentiation potential, however, is only achieved if the ESC are forced to differentiate both by morphological cues (embryoid body [EB] formation) as well as by growth- and differentiation-inducing factors. Steps for the induction of ESC differentiation include the production of morula-like aggregates, followed by the formation of blastula-like structures (cystic embryoid bodies) in suspension cultures and final differentiation in adhesion cultures. However, even under optimized conditions, only part of the ESC differentiate to cardiomyocytes[9,10] and even these cardiomyocytes are limited in their capability to proliferate.[11–13] Therefore, for the development of myocardial tissue engineering approaches it is important to establish controllable methods that are suitable for the large-scale production and differentiation of embryoid bodies.

Microencapsulation of animal cells into alginate hydrogels has been used with a large number of different cell types.[14–16] Immobilization of ESC into such gels, and their proliferation, should give rise to a large number of isolated ESC aggregates and later to embryoid bodies that might be able to differentiate to cells of all three germ layers. The number of equally developed embryoid bodies that could be generated by using this technology cannot be reached with any other current method. Here we describe such a large-scale production of EB by immobilization of ESC into alginate microbeads. Microencapsulated ESC can grow as compact colonies within the beads and give rise to morula- and subsequently to blastula-like structures. The ability to generate large number of EB by microencapsulation makes microbead-grown EB a potential *in vitro* source of cardiomyocytes for tissue engineering approaches. The differentiated EB can then easily be released from the beads by $Ca^{2+}$-depletion.

## MATERIAL AND METHODS

### *Culture and Microencapsulation of Embryonic Stem Cells*

Undifferentiated ESC of the mouse R1 cell line[17] were cultured on mouse feeder fibroblasts according to established procedures.[18] For microencapsulation, single cell suspensions of ESC were mixed with sterile filtered alginate (UP-LVG alginate; Pronova Biomedical A.S., Oslo, Norway) dissolved in Joklik medium (Cell Culture Technologies Inc., Zurich, Switzerland). Drops were formed from the alginate-ESC suspension using either the Nisco Var.A, laminar-jet-breakup microencapsulator (Nisco Engineering Inc., Zurich, Switzerland) or the Nisco Var.V high-voltage-driven microencapsulator (Nisco) into a hardening bath (100 mM $CaCl_2$, 10 mM morpholinoethanesulphonic acid (MOPS), pH = 7.4). After 10 minutes of hardening, beads were washed three times with Joklik medium and once with M199 medium (Amimed AG, Basel, Switzerland) and were cultured in M199 medium, supplemented with

10% FCS (PAA, Vienna, Austria), 1% penicillin/streptomycin (Gibco Laboratories, Grand Island, NY).

## Induction of Differentiation

Colonies of ESC, grown in 1.6% alginate microbeads were released by incubation of the beads in depolymerization buffer (50 mM Na-citrate, 77 mM NaCl, 10 mM MOPS, pH = 7.4) until the bead matrix was completely depolymerized. Bead-released ESC colonies were washed once with Joklik medium and once with M199 medium and plated onto gelatinized tissue-culture plates. Formation of spontaneously beating cardiomyocytes was promoted by supplementation of the medium with retinoic acid to a final concentration of $10^{-8}$ M[19] (RA; Sigma Chemical Co., St. Louis, MO). In case of ESC colonies grown in 1.1% alginate beads, differentiation within the beads was only promoted by supplementation of the medium with RA.

## Immunofluorescence Staining and Microscopic Analyzes

Fixation and immunostainings were performed as described previously.[20] Cells were monitored by staining of the DNA with Pico-green or by staining of the actin cytoskeleton with rhodamine-phalloidin (both from Molecular Probes Inc., Eugene, OR). For cardiomyocyte specific staining monoclonal mouse antibodies directed against sarcomeric $\alpha$-actinin (clone EA-53; Sigma) and for smooth muscle cell specific staining monoclonal mouse antibodies directed against $\alpha$-smooth muscle actin (clone 1A4; Sigma) or polyclonal rabbit antibodies against calponin (generously donated by Dr. Mario Gimona, Salzburg, Austria) were used. Optical analysis was performed by using a Leica TCS-NT confocal microscope (Leica, Mannheim, Germany) equipped with an argon-krypton mixed gas laser. Image analysis was performed using the Imaris software package (Bitplane AG, Zurich, Switzerland). Cellular and tissue contractions were documented using real-time videoimaging of beating or peristaltically contracting areas using a Zeiss Axiovert microscope (Zeiss, Oberkochen, Germany) combined with a CCD camera (C-5810; Hamamatsu Photonics K.K., Hamamatsu, Japan) and a video recorder (Panasonic AG-7350-E; Matsushita Electronics Co. Ltd., Kyoto, Japan).

## RESULTS

We have analyzed growth and differentiation of ESC inside alginate microbeads as a potential tool for large scale production of ESC derived cardiomyocytes. When encapsulated into 1.6% alginate beads, ESC grew to compact, lens-shaped colonies (see FIGURE 1A). The number of ESC per bead and the survival rate of the cells determined the number of embryoid bodies growing in the beads. Even extended culturing did not result in the development of blastula-like structures or in the differentiation to spontaneously beating cardiomyocytes and the lens-shaped morphology was retained in all preparations throughout the entire culturing period. Therefore, we released the ESC colonies from the alginate beads by calcium chelation. Freshly

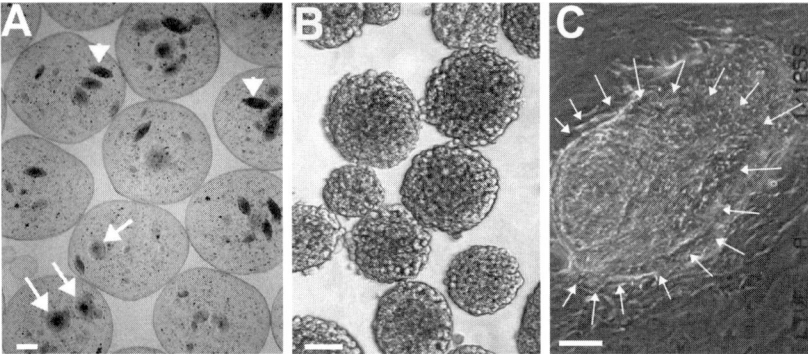

**FIGURE 1.** Morphology of bead-grown ESC colonies and EB. (**A**) Phase contrast image of ESC colonies grown in 1.6% alginate microbeads. Note that the oval appearance of the colonies is a chance result of the adjusted lateral view (*arrowheads*). A spherical appearance of colonies is due to the perpendicular view angle (*arrows*). (**B**) Freshly released ESC colonies have an apparent spherical form, whereas this is only due to the fact that the lens-shaped colonies lie on their broad side. (**C**) Beating area in a differentiated EB. Boundary of the area is depicted by *arrows* pointing toward its center.

released colonies remained compact and retained their lens-shaped morphology. Culture of these colonies in suspension in bacterial dishes resulted in the formation of spheroid, morula-like structures within one to two days. Additional culture for one to two days led to the differentiation to blastula-like structures (cystic embryoid bodies) in the vast majority of the colonies. On further culturing in gelatin-coated tissue culture dishes, these structures adhered to the substratum and differentiated into various cell types, as judged by the multiform appearance of the colonies. A varying number of these colonies showed regions that differentiated into cardiomyocytes, as judged by the spontaneous periodic beating of the cells.

Since our aim was to establish a method suitable for the large-scale differentiation of ESC to EB and to EB with spontaneously beating cardiomyocytes, we tested whether a minimization of alginate concentration would permit a differentiation already inside the beads. Due to the weak mechanical resistance of these beads during the hardening process, microencapsulation of ESC into monodisperse and spherical 1.1% alginate microbeads was only possible using a high-voltage-driven microencapsulator. Similarly to ESC colonies grown in 1.6% alginate microbeads, in 1.1% alginate gels the initial form of the colonies was lens-shaped. After four days in culture, however, some of the ESC colonies became cystic, indicating that differentiation could proceed further than in 1.6% alginate beads. Cystic colonies also developed spontaneously beating areas, similarly to adherent cultures of 1.6% alginate bead-grown EB on gelatinized tissue culture dishes. Therefore, microencapsulation of ESC into 1.1% alginate microbeads allowed the generation of a large number of differentiated EB with spontaneously beating areas in a small culture volume.

In long-term (more than 10 days) cultures of adherent EB in the presence of RA showed large areas of slow, spontaneous, wave-like contractions. If analyzed by smooth muscle cell-specific immunostaining (see FIGURE 2 B, C, and D), these areas contained large numbers of smooth muscle cells, aligned in an organized, parallel

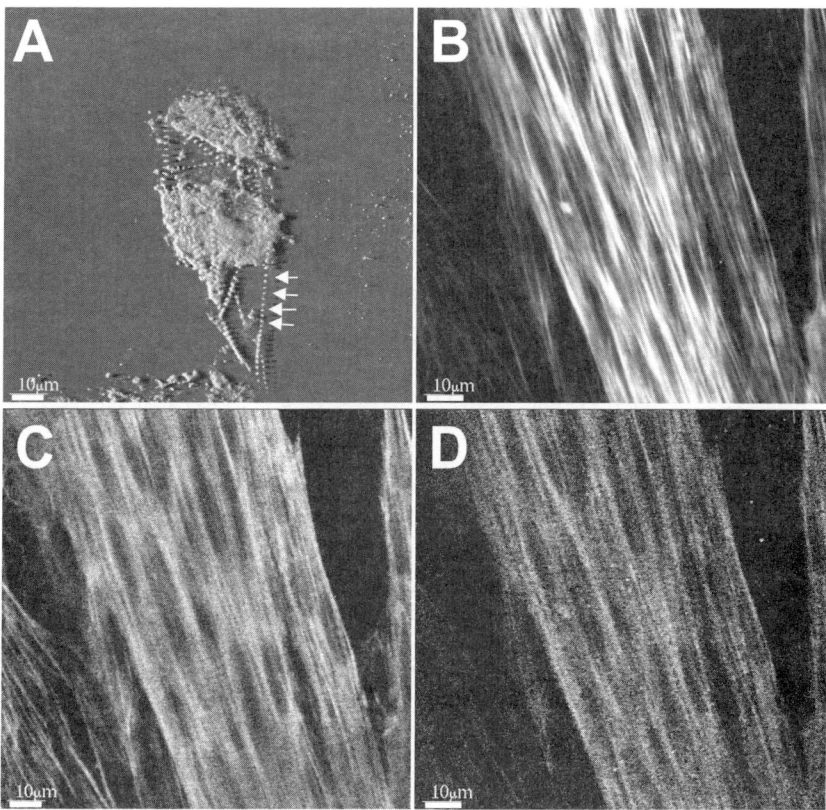

**FIGURE 2.** Differentiation of bead-grown EB to cardiomyocytes and smooth muscle cells. (**A**) Immunofluorescence staining of differentiated EB, grown in 1.6% alginate beads and differentiated in adherent cultures on gelatin-coated cell culture dishes. Striated appearance of the staining and expression of sarcomeric α-actinin clearly identifies cardiomyocytes in a region that was selected based on the basis of beating activity before fixation. (**B**, **C**, and **D**) Smooth muscle cells differentiated in the same culture were also identified by their slow contractions. Coimmunostaining for α-smooth muscle actin (**C**), and calpain (**D**) confirmed the presence of smooth muscle-specific proteins in these cells. Note the self-organization of the smooth muscle cells into parallel strands, best visualized by staining for f-actin (**B**: phalloidin stain).

fashion. Interestingly, these smooth muscle cells expressed, in addition to the smooth muscle actin α-isoform (FIG. 2C), calponin (FIG. 2D), a marker protein for smooth muscle cells that is normally rapidly downregulated in culture.[21] Therefore, the presence of calponin likely indicates the high degree of differentiation of these cells. The respective areas were much larger than the areas comprising of cardiomyocytes, indicating that the ESC derived smooth muscle cells could either be faster or longer proliferation competent than ESC derived cardiomyocytes. Indeed, the number of beating areas, attributed to cardiomyocytes, seemed to decrease in long-term cultures, as had been similarly reported for systems not involving microencapsulation.[9,22]

## DISCUSSION

The capacity of ESC to form embryoid bodies and to differentiate *in vitro* to all three germ layers has been demonstrated in rodents[23] as well as in humans.[24] A full differentiation range can only be achieved by the generation of EB. These can be generated by either using "hanging drop" technology,[19] by culturing ESC colonies detached from cultures grown without a feeder cell layer,[25,26] or by the spontaneous aggregation of ESC in suspension culture without[22] or with spinning[27] or with a combination thereof.[28] Therefore, it seems that the formation of cystic EB may be a prerequisite for differentiation into cardiomyocytes. Applying a large scale approach, it is important that the variability in the differentiation state of the EB is minimal. Although, depending on the concentration of the ESC in the encapsulation matrix, the number of cells per microbead varies, we assume that at a reasonable high dilution almost all of the EB is derived from a single cell, which ensures a relatively narrow distribution in size and differentiation state of the EB. (This statement does not imply that a single cell colony is produced in the microcapsule.) Using microencapsulation, one ESC is assumed to give rise to one EB, which offers significant advantages over the hanging drop technology, where typically 500 cells are used for the formation of a single EB, or over spontaneous aggregation, where an unknown amount of ESC aggregate to EB. In addition, the monoclonality of bead-grown EB offers the possibility to test large scale gene-trap approaches[29] in ESC for the identification of tissue specific genes.

Out of an ESC line it is possible to generate *in vitro* a tissue-specific stem cell lineage.[30] Using our microencapsulation system it is possible to culture a large number of cells, well separated from each other, within a small volume or area. Therefore, microencapsulation of a single cell suspension of an EB containing beating structures might allow the isolation of a mesenchymal stem cell line with an increased potential to differentiate into the cardiomyocytic lineage.

The number of EB displaying spontaneously beating areas can vary (91%,[9] 70%,[31] or less). Factors potentially responsible for these differences might include (1) ESC line-specific differences, (2) differences in the medium composition, and (3) differences in the serum composition. This variability and the finding that only a part of an EB differentiates to cardiomyocytes points to the importance of the identification of cardiomyocyte stem cells. Since 80% of the myocardial volume is made up by cardiomyocytes but only 25% of all cells are cardiomyocytes, unequivocal identification of these cells within the myocardium has always been a controversial issue (Field, 1997). Therefore, reports describing the ability of bone marrow-derived mesenchymal stem cells to differentiate to cardiomyocytes[32] needs to be carefully revised.

We have tested the microencapsulation of ESC into alginate microbeads. Our results show that immobilization of ESC into hydrogel microbeads allows the mass production of EB. This process will need to be optimized in order to (1) increase the number of EB with beating areas, (2) increase the number of cardiomyocytes within a given EB, and (3) increase the survival of the EB-derived cardiomyocytes. Our data indicate that the bead matrix has an influence on the ability of the bead-grown ESC colonies to differentiate to EB and we believe that the influence of the matrix composition needs to be analyzed by a systematic testing of different alginate preparations as well as by the use of other matrices like sulfocellulose.[33] Since a large number of factors and substances have been described that promote ESC differentiation towards cardiomyocytic lineage, evaluation of combinations of these is of great importance and might include: RA,[34] DMSO,[35] $H_2O_2$, menadione,[27] activin A,[36] and bone morphogenic protein 2 (BMP-2), together with fibroblast growth factor-4 (FGF-4),[37] insulin, fibroblast growth factor-2 (FGF-2),[38] insulin-like growth factor-1 (IGF-I)[38,39] serum-responsive factor (SRF),[40,41] and a high glucose content of the medium.[9]

In this paper we have shown the feasibility of a large scale production of equally developed embryonic bodies in a scale most likely suitable for tissue engineering approaches. Future work will need to optimize the condition to obtain the outmost number of differentiated cells.

## ACKNOWLEDGMENTS

Thanks to Dr. Christian Zuppinger (University Hospital Berne, Switzerland) for the digitalization of real-time video films and to Dr. Mario Gimona (Salzburg, Austria) for providing anti-calponin antisera.

## REFERENCES

1. EAGLSTEIN, W.H. & V. FALLANGA. 1998. Tissue engineering for skin: an update. J. Am. Acad. Dermat. **39:** 1007–1010.
2. KIM, W.S., et al. 1994. Cartilage engineered in predetermined shapes employing cell transplantation on synthetic biodegradable polymers. Plast. Reconstr. Surg. **94:** 233–240.
3. VACANTI, C.A. & L.J. BONASSAR. 1999. An overview of tissue engineered bone. Clin. Orthop. **367**(Suppl): S375–S381.
4. BRUDER, S.P. & B.S. FOX. 1999. Tissue engineering of bone. Cell based strategies. Clin. Orthop. **367**(Suppl): S68–S83.
5. HUNKELER, D. 1999. Bioartificial organs transplanted from research to reality. Nat. Biotechnol. **17:** 335–336.
6. MAGYAR, J.P. & H.M. EPPENBERGER. 1999. Factors involved in the cell cycle arrest of adult rat cardiomyocytes. Cell Engineering **1:** 239–254.
7. DOETSCHMAN, T.C., et al. 1985. The in vitro development of blastocyst-derived embryonic stem cell lines: formation of visceral yolk sac, blood islands and myocardium. J. Embryol. Exp. Morphol. **87:** 27–45.
8. KELLER, G.M. 1995. In vitro differentiation of embryonic stem cells. Curr. Opin. Cell Biol. **7:** 862–869.
9. GUAN, K., et al. 1999. Modulation of sarcomere organization during embryonic stem cell-derived cardiomyocyte differentiation. Eur. J. Cell Biol. **78:** 813–823.
10. KLINZ, F., et al. 1999. Inhibition of phosphatidylinositol-3-kinase blocks development of functional embryonic cardiomyocytes. Exp. Cell Res. **247:** 79–83.
11. MEYER, N., et al. 2000. A fluorescent reporter gene as a marker for ventricular specification in ES-derived cardiac cells. FEBS Lett. **478:** 151–158.
12. KLUG, M.G., et al. 1995. DNA synthesis and multinucleation in embryonic stem cell-derived cardiomyocytes. Am. J. Physiol. **269:** H1913–H1921.
13. HESCHELER, J., et al. 1997. Embryonic stem cells: a model to study structural and functional properties in cardiomyogenesis. Cardiovasc. Res. **36:** 149–162.
14. SUN, A.M. 1997. Microencapsulation of cells. Medical applications. Ann. N.Y. Acad. Sci. **831:** 271–279.

15. CHANG, P.L. 1996. Microencapsulation—an alternative approach to gene therapy. Transfus. Sci. **17:** 35–43.
16. TYLER, J.E. 1990. Microencapsulation of mammalian cells. Bioprocess. Technol. **10:** 343–361.
17. NAGY, A., *et al.* 1993. Derivation of completely cell culture-derived mice from early-passage embryonic stem cells. Proc. Natl. Acad. Sci. USA **90:** 8424–8428.
18. SORIANO, P., *et al.* 1991. Targeted disruption of the c-src proto-oncogene leads to osteopetrosis in mice. Cell **64:** 693–702.
19. MALTSEV, V.A., *et al.* 1999. Establishment of beta-adrenergic modulation of L-type $Ca^{2+}$ current in the early stages of cardiomyocyte development. Circ. Res. **84:** 136–145.
20. EHLER, E., *et al.* 1999. Myofibrillogenesis in the developing chicken heart: assembly of Z-disk, M-line and the thick filaments. J. Cell Sci. **112:** 1529–1539.
21. GIMONA, M., *et al.* 1990. Smooth muscle specific expression of calponin. FEBS Lett. **274:** 159–162.
22. SCHREIBER, K.L., *et al.* 2000. Distant upstream regulatory domains direct high levels of beta-myosin heavy chain gene expression in differentiated embryonic stem cells. J. Mol. Cell. Cardiol. **32:** 585–598.
23. ROBBINS, J., *et al.* 1990. Mouse embryonic stem cells express the cardiac myosin heavy chain genes during development *in vitro*. J. Biol. Chem. **265:** 11905–11909.
24. ITSKOVITZ-ELDOR, J., *et al.* 2000. Differentiation of human embryonic stem cells into embryoid bodies compromising the three embryonic germ layers. Mol. Med. **6:** 88–95.
25. CHEN, Y., *et al.* 2000. Fibroblast growth factor (FGF) signaling through PI 3-kinase and Akt/PKB is required for embryoid body differentiation. Oncogene **19:** 3750–3756.
26. MARTIN, G.R., *et al.* 1977. The development of cystic embryoid bodies *in vitro* from clonal teratocarcinoma stem cells. Dev. Biol. **61:** 230–244.
27. SAUER, H., *et al.* 2000. Role of reactive oxygen species and phosphatidylinositol 3-kinase in cardiomyocyte differentiation of embryonic stem cells. FEBS Lett. **476:** 218–223.
28. DOEVENDANS, P.A., *et al.* 2000. Differentiation of cardiomyocytes in floating embryoid bodies is comparable to fetal cardiomyocytes. J. Mol. Cell Cardiol. **32:** 839–851.
29. CANNON, J.P., *et al.* 1999. Gene trap screening using negative selection: identification of two tandem, differentially expressed loci with potential hematopoietic function. Dev. Genet. **25:** 49–63.
30. PALACIOS, R., *et al.* 1995. *In vitro* generation of hematopoietic stem cells from an embryonic stem cell line. Proc. Natl. Acad. Sci. USA **92:** 7530–7534.
31. BADER, A., *et al.* 2000. Leukemia inhibitory factor modulates cardiogenesis in embryoid bodies in opposite fashions. Circ. Res. **86:** 787–794.
32. LIECHTY, K.W., *et al.* 2000. Human mesenchymal stem cells engraft and demonstrate site-specific differentiation after in utero transplantation in sheep. Nat. Med. **6:** 1282–1286.
33. MERTEN, O.W., *et al.* 1991. A new method for the encapsulation of mammalian cells. Cytotechnology **7:** 121–130.
34. WOBUS, A.M., *et al.* 1997. Retinoic acid accelerates embryonic stem cell-derived cardiac differentiation and enhances development of ventricular cardiomyocytes. J. Mol. Cell Cardiol. **29:** 1525–1539.
35. MCBURNEY, M.W., *et al.* 1982. Control of muscle and neuronal differentiation in a cultured embryonal carcinoma cell line. Nature **299:** 165–167.
36. SCHULDINER, M., *et al.* 2000. From the cover: effects of eight growth factors on the differentiation of cells derived from human embryonic stem cells. Proc. Natl. Acad. Sci. USA **97:** 11307–11312.
37. LOUGH, J., *et al.* 1996. Combined BMP-2 and FGF-4, but neither factor alone, induces cardiogenesis in non-precardiac embryonic mesoderm. Dev. Biol. **178:** 198–202.
38. ANTIN, P.B., *et al.* 1996. Regulation of avian precardiac mesoderm development by insulin and insulin-like growth factors. J. Cell Physiol. **168:** 42–50.

39. FISHMAN, M.C. & K.R. CHIEN. 1997. Fashioning the vertebrate heart: earliest embryonic decisions. Development **124:** 2099–2117.
40. WEINHOLD, B., *et al.* 2000. Srf(-/-) ES cells display non-cell-autonomous impairment in mesodermal differentiation. EMBO J. **19:** 5835–5844.
41. ARSENIAN, S., *et al.* 1998. Serum response factor is essential for mesoderm formation during mouse embryogenesis. EMBO J. **17:** 6289–6299.

# Soft, Porous Poly(D,L-lactide-co-glycotide) Microcarriers Designed for *Ex Vivo* Studies and for Transplantation of Adherent Cell Types Including Progenitors

ARRON S.L. XU AND LOLA M. REID

*Department of Cell & Molecular Physiology and Program in Molecular Biology and Biotechnology, CB 7038, School of Medicine, University of North Carolina, Chapel Hill, North Carolina, USA*

ABSTRACT: Our laboratory is undertaking tissue engineering of liver using enriched liver progenitor cells. We report here our ongoing study to design biodegradable and biocompatible three-dimensional substratum supports of both natural and synthetic polymeric materials suitable to the adhesion, growth, and differentiation of adult and progenitor liver cells for their transplantation, and for the development of a bioartificial liver assist device. Porous biocompatible and biodegradable microcarriers of diameter 20–40 μm and 100–300 μm were prepared from (α-hydroxy) acid family of polymers. Human hepatoma cell line HepG2 and adult rodent liver cells were found to attach to collagen-coated surface of poly(D,L-lactide-co-glycotide) microcarriers. HepG2 cells attached to the degradable microcarriers remained viable and underwent growth expansion, forming three-dimensional cell-degradable microcarrier colonies in culture. These cell-degradable microcarrier colonies may undergo further growth expansion, thus providing a viable approach for three-dimensional organogenesis of tissue.

KEYWORDS: poly(lactide-co-glycotide); microcarriers; biodegradable beads; liver cells; progenitor cells; tissue engineering; cell therapies

## INTRODUCTION

Cell therapies and bioartificial organs are emerging as potential therapeutic approaches to tissue and organ disorders. The optimal class of cells for both cell therapies and bioartificial organs is hypothesized to be progenitor cells and diploid adult cells based on their extraordinary expansion and differentiation potential.[1,2] Although biologically relevant synthetic or hybrid substrata have been proposed for many types of mature cells in culture,[3–5] there are none for three-dimensional culture systems involving progenitor cells that are anchorage-dependent but require flexible,

Address for correspondence: Dr. Arron S.L. Xu and Dr. Lola M. Reid, Department of Cell & Molecular Physiology and Program in Molecular Biology and Biotechnology, CB 7038, School of Medicine, University of North Carolina, Chapel Hill, NC 27599-7038, USA. Voice: 919-966 0346; fax: 919-966 6112.
Dr. Arron S.L. Xu: axu@med.unc.edu
Dr. Lola M. Reid: stemcell@med.unc.edu

porous substrata for survival, growth, and differentiation. Ongoing liver studies are representative. Under *in vivo* conditions hepatic progenitors, located in the vicinity of the portal triads,[6] are attached to an extracellular matrix similar to basement membranes and consisting primarily of soft and flexible collagen type IV, laminin, hyaluoronates, and liver-specific forms of heparan sulfate proteoglycan.[7] The progenitors give rise to daughter cells undergoing a maturation that is coordinate with a gradient in extracellular matrix chemistry in which the laminins, type IV collagen, and hyaluronates are eliminated and there is conversion to predominantly fibrillar collagens, fibronectins, and highly sulfated species of proteoglycans, such as heparin proteoglycan.[7]

Cell morphology is influenced by the chemistry and physical features of extracellular matrix (ECM) forming the cellular substratum. Extracellular matrix is known to regulate the gene expression.[2,8-15] Tissue-specific ECM has been shown to regulate hepatocyte aggregate morphology[15-18] and growth versus differentiation.[14,19,20] Achieving tissue histological structure and possibly organotypic functions are important for expression of tissue-specific functions of cells cultured under *ex vivo* conditions.

In comparison with attachment of adherent cells to a rigid and smooth surface, greater extent of attachment, survival, and function can be achieved on soft and porous substratum that resembles the macromolecular structure of extracellular matrix (see, for example, Refs. 2, 10, 19, 21) with their texture morphology in the magnitude order of the physical dimension of the cells.[12] Attachment to highly porous surface is also thought to be important to encourage the ingrowth of cells into extracellular matrix and synthetic matrix scaffolds, a critical aspect in the design of implantable tissue engineering scaffolds. Many different forms of three-dimensional matrix scaffolds have been investigated for *ex vivo* culture of liver cells for expressing and maintaining liver differentiated functions. Hepatocytes encapsulated in collagen matrix,[22,23] embedded in collagen gel or matrix gel,[24] aggregated as spheroids,[25] and attached to porous degradable sponge, fiber mesh[26,27] have been reported for live cell transplantation and development of bioartificial liver assist devices (LAD). Despite the difference in their physical appearances, degradable scaffolds aim to provide liver cells with substrata suitable for cell attachment, and to maintain cell–matrix as well as cell–cell interactions that are critical for cell signaling and the expression of their differentiated functions.[9,12,14,15,27] Controllable degradation of substratum scaffold is important to the ingrowth and ultimate clearance of the synthetic implant materials during organogenesis of engineered tissue.

Non-degradable beads that are rigid and non-porous have been used as anchorage supports for transplantation of hepatocytes in experimental studies underpinning future plans for cell therapy (see Ref. 28 and reference therein) or development of bioartificial liver assist devices currently in clinical trial.[29] Commercially available microbeads at present consist of non-degradable materials (e.g., polystyrene, polyacrylamide, and dextrane) coated with denatured matrix proteins (e.g., cross-linked collagen type I or gelatin). These beads are typically non-porous with rigid structure (e.g., RapidCell of ICN Chemical, see FIGURE 1B). They are designed primarily for limited short-term *ex vivo* maintenance of the freshly isolated cells or transformed cell lines. Their rigidity and lack of porosity make them unsuitable as substrata for

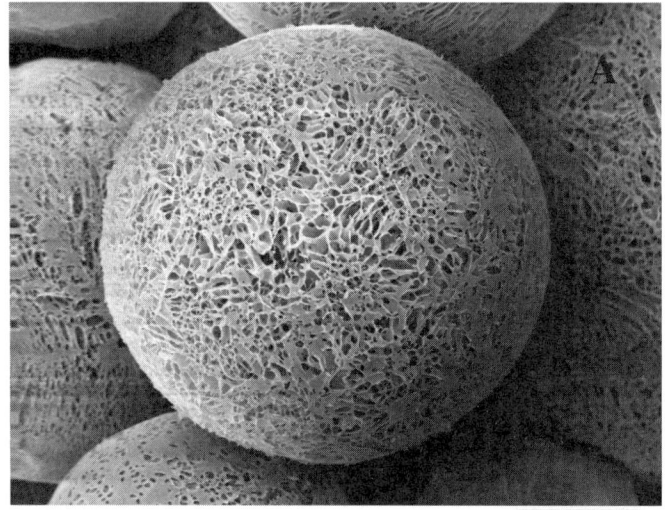

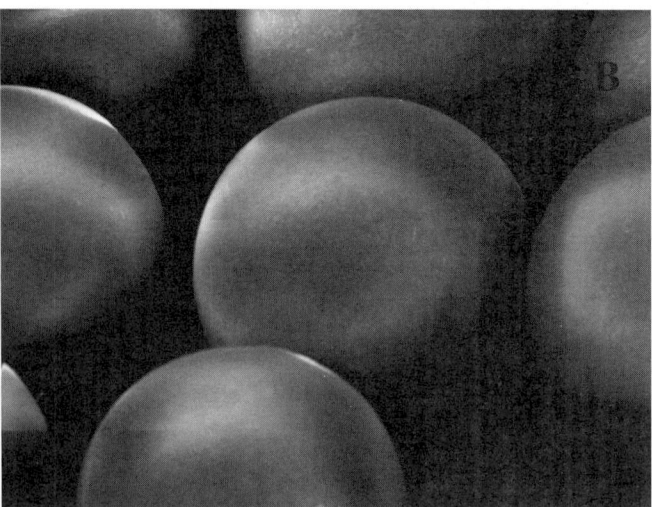

**FIGURE 1.** Scanning electron micrographs (SEM) showing the surface structure of (**A**) porous degradable poly(D,L-lactide-co-glycolite) microbeads and (**B**) non-porous RapidCell® beads obtained from ICN Biochemical.

culture of progenitor cells that die within hours on such substrata.[1,13,30,31] However, highly porous and degradable beads are not commercially available at present.

Polylactide (PLA), polyglycolite (PGA) and their copolymer poly(D,L-lactide-co-glycolite) (PLGA) and analogs are among the most widely used biocompatible and biodegradable polymers in clinical applications at present. A variety of analogs with different chemical and physical properties have been developed and fabricated into scaffolds (e.g., fibers, mesh, membranes, and sponge) and carriers for controlled release of pharmaceutics (e.g., see reviews in Refs. 32 and 33). To provide porous biocompatible and biodegradable substrata that offer larger specific surface area for cell attachment, porous degradable beads are more advantageous than degradable substrata, such as fiber, mesh, and sponges. In addition, porous beads can be readily adapted for *ex vivo* studies in either conventional cell cultures or novel bioreactors of various physical settings and used as carriers of cells and therapeutic agents in surgical implantation. Our laboratory is developing biocompatible and biodegradable porous beads or microcarriers as suitable matrix scaffolds for hepatic progenitors enabling them to survive, grow, and mature through the entire liver lineage. We report here the preparation of porous degradable PLGA beads. The conditions of matrix coating to the polymer beads and hepatocyte attachment were investigated. Analysis of the attachment of HepG2 cells and normal rodent primary liver cells to the porous degradable PLGA beads was carried out to evaluate the suitability of the degradable beads. The study using HepG2 cells, a transformed hepatic progenitor cell model, is particularly relevant to other progenitor cells.[34]

## EXPERIMENTAL SECTION

### *Preparation of Degradable Beads*

PLGA microcarriers with diameters less than 100 μm were prepared using an ultrasonic liquid atomization procedure adopted from that reported elsewhere.[35] In brief: a PLGA solution of dioxane, or other solvents where specified, was dispersed by probe ultrasonication into fine polymer droplets. The fine droplets were solidified and collected immediately into sufficient volume of liquid nitrogen overlaid on frozen ethanol. The polymer solvent was then extracted into the slowly melting ethanol at −76°C. This was followed by further extraction with cold hexane at −76°C. The remaining small amount of solvent was removed by lyophilization.

Larger PLGA mesobeads with approximate diameters of 100–300 μm were prepared by forming small droplets of water–polymer emulsion in 0.1% polyvinyl alcohol (PVA) solution. Briefly, PLGA was dissolved in dichloromethane followed by addition of approximate water or aqueous buffer desired. The emulsion was then formed by probe-ultrasonication in an ice bath. Fine droplets of polymer emulsion were formed in PVA solution by rapid injection of the emulsion into a stirred surfactant PVA solution. Dichloromethane was slowly evaporated from the PVA solution while the polymer beads were solidified during one day. The remaining solvent in the beads was finally removed by lyophilization during two days, and the dry beads were then stored at 4°C.

## Physical Analysis of Degradable Beads

The surface morphology of the degradable beads was examined by scanning electron microscopy (SEM) using a Cambridge S200 (LEO Electron Microscopy Inc., Thornwood, NY), operating at the accelerating voltage of 5 kV. The beads were sputter-coated with gold-paladium (60% and 40%) at a thickness of about 15 nm prior to acquisition of SEM images. The size distribution of degradable beads was determined by analyzing the SEM images. Alternatively, size distribution of the degradable beads was determined by laser-diffraction particle-size analysis on a Malvern Particle Analyzer (Malvern Instruments Inc., Southborough, MA).

## Collagen Coating of the Degradable Beads

Typically, dry PLGA beads were prewetted by dispersion into ethanol solution (10–25%) before being rinsed and then fully dispersed in coating buffer. Collagen was incubated with prewetted beads in either 10 mM acetic acid, PBS (pH 7) or carbonate buffer (pH 9.4) at 4°C or 37°C where indicated. The extent of collagen I coating on the polymer surface was determined by the immunochemical analysis of the binding of a monoclonal antibody against the triple helix of native collagen I (COL-1, C2456, Sigma Chemical, St Louis, MO.). This was followed by fluorescent staining with the binding of IgG-Alexa594 to the primary antibody (Molecular Probes, Eugene, OR). Cytodex-3® (Pharmacia) or RapidCell® (ICN Chemical) beads were used as controls with or without being coated further with collagen using the procedures of PLGA beads.

## HepG2 Cells and Adult Rodent Liver Cells

HepG2 cells were cultured on tissue culture flasks (T-75) until the cell density reached about $5 \times 10^6$ in a basal culture media (RPMI-1640, 5% fetal calf serum, penicillin, and streptomycin). The HepG2 cells at confluency were collected from the tissue culture plates by trypsin digestion. Adult rodent liver cells were isolated from adult male Sprague-Dawley rats (200–250 gms) by perfusion of collagenase using a protocol reported elsewhere.[36,37] Freshly isolated, unfractionated liver cells were resuspended in the basal culture media (RPMI-1640, 5% FCS, penicillin, and streptomycin) prior to being seeded with the PLGA beads or control beads. For monolayer cultures of adult rat liver cells, 35-mm tissue culture dishes were coated with type I collagen at a concentration of about $10 \,\mu g/cm^2$ prior to being used for cell seeding. The cell densities were about $5 \times 10^5$ ($5 \times 10^4/cm^2$) to $5 \times 10^6$ ($2.5 \times 10^5/cm^2$) cells per dish. The cells were typically suspended in the basal seeding media unless otherwise indicated. The basal seeding medium was replaced after 24 h with a serum-free hormonally defined media (HDM) containing: RMPI-1640, 100 µg/L penicillin, 100 µg/L streptomycin, 5 µg/ml insulin, 10 µg/ml high density lipoprotein, $1 \times 10^{-7}$ M selenium, 25 ng/ml EGF, and 10 µg/ml transferrin. The freshly isolated liver cells and HepG2 cells showed viabilities that routinely exceeded 90% as determined by Trypan blue exclusion assay.

## Seeding and Culture of Freshly Isolated Liver Cells with Degradable Beads

For seeding and culture of liver cells on collagen-coated degradable microbeads under stationary culture conditions, where specified, approximately $5 \times 10^5$ to $1 \times 10^6$ beads were incubated with about $1 \times 10^6$ to $2.5 \times 10^6$ liver cells in a 35-mm, uncoated bacterial culture dish first with the basal seeding media at 37°C, 5% $CO_2$ overnight. The media were then changed to HDM after 24 h. Cell viability was analyzed typically after the initial 24 h of seeding, and on the second day of culture where stated. Seeding of liver cells to collagen-coated degradable mesobeads was either in a 35-mm bacterial culture dish, using procedures similar to those described above, or in a orbital incubator-shaker as described below.

In the alternative, dynamic seeding procedure, seeding of liver cells to collagen-coated mesobeads was also carried out in an orbital incubator-shaker. The tissue culture flasks (T-25) were pretreated with 0.1% bovine serum albumin (BSA) to block cell adhesion to the culture flasks. Typically, cells and beads in basal seeding media were inoculated into the BSA-coated T-25 flasks. Seeding was allowed to proceed at 37°C overnight with continue orbital rotation at 25–35 rpm and inflow of humidified air mix of 15–20% $O_2$, 5% $CO_2$, and 75–80% $N_2$. Attachment of liver cells to the beads and cell viability were analyzed on the second day of culture.

## RESULTS

### Preparation and Physical Analysis of the Polymer Beads

At present commercially available microcarriers (e.g., Cytodex® of Pharmacia and Cultispher® of Percell Biolytica) are typically non-degradable and structurally rigid. They are suitable for three-dimensional culture of adherent dependent cells, such as cell lines and primarily adult cells, but not suitable for *ex vivo* culture of progenitor cells because of the rigid nature of the material and their non-porous surface morphology. They are not suitable for implantation of cells or for tissue organogenesis because of the non-degradable characteristics of the materials. To this end, porous PLGA microbeads and mesobeads were prepared by an ultrasonic atomization technique and by dispersion of polymer emulsion droplets in the presence of surfactant. Under the present protocols, more than 70% polymer mass was recovered typically from the preparation. PLGA beads prepared were amorphous. FIGURE 1A shows the scanning electron micrographs (SEM) of a representative population of porous degradable PLGA microbeads. The SEM micrograph shows the porous sur-

TABLE 1. Size distribution PLGA microbeads determined by electrozone sensing technique[a]

| Size range (μm) | 4.25–100 | 4.25–10 | 10–20 | 20–40 | 40–70 | 70–100 |
|---|---|---|---|---|---|---|
| Percentage of total count± SD ($n = 3$) | 94 ± 3 | 23 ± 6 | 10 ± 1 | 30 ± 1 | 19 ± 3 | 4 ± 1 |

[a]PLGA microbeads were prepared by ultrasonic atomization. The dry beads were rehydrated and suspended in isotonic buffer, Isoton. Particle counting was carried out with a Coulter Multisizer II. The suspension was continuously stirred to minimize the microbead sedimentation and clogging of a 200 μm-orifice tube during particle counting.

face of PLGA beads. However, surface pores are highly heterogeneous in size and shape. Confocal microscopy studies revealed the presence of both interconnecting and isolated internal pores (data not shown). In contrast to the porous structures of the PLGA beads, commercially available beads are typically non-porous (FIG. 1B).

TABLE 1 summarizes a representative size analysis of the PLGA microbeads prepared by the ultrasonic atomization procedure. This preparation yielded the major population within a range of diameters of 20–40 μm. The second largest population was within the diameter range of 2–10 μm. Note that the sum of fractional distribution for beads within the size of 4–100 μm was less than 100%. This is attributed to the presence of small debris of size less than 4 μm that were excluded from the total count by the instrument because of size sensitivity range limited by the aperture of the instrument.

### Degradation of PLGA Beads

We examined the macroscopic degradation of the PLGA (RG504) microbeads in solution. FIGURE 2 shows the SEM images of PLGA microbeads incubated in PBS at 37°C over: (A) 4.5 days, (B) 9.5 days, (C) 20 days, and (D) 28 days, respectively. The porous surface structure was clearly evident after 4.5 days in aqueous incubation, but become gradually less evident as a result of increased surface erosion upon prolonged hydrolytic degradation. The initial surface erosion was followed by major structural degradation as shown by the *melting* of the partially degraded polymer on day 28 of incubation. This is consistent with studies of the degradation of PLGA scaffolds in other physical forms.[38,39] In comparison with the degradation of the PLGA (RG504) beads shown above, the degradation of microbeads of an analogous polymer containing terminal carboxylation (RG504H) showed a marked acceleration of the degradation shown by the surface erosion on day 5, followed by complete *melting* of the polymer beads on day 20 (data not shown). The accelerated degradation is consistent with earlier studies of the polymer in powder form.[40] This is attributed to the increase in acid catalysis upon terminal carboxylation.[40]

### Coating of Collagen on Surface of the Degradable Beads

In the present study, the degradable beads were incubated with either collagen type I or IV in acidic solution to allow adsorption of soluble collagen onto the surface of polymer beads. Alternatively, beads were incubated with the collagen in neutralized solution in which collagen formed a gel in solution and on the surface of degradable beads. Immunochemical staining of collagen-coated beads by a monoclonal antibody against the native form of collagen in conjunction with a secondary antibody, IgG-Alexa594, showed intense fluorescence (image not shown here), indicating the presence of the native collagen I on the polymer surface. In addition, collagen-coated beads appeared to disperse well in comparison with a suspension of uncoated PLGA beads. The protein *reconditioning* of the polymer surface by collagen coating might have altered the surface hydrophobic properties of PLGA beads, resulting in a more hydrophilic surface and better dispersion of the coated beads in aqueous solution.

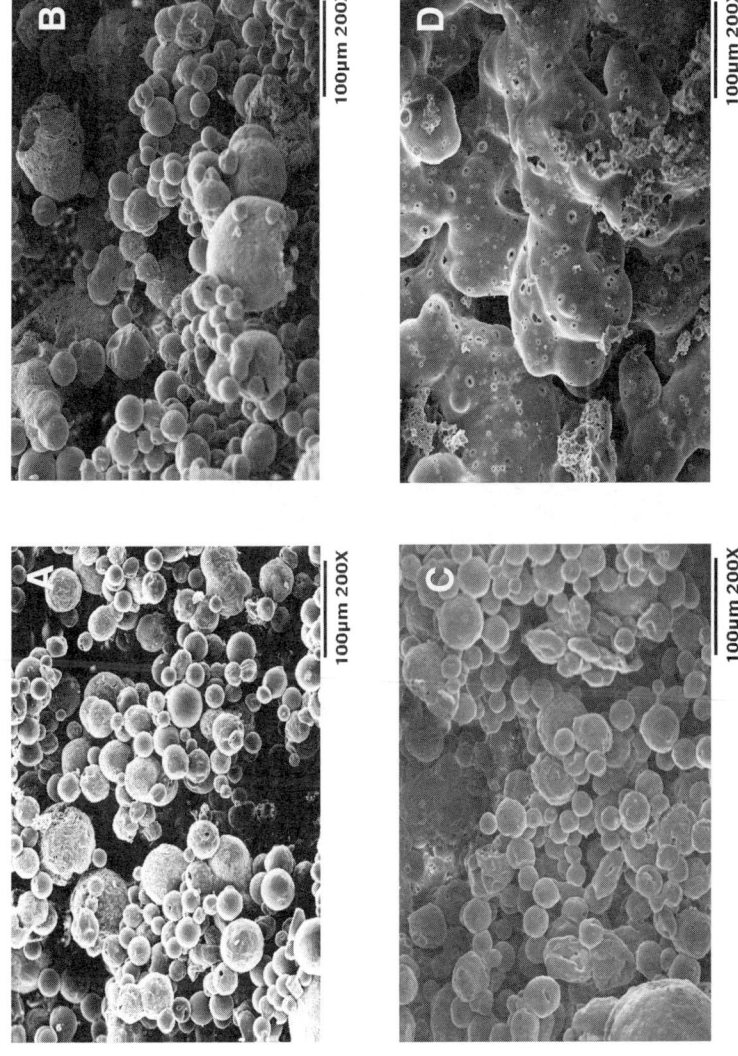

**FIGURE 2.** SEM images of the poly(D,L-lactide-co-glycolite) microbeads incubated in phosphate-buffered saline at 37°C over (**A**) 4.5 days, (**B**) 9.5 days, (**C**) 20 days, and (**D**) 28 days.

## Culture of Liver Cells Using Degradable Beads

To evaluate the suitability of the degradable microbeads as a substratum support for *ex vivo* culture of liver cells, we investigated the attachment of HepG2 cells and adult rodent liver cells to collagen-coated degradable beads. FIGURE 3 shows the phase contrast image of HepG2 cells cultured with type IV collagen-coated degradable microbeads. The extensive attachment of the HepG2 cells to the collagen-coated beads is evident. Note that the bright images are those of HepG2 cells, whereas the dark images are those of the degradable beads resulting from the amorphous characteristics of the beads. Not only did the HepG2 cells attach extensively to the beads, but they also appeared to spread on the bead surface. Staining with the viability dye Calcein AM showed intense green fluorescence within the cells, indicating that the cells attached to the beads were mostly viable cells (image not shown). This is consistent with the 70–80% viability determined by using Trypan exclusion assay of trypsin-digested cells. HepG2 cells attached to the beads and continued to grow, forming aggregates consisting of multiple beads plus HepG2 cells by the third day of culture (image not shown). By providing the HepG2 cells with three-dimensional substrata in the form of collagen-coated beads, the formation of three-

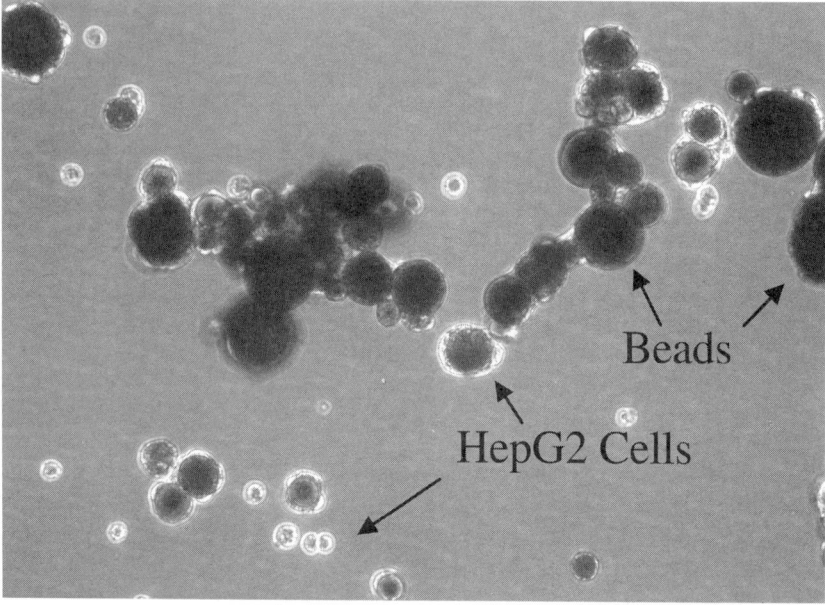

**FIGURE 3.** Phase contrast micrographs showing HepG2 cells cultured with collagen type IV-coated poly (D,L-lactide-co-glycolite) microbeads. The type IV collagen was derived from the EHS tumor. The microbeads were incubated with about 22-μg collagen IV/mg beads at 4°C and neutral pH. The ratio of HepG2:beads was about $3.3 \times 10^4$ HepG2/mg beads. The *darker images* are those of the beads, whereas the *bright contrasts* are the images of HepG 2 cells. The micrograph was taken at approximately 24 h after seeding of HepG2 cells with the beads.

dimensional aggregates of cells and substrata is facilitated. In contrast, culturing of HepG2 cells in the conventional two-dimensional tissue culture dish resulted in formation of monolayers of HepG2 cells with little evidence of formation of three-dimensional cell aggregates.

To determine whether the collagen-coated degradable beads are suitable for culture and expansion of primary liver cells, we first investigated the adhesion of unfractionated adult rodent liver cells to collagen-coated PLGA beads. Type I collagen (about 22 µg/mg) formed a gel in a suspension of degradable mesobeads at pH of about 7, at 37°C overnight, leaving a collagen coating on the surface of the beads. Excess collagen gelled in solution was routinely rinsed off before the beads were used for culture with rodent liver cells.

Seeding of cells onto a tissue culture plate puts the cells into direct physical contact with the plate or coated matrix, once cells sediment onto the plate surface. However, seeding of cells onto beads or other three-dimensional scaffolds requires facilitated initial physical contact between cells and the scaffold substrata.[41–43] To increase and facilitate the initial physical contact of the liver cells to the type I collagen gel-coated beads, seeding was carried out with constant gentle rocking of the

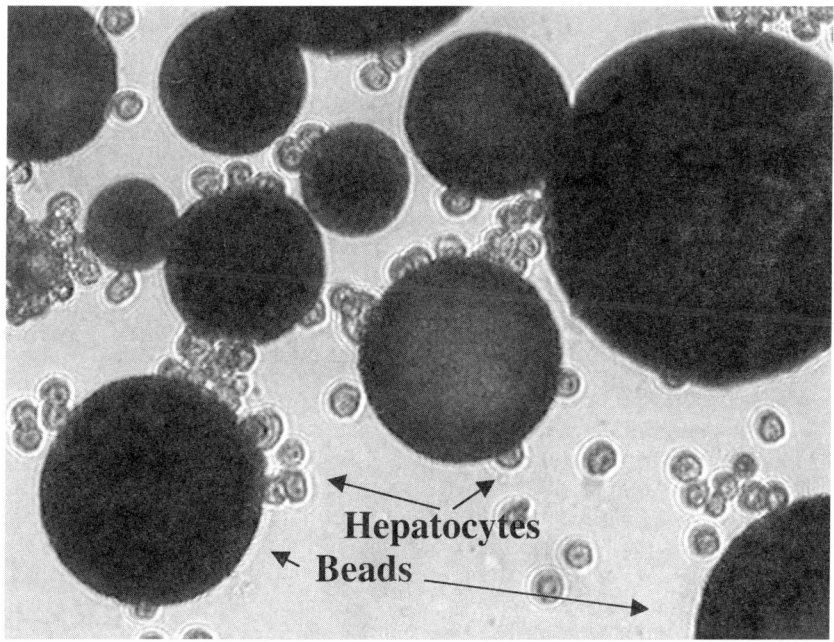

**FIGURE 4.** Phase contrast micrograph of adult rodent liver cells cultured in collagen type I-coated poly (D,L-lactide-co-glycolite) mesobeads. The degradable beads were preincubated with rat tail collagen type I (about 25 µg collagen/mg beads) at pH 7 and 37°C overnight before seeding with liver cells. Initial seeding and cell attachment were carried out at 37°C with 15% $O_2$, 5% $CO_2$, and 80% $N_2$ with rotary mixing at 35 rpm. The image was obtained at about 24 h after seeding of liver cells with the beads.

culture vessels. This is achieved in a 0.1% BSA-treated tissue culture T-25 flask placed in a continuous rotational shaker operating at 25–35 rpm. Humidified gas mix of 15–20% $O_2$, 5% $CO_2$, and 75–80% $N_2$ was supplied continuously to the flasks. FIGURE 4 shows phase contrast image of the rodent hepatocytes seeded with collagen I-coated PLGA mesobeads. It is evident the liver cells attached to the collagen-coated surface with some cells appearing to spread. However, attachment was heterogeneous with respect to the number of cells attaching to each bead. Furthermore, there was also attachment of liver cells to each other, forming multicell aggregates with or without attachment to the beads. Viability staining using Calcein AM revealed the attached cells mostly as viable cells (fluorescent image not shown).

## DISCUSSION

Extant forms of microcarriers used for culture of adherence-dependent cells are typically rigid and non-degradable (e.g., Cytodex-3®, RapidCell®, and Cytospheres® beads). These non-degradable beads have proven successful for mature cell types such as liver cells,[28] but do not work for progenitors and are, in general, not designed for tissue organogenesis and tissue engineering application. The use of porous degradable beads as synthetic substrata for liver cell cultures has not been thoroughly explored. We hypothesize that a soft and porous degradable scaffold coated with suitable natural matrix components may resemble more the physicochemical properties of a natural substratum for the cells. Hence, it might be a more suitable hybrid substratum for *ex vivo* growth of adherent cells, for example liver cells and especially liver progenitor cells. With the controllable degradation of biodegradable scaffolds, it is postulated that culturing of liver cells or liver progenitor cells (or other adherent cell types) on degradable beads may allow the aggregates of cells–substratum–beads to be transplanted into recipients without the need to isolate the cells from substratum or to remove the synthetic materials. The use of biocompatible and biodegradable materials may also provide an important avenue for incorporating and controlling released proteins and other bioactive factors (e.g., vascular endothelial growth factors, VEGF) critical to the formation of tissue vasculature.[32]

Under the present conditions, degradable microcarriers formed show heterogeneous morphology of porous surface. The mechanism for the formation of the pores was not investigated in this study. However, it is suspected that the pores formed during the melting of the non-polymer solvent and the extraction of the frozen polymer solvent, leaving behind pores of various dimensions in the microbeads prepared by the ultrasonic atomization method. Where the degradable beads were formed by extraction of melting polymer solvent from droplets of polymer emulsion, the pores formed probably as the void volume of the solvent. Since the emulsion droplets were not hardened instantly when they came in contact with the PVA solution, concentration and solidification of the polymer in the emulsion droplets may have occurred during the slow extraction of solvent from the polymer emulsion, thus leaving behind smaller pores throughout the mesobeads. Further study is needed to ascertain the exact mechanisms behind the formation of the porous structures.

The hydrolytic degradation of PLGA polymers is an acid-catalyzed reaction by which the ester bonds linking the monomer lactic and glycolic monomers are hydrolyzed.[38,39]

The rate of PLGA degradation depends on the fractional composition of the two monomers, lactic acid, and glycolic acid, with faster degradation of the copolymer with an increase of the fractional composition of glycolic acid.[38,39] Environmental factors such as pH and temperature are also critical to the degradation. Low pH and higher temperature often leads to increased rate of degradation. Furthermore, it also depends on the physical properties of the polymer scaffolds: greater surface area and thus exposure of the polymeric materials in aqueous solution often leads to greater surface erosion and overall degradation. The degradation of the present porous microcarriers in a period up to 28 days was consistent with other studies reported elsewhere.[38,39] Terminal carboxylation led to a marked acceleration of the degradation, similar to that of the polymer in powder form.[40]

PLGA polymers are non-charged and hydrophobic. Synthetic surfaces of PLGA typically interact unfavorably for cell adhesion primarily because of the lack of cell binding, matrix domains (e.g., peptides containing an RGD sequence) to associate with cell surface receptors. Seeding of HepG2 and unfractionated rodent-primary-liver cells on uncoated PLGA microcarriers did not lead to significant attachment of the cells (results not shown). Coating of polyvinyl alcohol has been used to improve the hydrophilicity and attachment by liver cells.[27] To provide a scaffold surface favorable for cell adhesion, synthetic surfaces are often coated physically or chemically with a layer of natural matrix components or presented with peptides with cell binding domains and derived from natural matrix components to facilitate association with cell surface receptors. Those approaches create hybrid surfaces that may possess not only desirable surface physical properties, such as surface area and pore volume of a synthetic scaffold, but also the matrix chemistry suitable for cell adhesion, survival, and growth or differentiation under defined conditions. Immunochemical staining using an antibody against native form of type I collagen showed the presence of collagen coating of the surface of microcarriers. Gelling of type I collagen on the polymer surface only led to presence of highly uneven coating of the collagen. Physical adsorption of soluble collagen in acidic solution resulted in the formation of a more uniform layer of collagen. No further chemical crosslinking of the adsorbed collagen was necessary prior to attachment of the HepG2 or adult rodent liver cells to the collagen-coated microcarriers under the present condition.

To evaluate suitability of the porous degradable beads for three-dimensional culture and expansion of progenitor liver cells, transformed cell lines, such as HepG2, were used as models of transformed progenitor cells in this study. HepG2 cells are capable of expansion under *in vitro* conditions.[30] Mature adult liver cells, especially the polyploid liver cells, have little growth potential under normal culture conditions and are used to study highly differentiated functions (reviewed in Refs. 2 and 13). Only diploid adult cells are capable of extensive hyperplastic growth and only under highly specific *ex vivo* culture conditions.[1] The HepG2 cells seeded on the degradable microcarriers underwent extensive growth, forming colonies or aggregates of multiple cells and microcarriers. The collagen-coated microcarriers provided the three-dimensional substratum support critical to the formation of the three-dimensional aggregates.

Unfractionated cell suspensions of rodent liver cells have been seeded onto collagen-coated degradable PLGA sponges[27] where limited differentiated functions were observed under *in vitro* conditions. Primary cultures of porcine liver cells attached to non-degradable Cytodex-3 beads have been inoculated into bioreactors to form bioartificial liver assist devices.[28,29] With the use of intermittent shaking during cell seeding with the beads, Foy et al.[41] reported attachment efficiency for rodent liver cells to Cytodex-3 beads close to 100 cells per bead. Stockmann et al.[42] were able to establish the attachment at about 130 hepatocytes per Cytodex-3 bead under similar conditions. The density of cells and beads, oxygen diffusion, and conditions of shaking are all critical to the cell attachment with Cytodex-3 beads.[41] In the present study, the density of liver cells at seeding ranged from approximately $6 \times 10^4/cm^2$ to $3 \times 10^5/cm^2$, a density significantly lower than the about $5 \times 10^5$ cells/cm$^2$ reported. The fewer attachments found under the present seeding density is consistent with those shown by Foy et al.,[41] where under their conditions of optimal oxygen concentration and shaking, there were very few attached cells at a seeding density below about $3 \times 10^5/cm^2$. In the present study, oxygen concentrations varied from 15% to 20%, a concentration substantially lower than that (75%) used in an early study.[41] A decrease of oxygen concentration leads to substantially fewer attachments of cells to Cytodex-3 beads.[41] Thus, the supply of oxygen at lower concentration in the present study might have been another factor for optimization to increase the number of cells attached to the beads.

In comparison with the number of liver cells attached to the PLGA beads, more liver cells appeared to attach to type I collagen-coated Cytodex-3 beads under the same dynamic seeding conditions (image not shown). However, very few liver cells were found to attach to Cytodex-3 beads without being further coated with collagen. One likely explanation for this discrepancy between the results of Cytodex-3 and PLGA beads is the quantitative difference of collagen available on the surface of the beads. It is possible that more collagen might be deposited on the surface of Cytodex-3 beads under the present coating conditions given the presence of crosslinked collagen on the untreated Cytodex-3 surface. This might explain the greater number of cells attached to the coated Cytodex-3 beads than either collagen-coated PLGA or untreated Cydex-3 beads.

Adsorption of a thin layer of type I collagen at alkali pH (pH > 9) has been used to coat polylactide polymeric matrixes for seeding of liver cells.[26] In this study, a similar protocol was used to coat the PLGA and Cytodex-3 beads. However, there was little attachment of viable liver cells to the degradable beads. In contrast, relatively more liver cells were found to attach to the Cytodex-3 beads coated under the conditions specified in the methods. A likely explanation for this discrepancy is that possibly little, if any, collagen was adsorbed by the degradable beads under the present coating conditions. The attachment of the liver cells to the Cytodex-3 beads was most likely through attachment to the collagen I covalently presented on the surface of Cytodex-3 beads.

In summary, we have successfully prepared porous degradable PLGA microbeads and mesobeads, and here explored preliminarily several conditions for attachment of cells of a cell line, HepG2, and freshly isolated rat liver cells to collagen-coated PLGA beads. Although liver cells were found to attach to the PLGA beads and remained viable during the course of seeding, the overall efficiency of liver cell attachment can be improved. A number of factors might be optimized further to achieve this goal. These are: (1) a stable layer adsorbed/coated collagen on the surface of hydrophobic polymer beads, (2) optimization of seeding density cells and beads, (3) oxygen concentration, and (4) use of intermittent shaking or other physical methods to improve initial physical contact between cells and matrix. Studies are ongoing to finalize the development of the microcarriers and optimal coating with appropriate extracellular matrix components prior to testing their efficacy with normal hepatic progenitors of rodent and human origin.

## ACKNOWLEDGMENTS

This work is supported, in part, by a grant to LMR (NIH 1-RO1-DK52851) from the National Institute of Diabetes and Digestive and Kidney Diseases (NIDDK) and a sponsored research grant from Renaissance Cell Technology, Inc, a wholly owned subsidiary of Incara Pharmaceuticals, Inc. We thank Dr. J.J. LeMasters and Sherry Franklin of the Center for Gastrointestinal and Biliary Disease Biology (CGIBD) for generously providing the isolated rodent liver cells. We thank Drs. Anthony Hickey, Tom Luntz and Nicholas Moss for fruitful discussions and Jane Bowen for technical assistance in some of the experiments. Jane Bowen was supported in part by a training grant (5 T35 DK07386) from the NIDDK. We also thank Dr. B. Bagnell for expert assistance with the SEM study, Dr. M. Louey for assistance with the laser diffraction experiments, and Cynthia Lodestro for lab management assistance.

## REFERENCES

1. KUBOTA, H. & L.M. REID. 2000. Clonogenic hepatoblasts, common precursors for hepatocytic and biliary lineages, are lacking classical major histocompatibility complex class I antigen. Proc. Natl. Acad. Sci. USA **97:** 12132–12137.
2. XU, A.S., T.L. LUNTZ, J.M. MACDONALD, et al. 2000. Lineage biology and liver. In Principles of Tissue Engineering. R. Lanza, R. Langer & J. Vacanti, Eds.: 559–598. Academic Press, San Diego.
3. LANGER, R. 1999. Selected advances in drug delivery and tissue engineering. J. Control Release. **62:** 7–11.
4. MARLER, J.J., J. UPTON, R. LANGER & J.P. VACANTI. 1998. Transplantation of cells in matrices for tissue regeneration. Adv. Drug Del. Rev. **33:** 165–182.
5. PETERS, M.C. & D.J. MOONEY. 1997. Synthetic extracellular matrices for cell transplantation. Mater. Sci. Forum. **250:** 43–52.
6. THEISE N.D., R. SAXENA, B.C. PORTMANN, et al. 1999. The canals of Hering and hepatic stem cells in humans. Hepatology **30:** 1425–1433.
7. MARTINEZ-HERNANDEZ, A. & P.S. AMENTA. 1993. Morphology, localization and origin of the hepatic extracellular matrix. In Extracellular Matrix: Its Chemistry, Biology and Pathobiology. M. Zern & L.M. Reid, Eds.: 255–330. Marcel Dekker, Inc., New York.
8. SPRAY, D.C., M. FUJITA, J.C. SAEZ, et al. 1987. Proteoglycans and glycosaminoglycans induce gap junction synthesis and function in primary liver cultures. J. Cell. Biol. **105:** 541–551.
9. INGBER, D.E. & J. FOLKMAN. 1989. Mechanochyemical switching between growth and differentiation during fibroblast growth factor-stimulated angiogenesis in vitro: role of extracellular matrix. J. Cell Biol. **109:** 317–330.
10. REID, L.M. 1990. Stem cell biology, hormone/matrix synergies and liver differentiation. Curr. Opin. Cell Biol. **2:** 121–130.
11. ZVIBEL, I., E. HALAY & L.M. REID. 1991. Heparin/hormonal regulation of autocrine growth factor mRNA synthesis and abundance: relevance to clonal growth of tumors. Mol. Cell. Biol. **11:** 108–116.

12. SINGHVI, R., G. STEPHANOPOULOS & D.I.C. WANG. 1993. Review: effects of substratum morphology on cell physiology. Biotech. Bioeng. **43:** 764–771.
13. BRILL, S., I. ZVIBEL & L.M. REID. 1995. Maturation-dependent changes in the regulation of liver-specific gene expression in embryonal versus adult primary liver. Differentiation **59:** 95–102.
14. MOONEY, D., L. HANSEN, J. VACANTI, et al. 1992. Switching from differentiation to growth in hepatocytes: control by extracellular matrix. J. Cell. Physiol. **151:** 497–505.
15. POWERS, M.J., R.E. RODRIGUEZE & L.G. GRIFFITH. 1997. Cell-substratum adhesion strength as determinant of hepatocyte aggregate morphology. Biotech. Bioeng. **53:** 415–426.
16. POWERS, M.J. & L. GRIFFITH-CIMA. 1996. Motility behavior of hepatocytes on extracellular matrix substrata during aggregation. Biotech. Bioeng. **50:** 392–403.
17. POWERS, M.J. & L.G. GRIFFITH. 1998. Adhesion-guided *in vitro* morphogenesis in pure and mixed cell culture. Microscopy Res. Tech. **43:** 379–384.
18. RANUCCI, C.S. & P.V. MOGHE. 1999. Polymer substrate topography actively regulated the multicellular organization and liver-specific functions of cultured hepatocytes. Tissue Eng. **5:** 407–419.
19. ENAT. R., D.M. JEFFERSON, N. RUIZ-OPAZO, et al. 1984. Hepatocyte proliferation *in vitro*: its dependence on the use of serum-free, hormonally defined medium and substrata of extracellular matrix. PNAS USA **81:** 1411–1415.
20. DOERR, R., I. ZVIBEL, D. CHIUTEN, et al. 1989. Clonal growth of tumors on tissue-specific biomatrices and correlation with organ site specificity of metastases. Cancer Res. **49:** 384–392.
21. ROJKIND, M., Z. GATMAITAN, S. MACKENSEN, et al. 1980. Connective tissue biomatrix: its isolation and utilization for long-term cultures of normal rat hepatocytes. J. Cell Biol. **87:** 255–263.
22. SIELAFF, T.D., S.L. NYBERG, M.D. ROLLINS, et al. 1997. Characterization of the three-compartment gel-entrapment procine hepatocyte bioartificial liver. Cell Biol. Toxic. **13:** 357–364.
23. NYBER, S.L., SHIRABE, K., M.V. PESHWA, et al. 1993. Extracorporeal application of a gel-entrapment, bioartificial liver: demonstration of drug metabolism and other biochemical functions. Cell Transplant. **2:** 441–452.
24. MOGHE, P.V., R.N. COGER, M. TONER & M.L. YARMUSH. 1997. Cell-cell interactions are essential for maintenance of hepatocytes' function in collagen gel but not on matrigel. Biotech. Bioeng. **56:** 706–711.
25. LECLUYSE, E., A. MADAN, G. HAMILTON, et al. 2000. Expression and regulation of cytochrome P450 enzymes in primary cultures of human hepatocytes. J. Biochem. Mol. Toxic. **14:** 117–188.
26. KAUFMANN, P.M., S. HEIMRATH, B.S. KIM & D.J. MOONEY. 1997. Highly porous polymer matrices as three-dimensional culture system for hepatocyte. Cell Transplant. **6:** 463–468.
27. MOONEY, D.J., K. SANO, P.M. KAUFMANN, et al. 1997. Long-term engraftment of hepatocytes transplanted on biodegradable polymer sponges. J. Biomed. Mater. Res. **37:** 413–420.
28. DEMETRIOU, A.A., A. REISNER, J. SANCHEZ, et al. 1988. Transplantation of microcarrier-attached hepatocytes into 90% partially hepatectomized rats. Hepatology **8:** 1006–1009.
29. MULLON, C. & B.A. SOLOMON. 2000. HepatAssist liver support system. *In* Principles of Tissue Engineering. R. Lanza, R. Langer & J. Vacanti, Eds.: 553–558. Academic Press, San Diego.
30. SIGAL, S.H., S. BRILL, L.M. REID, et al. 1994. Characterization and enrichment of fetal rat hepatoblasts by immunoadsorption ("panning") and fluorescence-activated cell sorting. Hepatology **19:** 999–1006.
31. SIGAL, S.H., S. GUPTA, D.F. GEBHARD, JR., et al. 1995. Evidence for a terminal differentiation process in the rat liver. Differentiation **59:** 35–42.

32. SHERIDAN, M.H., L.D. SHEA, M.C. PETERS & D.J. MOONEY. 2000. Bioadsorable polymer scaffolds for tissue engineering capable of sustained growth factor delivery. J. Control Release **64:** 91–102.
33. GRIFFITH, L.G. 2000. Polymeric Biomaterials. Acta Mater. **48:** 263–277.
34. ZVIBEL, I., A. FIORINO, S. BRILL & L.M. REID. 1998. Phenotypic characterization of hepatoma cell lines and lineage-specific regulation of gene expression by differentiation agents. Differentiation **63:** 215–223.
35. KHAN, M.A., M.S. HEALY & H. BERNSTEIN. 1992. Low temperature fabrication of protein loaded micropheres. Proceed. Intern. Symp. Control. Rel. Bioact. Mater. **19:** 518–519.
36. HERMAN, B., A.-L. NIEMINEN, G.J. GORES & J.J. LEMASTERS. 1988. Irreversible injury in anoxic hepatocytes precipitated by an abrupt increase in plasma membrane permeability. FASEB J. **2:** 146–151.
37. NIEMINEN, A.-L., A.K. SAYLOR, B. HERMAN & J.J. LEMASTERS. 1994. ATP depletion rather than mitochondrial depolarization mediates hepatocyte killing after metabolic inhibition. Am. J. Physiol. **267:** C67–C74.
38. PARK, T.G. 1995. Degradation of poly(lactic-co-glycolic acid) microspheres: effect of copolymer composition. Biomaterials **16:** 1123–1130.
39. GRIZZI, I., H. GARREAU, S. LI & M. VERT. 1995. Hydrolytic degradation of devices based on poly(DL-lactic acid) size-dependence. Biomaterials **16:** 305–311.
40. TRACY, M.A., L. FIROUZABADIN & Y. ZHANG. 1995. Effects of PLGA end groups on degradation. Proc. Intern. Symp. Control. Rel. Bioact. Mater. 786–787.
41. FOY, B., J. LEE, J. MORGAN, *et al.* 1993. Optimization of hepatocyte attachment to microcarriers: importance of oxygen. Biotech. Bioeng. **42:** 579–588.
42. STOCKMANN, H., R.G. TOMPKINS & F. BERTHIAUME. 1997. Expression of long-term liver-specific function by adult rat hepatocytes cultured on microcarriers. Tissue Eng. **3:** 267–279.
43. KIM, S.S., C.A. SUNDBACK, S. KAIHARA, *et al.* 2000. Dynamic seeding and *in vitro* culture of hepatocytes in a flow perfusion system. Tissue Eng. **6:** 39–44.

# Pectin-Based Microspheres

## A Preformulatory Study

ELISABETTA ESPOSITO,[a] RITA CORTESI,[a] GIOVANNI LUCA,[b] AND CLAUDIO NASTRUZZI[b]

[a]*Dipartimento di Scienze Farmaceutiche, Università di Ferrara, Ferrara, Italy*

[b]*Dipartimento di Chimica e Tecnologia del Farmaco, Università di Perugia, Italy*

> ABSTRACT: This paper reports on (a) the production of pectin microspheres and (b) the influence of different experimental parameters and ionic crosslinking on morphological and dimensional characteristics of pectin microspheres. Morphological and dimensional characteristics of pectin were analyzed as a function of the type of pectin, the dispersing phase, the stirring speed, and the emulsifying agent. Crosslinking by calcium chloride and the encapsulation of antibiotics (i.e., metronidazol and tetracycline) gave particles morphologically similar to empty particles but with slower swelling kinetic.
>
> KEYWORDS: pectin; microspheres; morphology; dimension

## INTRODUCTION

Microsphere-based formulations have been proposed for the treatment of several diseases that require either a constant drug concentration in the blood or drug targeted to specific cells or organs.[1] Additionally, microspheres can be used to treat diseases that require a sustained concentration of the drug at several anatomical sites. In this respect, the direct relationship between route of administration and particle size needs to be considered.[2] For instance, microspheres with diameters in the range 20–100 μm can be optimally employed for subcutaneous or intramuscular administration since they are retained in the interstitial tissue, acting as sustained release depots. Smaller microparticles have been proposed for the treatment of infection, allergy, and arthritis because of their capability of achieving discrete compartments (e.g., eye, lung, and joints).[2]

Natural polymers, such as pectin and gelatin, can be used to produce biocompatible and biodegradable microparticles, obviating the toxicity or biodegradability problems (i.e., formation of localized granulomatous inflammation) possibly related to the use of synthetic materials.[3] Pectin in particular, due to its interesting features, such as hydrophilicity, biocompatibility, and biodegradability, has been proposed for the production of pharmaceutical formulations intended for controlled drug delivery.[4–6]

---

Address for correspondence: Prof. Claudio Nastruzzi, Ph.D., Associated Professor in Pharmaceutics, University of Perugia, Dipartimento di Chimica e Tecnologia del Farmaco, via del Liceo, 06100 Perugia, Italy. Voice: +39-075-5852057; fax: +39-075-5847469.

nas@unipg.it <web www.unipg.it>

Pectin is a polysaccharide obtained by aqueous extraction from citrus peel or from apple pomace. It mainly consists of galactopyranosyluronic units partially esterified with methanol. The ratio between esterified and free acid groups of pectin, defined as *degree of esterification* (DE), is an important factor influencing different properties of pectin, such as solubility and ability to form gels. As a function of DE, pectin can be classified as *high methyl* (HM) or *low methyl* (LM) according to whether the DE is higher or lower than 50%, respectively. Pectin was recently proposed as biopolymer for the production of colonic drug delivery devices. For instance, pectin-based matrix tablets and the combination of pectin with commercially available aqueous polymer dispersion have recently been described as formulations for colonic drug delivery.[7-10]

Pectin has the disadvantage of swelling and dissolving rather rapidly in aqueous environments, making difficult the use of this polymer for the production of long-acting delivery systems. This adverse aspect requires the use of crosslinking procedures (e.g., calcium chloride) able to reduce polymer dissolution and drug release at body temperature. Pectin gelation is based on the formation of a three-dimensional network. In particular, HM pectins produce gel in acid- and sugar-containing systems, whereas LM pectins form gels with divalent cations, like calcium, through the formation of "egg-box" structures.[11]

The aims of this paper were to explore (1) the production of microspheres based on different pectins by an emulsion–dehydration procedure, (2) the influence of experimental parameters on morphological and dimensional characteristics of microspheres, (3) the evaluation of the effect of chemical crosslinking on microsphere morphology, and (4) the evaluation of drug encapsulation in pectin microspheres, using metronidazol or tetracycline as model antibiotics.

## MATERIALS AND METHODS

### Materials

Tetracycline hydrochloride and metronidazol were obtained from Sigma Chemical Co. (St. Louis, Missouri, USA) and from Fluka Chemical Co. (Buchs, Switzerland). Microspheres were prepared using various pectins (see TABLE 1). Sorbitan monolaurate (Span 20), sorbitan monooleate (Span 80), and sorbitan trioleate (Span 85) were purchased from Fluka. All other materials and solvents were from Fluka and were of the highest purity available.

### Microsphere Preparation

Empty pectin particles were produced by an emulsion–dehydration technique. In brief: 10 ml of a 5% (w/v) aqueous pectin solution were added, at 70°C, to 40 g of an oil phase alternatively constituted of mineral oil, mais oil, or isostearylisostearate. In some cases surfactants were used. In particular, Span 20, 80, and 85 were added in different amounts to the oil phase. The mixture was mechanically stirred under turbulent flow conditions (stirring speed between 500 and 1,500 rpm) to form a water–oil emulsion; after five minutes the solution was rapidly cooled at 15°C and

TABLE 1. Type of pectin used to prepare microspheres

| Name | Trade Name | Producer[a] | Origin | DE (%) |
|---|---|---|---|---|
| PHM slow set | Unipectine SS 150 | SKW BIOSYSTEM | apple pomace | 60–66 |
| PHM rapid set | Unipectine RS 150 | SKW BIOSYSTEM | apple pomace | 70–74 |
| PHM medium rapid set | Unipectine MRS 150 | SKW BIOSYSTEM | apple pomace | 66–70 |
| PHM medium rapid set | Unipectine MRS 160 ND | SKW BIOSYSTEM | citrus peels | 66–70 |
| PLM | | SIGMA | apple pomace | 7.8 |
| PLM | | SIGMA | citrus peels | 10 |
| PLM | | SKW BIOSYSTEM | fruit | 34–40 |

[a]SKW BIOSYSTEM (Novate Milanese, Italy), SIGMA (St. Louis, Missouri, USA).

then, 50 ml of acetone were added in order to dehydrate the pectin droplets. The pectin particles were isolated from the suspension by filtration through a syntered glass filter. The removal of residual oil was performed by washing the microspheres with $3 \times 80$-ml aliquots of acetone. In the case of drug-containing particles, 100 mg of tetracycline hydrochloride or 40 mg of metronidazol were added to the aqueous pectin solution. The preparation of pectin particles was then performed as described above.

### Ionic Crosslinking of Pectin Particles

The microsphere crosslinking was performed by using two alternative procedures, as described below.

In Situ *Method*

In this case, the hardening was accomplished during microsphere production one minute after the formation of the emulsion. One ml of $CaCl_2$ (1 M or 2 M), added to the emulsion, was maintained, under stirring, for five minutes at 70°C. The preparation of pectin particles was then performed as described above.

*Postproduction Method*

Following isolation, dried particles were poured into 5 ml of $CaCl_2$ (1 M or 2 M) for 30 or 180 min. In order to reduce particle swelling, a mixture of ethanol and water 9:1 (w/w) was used to solubilize $CaCl_2$.

### Microsphere Morphological Analysis

The morphology of pectin particles was evaluated by optical microscopy (Nikon Diaphot inverted microscope, Tokyyo, Japan) and scanning electron microscopy (SEM) observations (360 Stereoscan Cambridge Instruments Ltd, Cambridge, UK). Microsphere size and volume distributions were determined by photomicrograph analysis.

## Swelling Tests

The swelling characteristics of untreated or ionically crosslinked pectin particles were determined in a hydrophilic gel prepared by dispersing carboxymethyl cellulose sodium salt (CMC) (4%, w/v) in water at room temperature. This process resulted in the formation of a homogeneous gel with a viscosity of 13,600 cps. The kinetics of the increase of the initial diameter of particles was studied by using an optical microscope equipped with a micrometric device. The swelling ratio $q$ was calculated according to Equation (1) by measuring the diameter of pectin particles, assuming a spherical geometry for each particle.

$$q = V_s/V_d, \tag{1}$$

where $V_s$ and $V_d$ are the volume of the swollen microspheres and of the dried microspheres, respectively.

## Drug Content of Pectin Particles

The amount of encapsulated tetracycline hydrochloride, or metronidazol, per mg of dried microspheres, was determined by suspending 100 mg of microspheres in 5 ml of water at room temperature under magnetic stirring for two hours. The solution obtained was filtered with a μStar filter 0.22 μm (Costar, Cambridge, UK) and then analyzed by UV at 357 and 276 nm determining the tetracycline hydrochloride and metronidazol content, respectively.

## RESULTS AND DISCUSSION

### Microsphere Preparation

Pectin particles were prepared via an emulsion–dehydration technique, as described in MATERIALS AND METHODS. Choice and adjustment of the manufacturing parameters for the production of microspheres of defined size were made in agreement with the following equation[12]

$$d \propto K \frac{D_v R v_a \gamma}{D_s N v_o C_s}, \tag{2}$$

where $d$ is the average particle size, $K$ is a variable depending on the apparatus geometry (e.g., type and dimension of stirrer), $D_v$ and $D_s$ are the diameter of the vessel and of the stirrer, respectively, $R$ is the volume ratio between aqueous and oil phases, $v_a$ and $v_o$ their respective viscosities, $N$ is the stirring speed, $\gamma$ is the surface tension between the two immiscible phases, and $C_s$ is the stabilizer concentration.

With the aim of producing microparticles with variable dimensions, able to regulate drug release through a differential dissolution rate, the effect of different experimental parameters on particle size were investigated. Overall, good results were obtained by using the following experimental parameters: a 50-mm diameter vessel, a 35-mm, 4-blade turbine rotor, and a volume ratio of pectin solution to oil phase of 0.2. Various pectins were considered for microparticle production, including both high and low methyl pectins as well as pectins extractated from apple and citrus (see TABLE 1 for the complete list of pectins employed). In addition, other variables, such as type of oil phase, stirring speed, and surfactant type and concentration were analysed. In the following sections the effects of these variables on morphological characteristics, and the recovery efficiency of pectin microspheres, are described.

### Type of Oil Phase

The choice of the oil phase was found to play an important role on both the dimensions of microspheres, their recovery, and on the prevention of aggregate formation. As is reported in TABLE 2, the use of isostearylisostearate (viscosity of 30 mPa.s at 20°C) resulted in the production of microparticles with no aggregation phenomena (see FIGURE 1), whereas the other external phases tested, such as mais or paraffin oil, caused the formation of large particle aggregates.

### Pectin Type and Concentration

Various pectins were considered for their ability to form particles for pharmaceutical applications. In general, high methyl pectins were found to be inadequate in forming particles, invariably resulting in the formation of (1) particles with very large size distribution, (2) large aggregates constituted of fused particles, and (3) an irregular surface. Among low methyl (LM) pectin, generally more convenient for particle preparation, the best results were obtained with pectin extracted from apple pomace. On the other hand, microparticles obtained with LM pectin from citrus or mixed sources were characterized by a more irregular surface and by lower recovery efficiencies (see TABLE 3 and FIGURES 2 and 3).

**TABLE 2. Effect of oil phase on pectin particle characteristics**

| Oil Phase | Mean Size (μm) | Recovery[a] (w/w) | Morphology | Note |
|---|---|---|---|---|
| High methyl (HM) | | | | |
| mais oil | n.d.[b] | 73 | rough surface | aggregation |
| paraffin oil | n.d.[b] | 75 | rough surface | aggregation |
| isostearyl-isostearate | 79.2 ± 10.9 | 75 | rough surface irregular shape | — |
| Low Methyl (LM) | | | | |
| mais oil | n.d.[b] | 76 | irregular shape | aggregation |
| paraffin oil | n.d.[b] | 73 | irregular shape | aggregation |
| isostearyl-isostearate | 103.8 ± 5.2 | 88 | porous surface spherical shape | large size distribution |

[a]Percentage (w/w) of microsphere production, with respect to pectin used for preparation. See FIGURE 1 (Panels C and F) for size distributions. Experimental parameters were a 50-mm diameter vessel, a 35-mm, four-blade turbine rotor, a volume ratio of pectin solution to oil phase of 0.2, and 1,000 rpm stirring speed.

[b]n.d., not determined.

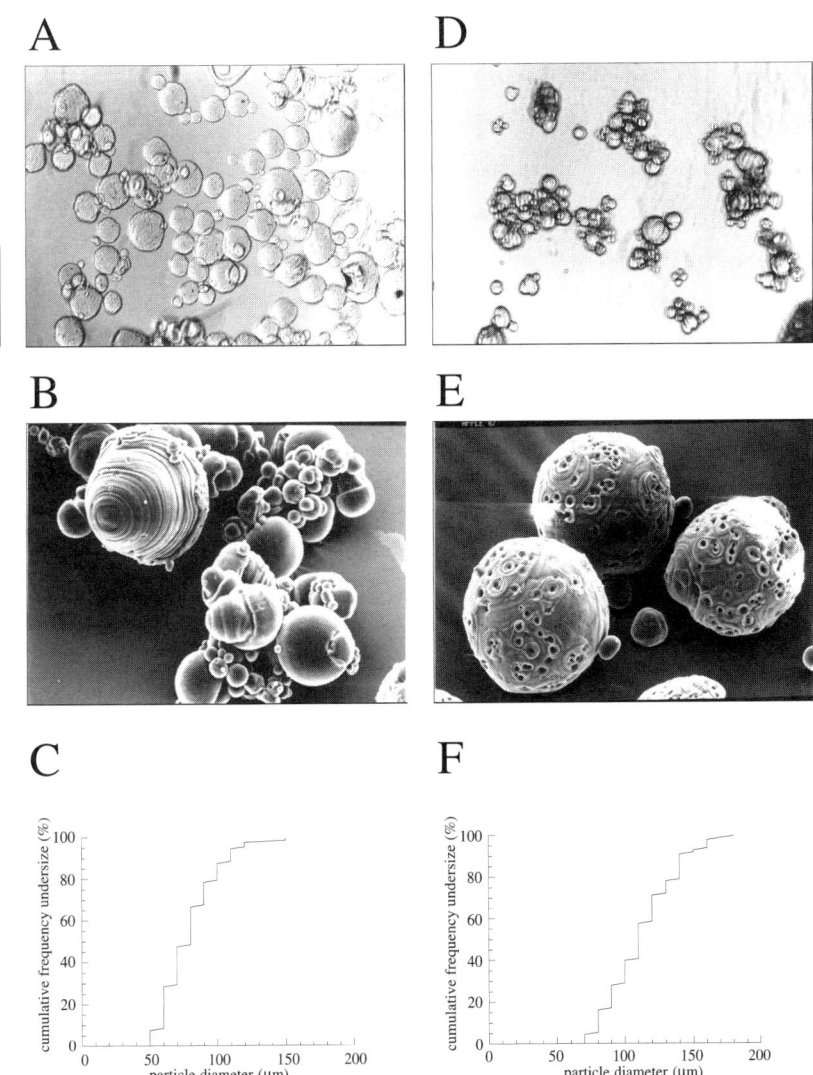

**FIGURE 1.** Effect of the oil phase on the morphology and size of pectin particles prepared with 5% solution of PHM medium rapid set (*Column 1*) and apple pomace PLM (*Column 2*) at 1,000 rpm and 0.2 water/oil volume ratio. **A** and **D**, optical micrographs of pectin particles; **B** and **E**, scanning electron micrographs of pectin particles; **C** and **F**, frequency distribution plot of pectin particles. The *bar* corresponds to 240, 96, 72, and 83 μm in panels **A**, **B**, **D**, and **E**, respectively.

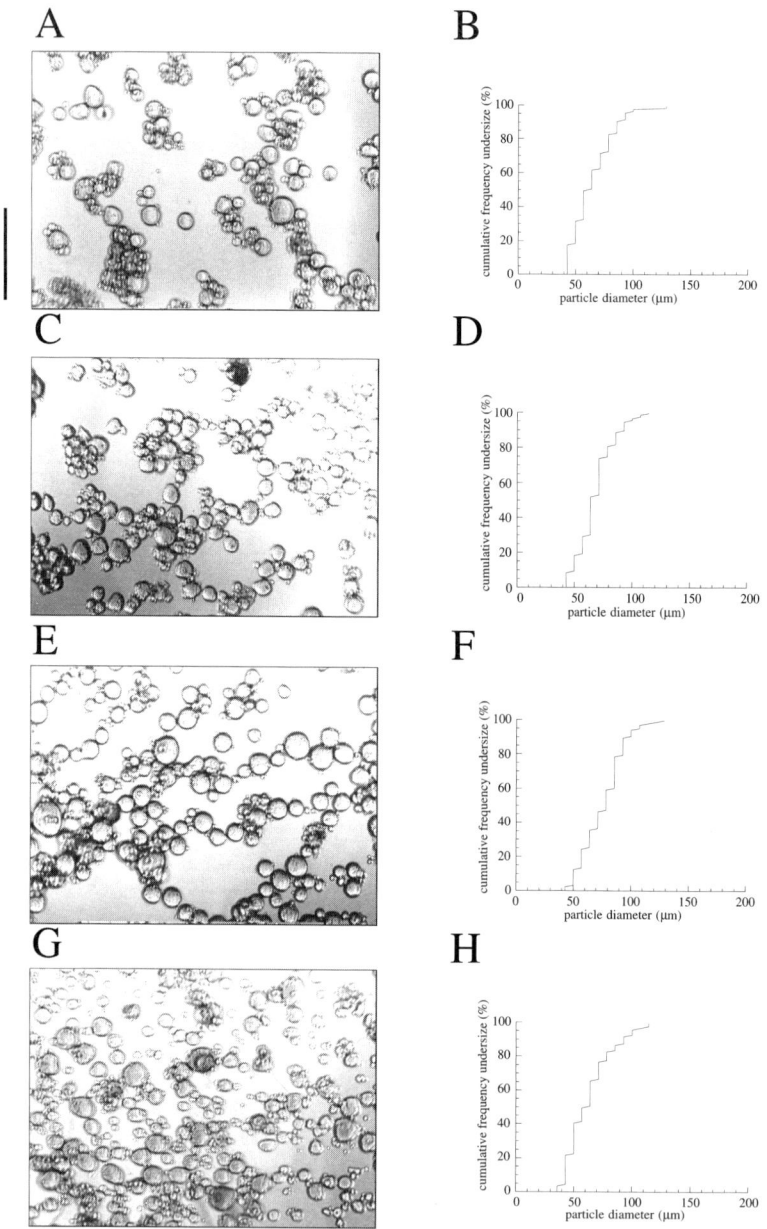

**FIGURE 2.** Effect of the type of HM pectin on the morphology and size of particles. Optical micrographs and frequency distribution plots of microspheres produced with PHM slow set (**A** and **B**), PHM rapid set (**C** and **D**), apple pomace PHM medium rapid set (**E** and **F**), and citrus PHM medium rapid set (**G** and **H**) pectin. The *bar* corresponds to 390, 420, 480, and 390 μm in panels **A**, **C**, **E**, and **G**, respectively.

TABLE 3. Effect of type of pectin on particle characteristics

| Type of pectin | Mean Size (μm) | Recovery[a] (w/w) | Morphology | Note |
|---|---|---|---|---|
| High Methyl (HM) | | | | |
| PHM slow set | 64.6 ± 18.3 | 76 | spherical | large size distribution |
| PHM rapid set | 79.2 ± 15.3 | 64 | irregular, rough surface | — |
| PHM medium rapid set (apple) | 75.7 ± 17.9 | 64 | spherical, rough surface | large size distribution |
| PHM medium rapid set (citrus) | 63.2 ± 19.5 | 78 | irregular, rough surface | large size distribution |
| Low Methyl (LM) | | | | |
| PLM (apple) | 103.8 ± 5.2 | 88 | spherical, porous surface | — |
| PLM (citrus) | 76.2 ± 19.2 | 84 | high surface roughness | — |
| PLM (fruit) | 40.3 ± 14.4 | 66 | irregular, rough surface | large size distribution |

[a]Percentage (w/w) of microsphere production, with respect to pectin used for preparation. See FIGURE 1 (Panel F), FIGURES 2 and 3 for size distributions. Experimental parameters were a 50-mm diameter vessel, a 35-mm, four-blade turbine rotor, a volume ratio of pectin solution to isostearyl-isostearate phase of 0.2, and 1,000 rpm stirring speed.


TABLE 4. Effect of pectin concentration on the characteristics of pectin particles

| Concentration[a] of Pectin (%) | Morphology | Mean Size (μm) | Recovery[b] (w/w) |
|---|---|---|---|
| 3 | spherical shape, smooth surface | 71.0 ± 11.9 | 60 |
| 5 | spherical shape, porous surface | 103.8 ± 5.2 | 88 |
| 7 | spherical shape, smooth surface | 198.0 ± 15.2 | 77 |

[a]Percentage (w/v) of pectin in the aqueous solution used in the emulsion-dehydration procedure.
[b]Percentage (w/w) of microsphere production, with respect to pectin used for preparation. See FIGURE 1 (Panel F) and FIGURE 4 (Panels C and F) for size distributions. Experimental parameters were a 50-mm diameter vessel, a 35-mm, four-blade turbine rotor, a volume ratio of LM pectin solution to isostearyl-isostearate phase of 0.2, and 1,000 rpm stirring speed.

By changing the amount of pectin used for microsphere preparation (3, 5, or 7% solution), a progressive increase in both mean size and size distribution was observed (see TABLE 4 and FIGURE 4). In addition, modifications of the surface characteristics of the microspheres were appreciable. For instance, the surface of microspheres prepared with a 5% pectin solution is characterized by a craterized surface as shown by the electron photomicrograph in FIGURE 1, panel E.

*Stirring Speed*

Since the aim of this investigation was to produce microspheres with various sizes, the influence of the stirring speed was analyzed (see TABLE 5 and FIGURES 5 and 6). Microspheres with dimensions between 77 and 156 μm were obtained by varying the stirring speed from 1,500 to 500 rpm. In particular, the particles obtained at 1,000 rpm, presented a spherical geometry with a narrow size distribution (FIG. 1). Aggregation phenomena were almost absent. Recovery was satisfactory, in many cases exceeding 80%, except for particles produced at the higher stirring speed, which resulted in a slightly lower recovery efficiency (73%).

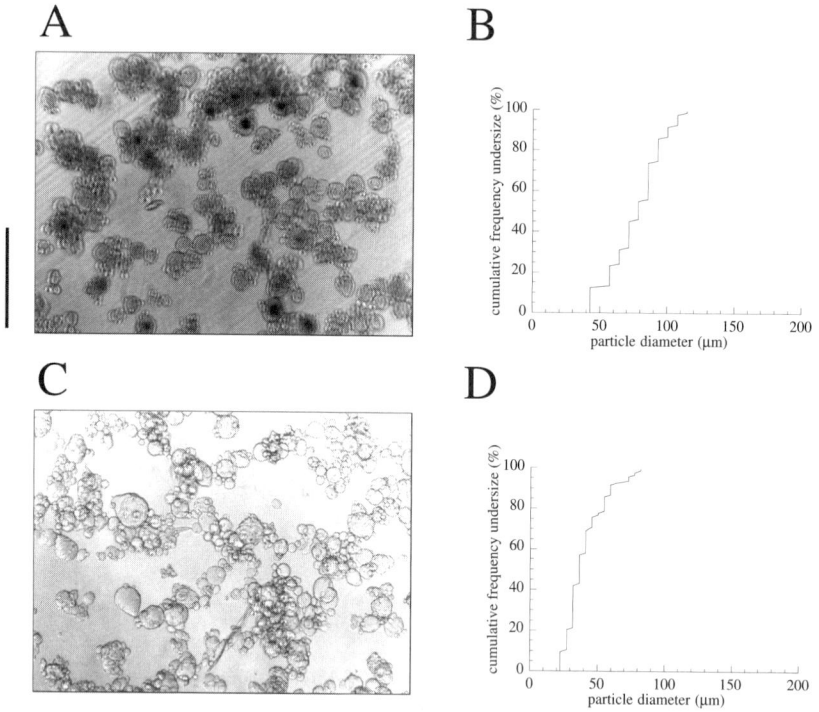

**FIGURE 3.** Effect of the type of LM pectin on the morphology and size of particles. Optical micrographs and frequency distribution plots of microspheres produced with citrus PLM (**A** and **B**) and mixed source PLM (**C** and **D**) pectin. The *bar* corresponds to 480 and 240 μm in panels **A** and **C**, respectively.

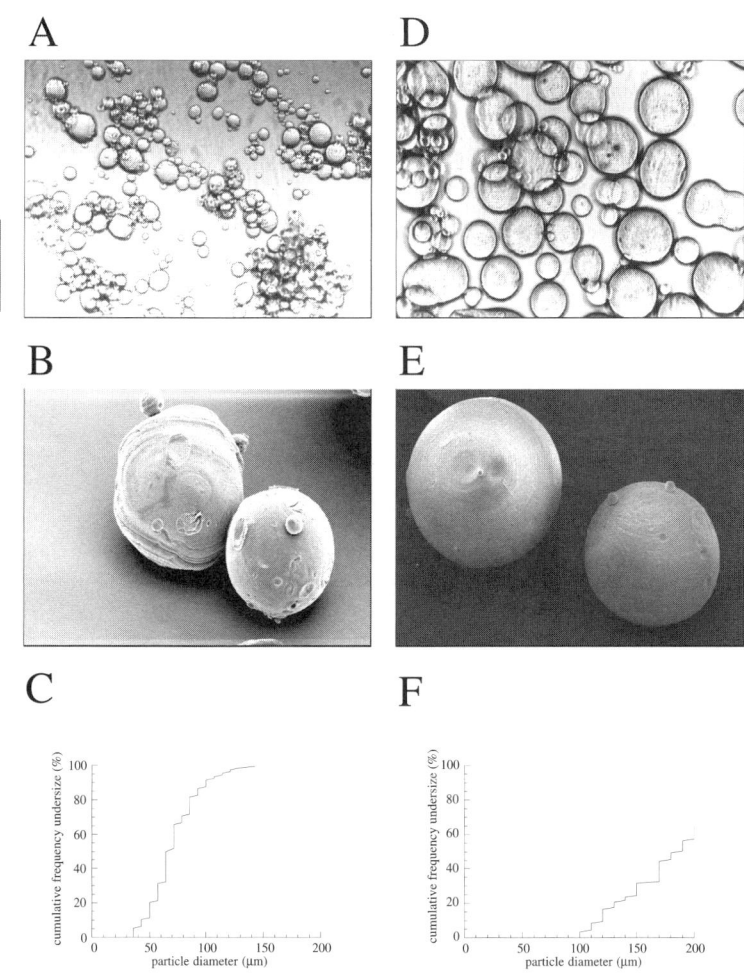

**FIGURE 4.** Effect of the amount of LM pectin on morphology and particle size of pectin particles. Particles were prepared using 3% (*left column*) and 7% (p/v) solution (*right column*) of apple PLM. **A** and **D**, optical micrographs of pectin particles; **B** and **E**, scanning electron micrographs of pectin particles; **C** and **F**, frequency distribution plot of pectin particles. The *bar* corresponds to 420, 63, 428, and 137 μm in panels **A**, **B**, **D**, and **E**, respectively.

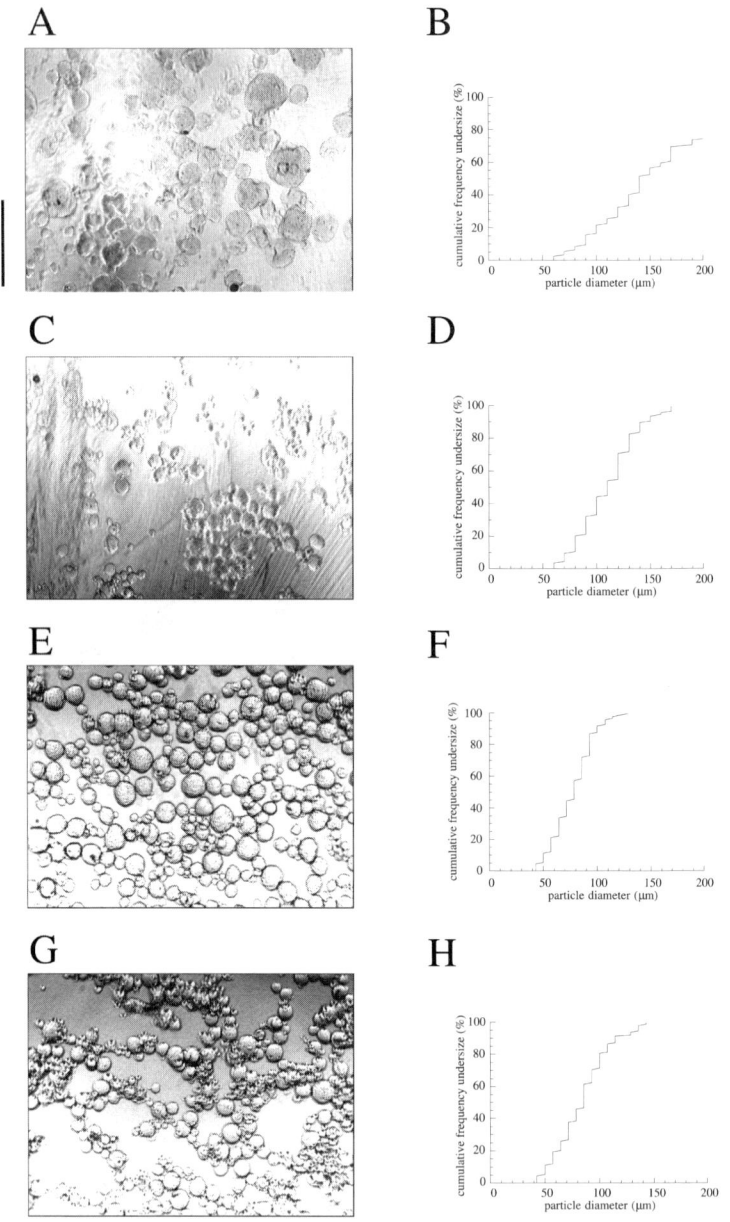

**FIGURE 5.** Effect of stirring speed on morphology and particle size of apple PLM particles. Optical micrographs and frequency distribution plot of microspheres produced at 500 rpm (**A** and **B**), 750 rpm (**C** and **D**), 1,250 rpm (**E** and **F**), and 1,500 rpm (**G** and **H**). The *bar* corresponds to 630, 720, 288, and 540 μm in panels **A**, **C**, **E**, and **G**, respectively.

TABLE 5. Effect of stirring speed on the characteristics of pectin particles

| Stirring Speed (rpm) | Mean Size (μm) | Recovery[a] (w/w) | Morphology | Note |
|---|---|---|---|---|
| 500 | 156.4 ± 25.2 | 85 | irregular, porous surface | large size distribution |
| 750 | 109.9 ± 17.2 | 83 | irregular, rough surface | large size distribution |
| 1,000 | 103.8 ± 5.2 | 88 | spherical, porous surface | narrow size distribution |
| 1,250 | 84.0 ± 14.5 | 82 | porous surface | narrow size distribution |
| 1,500 | 77.1 ± 8.9 | 73 | spherical | large size distribution |

[a]Percentage (w/w) of microsphere production, with respect to pectin used for preparation. See FIGURE 1 (Panel F) and FIGURE 5 for size distributions. Experimental parameters were a 50-mm diameter vessel, a 35-mm, four-blade turbine rotor, a volume ratio of LM pectin solution to isostearyl-isostearate phase of 0.2.

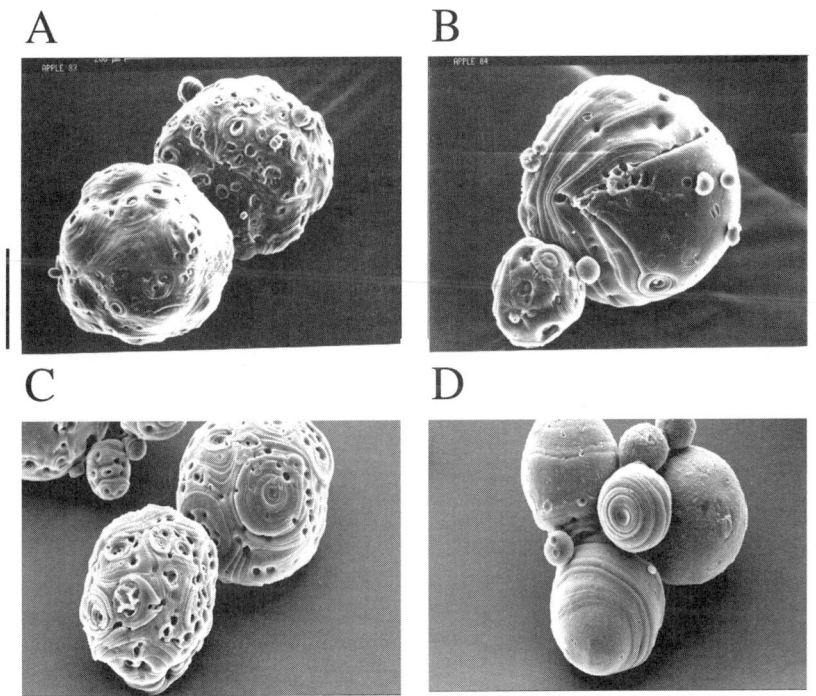

**FIGURE 6.** Scanning electron microscopy photographs of 5% apple PLM particles produced at 500 rpm (**A**), 750 rpm (**B**), 1250 rpm (**C**), and 1,500 rpm (**D**). The *bar* corresponds to 94, 66, 60, and 92 μm in panels **A**, **B**, **C**, and **D**, respectively.

## Surfactant Type and Concentration

The effect of the presence and concentration of various stabilizers was also tested. Span 20 (HLB 8.6), 80 (HLB 4.3), and 85 (HLB 1.8) were considered. As can be appreciated from the results obtained (see TABLE 6 and FIGURE 7), the addition of surfactants leads to a reduction of the size of the pectin droplets during the emulsification step, thus causing a significant reduction of the final microsphere size. In particular, microspheres obtained with 1% of Span 20 and 80 were smaller in size, with a mean diameter varying from 103.8 µm to 23.0 and to 79.5 µm, respectively. Microspheres with intermediate sizes, were produced by adjusting the concentration of stabilizer. For instance, in the absence of surfactants the microsphere size was 103.8 µm, whereas in the presence of 0.5, 1.0, or 1.5% of Span 85 the mean diameters of the microspheres were 110.3, 106.7, and 80.9 µm, respectively (see FIGURE 8). In addition the use of 0.5% of Span 85 allowed the formation of holed microparticles as is clearly appreciable from FIGURE 8B. It needs to be emphasized that in all cases particle recovery higher than 73% and spherical microparticles were obtained.

## Water/Oil Volume Ratio

As indicated by Equation (2), an increase of the volume ratio ($R$) between the droplet phase and suspension medium is expected to proportionally increase the particle size.[12] Experiments aimed at evaluating the influence of this parameter on particle dimension were performed. The results reported in TABLE 7 and FIGURE 9 indicate a progressive increase in pectin particle size when larger amounts of the droplet phase were employed. On the other hand, no significant changes in particle recovery was observed, being 80, 88, and 76% for 0.1, 0.2, and 0.3 water/oil ratio, respectively. Concerning the morphological characteristics of these pectin particles,

TABLE 6. Effect of the surfactant on the characteristics of pectin particles

| Surfactant | Concentration[a] (w/w) | Mean Size (µm) | Recovery[b] (w/w) | Morphology |
|---|---|---|---|---|
| Span 20 | 1.0 | 23.0 ± 8.5 | 76 | n.d. |
| Span 80 | 1.0 | 79.5 ± 9.2 | 74 | spherical |
| Span 85 | 0.5 | 110.3 ± 18.7 | 73 | spherical |
| Span 85 | 1.0 | 106.7 ± 15.1 | 77 | spherical, rough surface |
| Span 85 | 1.5 | 80.9 ± 11.9 | 83 | spherical, rough surface |

[a] Percentage (w/w) of surfactant, with respect to the total weight of oil and aqueous phases used for the microsphere preparation.

[b] Percentage (w/w) of microsphere production, with respect to pectin used for preparation. See FIGURES 7 and 8 for size distributions. Experimental parameters were a 50-mm diameter vessel, a 35-mm, four-blade turbine rotor, a volume ratio of pectin solution to isostearyl-isostearate phase of 0.2, and 1,000 rpm stirring speed.

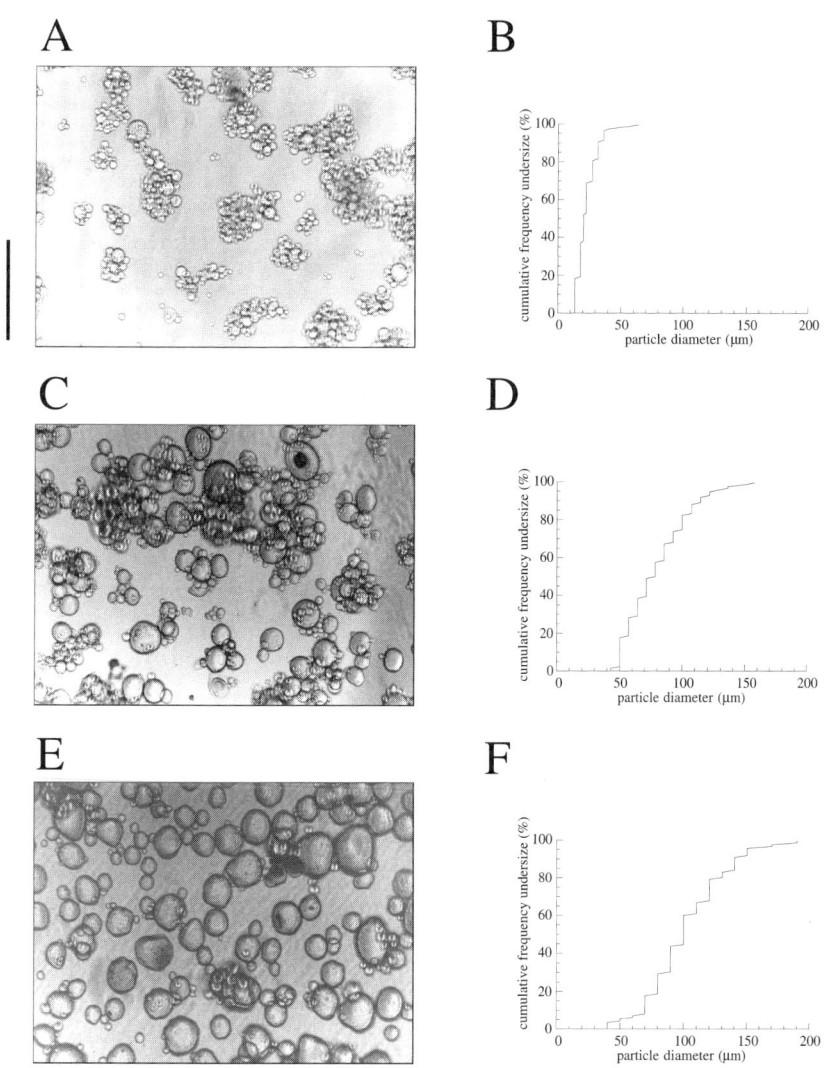

**FIGURE 7.** Effect of stabilizer (surfactant) on particle characteristics. Optical micrographs and frequency distribution plot of pectin microspheres prepared with 5% of pectin solution in the presence of 1% (w/w) Span 20 (**A** and **B**), Span 80 (**C** and **D**), or Span 85 (**E** and **F**). The *bar* corresponds to 225, 360, and 396 μm in panels **A**, **C**, and **E**, respectively.

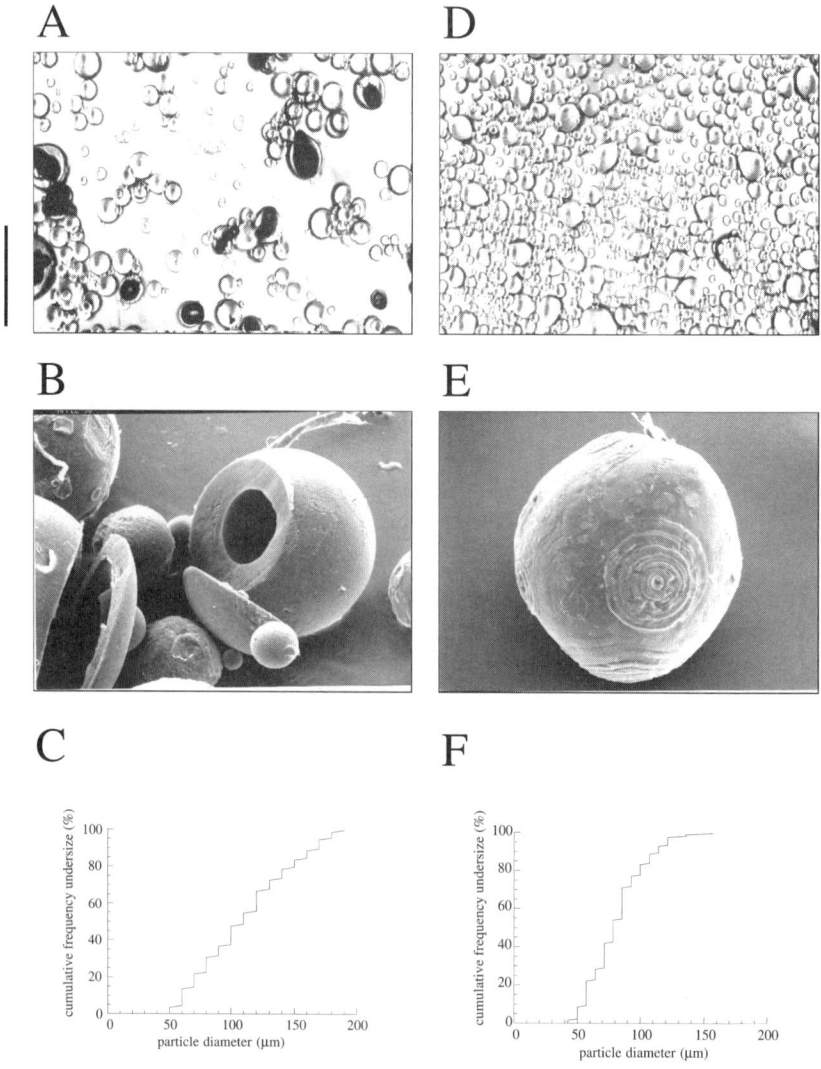

**FIGURE 8.** Effect of stabilizer concentration on the particle characteristics. Pectin microspheres were prepared using 5% of pectin at 1,000 rpm in the presence of 0.5% (*left column*) or 1.5% (w/w) (*right column*) Span 85. **A** and **D**, optical micrographs of pectin particles; **B** and **E**, scanning electron micrographs of pectin particles; **C** and **F**, frequency distribution plot of pectin particles. The *bar* corresponds to 720, 86, 360, and 36 μm in panels **A**, **B**, **D**, and **E**, respectively.

TABLE 7. Effect of the water/oil volume ratio on the characteristics of pectin particles

| Water/Oil Ratio[a] | Mean Size (μm) | Recovery[b] (w/w) | Morphology |
|---|---|---|---|
| 0.1 | 106.5 ± 14.8 | 80 | irregular, rough surface |
| 0.2 | 103.8 ± 5.2 | 88 | spherical, porous surface |
| 0.3 | 140.0 ± 9.4 | 76 | spherical, porous surface |

[a]Volumetric ratio between the volumes of the aqueous and the oily phase used to prepare pectin particles.
[b]Percentage (w/w) of microsphere production, with respect to pectin used for preparation. See FIGURE 1 (Panel F) and FIGURE 9 for size distributions. Experimental parameters were a 50-mm diameter vessel, a 35-mm, four-blade turbine rotor, a 5% LM pectin solution, and 1,000 rpm stirring speed.

an increase of the water/oil volume ratio induces the formation of spherical and porous microspheres.

## *Drug Encapsulation Efficiency*

With respect to the encapsulation efficiency of the pectin microspheres, the crucial role of the chemicophysical characteristics of the drug employed should be emphasized. In particular, the hydrophobic–hydrophilic balance of the drug was found to influence entrapment yield.[13] Indeed, hydrophilic drugs can be more efficiently incorporated in microspheres, whereas molecules with hydrophobic portions display a reduced trapping efficiency. For instance, tetracycline, being more hydrophilic with respect to metronidazol, displayed a higher encapsulation efficiency (11.5%), whereas compounds having greater lipophilic portions, such as metronidazol, showed lower entrapment yields (0.75%). This behavior can be attributed to the diffusion of drug molecules, from the aqueous droplets to the external continuous oil phase, during the emulsification step. From a morphological point of view, pectin particles containing antibiotics are similar to the correspondent empty beads.

## *Ionic Hardening of Pectin Microspheres*

Since pectin microspheres swell, and dissolve, quite rapidly in aqueous environments, they are not be suitable for sustained release of therapeutic agents requiring long release periods (up to eight hours) or for cell encapsulation strategies. In order to modify the microsphere swelling, solubility, and, consequently, the drug release profiles, the feasibility of a ionic crosslinking procedure of the pectin matrix was considered. Ionic crosslinking of microspheres with calcium chloride was accomplished following two alternative experimental procedures. The first (the *in situ method*) consists of the addition of calcium ions during the maintenance of the water/oil emulsion, generated for microsphere preparation. The second (the *postproduction method*) involves the isolation and dehydration of microspheres exposed to a solution of calcium chloride for 30 or 180 minutes. With both ionic hardening

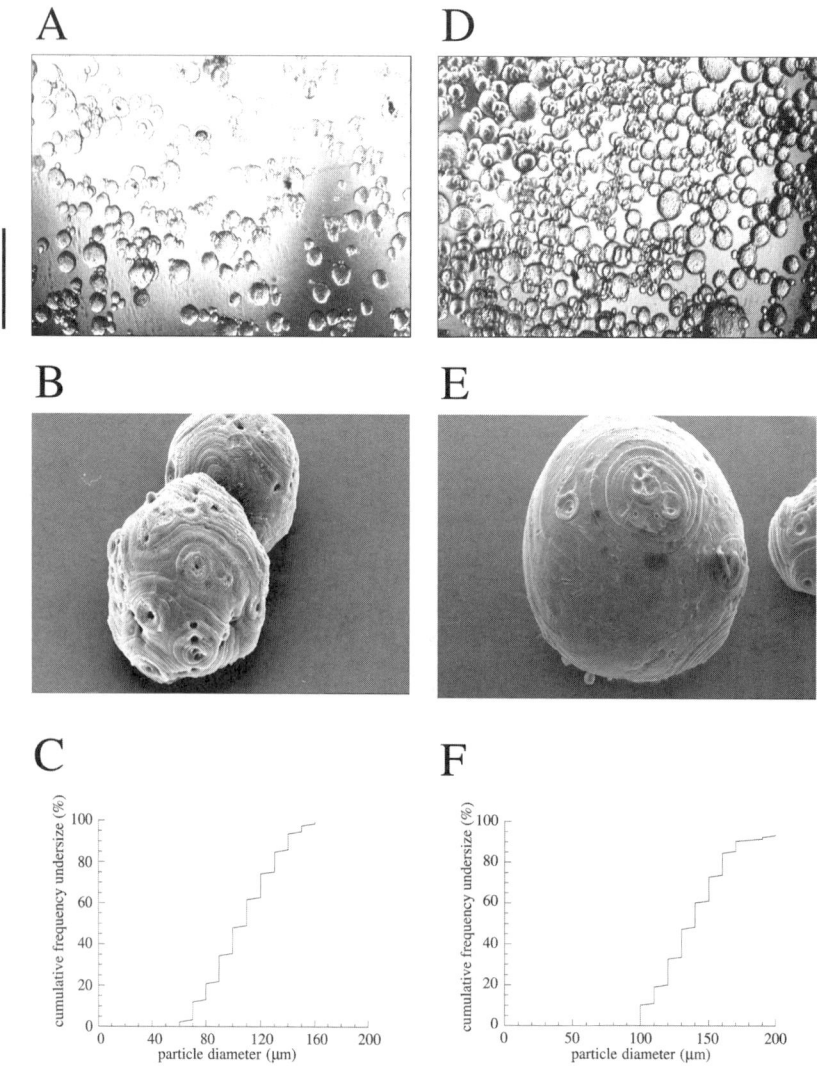

**FIGURE 9.** Effect of water/oil volume ratio on the morphology and particle size of apple LM particles. Pectin microspheres were prepared using 5% pectin at 1,000 rpm and 0.1 (*left column*) or 0.3 (*right column*) water/oil volume ratio. **A** and **D**, optical micrographs of pectin particles; **B** and **E**, scanning electron micrographs of pectin particles; **C** and **F**, frequency distribution plot of pectin particles. The *bar* corresponds to 660, 79, 840, and 63 μm in panels **A**, **B**, **D**, and **E**, respectively.

procedures, the particle morphology (i.e., size and general shape) does not substantially change (see FIGURE 10). In order to compare the effect of the two ionic hardening procedures on the swelling of the treated microspheres, a series of experiments were performed, as is described below.

Treated and untreated particles were dispersed in a CMC-based hydrophilic gel. The choice of this particular swelling medium was made since its viscosity enabled us to maintain the microspheres in fixed positions during microscopic observation. It should be emphasized that this method permits a study not only of the average swelling of a microsphere population, but also of the swelling of individual particles, allowing the analysis of the size influence on swelling and possible interparticle interactions. FIGURE 11 shows the microphotographs of untreated (Panel A) and ionically treated (Panels B and C) pectin particles by the *postproduction method* and swollen for four hours together with the swelling kinetics (Panel D).

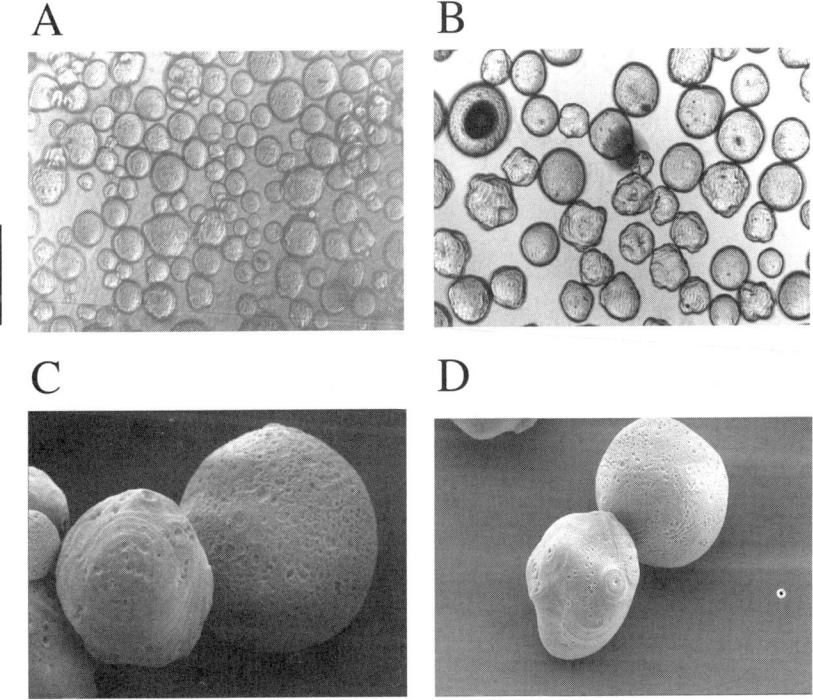

**FIGURE 10.** Effects of *in situ* ionic crosslinking on the morphology of apple LM particles. Pectin microspheres were prepared using 5% of pectin at 1,000 rpm, 0.2 water/oil volume ratio and 1 M (*left column*) or 2 M (*right column*) $CaCl_2$. **A** and **C**, optical micrographs of pectin particles; **B** and **D**, scanning electron micrographs of pectin particles. The *bar* corresponds to 378, 47, 236, and 94 μm in panels **A**, **B**, **C**, and **D**, respectively.

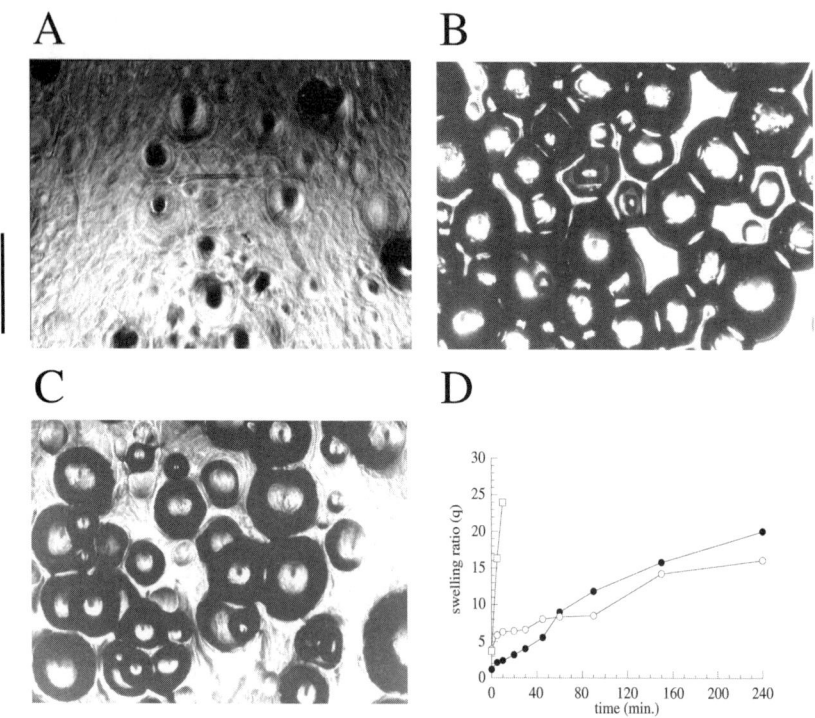

**FIGURE 11.** Effects of ionic treatment on the swelling of pectin microspheres. Optical photomicrographs of microspheres untreated (**A**) or treated by the *postproduction method* for 30 (**B**) or 180 (**C**) min. Photographs were taken after four hours of swelling. *Bar* corresponds to 380 μm. **D**, swelling profile of untreated microspheres (□) and of microspheres treated for 30 (●) or 180 (○) min. Data represent the average of three independent experiments on different microsphere batches.

## CONCLUDING REMARKS AND FUTURE WORK

The preformulatory study presented here enabled us to obtain important information about the production of pectin microspheres intended for controlled release of drugs. Isostearyl isostearate as oil phase and pectin from apple pomace were selected as raw materials, resulting in the formation of microparticles characterized by spherical shape, regular surface, absence of aggregates and narrow dimensional distribution. An increase in pectin concentration led to an increase in mean size and size distribution. As expected, the increase of the stirring speed (from 500 to 1,500 rpm) resulted in a progressive decrease of particle mean size, with diameters ranging from 156 to 77 μm, possibly useful for administration procedures such as those using an oral route. The use of Span 20, Span 80, or Span 85 led to a reduction of particle mean size as a function of surfactant concentration.

Concerning the volume ratio between aqueous phase and oil phase, the best results in term of particle morphology and recovery were obtained by the use of a 0.2 water/ oil volume ratio. In order to modify the rapid swelling and solubility in water of pectin microspheres, two different approaches were performed based on the use of calcium chloride as ionic crosslinker, and both methods enabled the hardening of particle matrix.

It has been demonstrated, by means of particle size modification and hardening procedures, that the possible pharmaceutical applications of pectin microcapsules can be varied. This broadens the potential for the administration of various compounds rendering pectin with the nature of a robust carrier.

With respect to ionically treated microspheres, experiments are in progress aimed to (1) better investigate the effect of the two alternative approaches of crosslinking (2) clarify the drug-release mechanism from ionically crosslinked particles, and (3) investigate the *in vivo* biocompatibility and degradability of hardened microspheres.

## REFERENCES

1. LEE, K.C., Y.J. LEE, W.B. KIM & C.Y. CHA. 1990. Monoclonal antibody-based targeting of methotrexate-loaded microspheres. Int. J. Pharm. **59:** 27–33.
2. TOMLINSON, E. 1987. Biological opportunities for site-specific drug delivery using particulate carriers. *In* Drug Delivery Systems. Fundamentals and Techniques. P. Johnson & J.G. Lloyd-Jones, Eds.: 32–65. Ellis Horwood Ltd., Chichester, UK.
3. MAJORS, K.R. & M.B. FRIEDMAN. 1991. Animal testing of polymer based systems. *In* Polymers for Controlled Drug Delivery. P.J. Tarcha, Ed.: 231–239. CRC Press Inc., Boca Raton.
4. NOVOSEL'SKAYA, I.L., N.L. VOROPAEVA, L.N. SEMENOVA & S.S. RASHIDOVA. 2000. Trends in the science and applications of pectins. Chem. Nat. Comp. **36:** 1–10.
5. MACLEOD, G.S., J.T. FELL & J.H. COLLETT. 1999. An *in vitro* investigation into the potential for bimodal drug release from pectin/chitosan/HPMC-coated tablets. Int. J. Pharm. **188:** 11–18.
6. SRIAMORNSAK, P. & J. NUNTHANID. 1999. Calcium pectinate gel beads for controlled release drug delivery: II. Effect of formulation and processing variables on drug release. J. Microencap. **16:** 303–313.
7. SEMDE, R., K. AMIGHI, M.J. DEVLEESCHOUWER & A.J. MOES. 2000. Studies of pectin HM/Eudragit® RL/Eudragit® NE film-coating formulations intended for colonic drug delivery. Int. J. Pharm. **197:** 181–192.
8. SEMDE, R., K. AMIGHI, M.J. DEVLEESCHOUWER & A.J. MOES. 1999. *In vitro* evaluation of pectin HM/ethylcellulose compression-coated formulations intended for colonic drug delivery. STP Pharma. Sci. **9:** 561–565.
9. ASHFORD, M., J. FELL, D. ATTWOOD, *et al.* 1994. Studies on pectin formulations for colonic drug delivery. J. Control Rel. **30:** 225–232.
10. SEMDÈ, R., K. AMIGHI, D. PIERRE, *et al.* 1998. Leaching of pectin from mixed pectin/insoluble polymer films intended for colonic drug delivery. Int. J. Pharm. **174:** 233–241.
11. SANOFI BIOINDUSTRIES. 1999. Thickening, Gelling and Stabilizing Effects with Hydrocolloids [manual].
12. ARSHADY, R. 1990. Albumin microspheres and microcapsules: methodology of manufacturing techniques. J. Control Rel. **14:** 111–131.
13. ESPOSITO, E., R. CORTESI & C. NASTRUZZI. 1996. Gelatin microspheres: influence of preparation parameters and thermal treatment on chemico-physical and biopharmaceutical properties. Biomaterials **17:** 2009–2020.

# Approaches to Development of Microencapsulated Form of the Live Measles Vaccine

E.A. NECHAEVA,[a] N. VARAKSIN,[a] T. RYABICHEVA,[a] M. SMOLINA,[a] T. KOLOKOLTSOVA,[a] A. VILESOV,[b] N. AKSENOVA,[b] R. STANKEVICH,[b] AND R. ISIDOROV[b]

[a]*State Research Center of Virology and Biotechnology "Vector," Koltsovo, Novosibirsk Region, 630559, Russia*

[b]*DELSI, St. Petersburg, Russia*

ABSTRACT: Development of delivery of antigens and antigenic complexes using microcapsules or microgranules made of pH-dependent polymers is one of several high priority directions of modern vaccinology. These polymers should protect the virus from acid gastric medium, dissolve or swell readily in weakly alkaline intestinal medium, in no way decrease the specific activities of viral antigens, promote their penetration into intestinal mucosa, and possess adjuvant properties. The State Research Center Vector and "DELSI" are developing the technology for production of microencapsulated form of the live measles vaccine L-16 viruses for oral administration. The authors have so far succeeded in selecting and characterizing a number of polymers that are promising for microencapsulated vaccine and for testing of virus titers and immune response of experimental samples of a new vaccine in animals. Control of samples in guinea pigs demonstrated that the encapsulated measles virus retained its specific activity and capability for inducing immune response in experimental animals.

KEYWORDS: microencapsulation; live measles vaccine

## INTRODUCTION

Development of non-injection methods for immunizing against measles is now of special importance. Despite the success in struggling with this disease, measles still present a serious problem, not only for developing, but also for industrial countries. According to WHO estimates, the annual measles morbidity rate is 67 million people. Each 15 seconds, one child dies of measles, 2 million children annually.[1,2] Therefore, the WHO Global Program of Measles Eradication requires widespread and, most likely, repeated immunization of both children and adults, necessitating, in turn, a simple and inexpensive technique of measles vaccine administration. Development of delivery of antigens and antigenic complexes using microcapsules or microgranules

---

Address for correspondence: Elena A. Nechaeva, SRC VB"Vector," Koltsovo, Novosibirsk Region, 630559, Russia. Fax: +007 (3832) 36 74 09.
nechaeva@vector.nsk.su

made from pH-dependent polymers is one of the high priority directions of modern vaccinology.

Mucosal vaccines containing soluble polymeric systems are now actively developed in the world. The polymer is prepared as spherical particles with size of 1 μm to 3 mm to incorporate virus particles. In the case of oral administration, the encapsulated virus is protected from low pH gastric juice and proteolytic enzymes of the gastrointestinal tract. Moreover, the polymeric capsule may play the role of adjuvant, increasing the immune response 10–100 times. For example, microencapsulated influenza virus antigen was shown to induce development of humoral and secretory immune responses; in these experiments, immunization with low doses of antigen resulted in higher protective antibody titers compared with high doses, the latter being potentially tolerogenic.[3] Offit et al.[4] were first to demonstrate the possibility of encapsulating the live virus. Microencapsulated preparations involving cytotoxic-T-lymphocyte (CTL) epitopes of measles virus and cholera toxin displayed pronounced immunogenicity.[5] However, the data on development of a microencapsulated form of the live measles vaccine are lacking at present. Therefore, the basic problem in developing this new vaccine form involving the live measles virus is preservation of its specific activity under conditions of microencapsulation or microgranulation and subsequent storage. There are grounds for believing that the unique packaging of the virus into microcapsules combined with a set of supplements, such as adjuvants, immunostimulators, antioxidants, stabilizers, and so forth, will provide virus delivery to M-cells from intestinal tissues and its subsequent release.

The goal of this work was to select the polymers showing promise for microencapsulating measles virus and to study their physicochemical properties, compatibility with measles virus, and immunostimulating activities in experimental animals.

## MATERIALS AND METHODS

Measles virus strain Leningrad-16 from the inoculation bank certified at the State Control Institution was used in the work. The virus was cultivated in Japanese quail embryo fibroblasts from a leukemia-free farm, SRC VB Vector. Sorbitol (ICN) sucrose (ICN), and gelatose (Vector, Novosibirsk region, Russia) with different extents of hydrolysis were used as stabilizers. To prepare microencapsulated forms of the vaccine, the polymers were added at various concentrations to either the maintenance medium during measles virus cultivation on the cell substrate or to vaccine stabilizer while pooling virus-containing material. The liquid semifinished product was frozen at $-55\pm5°C$ during 24 h and lyophilized for 48 h (the method of microencapsulation is now the subject of a patent application).

Specific activity of the virus-containing material determined by its cytopathic effect in Vero cell culture according to techniques approved by the Pharmacopoeial Committee of Russia[6] and presented in log tissue cytopathic infection doses (log $TCID_{50}$).

The following polymers were used as matrices for microencapsulation: polyacrylic acid (PAA) with a molecular weight of 31 kDa; copolymers of acrylic acid were produced by DELSI through etherification of the initial PAA (the characteristics of this synthesis were autocatalytic mode and high extent of PAA purification, providing for the absence of toxic admixtures and, consequently, good compatibility with biological objects); Eudragit EL-100; edible sodium alginate (viscosity of 1% solution amounting to 6.5°E at 20°C) (produced by the Experimental Plant of Algae Production, Archangelsk, Russia); chitosan with a molecular weight of 35 kDa, (produced by Bioprogress, Moscow Region, Russia); medical polyvinylpyrrolidone (PVP), 9.7 kDa; and low molecular weight spermidine ($N$-[3-aminopropyl]-1,4-butandiamine) (SIGMA). The polymers were characterized with respect to their boundaries of conformational transitions at various pH values, viscosities, toxicities for cells, and effects on specific activity of measles virus. Viscosity was measured using a capillary Ostwald viscometer with diameter 0.63 mm and temperature $25.0\pm0.05°C$, according to the established methods.[7] Toxicities were studied during cultivation of Vero cells with polymers and subsequent control of morphology of cells and index of cell proliferation. The index of cell proliferation was determined as the ratio of cell concentrations after and before cultivation of cells.

To evaluate toxicities and immunogenicities of microencapsulated vaccine samples *in vivo*, guinea pigs were immunized orally with different compositions of the virus and polymers; in parallel, the injection form of the vaccine was administered to the control animals either subcutaneously or orally. Blood was taken on day 28 postimmunization to study the sera using the hemagglutination inhibition test (HAIT) with four antigen units (AU) of measles virus Tween-ester antigen according to the Pharmacopoeial Article.[6]

## RESULTS AND DISCUSSION

To develop the new form of the live measles vaccine for oral administration, we applied microgranulation of viral particles in a matrix of pH-dependent polymers. In this process, the virus-containing material was united with the polymer in an alkaline pH range, wherein the polymer is in an unfolded state. A shift of the pH into the acid range results the polymer folding and phase separation according to coacervation mode. This material with a preformed microstructure can be further lyophilized. Thus, formation of virus-containing microcapsules under mild conditions requires the polymers to be maintained according to strict corresponding conditions (pH = 5.5–8.6) for their conformational transitions.

The results obtained are shown in FIGURE 1. This shows the results for relative viscosity (ordinal-axes) of various polymers (and concentration) depending on solution pH. The polymers studied fall into three groups with respect to their behavior in media with various pH values. The first group—polyacids, their substituted variants, and salts—exhibited pH dependence and included PAA, its substituted variants, EL-100, and sodium alginate (see the curves PAA 1%, PAA 5% vp3 0.2%, vp4 0.2%, vp8 0.1% in FIG. 1). They exist as polysalts in the basic medium where their molecules occur in an unfolded state due to mutual repulsion of ionized groups. On changing pH into acidic range, the number of undissociated carboxyl groups increases and the polymer molecule folds. Folding of the molecules may be assessed according to decrease in viscosity of polymer solution. Thus, the polyacids in question change from unfolded to folded conformations within the pH range 4.5–8.0, a range where

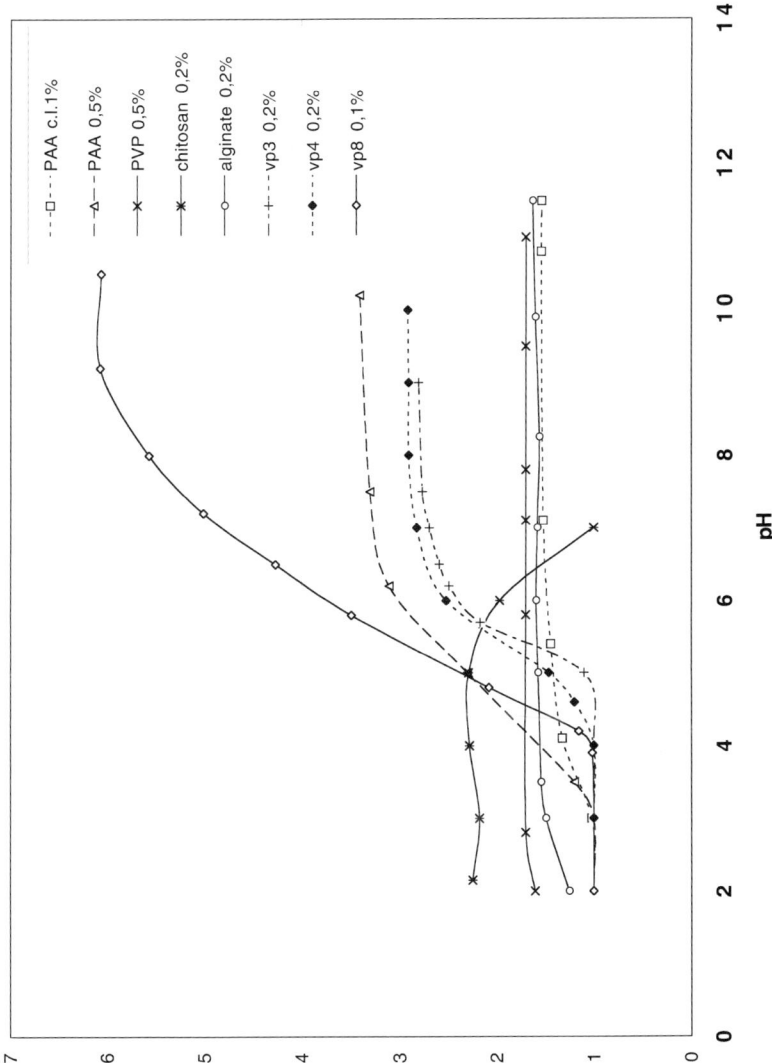

FIGURE 1. Relative viscosity.

measles virus specific activity is preserved. The second group—polybases—exhibit an opposite pattern, since they are ionized in acidic media (see the curve for chitosan 0.2% in FIG. 1). The third group—nonionogenic polymers, exemplified by PVP—is insensitive to changes in the pH (see the curve PVP 0.5% in FIG. 1).

We also tested microencapsulation of viral particles into different polymeric matrices. Several polyacids tested were found to interact with vaccine stabilizer (gelatose and peptone). No phase separation in the basic medium occurred when virus-containing material was united with PAA and copolymer No. 8 (containing 66% butyl groups) in the basic medium; a pH decrease to 4.35 or 4.60 for PAA and the copolymer, respectively, resulted in phase separation with the phase enriched with the polymer in a form of coagulate or coacervate. Thus, increasing the PAA degree of substitution shifted the coacervation pH slightly into the alkaline range; an increase in the concentration of polymer in solution gave a similar result. The material thus obtained and driven to phase separation may be further lyophilized. Dissolution of the material lyophilized restored the microparticles, which were stable in acid and neutral media.

TABLE 1. Data on specific activities and immunogenicities of live measles vaccine (LMV) samples containing various polymers

| No. | Composition | Specific activity, log $TCID_{50}$ | Hemagglutination inhibition test | | Seroconversion % |
|---|---|---|---|---|---|
| | | | Geometric mean antibody titer | Confidence interval of geometric mean | |
| 1 | LMV, subcutaneously | 3.3 | 13 | 2.8 | 100 |
| 2 | LMV, orally | 3.3 | 0 | 0 | 0 |
| 3 | LMV + 0.5% PAA | 4.95 | 3 | 3.8 | 40 |
| 4 | LMV + 0.75% PVP + 0.5% PAA | 4.0 | 4 | 2.45 | 50 |
| 5 | LMV + 0.1% vp 4 | 4.19 | 5.2 | 3.9 | 20 |
| 6 | LMV + 1% vp 8 | 3.36 | 37 | 1.97 | 100 |
| 7 | LMV + 0.1% vp 8 | 4.2 | 56 | 2.76 | 100 |
| 8 | LMV + 1% loosely crosslinked polymer | 3.7 | 7 | 6.75 | 60 |
| 9 | LMV + 0.1% Eudragit | 3.3 | 0 | 0 | 0 |
| 10 | LMV + 1% Na-alginate | < 3.2 | 16 | 8.95 | 75 |
| 11 | LMV + 0.5% Na-alginate + 0.5% spermidine | < 3.2 | 84 | 2.02 | 100 |
| 12 | LMV + 0.5% Na-alginate + 0.35% chitosan | 3.53 | 8 | 7.81 | 60 |

To test the compatibilities of polymers with measles virus, polymers at various concentrations were added to either the maintenance medium during measles virus cultivation on the cell substrate or to vaccine stabilizer while pooling the virus-containing material. The liquid semifinished product was frozen at $-55\pm5°C$ over 24 h and lyophilized for 48 h. Data relating to specific activity and immunogenicities of the live measles vaccine samples containing various polymers are listed in TABLE 1. The results indicate that addition of the majority of polymers under study allowed both the measles virus specific activity in lyophilized samples to be preserved and the virus to be protected from 0.1 N hydrochloric acid. Titers of viruses in samples were varied from 3.3 to 4.95. Analysis of the fraction composition of the samples produced demonstrated that spherical or irregular shaped particles with size 1–30 µm were predominant. Increase in the polymer concentration to 1–1.5% resulted in formation of heterogeneous particles with size 1–100 µm.

Oral immunization of guinea pigs with preparations containing various combinations of measles virus and polymers resulted in pronounced immunostimulating effects of PAA copolymer No. 8 at a concentration of 0.1–1.0% and complexes of sodium alginate with either chitosan or spermidine (see TABLE 1). In these cases, immunized pigs exhibited 100% seroconversion and the geometric mean antibody titer levels were 37, 56, and 84. In the last two variants, the recorded protective effect of the pairs sodium alginate–chitosan and sodium alginate–spermidine may result from formation of a polymer network structure involving polyacid salt (sodium alginate) and polybasic amine (chitosan and spermidine) that incorporates the virus particles. When these polymer pairs were used, the titers of hemagglutinating antibodies in animal blood sera one month post immunization significantly exceeded the immune response to injection form of the live measles vaccine.

## CONCLUSION

The research performed allowed us to select several polymers that are promising for the development of a microencapsulated form of the live measles vaccine. Supplementing the live measles vaccine stabilizer with a number of PAA copolymers, sodium alginate, chitosan, and so forth prior to lyophilization allowed both the measles virus specific activity in the lyophilized samples to be preserved and the virus to be protected from the acidic pH gastric juice. Further study of the preparations containing various polymers has demonstrated a significant increase in the antibody titers in a part of animals immunized orally with measles virus supplemented with several PAA copolymers and PAA–PVP, as well as pronounced immune response exhibited by guinea pigs immunized with measles virus supplemented with PAA copolymer No. 8, sodium alginate–chitosan, and sodium alginate–spermidine. Release of the virus from microcapsules, its penetration into the intestinal wall, and development of the immune response require further study. The proposed approach to developing a live measles vaccine might form the basis for developing vaccines against mumps, rubella, influenza, and other viral infections.

## REFERENCES

1. ORGANISATION MONDIALE DE LA SANTE (WHO). 1987 April. Journée mondiale de la Sante. Vaccination: chaque enfant sa chance. OMS.
2. MAHLER, H. 1987. Vaccination: a chaque enfant sa chance. Sante du Monde. Janv/fev. **3**.
3. MOLDOVEANU, Z. & M. NOVAK. 1993. Oral immunization with influenza virus in biodegradable microspheres. J. Infect. Dis. **167**(1): 84–90.
4. OFFIT, P.A., C.A. KHOURY & C.A. MOSER. 1994. Enhancement of Rotavirus immunogenicity by microencapsulation. Virology **203**(1): 6134–6143.
5. PARTIDOS, C.D. & P. VOHRA. 1997. CTL-responses induced by a single immunization with peptide encapsulated in biodegradable microparticles. J. Immunol. Meth. **195**(1–2): 135–138.
6. PHARMACOPOEIAL ARTICLE. 2000. Measles vaccine, culture, live, dried. FS 42-3092-00. Russia.
7. TVERDOCHLEBOVA, I.I. 1981. Konformatciya macromolecul. Himiya. Moskva, Russia.

# Purification of Polymeric Biomaterials

CHRISTINE WANDREY AND DIANELYS SAINZ VIDAL

*Laboratory of Polyelectrolytes and BioMacromolecules, Department of Chemistry, Swiss Federal Institute of Technology, CH-1015 Lausanne, Switzerland*

ABSTRACT: Employing a combined filtration and precipitation method, the endotoxin concentration in sodium alginate (SA) and sodium cellulose sulfate (SCS) was reduced to a value of 200 EU/g polymer. This is one tenth of the regulatory threshold calculated, for example, for an appropriate bioartificial pancreas that consists of approximately 420,000 encapsulated islets of Langerhans. The low endotoxin (ET) levels were maintained below this threshold during a six-month storage period. The purification procedure of the polymers did not negatively influence the final microcapsule properties. The mechanical stability of microcapsules from purified material is even slightly higher than that of microcapsules from the original polymers. A second approach to avoid endotoxin release from the device is its direct complexation during the bead or capsule formation process. The durability of endotoxin binding in binary, ternary, and quaternary complexes could be demonstrated for storage in culture medium and saline. Very low total endotoxin release from the complexes was detected after three months in culture medium and five months in saline. This complexation is primarily based on electrostatic interactions with the participating cationic components and provides additional security for the final bioartificial organ or delivery device.

KEYWORDS: purification; polymeric biomaterials; microcapsules

## INTRODUCTION

The application of polymeric materials for immunoprotection devices in bioartificial organs requires, in addition to their efficiency, that the appropriate devices are biocompatible and non-toxic. This implies the biocompatibility and non-toxicity for both the entrapped biological material and the recipient of the bioartificial organ. In addition to the chemical purity a harmless concentration of pyrogens such as endotoxins (ET) needs to be secured for the final application. Whereas chemical impurities, such as residual monomers, initiators, and other low molar mass additives, can in general easily be removed from synthetic or modified polymeric material, the removal of ET, in particular from polyanions, turns out to be much more complicated. This results, on the one hand, from their considerable chemical and physical heterogeneity.[1] On the other hand, they behave physicochemically in a similar way to polyanions in aqueous solutions.

Endotoxins are lipopolysaccharides by their chemical nature. They are an integral part of the outer cell membrane of the most gram-negative bacteria. FIGURE 1 shows,

---

Address for correspondence: Christine Wandrey, Laboratory of Polyelectrolytes and BioMacromolecules, Department of Chemistry, Swiss Federal Institute of Technology, CH-1015 Lausanne, Switzerland. Voice: +41-21-693 3672; fax: +41-21-693 5690.
Christine.Wandrey@epfl.ch

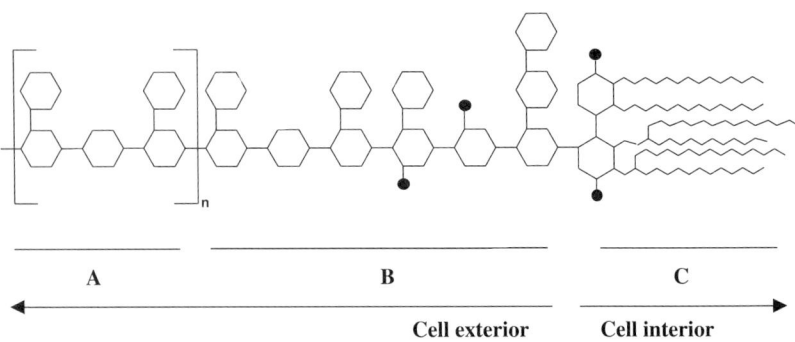

**FIGURE 1.** Principal chemical structure of endotoxin. **A**, O-antigen; **B**, core region; **C**, lipid A; • phosphorylated group.

schematically, the three main structural parts of endotoxins. In detail, these are: (A) a heteropolysaccharide with up to 40 units representing the surface antigen (O-antigen); (B) the so-called core oligosaccharide; and (C) a lipid component, called lipid A, consisting of a disaccharide of glucosamine covalently linked to aliphatic acid units with 12–16 carbon atoms.[1] Lipid A and the core region close to lipid A are partially phosphorylated. Therefore, endotoxin molecules exhibit a negative net charge in aqueous solutions of pH > 2.

General properties of endotoxins are listed below:

- Thermal stability up to 180–250°C.
- UV resistance.
- Ethylene oxide resistance.
- pH stability for pH > 2.
- Insolubility in methanol and ethanol.
- Molar mass of the single molecules in the range 2,500–25,000 g/mol.
- Aggregation in aqueous media in the presence of bivalent ions.
- Micelles $3\times10^5$–$1\times10^6$ g/mol and vesicles greater than $10^6$ g/mol of high stability.
- Aggregation and micellation are reversible.

There is no general method for the removal of endotoxin from aqueous solutions. Various techniques, described in particular in the patent literature, have been developed to solve specific product purification. These include ion-exchange,[2,3] two-phase extraction,[4–6] affinity separations,[7,8] and endotoxin-selective adsorber matrices.[9,10] Only some of the examples have been selected from a multitude of publications. However, all these techniques focus primarily on endotoxin removal from protein solutions. Several purification procedures, such as free flow electrophoresis[11] or multistep extractions consisting of more than 20 steps,[12,13] have been reported for alginate and also applied to other biopolymers.[13]

The system sodium alginate/sodium cellulose sulfate/poly(methylene-co-guanidine) hydrochloride/calcium chloride (SA/SCS//PMCG/CaCl$_2$) was found to be promising in order to develop the bioartificial pancreas.[14] Therefore, the purification and endotoxin removal studies have been focused on this quaternary system. Two approaches to avoid endotoxin release from the device are reported herein. These are, first, the purification of the polymeric components prior to microcapsule formation and, second, the complexation of endotoxin by the cationic components of the quaternary system.

There is no specific regulatory limit for endotoxin in a bioartificial pancreas, at least at present, where the "devices" or "biologies" are not yet in clinical studies. The threshold level of endotoxin for intravenous applications is set to five endotoxin units (EU) per kg body weight and hour.[15] Taking this value, the calculated endotoxin limit is approximately 2,000 EU/g dry polymer for the polymeric components in a bioartificial pancreas that consists of 420,000 islets encapsulated in microcapsules having a diameter of 0.4 mm.

## EXPERIMENTAL

### Materials

Sodium alginate (SA) (Keltone HV Kelco/NutraSweet, San Diego, CA, USA) and sodium cellulose sulfate (SCS) (Across Organics, Geel, Belgium) were used as polyanions. The polycation poly(methylene-co-guanidine) hydrochloride (PMCG) was purchased as 35% aqueous solution from Scientific Polymer Products, Inc. (Ontario, NY, USA).

### Endotoxin Removal from Polyanions

SA and SCS were dissolved in highly purified deionized water from a Milli-Q PF water purification system (Millipore, Switzerland). The solutions having concentrations of 1.5% (SA) and 2% (SCS) were successively filtered through filters with decreasing pore size in the range 30 to 0.22 μm. The filtration was followed by precipitation in solvent/non-solvent mixtures, polymer isolation, and drying (patent pending).

### Polymer Characterization

The intrinsic viscosity, [η], of SA and SCS was measured in 0.1 m NaCl solutions using an automatic viscosimeter, Viscologic TI1 (SEMATech, France). The kinematic viscosity of the polyanion solutions for microcapsule formation was measured with the same equipment. The degree of substitution (DS) of SCS and SA was determined by direct potentiometric complex titration (692 pH/Ion Meter, Metrohm, Switzerland) with poly(diallyldimethylammonium chloride) as polycationic component,[16] or was calculated from the partial specific volume, $\bar{v}$, applying the relationship

$$DS = 16.368 - 56.807\bar{v} + 49.87\bar{v}^2 \tag{1}$$

derived from recently published data.[17] The partial specific volume itself was calculated from a concentration series of density measurements carried out at 20°C using a Digital Precision Density Meter DMA60/DMA602 (Anton Paar, Graz, Austria).[17]

## Capsule Formation

Microcapsules were prepared by a two-step air-stripping droplet-generation method (patent pending). Droplets from 1.2% polyanion mixture (SA:SCS = 1:1) in PBS reacted in the first step with 1.5% calcium chloride/0.9% NaCl solution followed by a second reaction in 1.2% PMCG/0.9% NaCl solution and successive washing and storage in 0.9% NaCl solution.

## Complex Formation

Binary and ternary complexes have been produced by slight modifications of the capsule formation procedure. The appropriate polymer combination, consisting of two, three, or four components, was reacted. The complex formation included the following steps:

- Preparation of 2 ml sterile polyanion solution (1.2%),
- Precipitation in 75 ml cation/polycation solution,
- Washing with NaCl, and
- Storage in NaCl or culture medium.

## Endotoxin Test

The endotoxin content was determined by a standard kinetic turbidimetric method (LAL-5000 Series 2), and as recommended by the new FDA guidance from 1991.[18] Each test was performed in duplicate. The values presented in FIGURES 7 and 8 (see below) represent the average values. In general, for the endotoxin analysis a methodic error of 50% is accepted. However, it needs to be mentioned that this strongly depends on the total endotoxin content, with lower errors at higher concentrations.

## Mechanical Capsule Characterization

The mechanical resistance of microcapsules to compression was determined on a texture analyzer (Ta-XT2I, Stable Micro Systems, Godalming, U.K.). Each single capsule was compressed until it burst, at a rate of 0.4 mm/s. Force values at the bursting point were registered. The mechanical tests were performed after an equilibrium phase of five days.[19]

# RESULTS AND DISCUSSION

## Polyanion Purification and Storage

The previously described purification procedure delivered SA and SCS samples with endotoxin contents far below the FDA threshold. Repeating the precipitation step lead to further endotoxin decrease. The storage stability of the purified SA and SCS, having an initial endotoxin content ten times lower than the FDA threshold, was investigated during periods of six and five months, respectively. The results for these two polyanions are summarized in FIGURES 2 and 3.

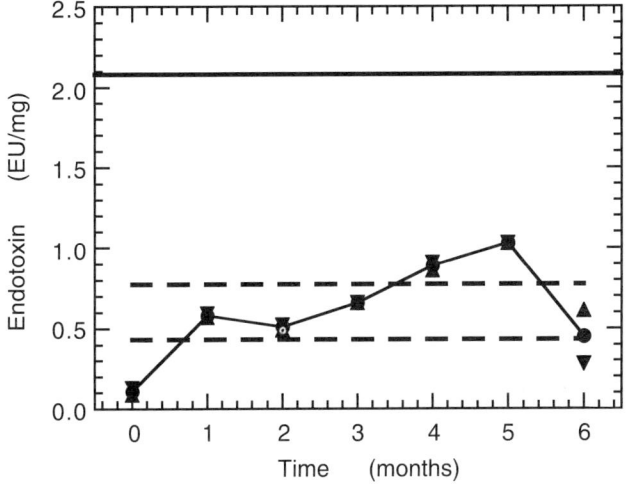

**FIGURE 2.** Storage stability of purified sodium alginate: ▲ first, ▼ second, ● mean value, --- confidence interval, — FDA threshold.

During the period of investigation the endotoxin content was maintained far below the FDA threshold. Whereas for SCS (FIG. 3), there is no significant time dependent variation in endotoxin concentration as seems to be the case for SA. The sample to sample variation for SA, however, may result from the relatively compact

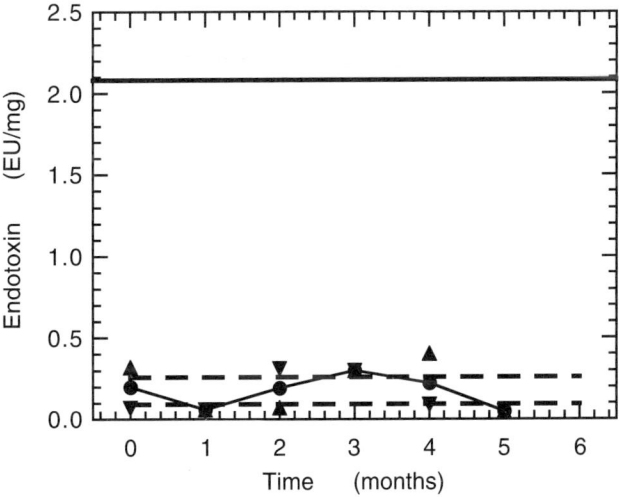

**FIGURE 3.** Storage stability of purified sodium cellulose sulfate: ▲ first, ▼ second, ● mean value, --- confidence interval, — FDA threshold.

TABLE 1. Influence of purification on macromolecular characteristics[a]

| | Sodium Alginate | | Sodium Cellulose Sulfate | |
|---|---|---|---|---|
| Parameter | Non-purified | Purified | Non-purified | Purified |
| $[\eta]$ (ml/g) in 0.1 m NaCl | 948 ± 28 | 904 ± 27 | 723 ± 22 | 793 ± 24 |
| DS | 1 | 1 | 2.5 ± 0.2 | 1.8 ± 0.2[b] |
| $\bar{v}$ (ml/g) | — | — | 0.359 ± 0.010 | 0.391 ± 0.012 |

[a] $[\eta]$, intrinsic viscosity; DS, degree of substitution; $\bar{v}$, partial specific volume.
[b] Calculated from $\bar{v}$ (see Ref. 18).

precipitation product investigated in the reported storage test. Such a compact precipitation may include endotoxin heterogeneously. The more homogeneous SCS precipitate did not exhibit this test to test variation. It was concluded from these results that SA precipitation had been improved.

The depyrogenation procedure did not influence the macromolecular characteristics significantly, as is summarized in TABLE 1.

For SA the intrinsic viscosity decreased by approximately 5%. An opposite change was found for SCS. Here the intrinsic viscosity increased by approximately 10% accompanied by a decrease of the degree of substitution from 2.5 to 1.8. However, these changes did not negatively influence the final microcapsule properties. Furthermore, no optical difference is visible in FIGURE 4 between capsules prepared from crude polymers and those from depyrogenated materials.

Measurement of the mechanical stability, five days after production, revealed a slightly higher stability for the pure materials. This is illustrated for three batches of each quality in FIGURE 5.

## Endotoxin Complexation

Based on the chemical structure of endotoxins, which possess a negative net charge, complexation with multivalent cations and polycations is expected. Since screening experiments detected very low endotoxin concentrations in the supernatant of the capsule, storage solutions detailed complex stability studies were performed to investigate separate complex combinations of the quaternary system. These are listed in TABLE 2.

The appropriate binary, ternary, and quaternary complexes from the combinations in TABLE 2 were stored, separately, in total volumes of 10 ml NaCl solution and 12 ml culture medium (RPMI). The photomicrographs of FIGURE 6 show selected complexes in NaCl and culture medium. It needs to be mentioned that SCS does not form a complex structure with calcium ions.

As it can be seen from FIGURE 6 the alginate complexes lead to a spherical geometry. Strong shrinking is evident for SCS.

Storage of endotoxin complexes in NaCl or culture medium did not indicate a remarkable endotoxin release after five months or three months, respectively. The total endotoxin concentration in the samples invariably remained far below the calculated FDA threshold. This is demonstrated in FIGURES 7 and 8 for storage at 4°C.

FIGURE 7 indicates, for all binary and ternary complexes of alginate, as well as the binary complex of SCS, after five months, even endotoxin levels below 1 EU/ml are detected. For these experiments the FDA threshold was estimated to be 5 EU/ml (not shown in FIG. 7). The more significant storage in culture medium was, additionally, extended to the quaternary complex and storage at 37°C. Under these conditions the endotoxin concentration exceeded 1 EU/ml only for SA in $CaCl_2$. The shaded

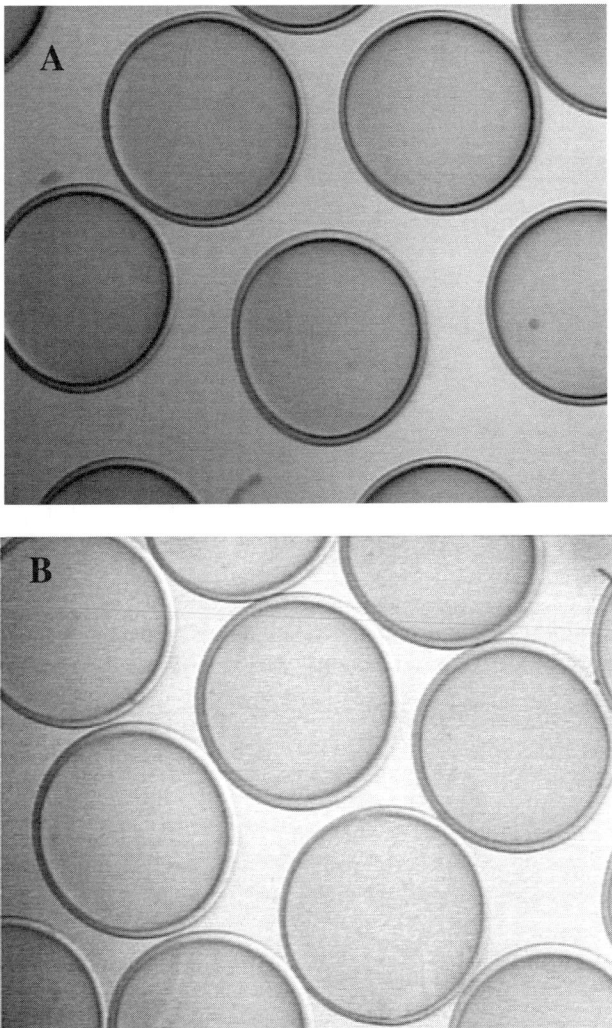

**FIGURE 4.** Capsules from non-purified (**A**) and purified (**B**) polyanions. 1.2% SA/SCS in PBS, viscosity: (**A**) 65.6 mPas, (**B**) 63.2 mPas. Receiving bath 1, 1.5% $CaCl_2$/0.9% NaCl. Receiving bath 2, 1.2% PMCG/0.9% NaCl. Capsule size, 1.0±0.1 mm.

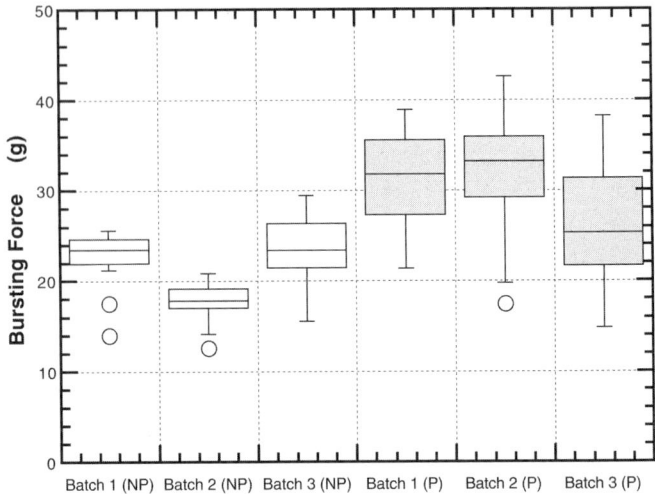

**FIGURE 5.** Influence of purification on the mechanical properties of microcapsules prepared from non-purified (*NP*) and purified polyanions (*P*), prepared as described in FIGURE 4, with membrane formation for 40 seconds. The experimental data are represented by a *box plot*. The *horizontal lines* inside the boxes represent the median values of the bursting force and the limits of the box denote the upper and lower quartiles. The maximum and minimum values delimit the *bars* and the *circles* are extremes.

columns in FIGURE 8 represent the endotoxin concentration after storage for four weeks at 4°C and additionally two weeks at 37°C. After this investigation period, and considering the error range, the endotoxin release did not change in comparison to that at 4°C. Long term investigations are now in progress.

The thresholds were calculated based on the assumption that a bioartificial pancreas consists of 420,000 islet-containing microcapsules having a diameter of 0.4 mm. These correspond to a pancreas volume of 14 ml with a total endotoxin limit release of 350 EU/h for a 70-kg patient. For the 2 ml of capsules produced for each experimental batch, the threshold is 50 EU/h and by considering the dilution by the supernatant (totally 10 or 12 ml) limits of 5 EU/ml (storage in NaCl) and 4.2 EU/ml

**TABLE 2. Chemical combinations for binary, ternary, and quaternary complexes**

| Complex Number | Complex Type | Polyanion Solution | Cation/Polycation Solution |
|---|---|---|---|
| 1 | binary | SA/ET | $CaCl_2$ |
| 2 | binary | SA/ET | PMCG |
| 3 | ternary | SA/ET | $CaCl_2$/PMCG |
| 4 | binary | SCS/ET | PMCG |
| 5 | quaternary | SA/SCS/ET | 1. $CaCl_2$, 2. PMCG |

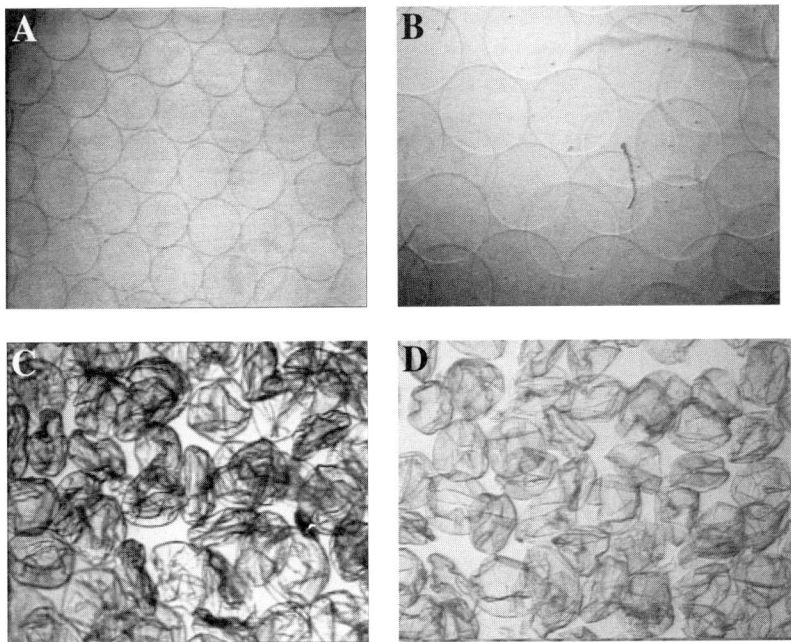

**FIGURE 6.** Selected complexes in NaCl and culture medium. (**A**) SA/CaCl$_2$ in NaCl and (**B**) in RPMI. (**C**) SCS/PMCG in NaCl and (**D**) in RPMI.

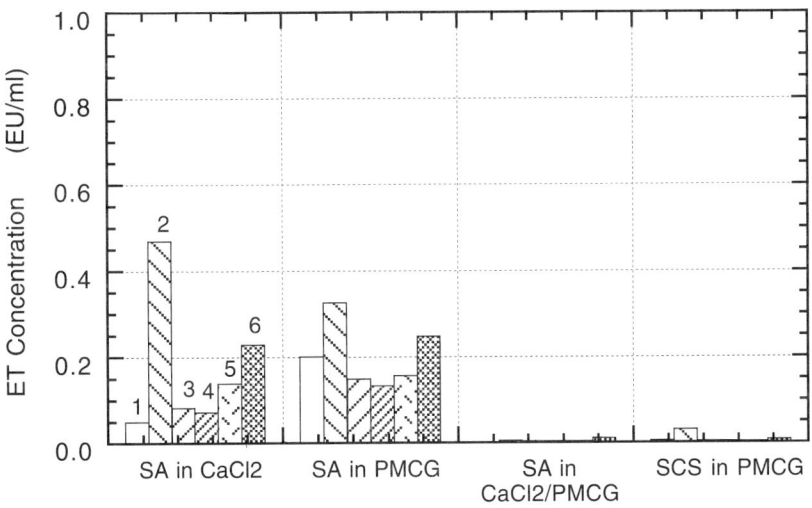

**FIGURE 7.** Storage stability of endotoxin complexes in NaCl at 4°C. *1*, 24 h; *2*, one month; *3*, two months; *4*, three months; *5*, four months; *6*, five months. FDA threshold at 5 EU/ml.

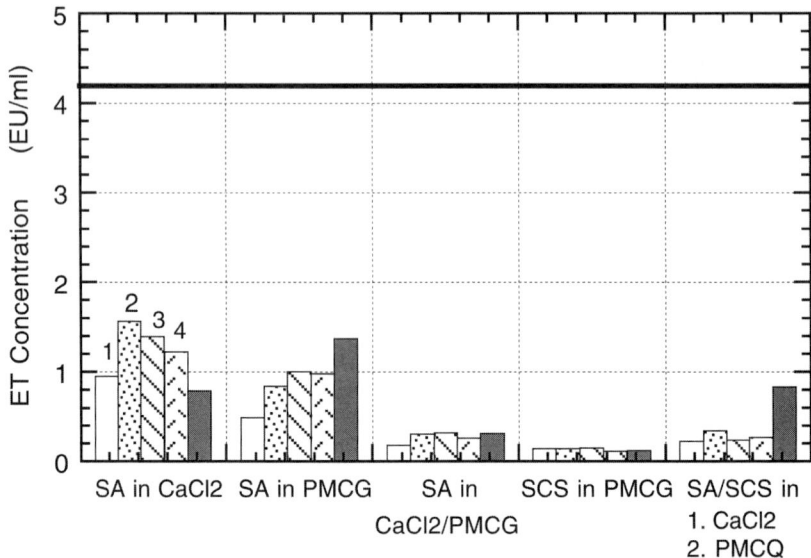

**FIGURE 8.** Storage stability of entotoxin complexes in culture medium (RPMI) at 4°C. *1*, 24 h; *2*, two weeks; *3*, one month; *4*, three months. *Shaded columns*, four weeks at 4°C and two weeks at 37°C.

(storage in culture medium) can be derived. A comparison with the initial endotoxin concentrations in the polyanions indicates that significant amounts of endotoxin are bound in the various complexes. Without any endotoxin complexation, for example, in the supernatant of Complexes 1–5 (TABLE 2) stored in the culture medium, the following endotoxin concentrations should be present:

- 16.8 EU/ml for Complexes 1–3,
- 36.4 EU/ml for Complex 4, and
- 26.6 EU/ml for Complex 5.

The endotoxin concentrations plotted in FIGURE 8 show, for all complexes, 10 to 100 times lower values and, therefore, prove that a stable complexation of endotoxin is obtained if the complexes are prepared from sterile polyanion solutions.

## CONCLUSIONS

The experimental studies described in this paper reveal that endotoxin can be reduced in sodium alginate and sodium cellulose sulfate to one order of magnitude below the regulatory threshold by procedures that are based on various solubilities in organic solvents. The low endotoxin content remains stable for at least six months. The purification process developed shows only minor influence on the macromolecular characteristics of the two polyanions employed and, as a consequence, on the microcapsule properties. Furthermore, it was proved that endotoxin forms stable complexes with the cationic components of the quaternary capsule system. Therefore, endotoxin release can, most likely, be excluded as a reason for the body response to transplanted microcapsules produced from the chemistry investigated.

## ACKNOWLEDGMENTS

D. Hunkeler is acknowledged for his critical and helpful discussions. D. Espinosa, B. Rochat, G. Grigorescu U. Schuldt, A. Rehor, and I. Ceausoglu are acknowledged for experimental support. The EPFL, FNS, and CTI supported the work financially.

## REFERENCES

1. PETSCH, D. & F.B. ANSPACH. 2000. Endotoxin removal from protein solutions. J. Biotechnol. **76:** 97–119.
2. HOU, K.C. & R. ZANIEWSKI. 1990. Depyrogenation by endotoxin removal with positively charged depth filter cartridge. J. Parenter. Sci. Technol. **44:** 204–209.
3. HEIDHARDT, E.A., M.A. LUTHER & M.A. RECNY. 1992. Rapid, two-step purification process for the preparation of pyrogen-free murine immunoglobulin G1 monoclonal antibodies. J. Chromatogr. **590:** 255–261.
4. BORDIER, C. 1981. Phase separation of integral membrane proteins in Triton X-114 solution. J. Biol. Chem. **256:** 1604–1607.
5. AIDA, Y. & M.J. PABST. 1990. Removal of endotoxin from proteion solutions by phase separation using Triton X-114. J. Immunol. Meth. **132:** 191–195.
6. LIU, S., R. TOBIAS, S. MCCLURE, et al. 1997. Removal of endotoxin from recombinant protein preparations. Clin. Biochem. **30:** 455–463.
7. KARPLUS, T.E., R.J. ULEVITCH & C.B. WILSON. 1987. A new method for reduction of endotoxin contaminations from protein solutions. J. Immunol. Meth. **105:** 211–220.
8. ANSPACH, F.B. & O. HILBECK. 1995. Removal of endotoxin by affinity sorbents. J. Chromatogr. A **711:** 81–92.
9. MATSUMAE, H., S. MINOBE, K. KINDAN, et al. 1990. Specific removal of endotoxin from protein solutions by immobilized histidine. Biotechnol. Appl. Biochem. **12:** 129–140.
10. MITZNER, S., J. SCHEIDEWIND, D. FALKENHAGEN, et al. 1993. Extracorporeal endotoxin removal by immobilized polyethylenimine. Artificial Organs **17:** 775–781.
11. ZIMMERMANN, U., G. KLÖCK, K. FEDERLIN, et al. 1992. Production of mitogen-contamination free alginates with variable ratios of mannuronic acid to guluronic acid by free flow electrophoresis. Electrophoresis **13:** 269–274.
12. KLÖCK, G., H. FRANK, R. HOUBEN, et al. 1994. Production of purified alginates suitable for use in immunoisolated transplantation. Appl. Microbiol. Biotechnol. **40:** 638–643.
13. PROKOP, A. & T.G. WANG. 1996. Purification of polymers used for fabrication of an immunoisolation barrier. Bioartificial organs I. Ann. N.Y. Acad. Sci. **831:** 223–231.
14. BARTKOWIAK, A., L. CANAPLE, I. CEAUSOGLU, et al. 1999. New multicomponent capsules for immunoisolation. Bioartificial organs II. Ann. N.Y. Acad. Sci. **875:** 135–145.
15. EUROPEAN PHARMACOPOEIA. 1997. Third edit. European Department for the Quality of Medicines within the Council of Europe, Strasbourg.
16. WANDREY, C., J. HERNANDEZ-BARAJAS & D. HUNKELER. 1999. Diallyldimethylammonium chloride and its polymers. Adv. Polym. Sci. **145:** 123–182.

17. WANDREY, C., A. BARTKOWIAK & D. HUNKELER. 1999. Partial molar and specific volumes of polyelectrolytes: comparison of experimental and predicted values in salt-free solutions. Langmuir **15:** 4062–4068.
18. FEDERAL DRUG ADMINISTRATION. 1987. FDA Guidelines 1991. USP: bacterial endotoxins test.
19. REHOR, A., L. CANAPLE, Z. ZHANG & D. HUNKELER. 2001. The compressive deformation of multicomponent microcapsules: influence of size, membrane thickness and compression speed. J. Biomat. Sci., Polym. Edit. **12:** 157–170.

# A Novel Class of Amitogenic Alginate Microcapsules for Long-Term Immunoisolated Transplantation

ULRICH ZIMMERMANN,[a] FRANK THÜRMER,[a] ANETTE JORK,[a] MEIKE WEBER,[a] SASKIA MIMIETZ,[a] MARKUS HILLGÄRTNER,[a] FRANK BRUNNENMEIER,[a] HEIKO ZIMMERMANN,[b] INES WESTPHAL,[b] GÜNTER FUHR,[b] ULRIKE NÖTH,[c] AXEL HAASE,[c] ANDRE STEINERT,[d] AND CHRISTIAN HENDRICH[d]

[a]*Lehrstuhl für Biotechnologie, Biozentrum, Universität Würzburg, D-97074 Würzburg, Germany*

[b]*Lehrstuhl für Membranphysiologie, Institut für Biologie, Humboldt-Universität zu Berlin, D-10115 Berlin, Germany*

[c]*Lehrstuhl für Biophysik, Physikalisches Institut, Universität Würzburg, D-97074 Würzburg, Germany*

[d]*Orthopädische Universitätsklinik, König-Ludwig-Haus, Universität Würzburg, D-97074 Würzburg, Germany*

ABSTRACT: In the light of results of clinical trials with immunoisolated human parathyroid tissue $Ba^{2+}$-alginate capsules were developed that meet the requirements for long-term immunoisolated transplantation of (allogeneic and xenogeneic) cells and tissue fragments. Biocompatibility of the capsules was achieved by subjecting high-M alginate extracted from freshly collected brown algae to a simple purification protocol that removes quantitatively mitogenic and cytotoxic impurities without degradation of the alginate polymers. The final ultra-high-viscosity, clinical-grade (UHV/CG) product did not evoke any (significant) foreign body reaction in BB rats or in baboons. Similarly, the very sensitive pERK assay did not reveal any mitogenic impurities. Encapsulated cells also exhibited excellent secretory properties under *in vitro* conditions. Despite biocompatible material, pericapsular fibrosis is also induced by imperfect capsule surfaces that can favor cell attachment and migration under the release of material traces. This material can interact with free end monomers of the alginate polymers under formation of mitogenic advanced glycation products. Smooth surfaces, and thus topographical biocompatibility of the capsules (visualized by atomic force microscopy), can be generated by appropriate crosslinking of the UHV/CG-alginate with $Ba^{2+}$ and simultaneous suppression of capsule swelling by incorporation of proteins and/or perfluorocarbons (i.e., medically approved compounds with high oxygen capacity). Perfluorocarbon-loaded alginate capsules allow long-term non-invasive monitoring of the location and the oxygen supply of the transplants by using $^{19}$F-MRI. Transplantation studies in rats demonstrated that these capsules were functional over a period of more than two years.

KEYWORDS: alginate; encapsulation; immunoisolation; mitogenicity; chondrocytes

Address for correspondence: Prof. Dr. U. Zimmermann, Lehrstuhl für Biotechnologie, Biozentrum, Am Hubland, D-97074 Würzburg, Germany. Voice: 0049 931 888 4508; fax: 0049 931 888 4509.
zimmerma@biozentrum.uni-wuerzburg.de

## INTRODUCTION

Immunoisolated allo- and xenotransplantation offer a promising way to overcome the limitations of current treatments of disorders that are closely coupled to deficient or subnormal metabolic or secretory cell functions. Various synthetic polymers and biopolymers are used for immunoisolation.[1,2] Among these, alginate has been and will continue to be one of the most important biomaterials. Recent pilot clinical trials have shown the feasibility of alginate-based microcapsules for immunoisolated transplantation.[3,4] Transplantation of $Ba^{2+}$-alginate–encapsulated, subclinical allogeneic parathyroid tissue into the non-dominant forearm muscles of two patients with hypoparathyroidism demonstrated normocalcemia and normal levels of parathormone, shortly after surgery. The patients did not receive any immunosuppressives. After about three months, graft failure occurred, but on reexamination about one year later, one of the patients was nearly normocalcemic and again free from symptoms (for details, see Zimmermann *et al.*[4]).

The first small-scale clinical studies were encouraging, but they also clearly demonstrated the need for engineering long-term functional, immunoprotective microcapsules. Research in our laboratories during the past three years has shown that several matrix-related factors were responsible for the functional loss of the parathyroid transplant. Consideration of these factors has resulted in novel alginate microcapsules that meet the requirements for long-term clinical applications.

### *Large-Scale Production of Clinical-Grade, Ultra-high-viscosity Alginate*

One of the major problems associated with alginate-based transplants is the mitogenic and cytotoxic impurities in the commercial alginates. Due to the industrial harvesting and extraction processes from brown algæ, commercial alginates are contaminated, not only with natural mitogenic impurities, but also by bacterial compounds of animal and human origin. Separation of commercial alginates by using free flow electrophoresis has shown (see FIGURE 1 A) that this material contains 10–20 mitogenic impurities (for details, see Zimmermann *et al.*[5]). Therefore, implantation of commercial alginate capsules (crosslinked with $Ba^{2+}$ by using a two-channel droplet generator) into rodents evokes heavy pericapsular fibrosis (FIG. 1 A).[6] Removal of the mitogenic (and cytotoxic) contaminants by free flow electrophoresis, or by chemical means, resulted in the absence of any significant fibrotic overgrowth, even when empty capsules were implanted in BB/OK rats (FIG. 1 B).[5,7] This strain exhibits—in contrast to other less immunoreactive rodents (such as, BALB and Lewis)—an elevated macrophage activity and is, therefore, a very good model system for the evaluation of possible immune reactions in human beings.

Amitogenic alginate purified from commercial alginate was used in the clinical trials mentioned above. Reproducible production of clinical-grade alginate from commercial products is, however, very difficult because of large variations in the initial composition of the raw algal material. Additionally, commercial alginates must be subjected to many extraction steps to purify to the level necessary for clinical applications and only relatively small amounts of amitogenic alginate are obtained.[7]

The problems of current purification methods can be circumvented by using clearly defined algal material instead of commercial alginate. Research in this direction has shown that fresh stipes of *Laminariales* (e.g., *Laminaria pallida* and *Lessonia*

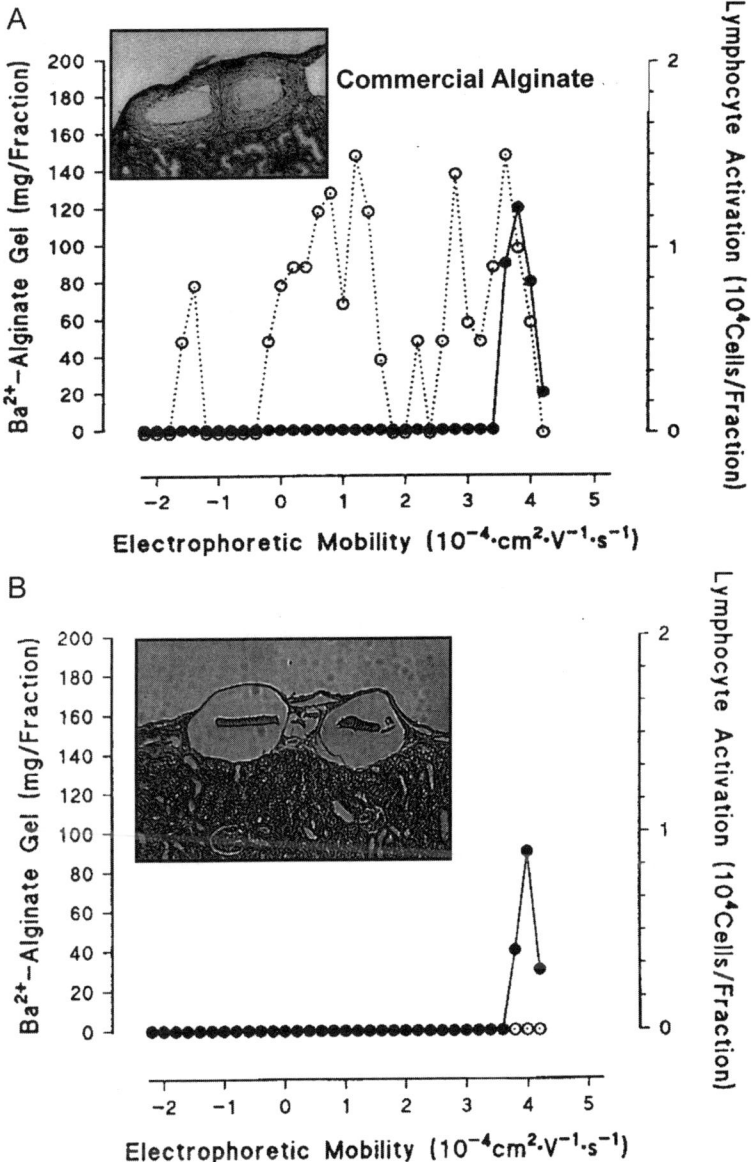

FIGURE 1. (A) Fractions of commercial alginate were separated by free flow electrophoresis and precipitated by $Ba^{2+}$ (*closed circles*). Mitogenic impurities (*open circles*) were detected when the 35 fractions were subjected to the "mixed lymphocyte assay" in $Ca^{2+}$-containing culture medium. When such alginate is implanted under the kidney capsule of BB/OK rats, pericapsular fibrosis is induced (*inset*). Removal of the mitogenic impurities by purification of the alginate (B) resulted in biocompatible implants (*inset*). (Taken from Zimmermann et al., Ref. 5, with permission.)

*nigrescens*) harvested directly from the sea or genetically defined sporophytes of these species (see e.g., Venegas *et al.*[8]) grown in bioreactors are ideal input sources. When using such material, the manufacturing process can be simplified considerably (see FIGURE 2), thus allowing not only a reproducible, but also a large-scale production of clinical-grade (CG) alginate.

Depending critically on the extraction and purification parameters, ultra-high-viscosity and clinical-grade (UHV/CG) alginate can be obtained. The dynamic viscosity of a 0.1% w/v solution of a typical batch was determined to be 20–40 cP (in contrast to 1–5 cP of a corresponding solution made up of commercial alginate). Analysis of the UHV/CG-alginate showed the absence of proteins, polyphenols, endotoxins (about 0.5 EU per ml of a 0.5% w/v alginate solution), and so forth, as well as very low levels of heavy metal ions and particularly of sulfur (less than 370 mg sulfur/kg alginate) indicating the complete removal of fucoidan and other related sulfated mitogenic compounds (unpublished data).[9]

### *Biocompatibility of UHV/CG-Alginate*

With increasing viscosity (i.e., with increasing molecular mass) toxicity of compounds generally decreases to negligible levels.[10,11] Furthermore, it is well known that saccharides can react non-enzymatically with proteins, nucleotides, and lipids resulting in advanced glycation products (AGEs) that can evoke an inflammatory response.[12,13] Alginates are composed of homo- and heteropolymeric blocks of 1,4-linked α-L-guluronic monomers and β-D-mannuronic monomers (G-G, M-M, and M-G blocks).[4,14] Due to its high molecular mass UHV-alginate contains less free sugar residues than low-viscosity alginate provided that the crosslinking process is performed properly (see below). Thus, it can be expected that formation of AGEs by reactions of $Ba^{2+}$-crosslinked UHV-alginate with blood components should be less

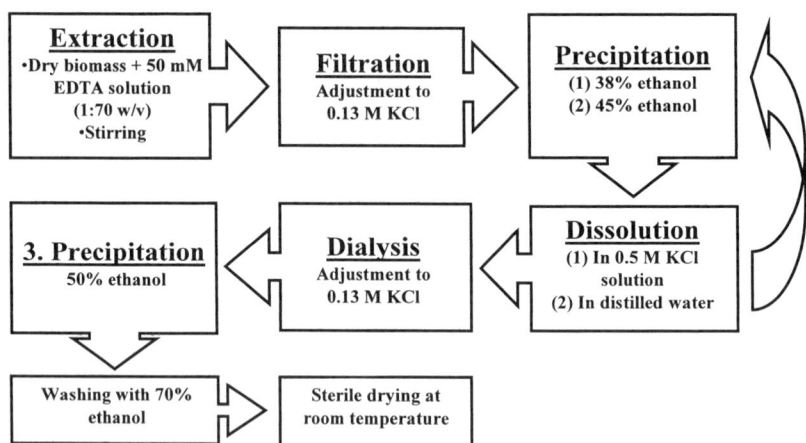

**FIGURE 2.** Flow chart for the purification of high-M, ultra-high-viscosity alginate extracted from fresh brown algae.

or even completely eliminated when vascularization of the transplanted microcapsules has occurred.

Consistent with this assumption, the "costimulated, mixed lymphocyte test" (for details, see Zimmermann et al.[14,15]) as well as the electronic determination of the number and the size of proliferating lymphocytes did not reveal any mitogenic impurity of UHV/CG alginate extracted from freshly collected stipes of L. pallida or L. nigrescens. An in vitro cell assay that responds extremely sensitively to the presence of mitogenic impurities yielded similar results (see FIGURE 3; Brunnenmeier et al., manuscript in preparation). This assay is based on the phosphorylation of ERK, a component of the MAPK signaling cascade.[16] Phosphorylated ERK (pERK) can accurately be determined by Western immunoblot. Furthermore, when UHV/CG alginate microcapsules crosslinked with $Ba^{2+}$ were implanted for three weeks under the kidney capsule of BB/OK rats, retrieval of the implants did not exhibit any significant foreign body reactions (see FIGURE 4 A and B). The small pericapsular fibrosis seen sometimes after a 12-week implantation in the muscle of baboons (FIG. 4C) was presumably induced by the surgery procedure, as suggested by recent animal studies (see also below).

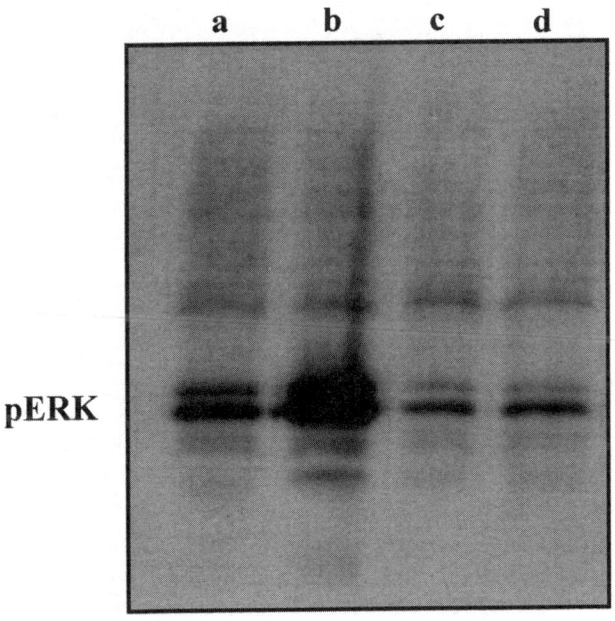

**FIGURE 3.** In vitro bioassay based on the phosphorylation of ERK (a component of the MAPK signaling cascade) induced by mitogenic impurities. Phosphorylated ERK (pERK) was determined by Western immunoblot. a, unstimulated Jurkat cells (negative control); b, cells stimulated with mitogenic phorbol-12-myristate-13-acetate (positive control); c and d, cells stimulated with UHV/CG alginate extracted and purified from L. pallida and L. nigrescens, respectively, according to the flow chart in FIGURE 2. Note that the formation of pERK in the presence of UHV/CG alginate is weaker than the negative control. This could be a hint for immunosuppressive properties of the alginate.

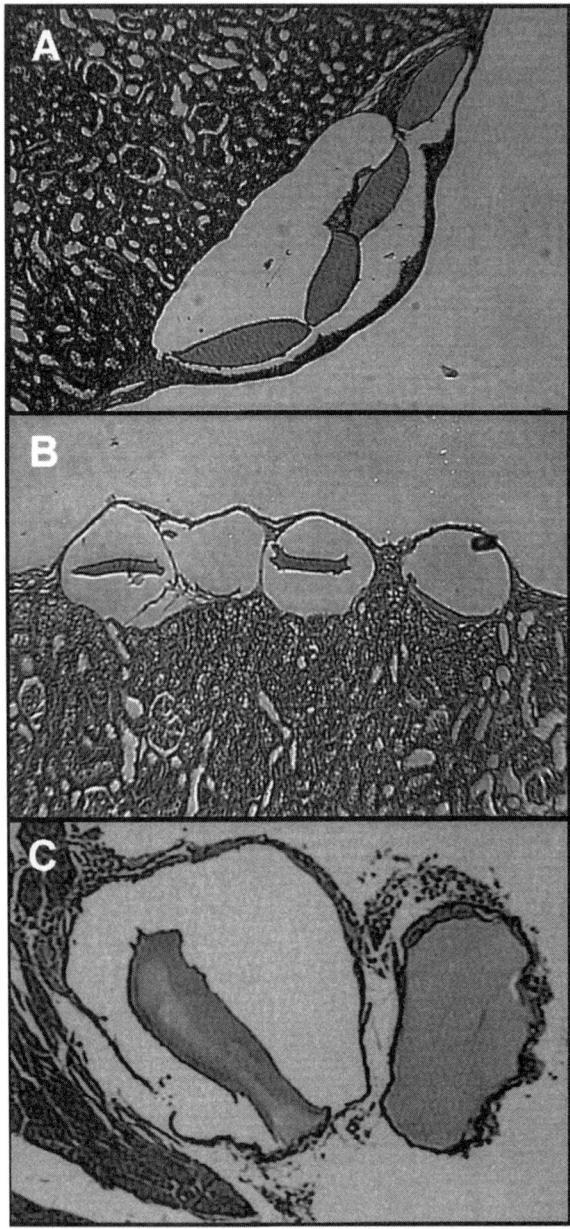

**FIGURE 4.** $Ba^{2+}$-alginate microcapsules made up of UHV/CG alginate extracted from *L. pallida* (**A** and **C**) and *L. nigrescens* (**B**) and implanted under the kidney capsules of BB/OK rats (**A** and **B**) and in the muscle of a baboon (**C**). Capsules were retrieved four weeks (**A** and **B**) and 12 weeks (**C**) after implantation. Note that because of the fixation process, the alginate capsules may collapse or become deformed. For further details, see text.

The biocompatibility of the UHV/CG alginate was also tested by encapsulation of different human and murine cell lines and by subsequently monitoring their secretory functions (e.g., monoclonal antibodies, TNF-α, and collagen secretion). These experiments demonstrated that ultra-high-viscosity alginate is advantageous for cell encapsulation because it allows optimum adaptation of permeation properties (while maintaining immunoprotection) to the desired needs by delicate adjustment of the concentration of the alginate. Due to the extremely high viscosity, only alginate solutions of 0.5 to 1% w/v can be used (in contrast to 2–3% in the case of commercial alginate solutions). An example for cell encapsulation is shown in FIGURE 5. C3H10T1/2-BMP-2 or BMP-4 is a murine mesenchymal progenitor cell line in which cDNA encoding the human bone morphogenetic protein BMP-2 or BMP-4 was permanently transferred.[17] Therefore, this adherent cell line is a realistic model system for investigation of restoration of cartilage. In contrast to monolayer cultures, cell proliferation was prevented in the three-dimensional matrix made up of $Ca^{2+}$-UHV/CG alginate (FIG. 5A). Immunochemistry carried out two weeks after addition of differentiation medium demonstrated that the cells did not secrete collagen I (FIG. 5C; as the proliferating monolayer cultures), but collagen II (FIG. 5B), one of the main components of functional cartilage.

## *Performance of Biocompatible $Ba^{2+}$-Alginate Microcapsules for Long-Term Transplantation*

Amitogenic properties of the capsule matrix material is not the only obligatory requirement for immunoisolated transplantation. Capsule stability and particularly topography are equally important as indicated by the clinical studies with encapsulated human parathyroid tissue (see above). Studies with biomaterial-based or synthetic implants have also shown that the immune response of the host to the implant is not only determined by the chemical reactivity, but also by the topography of its surface.[18,19] The topography is closely linked with the swelling properties of the polyelectrolyte gel and depends, therefore, on a delicate balance between several competing thermodynamic forces.[20] These include (1) osmotic pressure of free ions in the gels, (2) Debye-Hückel interaction of ions, (3) molecular interactions between water and the polymeric chains, and (4) network elasticity. Network elasticity is not a problem when high-M or—even better—high-M, ultra-high-viscosity alginate with $Ba^{2+}$ as a crosslinking agent is used.[3,5–7,21] The alginates extracted from *L. pallida* and *L. nigrescens* contain about 60–70% M and, therefore, meet these requirements.[22–24] Removal of excessive $Ba^{2+}$-ions within the matrix can easily be achieved by washing the microcapsules after formation with a 6 mM sodium sulfate solution. In this way, the osmotic pressure of free ions, as well as Debye-Hückel interactions of mobile and fixed ions, are reduced significantly. As depicted in FIGURE 6, this treatment delays the swelling of the capsules under *in vitro* conditions, but does not prevent burst. The reason for this is the binding of the water molecules to the polymeric chains of the alginate—an effect that was not taken into account in the past when microcapsules with different features were designed. Electrorotation studies have revealed that the aqueous environment within the capsules is completely different to that of the bulk solution.[25,26] As shown in FIGURE 7 the dispersion of water centered around 20 GHz for free water is shifted to about

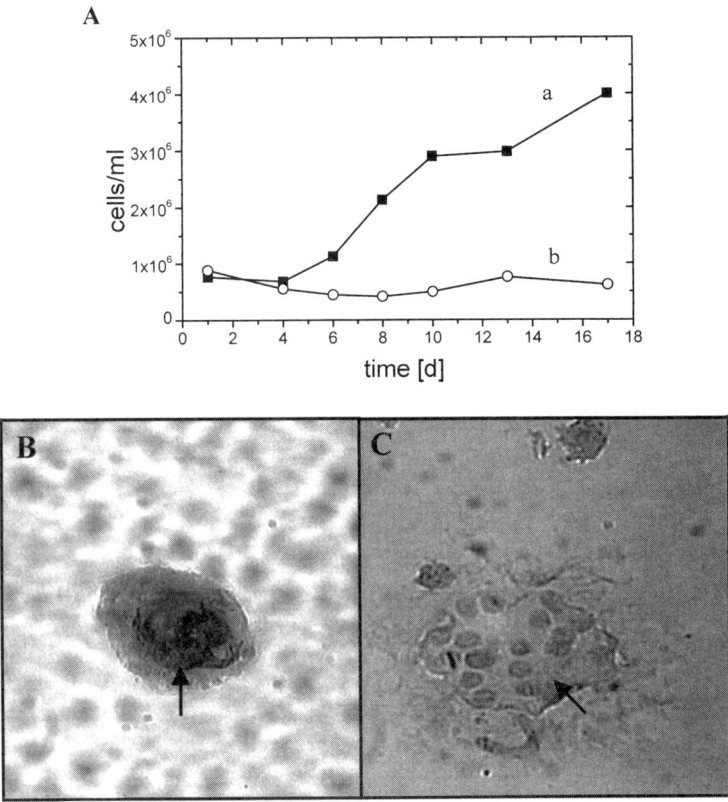

**FIGURE 5.** (**A**) Typical growth curves of the adherent cell line C3H10T1/2 transfected permanently with a gene encoding for bone morphogentic protein BMP-2 (similar curves were obtained for cells transfected with BMP-4). Cells were grown (at an initial density of $1 \times 10^6$/ml) for 17 days in monolayers (*a*) and in microcapsules (*b*) made up of a 0.5% w/v UHV/CG alginate solution that was crosslinked with $Ca^{2+}$. On day three, the culture medium was replaced by differentiation medium (supplemented with ascorbic acid and β-glycerophosphate). Subsequently, half of the differentiation medium was exchanged by fresh medium every three days. After trypsin treatment and dissolution of the capsules with a 50 mM EDTA solution, respectively, the number of viable cells was counted with an electronic cell analyzer. Note that some cells were lost by the suspension procedures of the cells. (**B** and **C**) The three-dimensional matrix apparently suppressed growth but stimulated the secretory function of the encapsulated cells. Evidence of collagen II (*arrow* in **B**), but not of collagen I (*arrow* in **C**) production of encapsulated C3H10T1/2-BMP-4 cells 17 days after cultivation in differentiation medium (for conditions, see **A**). Immunostaining was performed on 50-μm-thick cryosections of beads embedded in Tissue-Tek (Sakura, Zoeterwoude, the Netherlands). The sections (stained with Mayers Hämalaun for 5 min) were treated with pepsin (8 g/l in 0.1 N HCl) prior to incubation with the specific anticollagen II antibody (1:100 mouse anticollagen type II monoclonal antibody, Chemicon International Inc., Temecula, USA). In the case of collagen I (1:50 rabbit mouse anti-collagen type I polyclonal antiserum) predigestion was not necessary.

20 MHz—a clear indication that most of the water is bound in alginate-based microcapsules (independent of the crosslinking divalent cation).

Bound water not only induces capsule swelling of the three-dimensional matrix, but could also have extremely important consequences on the viability, proliferation, and secretory properties of the encapsulated cells and tissues.[15] For example, water of high structural order may be the cause for the greatly improved viability of encapsulated cells when compared with freely suspended cells (e.g., Schnabl et al.[27]). Because of the high level of bound water in the three-dimensional matrix, it is conceivable that (protein- and lipid-degrading) enzymes released from dead cells are not developing full activity or are completely inactive, thus protecting other cells against enzymatic degradation. At the present state of the art the information about possible effects of bound water on the transplant is too rudimentary in order to arrive at a safe conclusion (see Webb[28]). Other factors such as stagnant water may be of equal importance. In the case of encapsulated cells (such as chondrocytes or C3H10T1/2-BMP fibroblasts, see above) it is even more difficult to predict "bound water" effects on

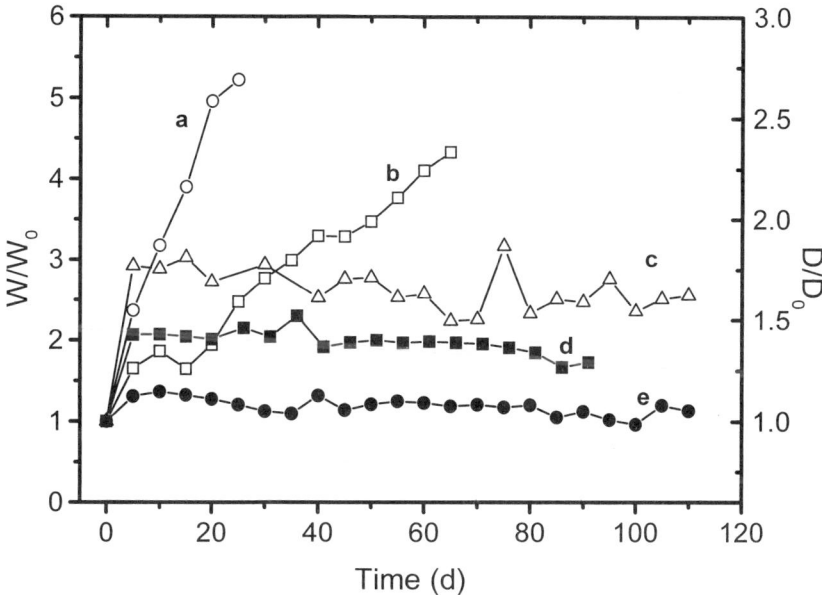

**FIGURE 6.** Typical swelling (stability) curves of microcapsules made up of UHV/CG alginate and crosslinked with $Ba^{2+}$. The capsules were kept in an iso-osmolar NaCl solution and their (increase in) weight was measured regularly by using a balance. In the graph (*open symbols*) the weight ($W$) is plotted normalized to the initial weight ($W_0$). Measurements of the diameter ($D$ normalized to the initial diameter $D_0$; *closed symbols*) under the microscope yielded similar results. (*a*) controls, (*b*) treated with 6 mM $Na_2SO_4$, (*c*) and (*d*) 6 mM $Na_2SO_4$ + incorporation of 10% human serum proteins and of FCS, respectively, (*e*) 6 mM $Na_2SO_4$ + incorporation of 10% FCS and perfluorocarbon (alginate : Fluosol® = 1 : 1). For further details, see Hillgärtner et al.[30] Note that only a part of the swelling curves is shown. Serum-alginate capsules were stable for about two years.

secretion of hormones, collagen and other factors because the matrix barrier may force the cells to adapt their morphology and shape. Such changes can be coupled with the secretory function of these cells.[29]

The compromising effect of bound water on capsule swelling can be eliminated (while preserving the obviously beneficial effect of bound water on transplant function) when proteins (e.g., FCS or serum proteins of the patients) and/or hydrophobic (medically approved) perfluorocarbons are incorporated into the microcapsules (see FIG. 6).[4,15,30] Proteins shift the water dispersion to about 110 MHz (FIG. 7), that is, to a frequency range where part of the water is mobile. Perfluorocarbons lowered the concentration of bound water by half, as indicated by a decrease in the relative permittivity of the capsule (FIG. 7). These treatments together with the use of high-M and ultra-high-viscosity alginate result in capsules that are stable under *in vitro* and *in vivo* conditions for more than two years (the experiments and the animal studies are still going on; see below).

The suppression of swelling has a positive effect on the nano/microscale topography of the microcapsules. Atomic force microscopy (AFM) images of $Ba^{2+}$-alginate capsules of 1 mm diameter made up of UHV/CG alginate and stabilized with sulfate and protein look quite homogeneous, except for some wrinkles. Cap-

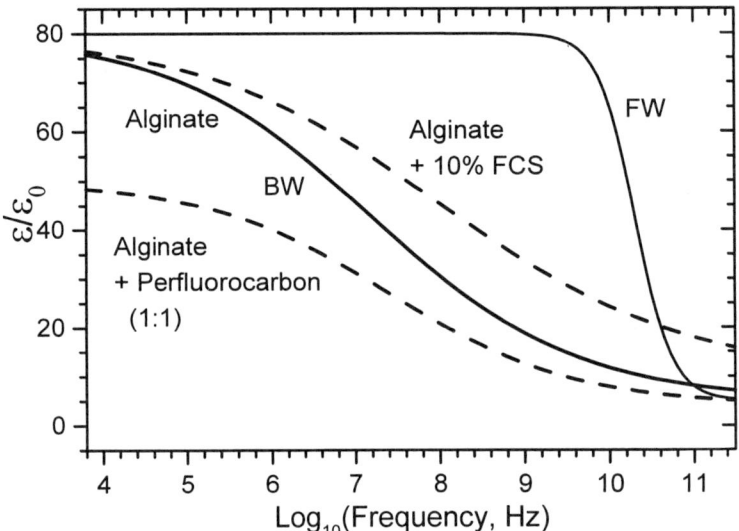

**FIGURE 7.** Frequency dependence of the relative permittivity $\varepsilon/\varepsilon_0$ of free water (*FW*) and of alginate hydrogel capsules (*BW*) derived from electrorotation spectra. The dispersion of free water occurs at about 20 GHz whereas the dispersion of the water in the alginate capsules is smeared and centered around 20 MHz, indicating a tightly bound water structure within the gel. Incorporation of proteins into the alginate capsules shifts the dispersion back to higher frequencies (about 106 MHz), whereas perfluorocarbons (Fluosol®) reduce the concentration of bound water as indicated by a decrease in the relative permittivity of the capsules (alginate : Fluosol® = 1 : 1). For further details, see Esch *et al.*[25]

sules retrieved after a four-week implantation in the peritoneum of a rat show no significant changes in the topography of their surfaces (see FIGURE 8A). In contrast, AFM images of perfluorocarbon-alginate capsules implanted for 15 months show deposition of fibrils on their surfaces (FIG. 8B). The deposition of the material may be due to crevices in the capsule surfaces generated by mechanical shearing forces exerted on the relatively large capsules during implantation. This assumption is supported by *in vitro* experiments performed in the meantime, calling for an improvement of the implantation techniques. However, the possibility cannot be excluded that, during the long implantation period, imperfections in the microarchitecture of the capsule surface occurred due to mechanical stress. Formation of AGEs may also be a possible cause for the occurrence of material deposition on the capsule surface. These reactions will depend on the vascularization and, thus, on the transplantation site.

In any case, these findings and other evidence suggest that the cascades of fibrotic overgrowth must be studied in more depth with respect to dependence on the transplantation site.[18,19] Model experiments performed in the last two years in the laboratories of the authors have given some insight into the initial processes that may be involved in fibrotic overgrowth. Fibroblasts, antigen-presenting cells (APCs) and other anchorage-dependent cells cannot use UHV/CG alginate as a substratum for attachment as well as subsequent spreading and migration. This can be demonstrated (H. Zimmermann, I. Westphal, and G. Fuhr, manuscript in preparation) when attachment and migration of fibroblasts were studied by *in vitro* experiments in which the mechanical and/or chemical imperfections in the surface of implanted microcapsules were modeled by a planar $Ba^{2+}$-UHV/CG alginate film of very smooth topography (see FIGURE 9A) that only partly covered a glass surface (FIG. 9B). It is evident that cell adhesion and migration only occurred on the alginate-free surface—despite some efforts of the cell to crawl over the alginate film (FIG. 9B). These findings indicate that smooth $Ba^{2+}$-UHV/CG alginate surfaces prevent cell adhesion and migration. During crawling on the alginate-free surface cells regularly release material traces (FIG. 9B) that can be visualized by AFM, electron scanning, interference reflection, or confocal laser scan microscopy.[31–33] These material traces can be grouped in two main classes: (1) discrete, high-ordered dendritic structures (FIGS. 9B and C) that contain filamentous actin and are enveloped by membranes and (2) smaller, non-organized traces that randomly cover the migration area of the crawling cell and are apparently made up of collagen.[4] Collagen is an ideal substratum for adhering cells (FIG. 9C), thus facilitating attachment and migration of further cells under increased release of cellular material.[34]

In the light of these model experiments, it seems likely that pericapsular fibrosis around UHV/CG microcapsules can be initiated by deposition of cellular material and serum proteins on the outer surface due to topographical roughness, leading to changes of its adhesion and AGE–reactivity properties. If necessary, production of extremely smooth and long-term stable surfaces of UHV/CG alginate microcapsules can be achieved when the crosslinking process of the alginate is performed by internal gelation, for example, by use of caged $Ca^{2+}$ and/or caged $Ba^{2+}$. Upon formation of the capsules, the divalent, reactive cations are released from the "cage" by UV-irradiation.[30] This results in a uniform crosslinking throughout the bead that is

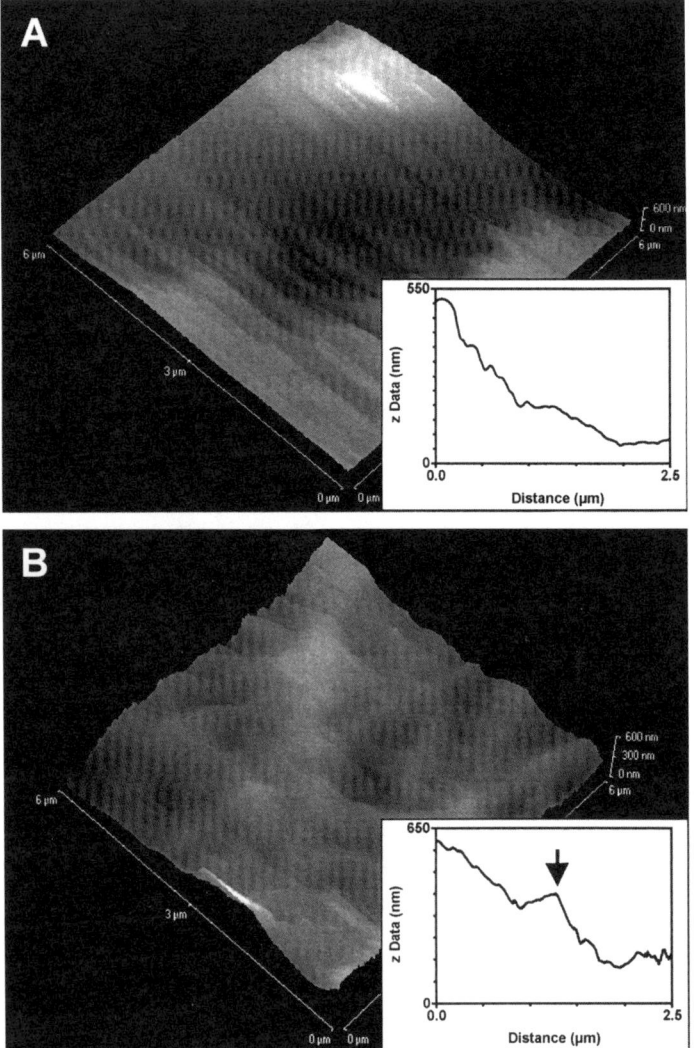

**FIGURE 8.** Three-dimensional view of the surface of a $Ba^{2+}$-alginate microcapsule (in 0.9% NaCl solution) acquired with an atomic force microscope using the non-contact mode. The capsules were stabilized by treatment with sulfate and incorporation of proteins or perfluorocarbon (see legend to FIG. 6) before implantation into the peritoneal cavity of a rat. (**A**) Surface of a protein-alginate capsule retrieved after four-week implantation. The scan range is $6 \times 6$ µm$^2$; the height scale is 0–600 nm. (**B**) Surface of a perfluorocarbon-alginate capsule prepared from commercial purified alginate and retrieved 15 months after implantation. The scan range is $6 \times 6$ µm$^2$; the height scale is 0–600 nm. Note that, in contrast to (**A**), the surface appears less smooth caused by fibrils. This is emphasized by the line scans depicted in the *insets*. The line-scans were taken from the maximum to the minimum height and show that the total change in height is with 462 nm (**A**) and 493 nm (**B**) comparable for both capsules (except for the cross-section of the fibril; see *arrow*)

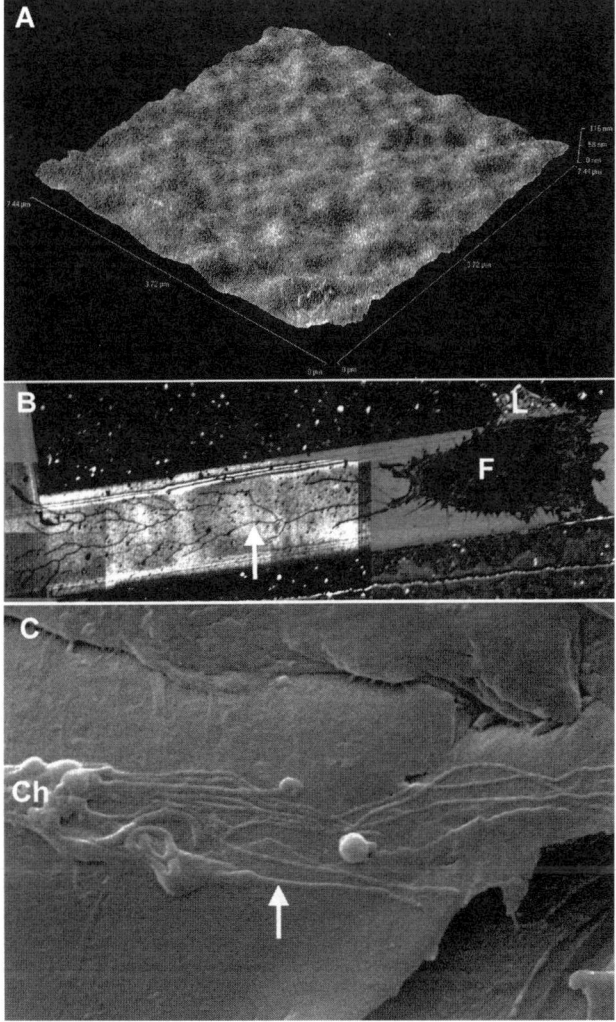

**FIGURE 9.** (**A**) Three-dimensional view of the surface of an alginate film (in 0.9% NaCl solution) on a glass substrate acquired with an atomic force microscope using the non-contact mode. The scan range is $7.44 \times 7.44$ µm$^2$; the height scale is 0–116 nm. A very smooth surface with homogenous small corrugations can be seen. (**B**) Cell trace (*arrow*) of a mouse fibroblast (*F*) on a microstructured alginate film. The image was acquired with a confocal laser scan microscope in the reflection mode (depicted area, $140 \times 50$ µm$^2$); the image area with the trace is computer-processed for enhanced contrast. The material released from the cells during migration (*arrow*) indicates that the fibroblast moved exclusively on the alginate-free "street", even though parts of the lammellipodium of the cell touch the alginate film (*L*). (**C**) Near-field traces (*arrow*) of a human primary chondrocyte on the surface of a piece of cartilage; part of the cell (*Ch*) migrating to the left-hand side is also seen. The image was taken with a scanning electron microscope. The depicted area is $11.1 \times 7.5$ µm$^2$. For further details, see Fuhr *et al.*[31] and H. Zimmermann, I. Westphal and G. Fuhr, manuscript in preparation.

simultaneously beneficial for the diffusion of nutrients and oxygen to the encapsulated cells or tissue fragments.

### Non-Invasive Monitoring of the Transplantation Site, the Functional Integrity, and the Oxygen Supply of the Transplants

A prerequisite for large-scale clinical trials is the selection of an appropriate transplantation site as well as the continuous, non-invasive monitoring of the location and function of the transplant after surgery. These requirements can be met by $^{19}$F-nuclear magnetic resonance imaging (MRI). Currently, most MRI studies are based on $^1$H-MRI. However, because of the high water content of alginate microcapsules (about 98%), the $^1$H-MRI signal of the alginate cannot be distinguished from that of the surrounding host tissue (see FIGURE 10A). In contrast, fluorine is only present in bones and teeth. Thus, perfluorocarbons that suppress capsule swelling (see above) are ideal MRI contrast agents to resolve the capsules clearly even after long implantation periods. A typical example is shown in FIGURE 10B.[35,36] Apart from these beneficial effects, perfluorocarbons are also known for their high oxygen capacity and enhanced oxygen transfer rates, thus solving the problem of sufficient oxygen supply to the encapsulated cells/tissues.[37] Moreover, the partial pressure of oxygen within the capsules can be estimated by changes in the fluorine spin-lattice relaxation time.[35] Graft failure due to breakage or migration of capsules can, therefore, easily be detected by the disappearance of the $^{19}$F-signal in the MRI cross-section, in particular when relatively large-sized immunoisolated tissues (e.g., parathyroid glands) are transplanted. Similarly, changes in the $^{19}$F-signals are

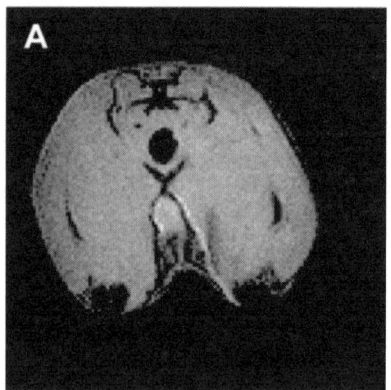 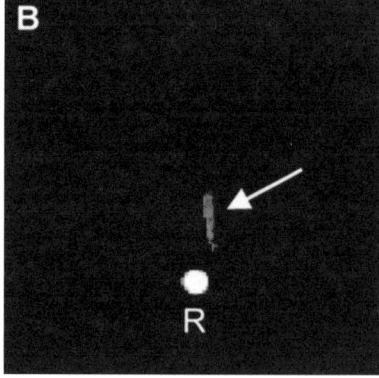

**FIGURE 10.** $^1$H-MR (**A**) and $^{19}$F-MR (**B**) images of a 3-mm-thick transaxial slice through a female Wistar rat. The images were acquired about one year after implantation of perfluorocarbon-loaded Ba$^{2+}$-alginate capsules (350 μm in diameter) in the muscle of the rat. The in-plane resolution was 0.5 × 0.5 mm$^2$. The *arrow* marks the location of the implanted $^{19}$F-labeled beads. The letter *R* denotes a glass capillary (5 mm in diameter) filled with pure perfluorocarbon placed under the rat during the experiment as an external reference. For further details, see Nöth *et al.*[35]

expected when fibrotic overgrowth restricts oxygen transfer to the enclosed perfluorocarbon and the cells. Even though some technical problems have to be solved before this technique can be applied to patients, it seems to be clear that $^{19}$F-MRI provides an early warning signal for the necessity of reexamination of the transplantation site.

## CONCLUSIONS

Retrospectively, the use of low-viscosity alginate, the chemical impurities of the commercial alginates as well as thermodynamic instabilities of the microcapsules, imperfect capsule surfaces and inappropriate oxygen supply, are the most likely reasons for early graft failure in many animal studies reported in the literature. Solutions to these problems were presented in this paper. Clinical allotransplantations are planned to begin shortly in a group of patients with hypoparathyroidism to realize the potential of the novel microcapsule configurations described here and tested successfully in animal studies during the past two years. Over the next years, as our knowledge of the novel capsule–cell systems increases, we can expect to see many new areas of applications of this technology. However, the enormous need for "spare parts" for the human body requires still further innovative techniques and creative solutions. A successful development of well documented, medically approved immunoisolated transplants necessitates close interdisciplinary collaboration among scientists with different areas of expertise such as biophysics, biotechnology, molecular biology, and medicine.

## ACKNOWLEDGMENTS

We are very grateful to P. Amersbach, S. Schmitt, P. Gessner, and J. Pfeuffer for skillful technical assistance. Furthermore, we would like to acknowledge B. Kuttler for implantation of microcapsules into BB/OK rats. This work was supported by grants from the BMBF (0311716) and from the Deutsche Bundesstiftung Umwelt (13019) to U. Z., by grants from the Deutsche Forschungsgemeinschaft (NMR-Graduierten-Kolleg NMR HA 1232/8-1) to A. H. and U. Z., by grants from the Deutsche Forschungsgemeinschaft (HA 2611/1-1) to the Lehrstuhl für Membranphysiologie, and by grants to C. H. from the Erweiterte Forschungsförderung des Freistaates Bayern.

## REFERENCES

1. HUNKELER, D. 1997. Polymers for bioartificial organs. Trends Polym. Sci. **5:** 286–293.
2. ANGELOVA, N. & D. HUNKELER. 1999. Rationalizing the design of polymeric biomaterials. TibTech. **17:** 409–421.
3. HASSE, C., G. KLÖCK, A. SCHLOSSER, et al. 1997. Parathyroid allotransplantation without immunosuppression. Lancet **350:** 1296–1297.
4. ZIMMERMANN, U., S. MIMIETZ, H. ZIMMERMANN, et al. 2000. Hydrogel-based nonautologous cell and tissue therapy. BioTechniques **29:** 564–581.
5. ZIMMERMANN, U., G. KLÖCK, K. FEDERLIN, et al. 1992. Production of mitogen-contamination free alginates with variable ratios of mannuronic acid to guluronic acid by free flow electrophoresis. Electrophoresis **13:** 269–274.

6. KLÖCK, G., A. PFEFFERMANN, C. RYSER, et al. 1997. Biocompatibility of mannuronic acid-rich alginates. Biomaterials **18:** 707–713.
7. KLÖCK, G., H. FRANK, R. HOUBEN, et al. 1994. Production of purified alginates suitable for use in immunoisolated transplantation. Appl. Microbiol. Biotechnol. **40:** 638–643.
8. VENEGAS M., F. TALA, E. FONCK & J. VASQUEZ. 1992. Sporangial sori on stipes of *Lessonia nigrescens* Bory (Laminariales, Phaeophyta): a high frequency phenomenon in intertidal populations of northern Chile. Botanica Marina **35:** 573–578.
9. ARFORS, K.E. & K. LEY. 1993. Sulfated polysaccharides in inflammation. J. Lab. Clin. Med. **121:** 201–202.
10. MATTIASSON, B. 1982. Immobilization methods. In Immobilized Cells and Organelles, Vol. I. B. Mattiasson, Ed.: 3–26. CRC Press, Boca Raton.
11. GACESA, P. 1998. Bacterial alginate biosynthesis—recent progress and future prospects. Microbiology **144:** 1133–1143.
12. WESTWOOD, M.E. & P.J. THORNALLEY. 1997. Glycation and advanced glycation endproducts. In The Glycation Hypothesis of Atherosclerosis. C. Colaco, Ed.: 57–87. Landes Bioscience.
13. HOFMANN, M.A., S. DRURY, C. FU, et al. 1999. RAGE mediates a novel proinflammatory axis: a central cell surface receptor for S100/Calgranulin polypeptides. Cell **97:** 889–901.
14. ZIMMERMANN, U., C. HASSE, M. ROTHMUND & W. KÜHTREIBER. 1999. Biocompatible encapsulation materials: fundamentals and application. In Cell Encapsulation Technology and Therapeutics. W.M. Kühtreiber, R.P. Lanza & W.L. Chick, Eds.: 40–52. Birkhäuser. Boston.
15. ZIMMERMANN, U., H. CRAMER, A. JORK, et al. 2001. Microencapsulation-based cell therapy. In Biotechnology G. Reed & H.-J. Rehm, Eds. Wiley-VCH. Weinheim, Germany. **10:** 547–571.
16. SEGER, R. & E. G. KREBS. 1995. The MAPK signaling cascade. FASEB J. **9:** 726–735.
17. AHRENS, M., T. ANKENBAUER, D. SCHRÖDER, et al. 1993. Expression of human bone morphogenetic proteins-2 or -4 in murine mesenchymal progenitor C3H10T1/2 cells induces differentiation into distinct mesenchymal cell lineages. DNA Cell Biol. **12:** 871–880.
18. CURTIS, A. & C. WILKINSON. 1999. New depths in cell behaviour: reactions of cells to nanotopography. Biochem. Soc. Symp. **65:** 15–26.
19. SKALAK, R. & C.F. FOX. 1988. Tissue Engineering. Alan R. Liss Inc., New York.
20. RYDZEWSKI, R. 1990. Swelling and shrinking of a polyelectrolyte gel induced by a salt solution. Continuum Mech. Thermodyn. **2:** 77–97.
21. HASSE, C., A. ZIELKE, G. KLÖCK, et al. 1997. First successful xenotransplantation of microencapsulated human parathyroid tissue in experimental hypoparathyroidism: long-term function without immunosuppression. J. Microencapsulation **14:** 617–626.
22. SKJÅK-BRÆK, G. & A. MARTINSEN. 1991. Applications of some algal polysaccharides in biotechnology. In Seaweed Resources in Europe: Uses and Potential. M.D. Guiry & G. Blunden, Eds.: 219–257. John Wiley & Sons, New York.
23. FUJIKI, K., H. MATSUYAMA & T. YANO. 1994. Protective effect of sodium alginates against bacterial infection in common carp, *Cyprinus carpio* L. J. Fish Dis. **17:** 349–355.
24. JORK, A., F. THÜRMER, H. CRAMER, et al. 2000. Biocompatible alginate from freshly collected *Laminaria pallida* for implantation. Appl. Microbiol. Biotechnol. **53:** 224–229.
25. ESCH, M., V.L. SUKHORUKOV, M. KÜRSCHNER & U. ZIMMERMANN. 1999. Dielectric properties of alginate beads and bound water relaxation studied by electrorotation. Biopolymers **50:** 227–237.
26. ZIMMERMANN, U. & G.A. NEIL. 1996. Electromanipulation of Cells. CRC-Press, Boca Raton, New York, London, Tokyo.
27. SCHNABL, H., R.J. YOUNGMAN & U. ZIMMERMANN. 1983. Maintenance of plant cell membrane integrity and function by the immobilization of protoplasts in alginate matrices. Planta **158:** 392–397.
28. WEBB, S.J. 1965. Bound Water in Biological Integrity. Charles C Thomas, Springfield.

29. FRIEDL, P. & E.-B. BRÖCKER. 2000. The biology of cell locomotion within three-dimensional extracellular matrix. Cell. Mol. Life Sci. **57:** 41–64.
30. HILLGÄRTNER, M., H. ZIMMERMANN, S. MIMIETZ, et al. 1999. Immunoisolation of transplants by entrapment in $^{19}$F-labelled alginate gels: production, biocompatibility, stability, and long-term monitoring of functional integrity. Mat.-wiss. u. Werkstofftech. **30:** 783–792.
31. FUHR, G., E. RICHTER, H. ZIMMERMANN, et al. 1998. Cell traces—footprints of individual cells during locomotion and adhesion. Biol. Chem. **379:** 1161–1173.
32. ZIMMERMANN, H., R. HAGEDORN, E. RICHTER & G. FUHR. 1999. Topography of cell traces studied by atomic force microscopy. Eur. Biophys. J. **28:** 516–525.
33. RICHTER, E., H. HITZLER, H. ZIMMERMANN, et al. 2000. Trace formation during locomotion of L929 mouse fibroblasts continuously recorded by interference reflection microscopy (IRM). Cell Mot. Cytoskel. **47:** 38–47.
34. GRÖHN, P., G. KLÖCK & U. ZIMMERMANN. 1997. Collagen-coated $Ba^{2+}$-alginate microcarriers for the culture of anchorage-dependent mammalian cells. Biotechniques **22:** 970–975.
35. NÖTH, U., P. GRÖHN, A. JORK, et al. 1999. $^{19}$F-MRI *in vivo* determination of the partial oxygen pressure in perfluorocarbon-loaded alginate capsules implanted into the peritoneal cavity and different tissues. Magn. Reson. Med. **42:** 1039–1047.
36. ZIMMERMANN, U., U. NÖTH, P. GRÖHN, et al. 2000. Non-invasive evaluation of the location, the functional integrity and the oxygen supply of implants: $^{19}$F-nuclear magnetic resonance imaging of perfluorocarbon-loaded $Ba^{2+}$-alginate beads. Artificial Cells, Blood Substitutes, Immobilization Biotech. **28:** 129–146.
37. CHANG, T.M.S. 1993. Blood Substitutes and Oxygen Carriers. Marcel Dekker, Inc., New York.

# Transplantation of Alginate Microcapsules with Proliferating Cells in Mice

## Capsular Overgrowth and Survival of Encapsulated Cells of Mice and Human Origin

ANNE MARI ROKSTAD,[a] BÅRD KULSENG,[a] BERIT L. STRAND,[b] GUDMUND SKJÅK-BRÆK,[b] AND TERJE ESPEVIK[a]

[a]*Institute of Cancer Research and Molecular Biology, Norwegian University of Science and Technology, Trondheim, Norway*

[b]*Institute of Biotechnology, Norwegian University of Science and Technology, Trondheim, Norway*

> ABSTRACT: Alginate microcapsules may be used to encapsulate therapeutic cells and, thereby, to protect them from the host immune system. Both the biomaterial, as well as the therapeutic cells, may give rise to immunological reactions. We have developed methods that are useful in the study of capsule biocompatibility, as well as reactions against the grafts. These imply investigation of the survival of the encapsulated cells as well as fibrotic reactions against the microcapsules. Studies were performed in Balb/c mice with empty alginate–PLL–alginate microcapsules as well as microcapsules containing cells of human or mouse origin. Confocal laser scanning microscopy (CLSM) was used to visualize live and dead cells within the microcapsules and to define some of the cells involved in the fibrotic reaction against the microcapsules. In both grafts, live cells were detected seven days after transplantation. Minor fibrotic reactions were found against empty alginate–PLL–alginate microcapsules and to microcapsules containing mouse cells. An extensive fibrotic reaction was found one week after transplantation against microcapsules containing human cells, and the secretion of therapeutic protein endostatin had ceased. Fibroblasts and macrophages were involved in the fibrotic reaction against the xenograft.
>
> KEYWORDS: transplantation; alginate microcapsules; proliferating cells; capsular overgrowth

## INTRODUCTION

Transplantation of therapeutic cells is a potential strategy for the treatment of various neurodegenerative and hormone deficient diseases. Host reactions against therapeutic cells of foreign origin is postulated to be neutralized by encapsulation, thus preventing the ingress of high molecular mass substances, such as immune cells, and secretory substances, such as cytokines, immunoglobulins, and complement

---

Address for correspondence: Anne Mari Rokstad, Institute of Cancer Research and Molecular Biology, Olav Kyrresgt. 3, 7489 Trondheim, Norway. Voice: 47-73 59 86 66; fax: 47-73 59 88 01.

anne.m.rokstad@medisin.ntnu.no

factors. Therefore, microencapsulation technologies, using alginate, may provide a safe and simple technique for implanting cells into various sites of the human body.

The first successful transplantation in alginate capsules was reported by Lim and Sun 21 years ago.[1] Since then, alginate capsules have been proposed as an immune-protective barrier, particularly for pancreatic islets, and successful attempts in large animal models and in type I diabetic patients has been reported.[2-6] Other approaches have involved the use of genetically engineered cells delivering therapeutic proteins.[7-10] The type of biomaterial used for encapsulation appears to play a crucial role involving both immunological[11-15] as well as mechanical aspects.[16-18] The immune reaction against the capsules also varies according to the encapsulated material. Xenogeneic tissue has been proposed as an alternate source of therapeutic cells. Some groups report on an increase in graft failure when using xenogeneic tissue.[19,20] Therefore, further studies of the cellular reactions to the different alginate microcapsules, as well as microcapsules containing therapeutic cells, should be carried out.

Analysis of the cellular reactions against transplanted microencapsulated xenogeneic islets using FACS analysis has been described.[21] We have used confocal laser scanning microscopy (CLSM) to study the capsule biocompatibility of the alginate microcapsules themselves as well as alginate microcapsules containing cells of xenogeneic and isogeneic origin. This implies visualizing live and dead cells within the capsules and identifying cells involved in the fibrotic reactions to the capsules. Studies were performed in Balb/c mice with empty alginate microcapsules and alginate microcapsules with proliferating cells of human or mice origin.

## EXPERIMENTAL

Alginates were derived from Laminaria hyperborea stipe (Pronova, UP-LVG). The alginate used in the capsule core consisted of 63% α-L-guluronic acid (G) and 37% β-D-mannuronic (M) acid with an average molecular weight of 277 kDa. Alginate used for the outer coating consisted of 68% G and 38% M with an average molecular weight of 142 kDa. The PLL was purchased from Sigma and had an average molecular weight of 27.5 kDa.

Inhomogeneous alginate-poly-L-lysine-alginate microcapsules were formed by letting droplets of alginate (final concentration of 1.8% mannitol-alginate), with or without cells, gel in a 50 mM $CaCl_2$ (0,15 mM mannitol solution), as described elsewhere.[17] The concentration of cells was two million per milliliter of alginate. The beads were coated with 0.05% PLL for ten minutes and subsequently with alginate (0.01%, 10 min). By using an electrostatic bead generator, the final microcapsule diameter was 0.6–0.7 mm.

A mouse sarcoma cell line designated CF-WEHI 164 and a human embryonic kidney cell line (293-EBNA), transfected with the gene for endostatin,[22] were used as graft models. The 293-EBNA cells were generously provided by Dr. B.R. Olsen, Department of Cell Biology, Harvard Medical School, Boston. Encapsulated CF-WEHI cells were grown *in vitro* one day before implantation, whereas human 293 EBNA-cells were grown for 14 days before implantation. The medium consisted of RPMI-1640 with 10% fetal calf serum, 2 mM glutamin, and 100 units/ml penicillin/streptomycin. When used on 293 cells the medium was also supplemented with 0.5 µg/ml puromycin and 250 µg/ml geneticin.

Female mice of strain Balb/c derived from M&B (Denmark) were acclimatized four weeks before use. Mice were anesthetized subcutaneously in the neck with Hypnorm/Dormicum. A small incision was made through the abdominal skin and peritoneum. Approximately 0.4-ml capsules were deposited in the peritoneal cavity of six mice per group by using a sterile syringe (1 ml) and a needle (2.1 × 25 mm). Two and seven days after implantation three mice in each group were examined. Mice sera were collected from the *vena saphena magna* of anesthetized mice before they were killed and microcapsules retrieved. The secretion of human endostatin was measured in mice sera after transplantation of microencapsulated 293-EBNA cells, and from retrieved alginate capsules with 293-EBNA cells cultivated *in vitro* before medium was sampled. Human endostatin was detected by use of the accucyte human endostatin kit (Cytimmune Science Inc.) according to the described procedure.

Macrophages were identified by use of PE–anti-mouse CD14 (from PharMingen, 10 µg/ml). Fibroblasts were identified by use of rat–anti-mouse fibroblasts (from Biogenesis, diluted 1:25) and FITC-marked mouse–antirat antibodies (PharMingen, 10 µg/ml). The secondary antibody was used as control for fibroblasts, whereas PE–antihuman CD14 (Becton Dicson, 10 µg/ml) were used as control for CD14. Encapsulated cells were stained with a live/dead kit (Molecular Probes) with calcein AM and ethidium homodimer (EthD-1) to visualize live and dead cells respectively. The microcapsules were washed twice before they were subjected to optical sectioning in a Zeiss 510 LSM confocal microscope.

## RESULTS AND DISCUSSION

Fibrotic reactions were found, both against empty alginate–PLL–alginate microcapsules and microcapsules containing cells (see FIGURE 1). Approximately 10% of the empty microcapsules and microcapsules containing mouse cells were attacked by fibrotic cells. Of the empty microcapsules, some were completely covered by cells one week after implantation, whereas others were free from cells. A portion of the microcapsules containing human 293-EBNA cells were found freely floating in the abdomen and another portion were attached to the surface of the abdominal organs one week after implantation. Generally, the retrieved microcapsules that contained 293-EBNA cells were extensively covered with fibrotic cells, although microcapsules free from adhered cells were also found. Furthermore, clusters of alginate microcapsules adhered together by fibrotic cells were found within this group. Such clusters were not found in the group containing CF-WEHI cells. The encapsulated CF-WEHI cells proliferated *in vivo*, since the size of the cell clusters were increased about five-fold from two to seven days after implantation (FIGURE 1B and E).

Spheroids consisting of live and dead cells were found after *in vitro* cultivation (see FIGURES 3 and 4). The overgrown alginate capsules containing 293-EBNA cells retrieved from the peritoneal cavity were treated with trypsin before the encapsulated cells were stained. Both grafts contained live cells seven days after transplantation (FIGS. 3 and 4). The endostatin was secreted from retrieved microcapsules containing 293-EBNA cells two days after retrieval, but after seven days, only a

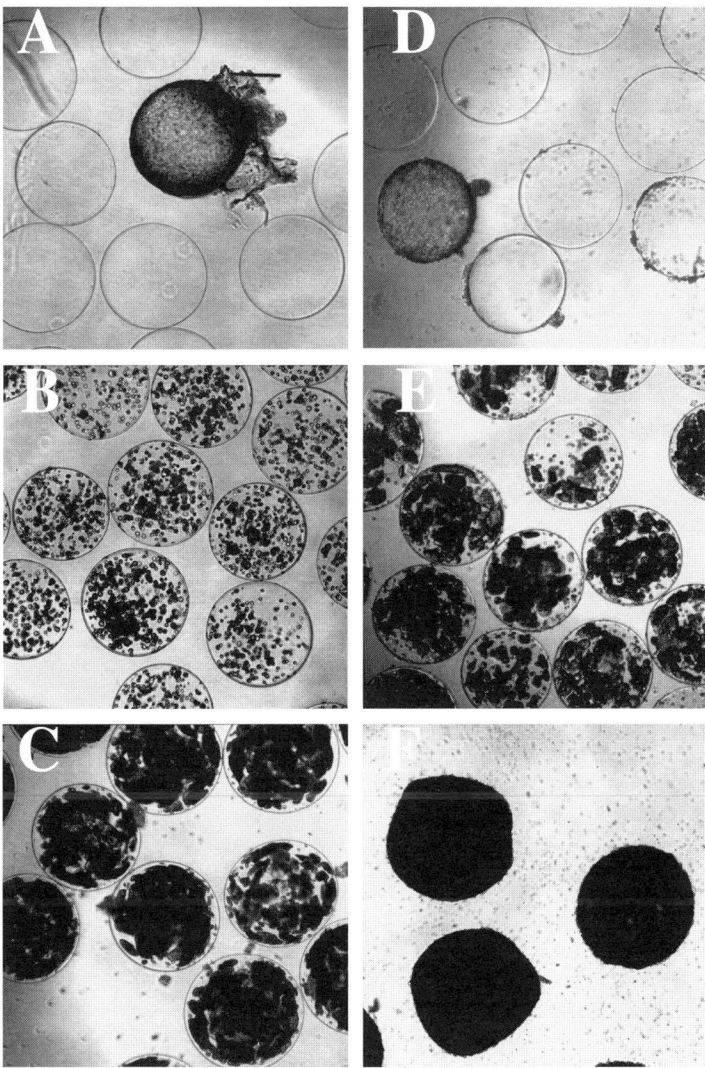

**FIGURE 1.** Alginate–PLL–alginate microcapsules retrieved from the peritoneal cavity of Balb/C mice two (**A–C**) and seven days (**D–F**) after implantation. Empty microcapsules (**A** and **D**), microcapsules with CF-WEHI cells (**B** and **E**), and microcapsules with 293-EBNA cells (**C** and **F**).

minor secretion was measured (see FIGURE 2B). In mice sera, endostatin was detected two days after transplantation, although not seven days post transplantation (FIG. 2A). This implies that the immune reactions against the xenograft were harmful to the 293-EBNA cells, despite the fact that the cells were still living one week after implantation.

The results from this study show that alginate capsules themselves, as well as the graft may give immunological reactions. We have recently shown that soluble PLL induce production of the proinflammatory cytokine TNF in human monocytes, and that exposed PLL on the surface of alginate capsule is a major contributor to the fibrotic reaction against empty capsules.[11] Although alginate–PLL capsules are covered with an outer layer of alginate to neutralize PLL, an insufficient coating of the polycation layer may explain the fact that some empty alginate capsules were covered by fibrotic cells, whereas others were free from fibrotic reactions. An extensive overgrowth was seen after transplantation of the human 293-EBNA cells, involving both fibroblasts and macrophages identified as CD14-positive cells (see FIGURES 5 and 6). This strong fibrotic reaction may be explained by its xenograft origin, since an immune response is possible against foreign proteins, including the therapeutic

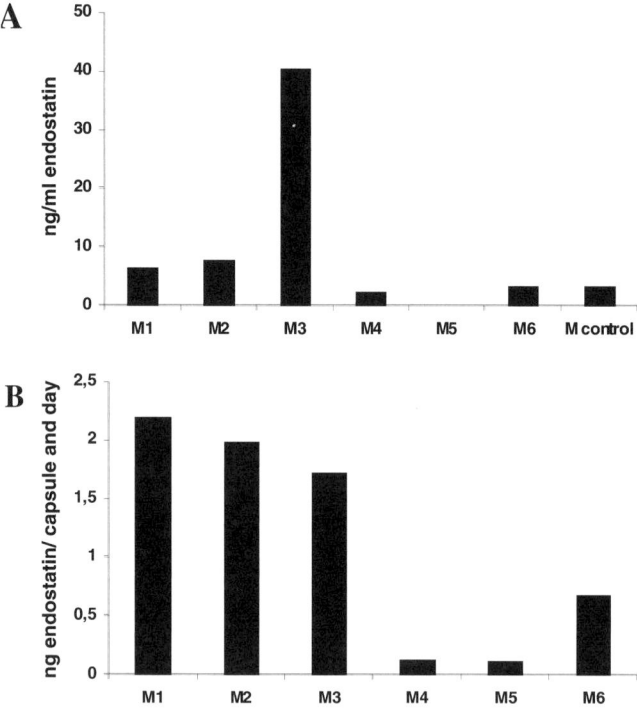

**FIGURE 2.** Endostatin secretion measured from 293-EBNA cells encapsulated in alginate–PLL–alginate microcapsules. **A.** Endostatin found in mice sera two (M1-3) and seven (M4-6) days after transplantation. **B.** Endostatin secreted from retrieved microcapsules after two (M1-3) or seven (M4-6) days in mice.

agent and cell surface molecules. Some alginate microcapsules containing xenografts were free from adherent cells. A question then arises as to whether there are some local variations in the peritoneal cavity according to immunological reactions. The CF-WEHI cell line is originally from Balb/c mouse, implying that the encapsulated mouse cells may function as an isograft. This may explain the lack of fibrotic reaction against most of the transplanted alginate capsules with mouse cells.

Components secreted upon cell death may also give rise to an immune reaction.[23] Both at the time of transplantation (not shown) and retrieval (FIGS. 3 and 4) dead 293-EBNA cells and CF-WEHI cells were observed inside the alginate microcapsules. This may have contributed to the fibrotic reactions observed in the xenografts and the minor reactions against some alginate microcapsules containing isografts.

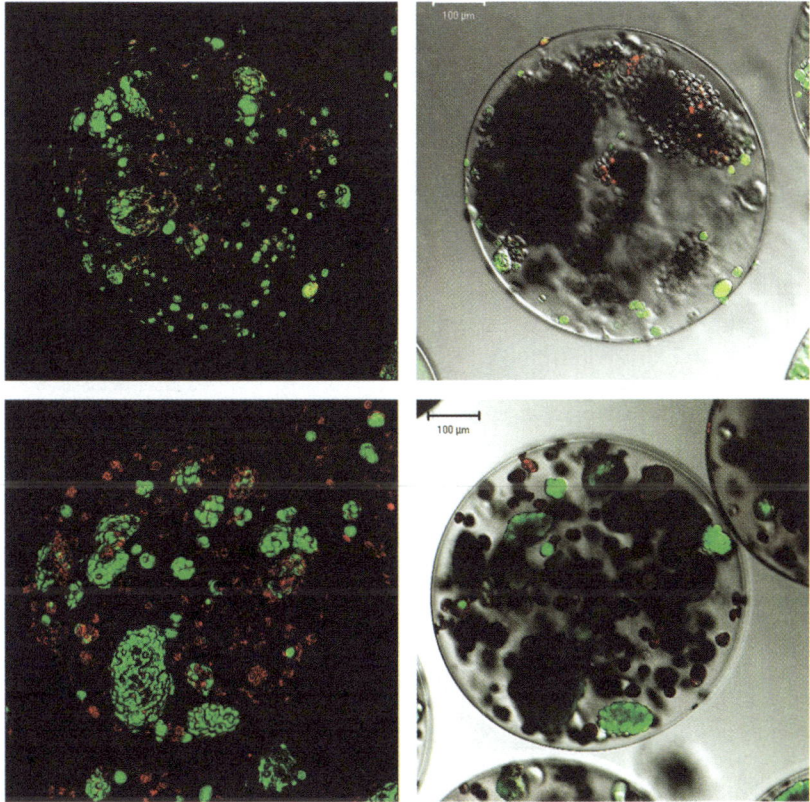

**FIGURE 3.** Live and dead CF-WEHI cells in alginate-PLL-alginate microcapsules. The *upper pictures* show capsules retrieved from the intraperitoneal cavity of Balb/c mice after seven days. The *lower pictures* reveal capsules with cells grown *in vitro* for the same period. *Green* designates live cells with *red* represent dead cells. The pictures on the *left* are three-dimensional reconstructions of optical sections taken from equator to the top of the capsule. On the *right* are examples of optical sections overlaid on the transmitted light micrographs.

The use of fetal calf serum in the culture medium also may introduce foreign proteins into the microcapsules, thus creating another source for the minor fibrotic reactions seen against the isograft.

Macrophages and fibroblasts have previously been shown to be involved in the cellular reactions both to empty alginate–PLL–alginate microcapsules and microcapsules containing xenografts.[21,24] TGFβ, a potent fibrinogenic cytokine, is also shown to be involved in the reaction against empty alginate–PLL–alginate microcapsules.[25] The host response to polymer microcapsules containing live cells may be viewed as an inflammatory response to the biomaterial and an immune response to the transplanted cells.[23] The fibrotic reactions toward alginate microcapsules with

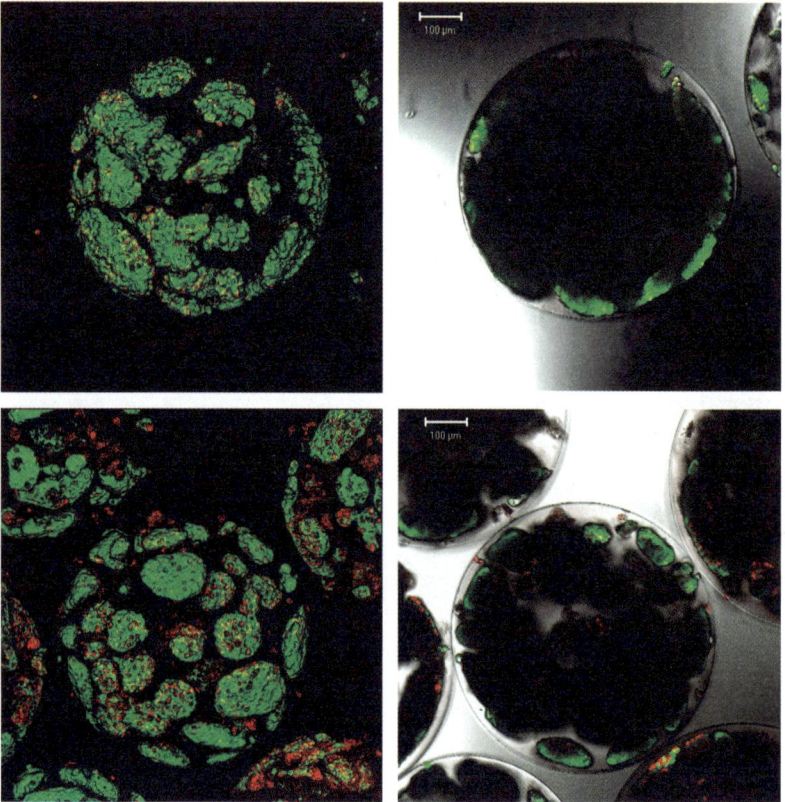

**FIGURE 4.** Live and dead 293-EBNA cells in alginate–PLL–alginate microcapsules. The *upper pictures* show capsules retrieved from intraperitoneal cavity of Balb/c mice after seven days. The *lower pictures* reveal capsules with cells grown *in vitro* for the same period. *Green* designates live cells with *red* representing dead cells. The pictures on the *left* are three-dimensional reconstructions of optical sections taken from equator to the top of the capsule. On the *right* are examples of optical sections overlaid on the transmitted light micrographs.

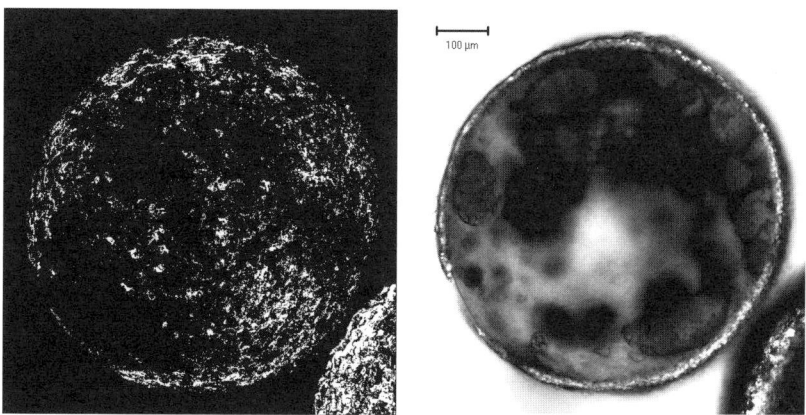

**FIGURE 5.** Alginate–PLL–alginate microcapsule with human 293 EBNA-cells retrieved from the peritoneal cavity of Balb/c mice seven days after implantation. *White/light gray* indicates the CD14 positive cells. The pictures on the *left* are three-dimensional reconstructions of optical sections taken from equator to the top of the capsule. On the *right* are examples of optical sections overlaid on the transmitted light micrograph.

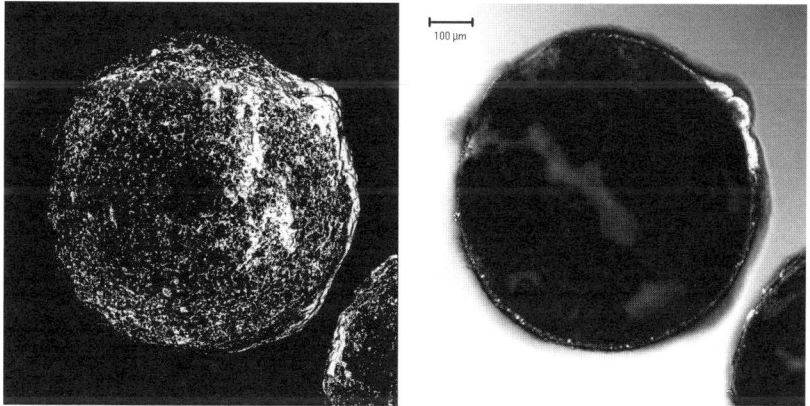

**FIGURE 6.** Alginate–PLL–alginate microcapsule with human 293 EBNA-cells retrieved from the peritoneal cavity of Balb/c mice seven days after implantation. *White/light gray* shows fibroblasts on the surface of the capsule. The pictures on the *left* are three-dimensional reconstructions of optical sections taken from equator to the top of the capsule. On the *right* are examples of optical sections overlaid on the transmitted light micrograph.

xenografts seem to vary depending on the chemical nature of the capsule materials as well as on the encapsulation methodology. Whether the host reactions will lead to fibrotic overgrowth likely depends on the chemical and physical properties of the capsule surface. Moreover, different cells may require different applications. The success of alginates as immobilization matrixes for transplantation of therapeutic cells will, therefore, rely on an appropriate choice of materials and methodology for each application.

## CONCLUSIONS

CLSM is useful for studying the biocompatibility of alginate microcapsules. This technique gives important information on the cell conditions inside the microcapsules as well as cell types adhering to the outer capsule membrane. Alginate–PLL–alginate microcapsules have promise in isograft applications. However, encapsulation of xenograft tissue may result in cellular overgrowth of the microcapsules, which may represent problems in applications.

## REFERENCES

1. LIM, F. & A.M. SUN. 1980. Microencapsulated islets as a bioartificial endocrine pancreas, Science **210:** 908–910.
2. SULLIVAN, S.J., T. MAKI, K.M. BORLAND, et al. 1991. Biohybrid artificial pancreas: long-term implantation studies in diabetic, pancreatectomized dogs. Science **252:** 718–721.
3. SOON-SHIONG, P., E. FELDMAN, R. NELSON, et al. 1992. Successful reversal of spontaneous diabetes in dogs by intraperitoneal microencapsulated islets. Transplantation **54:** 769–774.
4. SOON-SHIONG, P., E. FELDMAN, R. NELSON, et al. 1993. Long-term reversal of diabetes by injection of immunoprotected islet cells. Proc. Natl. Acad. Sci. USA **90:** 5843–5847.
5. SOON-SHIONG, P., R. HEINTZ, N. MERIDETH, et al. 1994. Insulin independence in a type I diabetic patient after encapsulated islet transplantation. Lancet **343:** 950–951.
6. LANZA, R., D.M. ECKER, W.M. KÜTHREIBER, et al. 1999. Transplantation of islets using microencapsulation: studies in diabetic rodents and dogs. J. Mol. Med. **77:** 206–210.
7. PEIRONE, M., C.J. ROSS, G. HORTELANO, et al. 1998. Encapsulation of various recombinant mammalian cell types in different alginate microcapsules. Biomed. Mater. Res. **42:** 587–596.
8. ROSS, C.J.D., M. RALPH & P.L. CHANG. 1999. Delivery of recombinant gene products to the central nervous system with nonautologous cells in alginate microcapsules. Human Gene Therapy **10:** 49–59.
9. JOKI, T., M. MACHLUF, A. ATALA, et al. 2001. Continuous release of endostatin from microencapsulated engineered cells for tumor therapy. Nat. Biotech. **19:** 35–39.
10. READ, T.A., D.R. SORENSEN, R. MAHESPARAN, et al. 2001. Local endostatin treatment of gliomas administered by microencapsulated producer cells. Nat. Biotech. **19:** 29–34.
11. STRAND, B.L., L. RYAN, P. IN'T VELD, et al. 2001. Poly-L-lysine induces fibrosis on alginate microcapsules via the induction of cytokines. Cell Transplant. **10:** 263–275.
12. OTTERLEI, M., K. ØSTGÅRD, G. SKJÅK-BRÆK, et al. 1991. Induction of cytokine production from human monocytes stimulated with alginate. J. Immunother. **10:** 286–291.
13. DE VOS, P., B. DE HAAN & R. VAN SCHILFGAARDE. 1997. Effect of the alginate compostion on the biocompatibility of alginate-polylysine microcapsules. Biomaterials **18:** 273–278.

14. DE VOS, P., B. DE HAAN, G.H.J. WOLTERS, et al. 1997. Improved biocompatibility but limited graft survival after purification of alginate for microencapsulation of pancreatic islets. Diabetologia **40:** 262–270.
15. KULSENG, B., G. SKJÅK-BRÆK, L. RYAN, et al. 1999. Transplantation of alginate microcapsules. Generation of antibodies against alginate and encapsulated porcine islet-like cell clusters. Transplantation **67:** 978–984.
16. THU, B., P. BRUHEIM, T. ESPEVIK, et al. 1996. Alginate polycation microcapsules I. Interaction between alginate and polycation. Biomaterials **17:** 1031–1040.
17. THU, B., P. BRUHEIM, T. ESPEVIK, et al. 1996. Alginate polycation microcapsules II. Some functional properties. Biomaterials **17:** 1069–1079.
18. CONSTANTINIDIS, I., I. RASK, R.C. LONG, et al. 1999. Effects of alginate composition on the metabolic, secretory, and growth characteristics of entrapped βTC3 mouse insuloma cells. Biomaterials **20:** 2019–2027.
19. IWATA, H., K. KOBAYASHI, T. TAKAGI, et al. 1994. Feasibility of agarose microbeads with xenogeneic islets as a bioartificial pancreas. J. Biomed. Mat. Res. **28:** 1003–1011.
20. LANZA, R., D. ECKER, W. KÜTHREIBER, et al. 1995. A simple method for transplanting discordant islets into rats using alginate spheres. Transplantation **59:** 1485–1487.
21. SIEBERS, U., A. HORCHER, H. BRANDHORST, et al. 1999. Analysis of the cellular reaction towards microencapsulated xenogeneic islets after intraperitoneal transplantation. J. Mol. Med. **77:** 215–218.
22. SASAKI, T., N. FUKAI, K. MANN, et al. 1998. Structure, function and tissue forms of the C-terminal globular domain of collagen XVIII containing the angiogenesis inhibitor endostatin. EMBO J. **17:** 4249–4256.
23. BABENSEE, J.E., J.M. ANDERSON, L.V. MCINTIRE & A.G. MIKOS. 1998. Host response to tissue engineered devices. Adv. Drug Delivery Rev. **33:** 111–139.
24. VANDERBOSSHE, G.M.R., M.E. BRACKE, C.A. CUVELIER, et al. 1993. Host reaction against empty alginate-polylysine microcapsules. Influence of preparation procedure. J. Pharm. Pharmacol. **45:** 115–120.
25. ROBITAILLE, R., F.A. LEBLON, N. HENLEY, et al. 1999. Alginate-poly-L-lysine microcapsule biocompatibility: a novel RT-PCR method for cytokine gene expression analysis in pericapsular infiltrates. J. Biomed. Mater. Res. **45:** 223–230.

# An Overview of the Immune System with Specific Reference to Membrane Encapsulation and Islet Transplantation

DEREK W.R. GRAY

*Nuffield Department of Surgery, University of Oxford, Oxford, United Kingdom*

ABSTRACT: The concept of immunoisolation by use of a bioartificial membrane is discussed, concentrating on the immunological mechanisms that are likely to be operative in the light of recent information on the workings of the immune system. Special attention is given to the use of encapsulation for the purpose of treating autoimmune diabetes by implantation of xenogeneic islet tissue. It is argued that the term immunoisolation is misleading because the immune system is always activated by the indirect pathway of antigen presentation and that the term immunomodulation would be more appropriate.

KEYWORDS: overview; immune system; membrane encapsulation; islet transplantation

## INTRODUCTION

For many years, the working hypothesis behind encapsulation technology and similar techniques was the concept termed *immunoisolation,* that is using a membrane prevented the immune system from detecting and reacting to the presence of foreign tissue within the encapsulation device. A large number of rodent and even large animal experiments have been performed with the aim of confirming this concept to be correct and producing functioning grafts of tissues, such as isolated islets. The author observes that each new conference on the topic brings a fresh batch of researchers claiming a new method of encapsulation with preliminary evidence of function in the rodent model. However, the techniques for encapsulation and similar approaches never seem to be reliably effective once an attempt is a made to move up to large animal studies or clinical transplantation. In this article, the author briefly reviews some fundamental concepts that have recently changed or consolidated our knowledge of the immune system. Subsequently, the relevance to encapsulation techniques for islet transplantation is discussed. Before commencing it is worth clarifying the terminology used to describe various types of transplantation as presented in the GLOSSARY of this volume. However, it should be noted that the terms (allograft, autograft, syngeneic graft, xenograft, concordant, and disconcordant grafts) still hide major variations in severity of the barrier being crossed. For example, a graft between rat and mouse is designated as a xenograft, but there are

Address for correspondence: Prof. D.W.R. Gray, D.Phil., F.R.C.P., F.R.C.S., The Nuffield Department of Surgery, John Radcliffe Hospital, Headington, Oxford, OX3 9DU, U.K. Voice: 44 1865 220145; fax: 44 1865 768876.
 derek.gray@nds.ox.ac.uk

relatively few differences in proteins other than the MHC, which is not the case when porcine tissue is transplanted to a human, for example. The crucial points to appreciate are, first, that rodent species are markedly less reactive to transplantation than humans, particularly with respect to the ability to wall off invaders, such as parasites, by production of dense fibrous tissue. Second, the immune barrier that is presented by transplantation between widely disparate xenografts is much greater than in an allograft, and still greater if the immune system has been preprimed, as is the case in autoimmune diabetes.

## THE IMMUNE SYSTEM: GENERAL POINTS RELEVANT TO ENCAPSULATION TECHNOLOGY

The mammalian immune system may be conveniently viewed as either a nonadaptive (innate) response that responds immediately to an invader, but with limited strength, or the adaptive immune system. The latter system separates further into antibody produced by the B cells and T-cell immunity which itself separates into CD8 T cells targeting peptides bound to MHC Class 1 and CD4 T cells targeting MHC Class II (see FIGURE 1). The major structural components of the immune system are outlined in FIGURE 2. From a point of view of encapsulation, without doubt it is the migratory dendritic cell that is the key player.[1,2] Other than the structural components of the immune system, we must also consider the signaling and adhesion molecules, named in FIGURE 2. It has recently become clear that the entire immune system is largely derived from a quite limited number of primordial

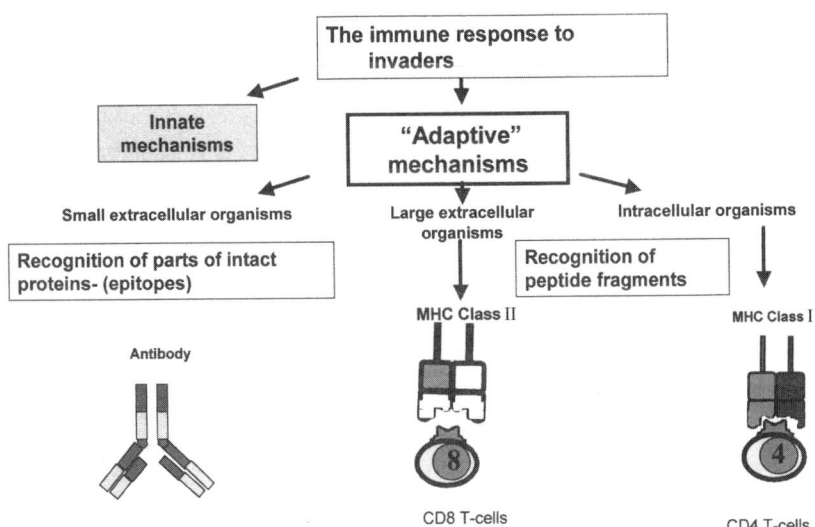

**FIGURE 1.** Two adaptive strategies for recognition of invaders.

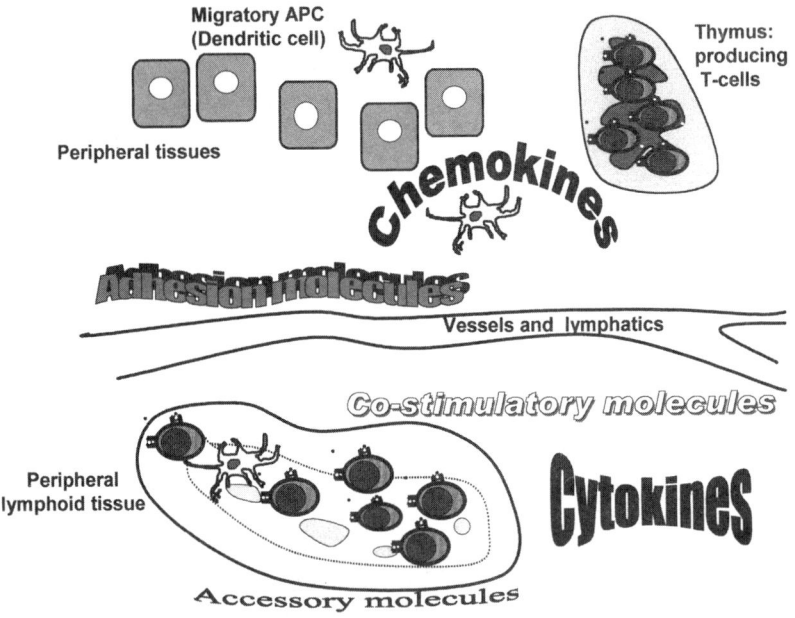

**FIGURE 2.** The components of the immune system summarized.

molecules that have mutated, duplicated, or become membrane-bound or soluble molecules (see TABLE 1). Some of these are large molecules, such as the derivatives of the Ig super-family, which are not likely to pass the pores of an encapsulation membrane, but other molecules, such as cytokines, are quite small.

A further basic concept to understand is that the strategy the immune system adopts for T-cell function is to have a highly variable set of T-cell receptors which will be able to identify virtually any peptide presented[3] (see TABLE 2). However, this implies that the number of cells that will initially respond to a foreign peptide is normally very low, of the order of one in $10^5$–$10^6$.[4,5] This means that rapid clonal expansion of the T cell once it has identified foreign peptide is crucial, and indeed this is precisely where most immunosuppression drugs are targeted, preventing rejection by stopping the necessary expansion. Despite the fact that the starting frequency of responding cells is so low, the response of the normal immune system to systemic infection is so rapid that within days a significant percentage of the total T cells in an individual may be targeted against a single virus.[6] However, the low starting frequency of T cells responding to a single foreign peptide contrasts strongly with the remarkable response of T cells that are exposed to allogeneic MHC molecules, as happens when an allograft is transplanted (see FIGURE 3) and then the number of responding cells may be 1,000-fold higher (see TABLE 3).[7] The exact mechanism by which this occurs is uncertain, since one might have expected a less good "fit" of the MHC molecule to result in non-recognition. The explanation put forward is that the combined allo-MHC + any peptide complex corresponds to a shape that

TABLE 1. Some basic immunology concepts relevant to encapsulation

**Concept 1.** The immune system has developed from relatively few "primordial molecules", some of which are large molecules, but some quite small (e.g., chemokines)

    Molecules binding to peptides with a variable binding site: *immunoglobulin superfamily*

    Molecules binding to sugars: *lectins*

    Molecules binding to structural proteins: *fibronectins*

    Signalling peptides and receptors: *chemokines*

    Growth hormones and receptors: *interleukins* and *cytokines*

**Concept 2.** The strategy for detecting and responding to novel invading organisms depends on detecting peptides derived from shed proteins

    Huge number of variant TCRs

    Number of T-cells responding to any single peptide low (precursor frequency not less than 1:100,000)

    Strategy critically dependent upon ability to rapidly proliferate responding cells

**Concept 3.** An allograft is an unexpected aberration that "catches out" the immune system

    A very complex situation arises as a consequence of MHC molecules "almost but not quite fitting"

    Between graft and host, most components of the immune system are the same or similar molecules which function normally

    Note that for xenografts more or less the opposite is true

**Concept 4.** Many phenomena in transplantation parallel those demonstrable in autoimmune disease/ regulation

    Susceptibility to immunosuppressive agents

    Role of peptides in immune response

    Th1 versus Th2 cytokines

    Development of anergy

    Role of regulatory cells

    *It is likely that the phenomenon of graft acceptance involves the mechanisms that normally control autoimmunity*

TABLE 2. How the immune system is switched on is largely understood, but we still do not understand how it is turned off

    Suggested mechanisms include:

        Th1 / Th2 hypothesis

        Microchimerism

        Anergy/apoptosis

        Danger hypothesis

        Regulatory cells

        Linked epitope suppression

        The authors hypothesis: MHC-based Suppression[27]

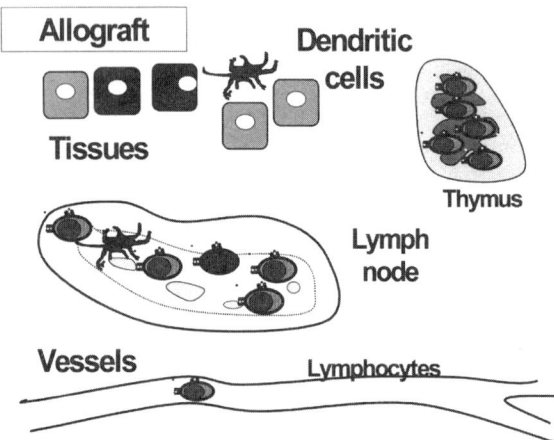

**FIGURE 3.** An allograft represents an expected and complex situation in which components of the immune system derived from the graft attempt to interact with the host. The result is an unexpectedly violent reaction, termed rejection.

is interpreted by the T cell as a self MHC molecule with a foreign peptide (see FIGURE 4).[8] The two responses of the T cell to transplanted tissue described above form the basis of what is termed the *indirect presentation* pathway,[9] corresponding to detection of peptide via what is essentially the normal route, and the so-called *direct presentation* pathway by which the mistaken recognition of the whole MHC occurs.[8] Understanding these two ways in which T cells may be activated by transplanted tissue is crucial to interpreting the effect of inserting a membrane barrier, and it is particularly important to understand that the two pathways have something of a reciprocal arrangement depending on whether the graft is an allograft or xenograft (see FIGURES 5 and 6).

**TABLE 3. Encapsulation technology and immunology: the author's advice**

| |
|---|
| Stop trying to do what is probably not achievable (e.g., molecular cut-off) |
| Drop the term immunoisolation—it is not |
| Use the term immunoprotection if you must |
| You cannot ignore the immunobiology—instead work with it |
| Exploit current niches |
| Define the secrets of biocompatibility |
| When the secrets of tolerance are unravelled, encapsulation technology may come to the fore as the best way of delivering appropriate membrane-bound biological signals |

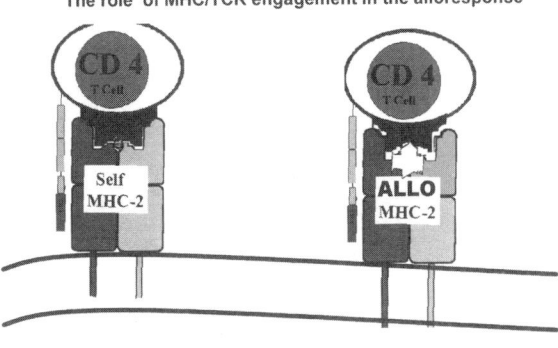

**FIGURE 4.** Allogeneic MHC molecules are reacted against by host T cells as though they all were self MHC molecules carrying an invader-derived peptide.

## POINTS RELATED TO ISLET TRANSPLANTATION AND ENCAPSULATION

Moving from more general concepts to the issues that specifically relate to transplantation of islets, there are a number of experimental models routinely used to ascertain the function of islet transplants and the effect of encapsulation. These are outlined in FIGURE 7, which emphasizes that there is an exponential increase in difficulty of these models as one approaches clinical transplantation. The commonly favored site for islet transplantation is into the portal vein,[10] where the islets have been shown to lodge in the terminal portal radicals[11] (see FIGURE 8).

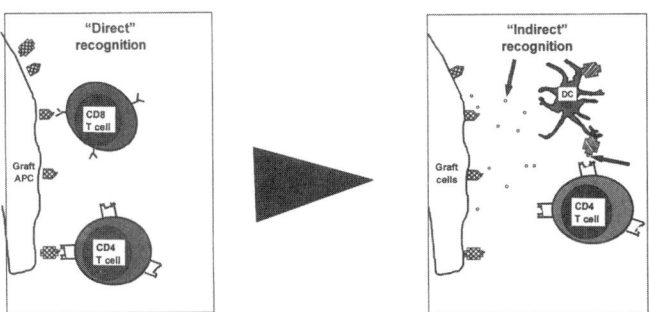

**FIGURE 5.** In an allograft situation, the major difference at the molecular level is in the MHC molecules and, therefore, the T cell response. Two ways in which this results in the graft being seen as "foreign" and attacked: the so-called *direct* and *indirect* pathways. The direct response predominates, at least in the early phase of vascularized graft rejection.

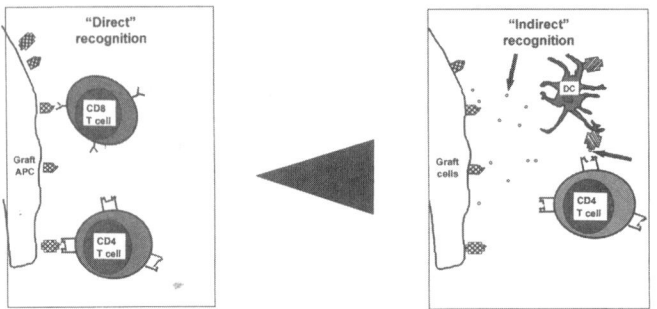

**FIGURE 6.** In the xenogeneic situation the MHC molecules may be so different that there is little direct T-cell response, but large numbers of different peptides derived from virtually every protein drive the indirect response.

There are three notable routes by which such transplanted islets may activate mechanisms that are harmful. FIGURE 9 relates to the first of these and describes the early, largely non-specific, inflammatory response to an islet transplant, part of which may in theory be modified by the presence of an encapsulation membrane barrier. However, there is little data specifically relating to the effect of encapsulation on these events, although there is an abundance of data concerning the effect of various individual cytokines on encapsulated islets.[12–15] Since many of the molecules involved have a molecular size close to the cut-off for membranes in common use, the exact effect achieved is likely to vary depending on the pore size of the membrane. The effect is also likely to be most striking for xenografts, particularly in

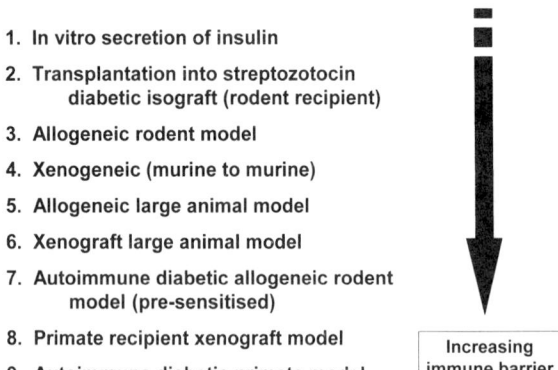

**FIGURE 7.** Models used for testing encapsulation devices containing insulin secreting tissue.

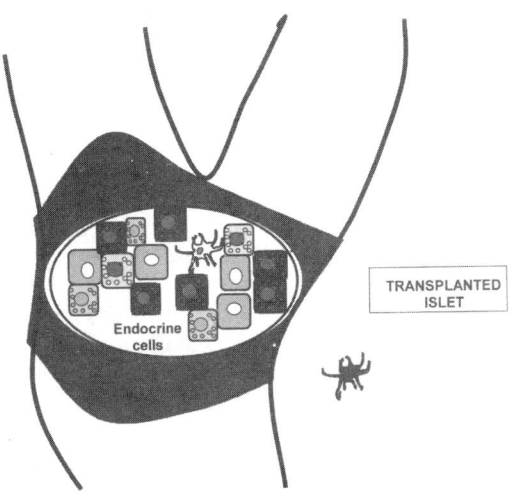

**FIGURE 8.** Cartoon representation of an islet transplanted into the liver, embolizing the terminal radicals of the portal vein, when it initially rests within a blind clot.

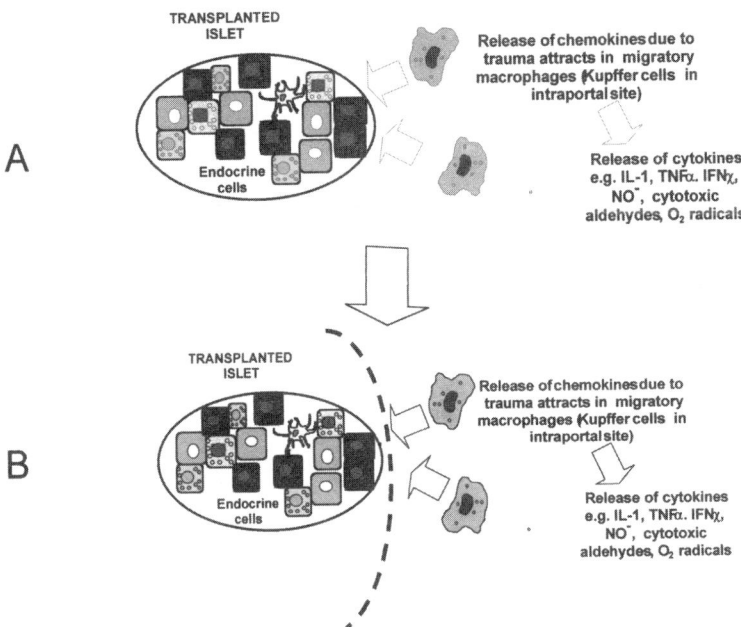

**FIGURE 9.** A representation of the early events that may influence islet graft implantation in the allogeneic situation (**A**) and the likely effect of introducing a membrane barrier as used in encapsulation of islets (**B**).

primate recipients, where the exposure of freshly isolated xenogeneic islets to human blood has been shown to result in rapid destruction of the graft. The ability of an encapsulation membrane to prevent this gross reaction is speculated as likely to be effective (see FIGURE 10), although the experiment has not been performed, to the author's knowledge.

The second route by which transplanted islets may activate mechanisms that are harmful is the now familiar *direct* pathway.[8] As shown in FIGURE 11, this depends critically on the migration of dendritic cells from within the graft to the recipient lymphoid tissue, where they present the allogeneic MHC molecules to the recipient T cells. The insertion of an encapsulation membrane prevents the dendritic cell migration (FIG. 11) and is therefore highly effective in preventing allograft rejection, in which the direct pathway is the most important mechanism.

The third route by which transplanted islets may activate mechanisms that are harmful is via the indirect pathway[9] (FIG. 11), and here the insertion of an encapsulation membrane is likely to be ineffective if the peptide and proteins shed by the graft are smaller than the pore size of the membrane.[16] The role of the indirect

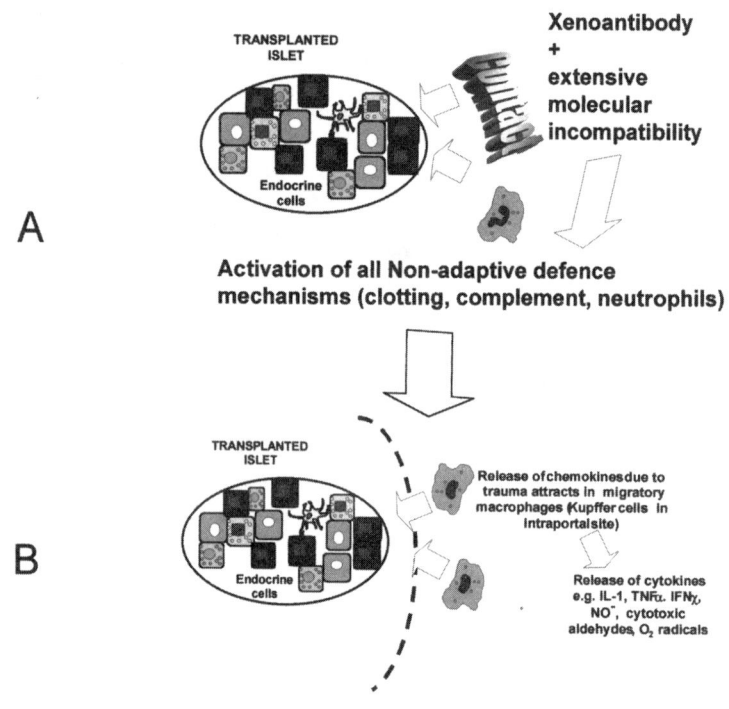

**FIGURE 10.** A representation of the early events that may influence islet graft implantation in the xenogeneic situation (**A**) and the likely effect of introducing a membrane barrier as used in encapsulation of islets (**B**).

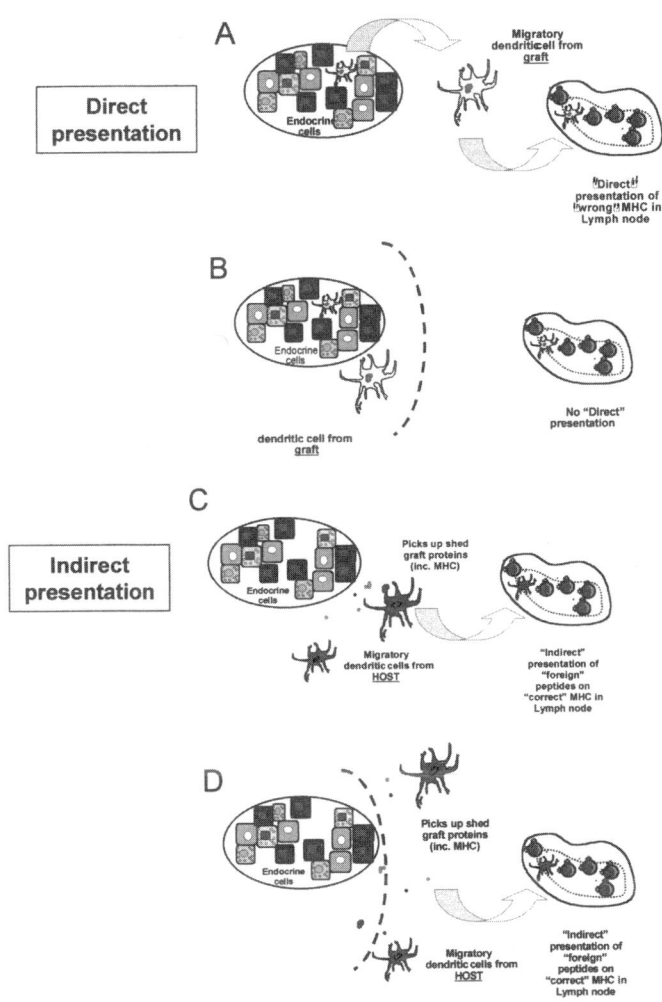

**FIGURE 11.** Series of diagrams to show how the migratory dendritic cell is crucial to the process of cellular rejection by direct presentation (**A**) and this is prevented by insertion of a membrane which prevents cell migration (**B**). However, the indirect pathway is driven by proteins and peptides diffusing out of the graft and picked up by host dendritic cells (depicted as *dark grey*) as in (**C**). A membrane will likely be largely ineffective against this pathway.

pathway in allograft rejection is relatively minor (at least in acute rejection, although chronic rejection may be a different matter). However, in xenotransplantation between disparate species the indirect pathway becomes dominant. In the hope that it may be possible to exclude such shed proteins it is, therefore, pertinent to ask what is their likely size, and unfortunately there is no data on this point. However, it is certain that sensitization does occur, as evidenced by antibody production following encapsulated islet xenotransplantation. It should also be pointed out that every cell inside an encapsulation membrane has the internal machinery for digesting proteins to peptides of 8–22 amino acids in length for the sole purpose of displaying them on the cell surface MHC molecules[17,18] (see FIGURE 12). It is known that these MHC/peptide complexes cycle, but what is not known is what eventually happens to the peptides. It would seem unlikely that they would be internalized and broken down further. Rather, it is likely they are lost into a surrounding tissue fluid and indeed this may be the route by which dendritic cells normally pick up antigen. If this were to be the case it would of course make the concept of a molecular cut-off untenable.

The final concept discussed here in relation to encapsulation technology is the question of induction of tolerance or, as it is less controversially described, donor-specific unresponsiveness. That such a phenomenon exists is clear from the clinical experience of reducing immunosuppression several weeks after transplantation, eventually reaching levels at which there is a return of relatively normal immune responses yet no graft rejection (see FIGURE 13). Interestingly, the effect appears to be more powerful the larger the graft. The parallels between many of the phenomena in transplantation and autoimmune disease leads to the conclusion that the same mechanisms are involved (TABLE 1), and extensive recent data has pointed to the critical role of regulatory (suppressor) cells.[19,20] The exact molecular mechanism by which T-cells are switched off remains uncertain. Some of the suggested mechanisms[21–27] are listed in TABLE 2. What is becoming certain is that the mechanism involves cell–cell contact and is, therefore, likely to be prevented by insertion of a membrane. However, once the mechanism is understood it should prove possible to produce membranes with the necessary molecules immobilized on the membrane surface.

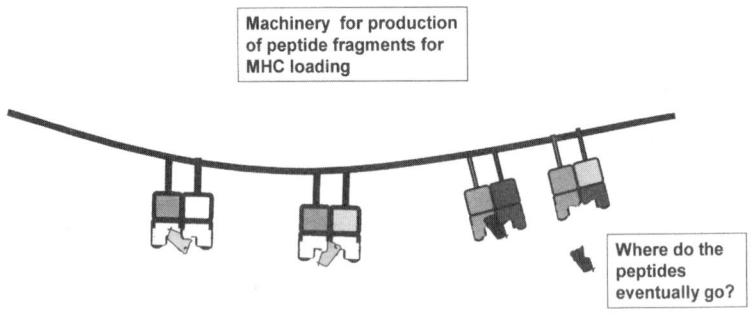

**FIGURE 12.** Question: Is the concept of a molecular cut-off realistic? How small are immunogenic peptides coming from the graft? Answer: Probably very small. Perhaps 8–15 amino acids.

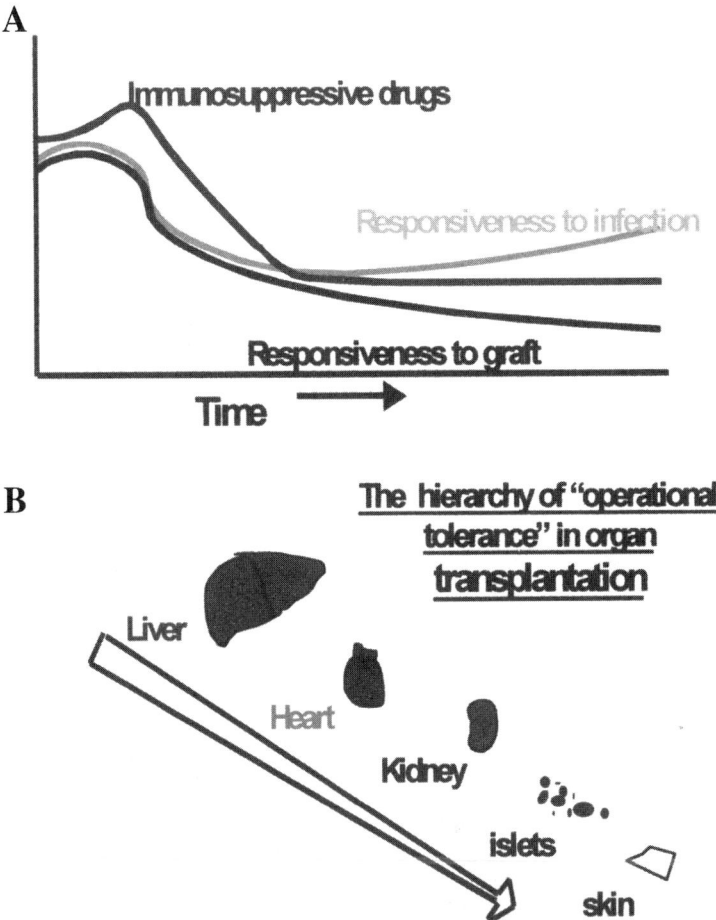

**FIGURE 13.** Two concepts that come from observation of clinical organ transplantation. **A.** The development of relative graft unresponsiveness while responsiveness to invaders returns almost to normal is crucial because it provides the therapeutic gap necessary for successful transplantation. **B.** The mechanism of graft acceptance appears to be easier to induce with increasing graft size.

## CONCLUSIONS

The author has looked at immune processes in islet transplantation from the point of view of encapsulation technology, and has a possible advantage of an "outside" point of view with no particular bias since he has never made a capsule of any form. For what they are worth, some suggestions that specialists in the field might like to consider are listed in TABLE 3.

## REFERENCES

1. LAFFERTY, K.J. & J. WOOLNOUGH. 1977. The origin and mechanism of the allograft reaction. Immunol. Rev. **35:** 231–262.
2. STEINMAN, R.M. & M.C. NUSSENZWEIG. 1980. Dendritic cells: features and functions. Immunol. Rev. **53:** 127–147.
3. FREMONT, D.H., W.A. REES & H. KOZONO. 1996. Biophysical studies of T-cell receptors and their ligands. Curr. Opin. Immunol. **8**(1): 93–100.
4. FORD, D. & D. BURGER. 1983. Precursor frequency of antigen-specific T cells: effects of sensitization *in vivo* and *in vitro*. Cell Immunol. **79**(2): 334–344.
5. JINGWU, Z., R. MEDAER, G.A. HASHIM, *et al.* 1992. Myelin basic protein-specific T lymphocytes in multiple sclerosis and controls: precursor frequency, fine specificity, and cytotoxicity. Ann. Neurol. **32**(3): 330–338.
6. MONGKOLSAPAYA, J., A. JAYE, M.F. CALLAN, *et al.* 1999. Antigen-specific expansion of cytotoxic T lymphocytes in acute measles virus infection. J. Virol. **73**(1): 67–71.
7. LOMBARDI, G. & R. LECHLER. 1991. The molecular basis of allorecognition of major histocompatibility complex molecules by T lymphocytes. Ann. Ist. Super Sanita **27**(1): 7–14.
8. LECHLER, R., R. BATCHELOR & G. LOMBARDI. 1991. The relationship between MHC restricted and allospecific T cell recognition. Immunol. Lett. **29**(1–2): 41–50.
9. AUCHINCLOSS, JR., H. & H. SULTAN. 1996. Antigen processing and presentation in transplantation. Curr. Opin. Immunol. **8**(5): 681–687.
10. KEMP, C.B., M.J. KNIGHT, D.W. SCHARP, *et al.* 1973. Effect of transplantation site on the results of pancreatic islet isografts in diabetic rats. Diabetologia **9:** 486–491.
11. GRIFFITH, R.C., D.W. SCHARP, B.K. HARTMAN, *et al.* 1977. A morphologic study of intrahepatic portal-vein islet isografts. Diabetes **26**(3): 201–214.
12. CAMPBELL, I.L., A. ISCARO & L.C. HARRISON. 1988. IFN-gamma and tumor necrosis factor-alpha: cytotoxicity to murine islets of Langerhans. J. Immunol. **141:** 2325–2329.
13. RABINOVITCH, A., W. SUMOSKI, R.V. RAJOTTE & G.L. WARNOCK. 1990. Cytotoxic effects of cytokines on human pancreatic islet cells in monolayer culture. J. Clin. Endocrinol. Metab. **71:** 152–156.
14. PUKEL, C., H. BAQUERIZO & A. RABINOVITCH. 1988. Destruction of rat islet cell monolayers by cytokines: synergistic interactions of interferon-γ, tumor necrosis factor, lymphotoxin, and interleukin 1. Diabetes **37:** 133–136.
15. POULSEN, T.M., K. BENDTZEN, J. NERUP, *et al.* 1986. Affinity-purified human interleukin I is cytotoxic to isolated islets of Langerhans. Diabetologia **29:** 63–67.
16. GRAY, D.W.R. 1997. Encapsulated islet cells: the role of direct and indirect presentation and the relevance to xenotransplantation and autoimmune recurrence. Brit. Med. Bull. **54:** 777–788.
17. PAMER, E. & P. CRESSWELL. 1998. Mechanisms of MHC class I—restricted antigen processing. Annu. Rev. Immunol. **16:** 323–358.
18. CHAPMAN, H.A. 1998. Endosomal proteolysis and MHC class II function. Curr. Opin. Immunol. **10**(1): 93–102.
19. SAKAGUCHI, S. 2000. Regulatory T cells: key controllers of immunologic self-tolerance. Cell **101**(5): 455–458.
20. ZHAI, Y. & J.W. KUPIEC-WEGLINSKI. 1999. What is the role of regulatory T cells in transplantation tolerance? Curr. Opin. Immunol. **11**(5): 497–503.
21. FRASCA, L., P. CARMICHAEL, R. LECHLER & G. LOMBARDI. 1997. Anergic T cells effect linked suppression. Eur. J. Immunol. **27**(12): 3191–3197.
22. MOSSMANN, T.R. 1987. Two types of mouse helper T cell clone: Implications for immune regulation. Immunol. Today **8:** 223–227.
23. LOMBARDI, G., S. SIDHU, R. BATCHELOR & R. LECHLER. 1994. Anergic T cells as suppressor cells *in vitro* [see comments]. Science **264**(5165): 1587–1589.
24. QIN, S., S.P. COBBOLD, H. POPE, *et al.* 1993. "Infectious" transplantation tolerance. Science **259**(5097): 974–977.
25. STARZL, T.E. & A.J. DEMETRIS. 1998. Transplantation tolerance, microchimerism, and the two-way paradigm [see comments]. Theor. Med. Bioeth. **19**(5): 441–455.

26. MATZINGER, P. 1994. Tolerance, danger, and the extended family. Annu. Rev. Immunol. **12**(991): 991–1045.
27. GRAY, D.W.R. 1998. Major histocompatibility complex-based suppression: a mechanism for T-cell control. Med. Hypotheses **50**(4): 289–302.

# Cellular Support Systems for Alginate Microcapsules Containing Islets, as Composite Bioartificial Pancreas

RICCARDO CALAFIORE,[a] GIOVANNI LUCA,[a] MARIO CALVITTI,[b] LUCA M. NERI,[c] GIUSEPPE BASTA,[a] SILVANO CAPITANI,[c] ENNIO BECCHETTI, AND PAOLO BRUNETTI[a]

[a]*Departments of Internal Medicine, Section of Internal Medicine, and Endocrine and Metabolic Sciences, and Consorzio Interuniversitario per i Trapianti d'Organo, University of Perugia, Perugia, Italy*

[b]*Department of Experimental Medicine and Biochemical Sciences, University of Perugia, Perugia, Italy*

[c]*Department of Morphology and Embryology, Section of Human Anatomy, University of Ferrara, Ferrara, Italy.*

ABSTRACT: To improve the functional performance of microencapsulated islets, we examined the effects of putative cellular support systems, consisting of rat purified Sertoli cells (SC) and astrocytes (AA), on coenveloped allogeneic islets. Coincubation of islets with SC but not AA, resulted in significant stimulation of β cell mitogenesis, coupled with a significant increase in *in vitro* glucose-stimulated insulin release. Preliminarily, the xenotransplantation of coencapsulated rat islets and homologous SC significantly prolonged remission of hyperglycemia in diabetic mice.

KEYWORDS: cellular support system; alginate microcapsules; islets; composite bioartificial pancreas

## INTRODUCTION

Human islet allografts have been recently reported by the University of Alberta, in Edmonton, Canada, to induce full and sustained remission of hyperglycemia, with normalization of metabolic parameters, thereby permitting withdrawal of exogenous insulin, in 7 of 7 patients with type I diabetes mellitus (IDDM), under general immunosuppressive regimens.[1] These results, for the first time have clearly proven the principle that islet transplantation (TX) may cure IDDM. However, at least two major issues still are pending: (1) the restricted availability of cadaveric human donor pancreases could never fulfill demand for islet tissue; (2) the newly available immunosuppressive agents adopted by the Edmonton protocol may be less harmful, as far as both islet-directed and general toxicity are concerned. Nevertheless, their

---

Address for correspondence: Ricardo Calafiore, Department of Internal Medicine and Endocrine and Metabolic Sciences, University of Perugia, 06126 Perugia, Italy. Voice: +39 075 578 3682; fax: +39 075 573 0855.
islet@unipg.it

long-term side effects are unknown. Ongoing clinical protocols, based on progressive discontinuation of the immunosuppressive agents, in an attempt to induce acquired immunotolerance are under way, although it is premature to anticipate the success of these efforts.

To surmount the hurdles mentioned above, both alternate tissues as a resource for donor islets, and alternate strategies for TX immunoprotection, with no general recipient immunosuppression, should be introduced. As to the former, adult, as well as neonatal porcine islets, could be readily available, whereas health authority approval for use of xenogeneic animal tissue sources in humans is still pending, primarily subject to safety requirements. In parallel, the development of engineered human/nonhuman β cells[2] or differentiation of nonengineered human/nonhuman stem cells[3,4] that originally derive from non-endocrine tissue (i.e., pancreatic ductal cell network), into functionally competent β cells, could permit access to virtually inexhaustible insulin-producing tissue procurement.

On the islet TX-directed immunity front, the new immunosuppressive agents (see TABLE 1), although apparently capable, within an allogeneic TX setting, of circumventing the host's immune response, including autoimmune recurrence of the disease,[1] have not been proved to be clearly effective thus far in obviating the islet xenograft-directed immune destruction. Although limited to few laboratories, microencapsulation technology, consisting of physical envelopment of the islets within highly biocompatible and selective permeable membranes, may fully protect islet xenografts, mainly in diabetic rodents, for very long periods of time.[5-8] However, the potential advantages associated with the use of microcapsules are shadowed by as many apparent pitfalls (see TABLE 2) that could attenuate the impact of this approach on islet transplantation in diabetic higher mammalians. In fact, with the exception of one relevant, yet isolated, report[9] no substantial evidence of function of microencapsulated allo/xenogeneic islet TX has been achieved by trials conducted in diabetic dogs or, preliminarily, in IDDM-patients that showed only partial and finite remission of hyperglycemia. In our own experience, diabetic patients undergoing complex vascular surgery were grafted with microencapsulated human islets embodied in a coaxial vascular chamber, directly anastomosed to blood vessels: insufficient islet cell mass was held responsible for clinical inconsistency of the results obtained,[10] although no evidence of immune rejection was observed. Finally, so far, of two patients with IDDM receiving intraperitoneal TX of microencapsulated neonatal porcine islets, neither one showed evidence of clinical correction of hyperglycemia, and only negligible raise in porcine C-peptide urinary levels was detected (unpublished data).

TABLE 1. General immunosuppression

| Old Agents | New Agents |
|---|---|
| cyclosporin | mycofenolate mofetil |
| FK 506 | rapamycin |
| antilymophocyte globulin (ALG) | anti-Tc MoAb |
| azathioprine | anti-IL2R MoAb |
| corticosteriods | |

The causes for the limited success so far achieved by microencapsulation as a physical immunobarrier strategy for islet TX may be multiple, although some issues deserve special attention. In particular:

*(1) Alginate Purification for Human Use.* Despite the recent introduction of validation procedures for alginate extraction, purification and endotoxin removal, there still is no certainty that the final product will comply with requirements of regulatory agencies for human application. For this purpose, special care should be taken in reducing the alginate (AG) protein content to minimal levels. Moreover, AG pharmacokinetics and pharmacodynamics as well as general toxicity should be investigated: a few studies on LD50 and, in general, on AG disposal, administered by various routes have been completed in several animal models, but never in humans. Furthermore, specifications for AG composition and storage also are necessary.

*(2) Immunobarrier Capacity.* Encapsulated islet allografts seem to be better protected than xenografts from the host's immune response. However, it is not clear whether this relates solely to substantial differences between allo- and xenogeneic immune reactivity. Initial reports[11] suggest that the microcapsules may be unable to prevent permeation of low molecular weight humoral molecules, released by xenogeneic islets. These could, in turn, trigger the host's immune attack, through indirect immune pathways. Furthermore, the eventual "helper" role of non-immunospecific environmental factors in promoting the islet xenograft destruction cannot be excluded.

*(3) Microcapsule Size and Configuration.* Starting from the original alginate/poly-L-lysine (AG/PLL) capsules generated by Sun,[12] which measured approximately 600–800 µ in diameter, other AG-based capsule prototypes have been developed, during the past two decades. The "newer" capsules, although basically formulated with the same polymers, have undergone progressive reduction in size, to an average 350–500 µ in diameter, and have been fabricated, in some instances, with various microdroplet generators, such as electrostatic devices.[13] In contrast to other laboratories, we selected poly-L-ornithine (PLO) instead of PLL, as an aminoacidic cation

TABLE 2. Alginate microcapsules for islet transplantation

| Strengths | Pitfalls |
|---|---|
| 1. Immunoisolation capacity for allo-/xenogeneic islet TX from the host's immune response shown in low as well as high mammals (Sun etc.) | 1. Clear evidence of success in small and large-size diabetic animals achieved in only few centers |
| 2. Long-term established procedure (1980) | 2. Techniques's reproducibility (raw materials, fabrication, etc.) difficult to achieve among and between different laboratories |
| 3. Material biocompatibility | 3. Inconsistency of pilot clinical trials |
| 4. Prevention on nonendocrine cell overgrowth | 4. Variable extent of immunobarrier competence (i.e., allo- vs. xenograft) |
|  | 5. Expected finite intracapsular islet cell survival (no reinnervation or revascularization at TX site) |

polymer coat, because of the higher reliability of PLO for ion/binding capacity.[14] Furthermore, we also developed a novel principle to prepare coherent microcapsules (CM), still formulated with AG/PLO, although based on completely different fabricative principle. CM, due to their constitution, form a skin-like hydrogel thin film that tightly adheres to each islet, with no dead space remaining between the capsule and the islet surface (average diameter 200 µ).[15] Whether small-size microcapsules can provide the encapsulated islet grafts with significant advantages, in terms of immunoisolatory capacity, as compared with larger-size spheres, remains controversial.[16] In our own system, although more suitable for nutrient/oxygen diffusion, CM have preliminarily been shown to provide a more vulnerable immunobarrier, in comparison with standard-size microcapsules (unpublished data). Consequently, an intermediate capsule size (350–500 µ) might represent a good compromise between large and small microspheres, at least for the peritoneal TX site.[14]

*(4) Site of TX.* The vast majority of the encapsulated islet TX trials has been conducted using the peritoneal cavity as an elective TX site, mainly due to the large final capsule TX volumes (exceeding 100 ml/dog or 180 ml/patient for standard capsules measuring more than 600 µ in diameter) employed in these studies. However, the smaller-size capsules could suit other sites within the mesenteric area, such as artificially constructed omental pouches or mesentery flaps. Since microencapsulated, unlike free islets, cannot be grafted intrahepatically, employment of alternate sites that are as close as possible to the liver should be pursued in order to enhance their metabolic performance. Additionally, the TX of "packed" microcapsules in a confined site, rather than freely located in the peritoneal cavity, could permit TX retrieval. With regard to CM, these smaller-size capsules could be considered for TX within a reasonable sized vascular chamber directly anastomosed to blood vessels as arterio–venous shunts. The concept of prevascularizing the TX site for microcapsules has already been indicated as a potential improvement for survival of the encapsulated islets.[17]

*(5) Intracapsular Environmental Conditions.* These conditions are critical for encapsulated islet TX longevity. The islets are comprised of both endocrine and nonendocrine cells, the latter including, for instance, fibroblasts that could thrive at expense of the β cells, in terms of oxygen and nutrient consumption. Moreover, if intrahepatically allografted free islets seem to survive for extraordinary long periods of time, it should be noted that free, unlike microencapsulated, islets are reinnervated and revascularized at the TX site. The encapsulated islets rely only on passive nutrient diffusion. Consequently, lifespan of the encapsulated islets likely is to be finite. Finally, neonatal islets could require the presence of factors that are known to implement their time-related maturation and acquisition of functional competence. In this respect, Sertoli cells (SC), which are originally situated in the testis, have been reported to possibly serve as "nursing" cells as well as an immunomodulatory system by the expression of immune-related molecules (i.e., FasL, TGFα, etc.) for the islets.[18] SC, by releasing a number of growth factors (see TABLE 3), could mimic effects of the extracellular pancreatic matrix from which the islets have been physically disconnected. These factors have been shown to enhance survival of fetal/neonatal[19] as well as adult[20] islets.

TABLE 3. Physiological properties

| Sertoli's Cells | Astrocytes |
|---|---|
| *Synthesis of growth factors* | *Synthesis of growth factors* |
| IGF (insulin-like gf I and II) | bFGF (basic fibroblast gf) |
| TGFα (transforming gf) | NGF (nerve gf) |
| EGF (endothelial gf) | CNTF (ciliary neurotrophic gf) |
|  | glial cell-line derived neurotrophic |
| *expression of FasL* |  |
| targeting CD8, DCD4-FasR |  |

## COMPOSITE BIOARTIFICIAL PANCREAS (CBP)

We have recently undertaken the task of developing CBP to implement islet TX survival and function within the special immunoisolatory microenvironment provided by AG/PLO microcapsules. CBP represents a hybrid entity in which the isolated allo- or xenogeneic islets are coenveloped within AG/PLO microcapsules, together with "nursing" cellular systems or possibly pharmacoactive substances that can prolong islet cell survival as well as retention of functional competence. In parallel, these systems also attenuate the impact of TX-directed immune or non-immunospecific destruction mechanisms. In order to develop a CBP prototype, standard AG/PLO microcapsules require specific size adjustments in order to host the islets together with other cells and, eventually, *ad hoc* formulated, packeted chemical molecules within the membranes. Initially, we examined coenvelopment of the islets with nursing cell systems in AG/PLO microcapsules.

## NURSING CELL SYSTEMS

### SC

The addition of SC has been reported to help survival and function of either free[21] or microencapsulated islet allografts in diabetic rats, and also to prevent recurrent autoimmune disease in syngeneic islet TX receiving NOD mice.[22] However, the basic mechanisms of action of these phenomena have not been clarified. We have recently observed[23] that SC, on coincubation with homologous adult rat islets, are associated with mitogenic effects on the β cells. This phenomenon appears to directly correlate with an increase of *in vitro* glucose-stimulated insulin release. TX of non-discordant AG/PLO microencapsulated xenogeneic rat SC + islets into diabetic mice resulted in longer remission of hyperglycemia in comparison with control mice receiving only encapsulated islet grafts. We wished to assess whether the SC-associated mitogenic effects on the islets depends on physical contact between SC and the islets or rather, on release of SC-related humoral factors affecting the islets.

## Astrocytes (AA)

Among additional cell types that can serve as putative nursing cellular systems we selected AA separated and purified from the adult rat brain. These cells release growth factors (TABLE 3) and cytokines that are associated with neurotrophic effects and take a major role in forming the blood/brain barrier. We employed AA as control cellular system for SC in terms of nursing effects on the islets.

## METHODOLOGY AND EXPERIMENTAL DESIGN

### Separation and Purification of SC from the Prepubertal Rat Testis

SC were separated from the testes of prepubertal Sprague Dawley (SD) rats and processed within 30 minutes of retrieval, according to methods described elsewhere,[18] and recently upgraded in our laboratory.[23] Briefly, each testicle pair, upon removal under sterile conditions, was stored in Eurocollins. The testes were finely minced and immediately incubated with an enzymatic solution comprising collagenase, trypsin, and DNAase. On termination of the digestion, the tissue was resuspended in RPMI medium, filtered through 500 µ stainless mesh, plated in $100 \times 15$ mm. Petri dishes, and culture maintained in HAM F12 supplemented with nicotinamide, 3-isobutylmethylxhantine (IBMX), 10% fetal calf serum and antibiotics at 37°C in air/CO2 95%. At 24 hours of culture, the tissue was treated with tris(hydroxymethyl)aminometane hydrochloride buffer in order to eliminate any residual germinal cells.[24] The latter could, in fact, create risks for tumors if not removed on exposure to higher temperatures (i.e., upon TX in the abdominal cavity).

### AA from SD Rat Brain

AA feature anatomic and functional properties, such as membrane receptors for most neurotransmitters and neuromodulators with functional signal transduction systems, aminoacidic neurotransmitter carriers, and ion channels that were once thought to be specific for neurons.[25] AA affect the neuronal excitability level and metabolically support the neurons, since glucose is taken up and stored in form of glycogen. Furthermore, AA are known to release growth factors (TABLE 4) that are involved with the control of cell developmental processes, like proliferation, differentiation, survival, migration, and maturation. We wished to assess if this cell type would improve survival and functional competence of the coincubated islet β cells. We, therefore, separated and maintained highly enriched AA from the brain cortex of adult SD rats in dissociated primary culture conditions, according to methods described elsewhere.[26] The preparations consisted of actively proliferating cells, one type of which could be immunocytochemically detected by A2B5 monoclonal antibody (MoAb), which specifically recognizes an extracellular ganglioside antigen.

### Islets from Adult SD Rats

The procedure was conducted according to the classic collagenase digestion method,[27] slightly modified in our laboratory. The final yield in pure islets per rat pancreas was close to 600. Care was taken to handpick the islets that entered *in vitro* coincubation and *in vivo* protocols.

## *In vitro* SC and AA/Islet Coincubation Studies

*Sample Preparation*

In brief: batches of 20 islets were coincubated with either 200,000 or 400,000 SC or AA in HAM F12, in quadruplicate. Isolated islets or SC or AA were incubated alone as controls. At 12 days of coculture, the study was terminated and the samples processed for confocal laser microscopy (CLM) examination. In order to assess whether potential beneficial effects on islet β cells were eventually associated with cell-to-cell contact with SC, or instead related to humoral factors released from SC, we also coincubated batches of 20 islets with dialyzed-concentrated supernatants collected from SC cultures (400,000 SC/microwell). 5-Bromodeoxyuridine (BrdU), a sensitive mitotic marker, was added to the culture medium, at the end of coculture, for 24 hours. The BrdU-labelled islets, after several process steps, were incubated with a mouse anti-BrdU MoAb conjugated with fluorescein isothiocyanate (FITC). For double staining purposes, the islets were finally incubated with mouse antiinsulin Ab conjugated with tetra-rhodamine isothiocyanate (TRITC).

*Sample Imaging*

The samples were imaged by a confocal system that revealed FITC signal with 488 nm and TRITC signal with 543 nm wavelenghts. Digitalized optical sections were transferred from the CLM to the graphics workstation. Colocalization of BrdU and insulin was analyzed to assess positivity of the BrdU-labelled nuclei, and at least 40 fluorescent spots, corresponding to DNA replicon clusters, were counted, regardless of the exhibited fluorescent morphology. To determine the percentage of the replicating cells, all the insulin-labelled cells were counted by reassembling the optical sections of CLM through the entire islet. Finally, the number of BrdU-labelled cells

TABLE 4. **Immunostaining with BrdU**

|  |  | Percent Viable (SC) Cells | BrdU-Positive β Cells |
|---|---|---|---|
| Sertoli cells (SC) | none | 91 ± 5 | 1 ± 1 |
|  | 200,000 | 93 ± 3 | 5.8 ± 1.3[a] |
|  | 400,000 | 92 ± 4 | 8.1 ± 1[a] |
| Medium from SC | none | 91 ± 4 | 1.5 ± 1 |
|  | 200,000 | 94 ± 3 | 4.6 ± 1.2[a] |
|  | 400,000 | 93 ± 4 | 7.4 ± 1.4[a] |
| Astrolgial cells | none | 91 ± 6 | 1.6 ± 1.1 |
|  | 200,000 | 92 ± 4 | 1.6 ± 1.3 |
|  | 400,000 | 93 ± 4 | 1.8 ± 1.4 |

[a] $p < 0.01$.

were ranked on the physical position that they occupied within the islet. The cells were counted only once.

In vitro *Functional Studies*

Immunoreactive insulin (IRI) levels were assayed by radioimmunoassay. To evaluate the islet functional competence, batches of either free or SC- or AA-coincubated islets were exposed to glucose at different concentrations (sequentially 50-300-50 mg/dl) during a two-hour static incubation time fractions.

In vivo *Studies*

Batches of SC + islets, similar to those employed for *in vitro* studies, but at 1:10000 islet:SC ratio, were transplanted, after envelopment in AG/PLO microcapsule in the peritoneal cavity of mice rendered diabetic by streptozotocin (STZ).

*Microencapsulation Procedure.* Tissue batches were encapsulated in AG/PLO following our original method.[28] Briefly, the tissue was suspended in 1.6% sodium alginate at an appropriate AG/tissue ratio, thoroughly mixed and mechanically pumped through an air-driven microdroplet generator. The microdroplets containing the tissue immediately turned into gel microspheres upon reaction on a $CaCl_2$ collection bath. The gel microbeads were sequentially coated with PLO twice, in order to saturate all the COO•alginate radicals, and finally with highly purified NAG to enhance the capsule biocompatibility (see FIGURE 1).

*Recipients and TX Procedure.* CD-1 mice, weighing approximately 25 g, were rendered diabetic by a single unit dose of intravenously administered STZ (150 mg/Kg), under fasting conditions. Only animals with blood glucose (BG) levels in excess of 400 mg/dl, on three different measurements, were enrolled in the TX study. TX success was associated with restoration and sustenance of BG levels lower than 150 mg/dl under postabsorptive conditions. On the other hand, recurrent hyperglycemia, above 250 mg/dl, indicated TX failure. The encapsulated islets were grafted, under general anesthesia, on small midline abdominal incision, freely in the peritoneal cavity.

*Experimental Design.* 10 diabetic mice were separated into two experimental groups: $n = 5$ animals received an intraperitoneal unit dose of 1,000 islets + 10,000 SC/islet within AG/PLO microcapsules; $n = 5$ controls were grafted with 1,000 microencapsulated islets alone. BG was determined by reflectometer at days three

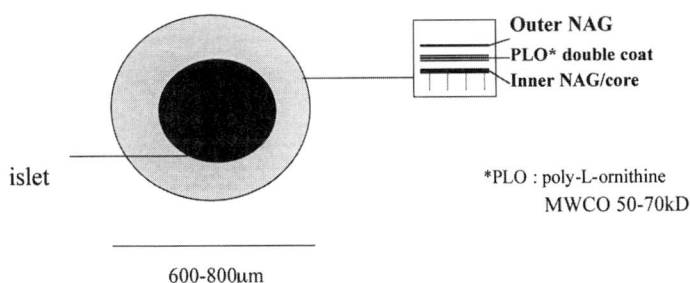

**FIGURE 1.** Schematic representation of AG/PLO microcapsules (University of Perugia).

and seven post-TX, and thereafter on a weekly basis. Data were expressed as mean ± SD; $p < 0.01$ in a Student's paired $t$ test was considered significant.

## RESULTS

### Morphological Studies

CLM examination was associated with BrdU-positive cells whose cytoplasms were strongly stained by the anti-insulin Ab. These findings applied to SC, but not to AA, only when the SC:islet coincubation ratio was 400,000:20. Quantification of the β cell mitotic figures was conducted by counting the FITC-labelled cells entering S-phase that were double-stained with TRITC. β cell mitotic rate, which was 1% for control islets, increased to 8.1% for islets + SC (400,000) and to 7.4% for islets + SC-concentrated supernatant, but it did not change for islets + AA.

In vitro *Functional Studies.* IRI levels, on static incubation with glucose, were significantly increased for islets+SC over islets alone, both in basal and after exposure to high glucose (see FIGURE 2). Addition of AA did not significantly affect the results obtained with free islets, thereby confirming the morphologic data.

In vivo *Studies.* All the encapsulated islet TX recipients, regardless of SC presence, showed full and rapid remission of hyperglycemia. The latter was sustained, however, for significantly longer periods of time in the animals receiving coencapsulated islets + SC, as compared to control islets alone (see FIGURE 3).

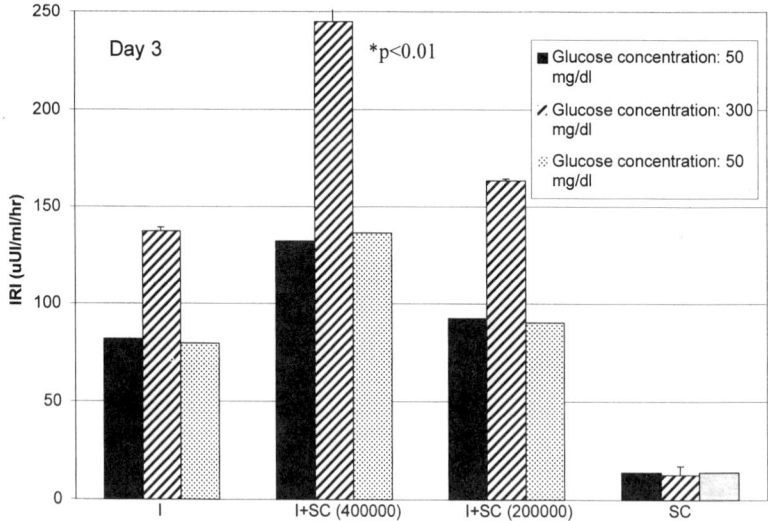

**FIGURE 2.** Static incubation of SC-islet co-cultures with glucose at various concentrations.

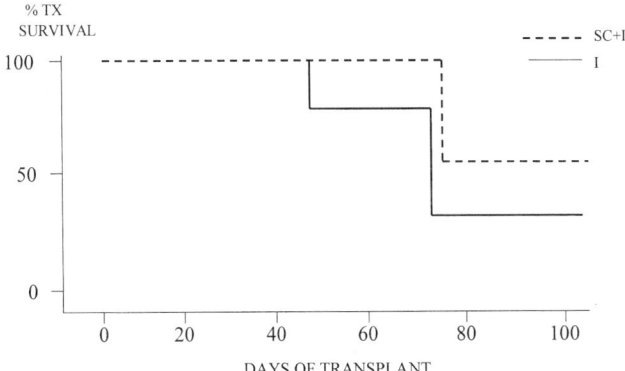

**FIGURE 3.** Xenotransplantation of microencapsulated rat islets ± SC into diabetic mice (SC, Sertoli cells with islets; I, islets alone)

## DISCUSSION

In order to expand clinical application, there certainly is a need to procure alternate islet sources, whether they be represented by nonengineered or engineered human/nonhuman insulin-producing cells. In this context, special attention is associated with pancreatic stem cells that can be committed to differentiate into functionally competent β cell lineages, thereby obviating need for use of cadaveric human islets. It would be then easy to grow insulin-producing cells in the laboratory. Regardless of the selected islet cell source, any TX immunoprotection strategy should obviate the host's pharmacological immunosuppression. This not only lacks specificity, but also is unpredictable in terms of morbidity, over long-term post-TX clinical follow-up periods. In this respect, islet TX immunoprotection by microcapsules that comprise biocompatible and immunoselective artificial membranes may represent an attractive alternative and is being pursued intensively at this time.

One aspect of this research has been and continues to be underscored: adult islet β cells are associated with an extremely limited mitotic rate (1%). It is even more unlikely that these cells will divide within the immunologically and metabolically complex TX set-up. Hence, any loss in the grafted islet β cell mass will be difficult to replace, which may adversely affect functional life span of the implanted tissue. Efforts to expand either fetal or adult islet β cells, in spite of initial encouraging observations, have never yielded substantial results. Nevertheless, methods to induce β cell expansion, irrespective of their origin, could significantly implement the TX functional performance. Toward this goal, we have studied the impact of nursing cell systems, such as SC and AA, coincubated and eventually (SC) comicroencapsulated with islets, in an attempt to unfold the involved mechanisms. Previous reports had in fact shown that SC indeed improved the functional performance of allogeneic rat islet grafts although no clear explanation as to how SC induced their beneficial effects on the islets were provided. Furthermore, unlike other SC preparations, our preparations were highly purified, thereby attenuating any possible immunological and metabolic interferences with the islet cell system. We have demonstrated that SC, but not other potential nursing cell systems, such as astroglial cells, significantly stimulate mitogenesis of homologous rat islet β cells. Looking at our data this effect seems to be dose dependent and apparently it is mediated by humoral factors, although further investigation is required to clarify the underlying molecular mechanisms.

Through preliminary studies, where SC-related mitogenic properties were investigated within AG/PLO microcapsules, we have shown that the islet TX function can significantly be prolonged in a nondiscordant xenogeneic setting. Additional study to confirm these initial data, and also to possibly suggest new engineering principles aimed at fabricating advanced bioartificial pancreas prototypes, is warranted.

In summary, on the basis of well-defined rationale, and on initial clarification of mechanisms of action, the idea of associating cellular support systems with islets in immunoisolatory microcapsules could positively have an impact on this field in the near future. In this respect, multifunctional microdevices, incorporating different cellular or even pharmacologic systems that synergistically interact between them can be envisioned. If successful, this new research could help to surmount some of the issues that have, so far, adversely affected biologic survival, but also immunoprotection of islet TX for the cure for IDDM.

## ACKNOWLEDGMENTS

The kind support of Telethon (Grant EC.0562) is thankfully acknowledged. We feel very grateful to Dr. Roberto Melcangi, University of Milano, Milano, Italy for providing us with the astroglial cells that were employed in our study.

## REFERENCES

1. SHAPIRO, A.M.J., J.R.T. LAKEY, E.A. RYAN, *et al.* 2000. Islet transplantation in seven patients with type I diabetes mellitus using a glucocorticoid-free immunosuppressive regimen. N. Engl. J. Med. **343**(4): 230–238.
2. EFRAT, S. 1999. Genetically engineered pancreatic β-cell lines for cell therapy of diabetes. *In* Bioartificial Organs II: Technology, Medicine & Materials. D. Hunkeler, A. Prokop, A. Cherrington, R.V. Rajotte & M. Sefton, Eds. Ann. N.Y. Acad. Sci. **875**: 286–293.
3. RAMIYA, V.K., M. MARAIST, K.E. ARFORS, *et al.* 2000. Reversal of insulin-dependent diabetes using islets generated in vitro from pancreatic stem cells. Nature Medicine **6**(3): 278–282.
4. BONNER-WEIR, S., M. TANEJA, G. WEIR, *et al.* 2000. *In vitro* cultivation of human islets from expanded ductal tissue. Proc. Natl. Acad. Sci. USA **97**(14): 7999–8004.
5. LANZA, R.P., A.M. BEYER, J.E. STARUK & W.L. CHICK. 1993. Biohybrid artificial pancreas: long-term function of discordant islet xenografts in streptozotocin-diabetic rats. Transplantation **56**: 1067–1072.
6. LANZA, R.P., R.M. BORLAND, J.E. STARUK, *et al.* 1992. Transplantation of encapsulated canine islets into spontaneously diabetic BB/Wor rats without immunosuppression. Endocrinology **131**: 637–642.
7. FAN, M.Y., Z.P. LUM, Z.W. FU & A.M. SUN. 1990. Reversal of diabetes in BB rats by transplantation of encapsulated pancreatic islets. Diabetes **39**: 519–522.
8. LUM, Z.P., I.P. TAI, M. KRESTOW, *et al.* 1991. Prolonged reversal of diabetic state in NOD mice by xenografts of microencapsulated rat islets. Diabetes **40**: 1511–1516.

9. SUN, Y., X. M.A, D. ZHOU, et al. 1996. Normalization of diabetes in spontaneously diabetic cynomologous monkeys by xenografts of microencapsulated porcine islets without immunosuppression. J. Clin. Invest. **98**: 1417–1422.
10. BRUNETTI P., G. BASTA, A. FALORNI, et al. 1991. Immunoprotection of pancreatic islet grafts within artificial microcapsules. Int. J. Artif. Organs 14: 789–791.
11. GILL, R.G. & L. WOLF. 1995. Immunobiology of cellular transplantation. Cell Trans. **4**(4): 361–370.
12. LIM, F. & A.M. SUN. 1980. Microencapsulated islets as bioartificial endocrine pancreas. Science **210**: 908.
13. WOLTERS, G.H., W.M. FRITSCHY, D. GERRITS & R. VAN SCHILFGAARDE. 1991. A versatile alginate droplet generator applicable for microencapsulation of pancreatic islets. J. Appl. Biomater. 3(4): 281.
14. CALAFIORE, R. & G. BASTA. Alginate/poly-L-ornithine microcapsules for pancreatic islet cell immunoprotection. *In* Cell Encapsulation Technology and Therapeutics. W.M. Kuhtreiber, R.P. Lanza & W.L Chick, Eds: 138–150. Birkhauser, Boston.
15. CALAFIORE, R., G. BASTA, G. LUCA, et al. 1997. Alginate/polyaminoacidic coherent microcapsules for pancreatic islet graft immunoisolation in diabetic recipients. *In* Bioartificial Organs I: Technology, Medicine & Materials. D. Hunkeler, A. Prokop, A. Cherrington, R.V. Rajotte & M. Sefton, Eds. Ann. N.Y. Acad. Sci. **831**: 313–322.
16. DE VOS, P. & R. VAN SCHILFGAARDE. 1999. Biocompatibility issues. *In* Cell Encapsulation Technology and Therapeutics. W.M. Kuhtreiber, R.P Lanza & W.L. Chick, Eds.: 63–75. Birkhauser, Boston.
17. DE VOS, P., J.L. HILLEBRANDS, B.J. DE HAAN, et al. 1997. Efficacy of a prevascularized expanded polytetrafluoroethylene solid support system as a transplantation site for pancreatic islets. Transplantation **63**(6): 824–830.
18. KORBUTT, G.S., J.F. ELLIOTT & R.V. RAJOTTE. 1997. Co-transplantation of allogeneic islets with allogeneic testicular cell aggregates allows long-term survival without systemic immunosuppression. Diabetes **46**: 317–322.
19. BEATTIE, G.M., J.S. RUBIN, M.I. MALLY, et al. 1996. Regulation of proliferation and differentiation of human fetal pancreatic islets by extracellular matrix, hepatocyte growth factor and cell to cell contact. Diabetes **45**: 1223–1228.
20. HAYEK, A., G.M. BEATTIE, V. CIRULLI, et al. 1996. Growth factor/matrix-induced proliferation of human adult β-cells. Diabetes **44**: 1458–1460.
21. KORBUTT, G.S., W.L. SUAREZ-PINZON, R.F. POWER, et al. 2000. Testicular Sertoli's cells exert both protective and destructive effects on syngeneic islet grafts in non-obese diabetic mice. Diabetologia **43**(9): 474–480.
22. SUAREZ-PINZON, W.L., G.S. KORBUTT, R. POWER, J. HOOTON, et al. 2000. Testicular Sertoli's cells protect islet β-cells from autoimmune destruction in NOD mice by a transforming growth factor β1-dependent mechanism. Diabetes **49**(11): 1810–1818.
23. LUCA, G., M. CALVITTI, L.M. NERI, et al. 2000. Sertoli's cells-induced reversal of adult rat pancreatic islet β-cells into foetal-like status: potent implications for islet transplantation in type I diabetes mellitus. J. Invest. Med. **48**(6): 441–448.
24. GALDIERI, M., E. ZIPARO, F. PALOMBI, et al. 1981. Pure Sertoli's cell cultures: a new model for the study of somatic-germ cell interaction. J. Androl. **5**: 249–259.
25. NORTON, W.T. & S.E. PODULO. 1970. Neuronal soma and whole neuroglia of rat brain: a new isolation technique. Science **167**: 1144–1146.
26. MELCANGI, R.C., F. CELOTTI, P. CASTANO & L. MARTINI. 1993. Differential localization of the 5α-reductase and the 3α-hydroxysteroid dehydrogenase in neuronal and glial cultures. Endocrinology **132**(3): 1252–1259.
27. LACY, P.E., O.H. HEGRE, A. GERASIMIDE-VAZEOU, et al. 1991. Subcutaneous xenografts of rat islets in acrylic copolymer capsules maintain normoglycemia in diabetic mice. Science **254**: 1782–1784.
28. CALAFIORE, R. 1998. Actual perspectives in biohybrid artificial pancreas for the therapy of type I, insulin-dependent diabetes mellitus. Diabetes Metab. Rev. **14**(4): 315–324.

# Preclinical Development of the Islet Sheet

RICHARD STORRS,[a] RANDY DORIAN,[a] SCOTT R. KING,[a]
JONATHAN LAKEY,[b] AND HORACIO RILO[c]

[a]*Islet Sheet Medical, LLC, 2180 Palou Ave. San Francisco, California, USA*

[b]*Surgical-Medical Research Institute, University of Alberta, Edmonton, Alberta, Canada*

[c]*Transplant Division, University of Cincinnati College of Medicine, Cincinnati, Ohio, USA*

ABSTRACT: The Islet Sheet is a thin planar bioartificial endocrine pancreas fabricated by gelling highly purified alginate and islets of Langerhans. Acellular alginate layers form a uniform immunoprotective barrier to host rejection of the encapsulated cells, with the tissue nourished by passive diffusion from adjacent host tissue. The overall thickness of the Islet Sheet, 250 μm, is chosen to maximize nutrient diffusion. In this paper we describe the early development of the Islet Sheet, including purification and fractionation of the alginates used, difficulties in maintaining sheet planarity, and preliminary metabolic studies in pancreatectomized dogs. In a key experiment, approximately 75,000 allogeneic islet equivalents in six Islet Sheets were sutured to the omentum of a 7-kg female beagle dog at the time of pancreatectomy. Fasting euglycemia was maintained for 84 days. Fed blood sugars were usually below 150 mg/dL. A single injection of 2 U insulin was administered on day 9, and antibiotics were administered for two weeks. No other drugs were used. IVGTT post implant was not normal, but seemed to improve between 30 and 60 days. Upon omentectomy and sheet removal the metabolic parameters deteriorated to a frankly diabetic state within seven days. The sheets did not remain flat, but fragments were recovered within hard, mostly acellular capsules. Dithizone staining showed islets within alginate sheets recovered from the interior of these capsules, suggesting that allogeneic islet tissue survived 84 days and was responsible for maintaining fasting euglycemia.

KEYWORDS: islet transplantation; bioartificial pancreas; microencapsulation; alginate; diabetes

## INTRODUCTION

The minimum criteria for a successful bioartificial pancreas are well known and fall in three general areas: preservation of viability and function of the donor tissue, prevention of destructive host response, and practical surgical implantation.[1,2] Unless all three criteria are met simultaneously the donor tissue will die, and the device will fail. For many years these criteria were addressed primarily using microencapsulation of individual islets[3] or with hollow fiber immunobarriers.[4]

Address for correspondence: Richard Storrs, Islet Sheet Medical, LLC, 2180 Palou Ave. San Francisco, CA 94131, USA
Rick@isletmedical.com

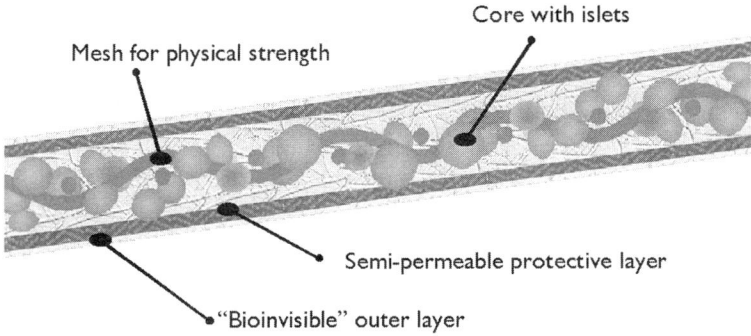

**FIGURE 1.** Diagram of an Islet Sheet, in cross-section. Alginate, containing up to 40% (v/v) islet tissue, is sandwiched between acellular alginate layers and gelled. A polymer mesh can be included in the islet-containing core to provide physical strength. Currently the semipermeable and bioinvisible layers are one and the same. Typical Islet Sheets measure 4 cm × 8 cm × 250 µm.

## THE ISLET SHEET: PREPARATION AND CHARACTERIZATION

The Islet Sheet follows a decade of experimentation with microencapsulation and responds to a number of shortcomings inherent to that approach. A broader range of polymer chemistries is available, and significantly less time is required for processing, boosting islet viability and function. The physical barrier between the islets and the host is more uniform and complete for better protection from destructive host response. Up to 40% of the sheet's implant volume is islet tissue, minimizing implant volume to a practicable size. Furthermore the Islet Sheet can be recovered intact, allowing for quantitative assessment of islet viability and function as well as host response, and conferring an additional advantage in clinical safety.

This article describes the development of the Islet Sheet to date.[a] For expediency in attaining this goal the data are not always rigorous or complete, and experimental design is often guided by impression and instinct rather than carefully controlled experimental analysis.

### Description of the Islet Sheet

The Islet Sheet is a multilayered construction of alginate where islets are cast as a thin flat sheet (optionally with a reinforcing polymer) which is completely sandwiched on both sides by an acellular immunoprotective alginate layer (see FIGURE 1). The entire construct is crosslinked throughout. Islet Sheets can be of any size; however, for ease of surgical manipulations, typical Islet Sheets measure approximately 4 cm × 8 cm × 250 µm.

---

[a]This research is entirely sponsored by Islet Sheet Medical LLC, and has the single-minded intent of demonstrating the *in vivo* efficacy of the thin sheet planar diffusion bioartificial pancreas.

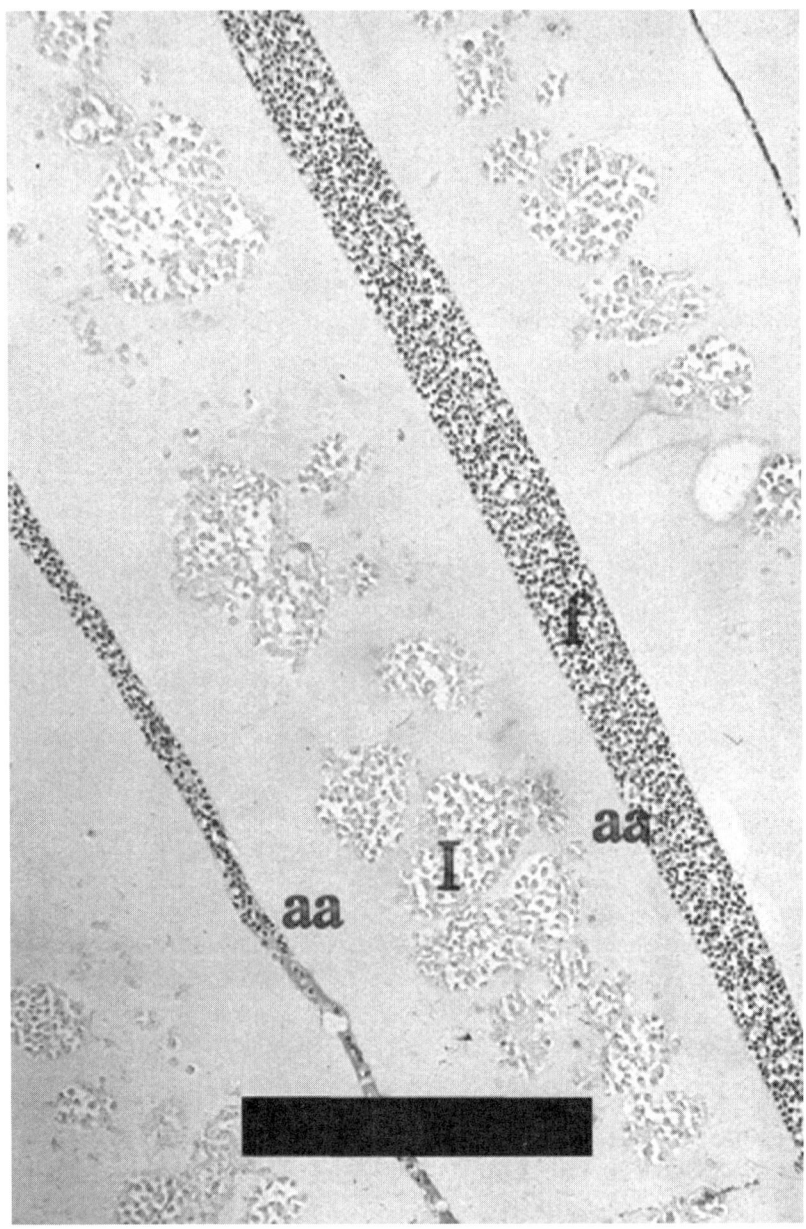

**FIGURE 2.** Micrograph of an Islet Sheet recovered from the peritoneum of a dog after three weeks. Islets were dead at implantation and the sheet rolled on itself *in vivo*. H & E staining shows the residual islet debris (I) in the center of three rolls of the Islet Sheet entirely separated from host fibroblasts (f) by a continuous acellular alginate layer (aa). *Bar*, 250 µm.

FIGURE 2 is a transverse section of an Islet Sheet that had been implanted in the peritoneal cavity of an adult female beagle dog for three weeks. Without an encapsulated reinforcing fabric this sheet rolled on itself. What appears in the micrograph are several turns of the same sheet, with a significant accumulation of fibroblasts between the rolls. The encapsulated islets did not survive because of an error during processing (the pH of one of the reagents was too low), but nonetheless this micrograph demonstrates achievement of a number of objectives for the Islet Sheet.

The overall thickness of the Islet Sheet is 250 µm, a thinner distance for oxygen flux than even the smallest microcapsules.[5] FIGURE 2 demonstrates that the overall thickness is unchanged after three weeks *in vivo* and no swelling or separation of the alginate layers is evident. Like microencapsulation, the Islet Sheet relies on passive diffusion for transport of glucose, insulin, and metabolites. To allow adequate flux of these essential nutrients the immunoprotecting barrier must be minimally thin. As shown by Colton[6] even a 25 µm thick barrier across which oxygen must diffuse reduces the oxygen tension available to an immunoisolated islet by 50%. A 200 µm barrier reduces oxygen flux to such an extent that insulin production substantially stops. The immunoprotecting layer of the Islet Sheet in FIGURE 2 is 50–75 µm.

Complete coverage of the islets is another requirement for successful immunoprotection from the host. This criterion is difficult to fulfill with microcapsules[7,8] but is virtually assured with the Islet Sheet because the islets are encapsulated in preformed, ultrathin crosslinked alginate layers. FIGURES 2 and 3 show islet tissue within the core completely protected from contact with the host cells.

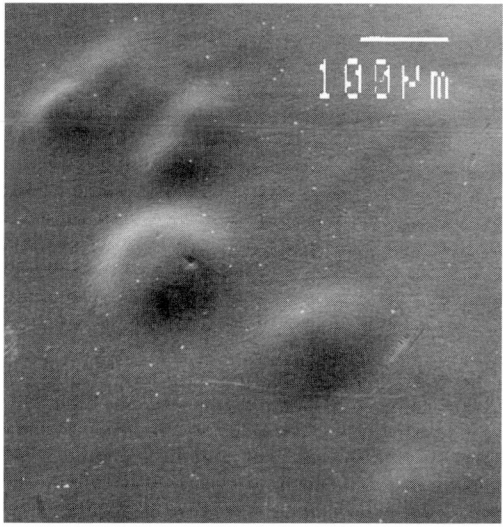

**FIGURE 3.** Scanning electron micrograph of an Islet Sheet. This Islet Sheet contained a minimal number of islets to demonstrate the complete coverage and smooth surface texture. The islets appear as mounds beneath the continuous acellular alginate layer. The alginate gel has shrunk during processing for electron microscopy.

High tissue density is another advantage of the Islet Sheet. The areas of islets evident in FIGURE 2 constitute 38% of the total area of the Islet Sheet, having a density of 50% (v/v) in the core alginate during fabrication. The completed sheet can contain 40% islets by volume. This reduces the theoretical volume of the implant needed to cure a human diabetic to less than 5 ml, or an Islet Sheet that measures roughly 200 $cm^2$.

Providing sufficient islet tissue to reverse the diabetes of a typical human thus requires ten 3 cm × 7 cm sheets. To accomplish this using microencapsulation would take more than 400,000 capsules for a 70 kg individual. Retrieval of a microencapsulated implant is not feasible in the clinical arena.

Surface properties are also important in preventing destructive host fibrotic response.[9,10] Irregularities in surface texture provide physical handles for fibroblast attachment, even in the absence of chemical triggers for fibrosis. FIGURE 3 shows a scanning electron micrograph of the surface of an Islet Sheet. Islets appear as raised mounds protruding from the otherwise smooth surface because of the shrinkage of the alginate hydrogel during dehydration for SEM. Evident from this micrograph is the continuity of smooth coverage of all encapsulated islets.

The process for manufacture of the Islet Sheet confers many advantages, since it was developed from the point of view of maximizing islet viability. Less than an hour is required for a single operator to encapsulate sufficient islets for a single patient. This minimizes the culture time for islets, improving implant viability. Furthermore, the islets are subjected to a minimum of shear stress further boosting implant viability. The process also allows for a broader range of alginate chemistries, in particular use of more viscous solutions of greater concentrations of higher molecular weight alginates. Because the immunoprotective layer is fabricated separately from the islet suspension layer, the process allows more flexibility in tailoring these layers to their separate functions. The process is reproducible and offers more opportunity for quality control measures, all of which will aid eventual clinical development.

## EXPERIMENTAL—SHEET CHARACTERIZATION

### *Alginate Purification*

The Islet Sheet is made from highly purified alginates using standard and well-defined chemistry. Beginning with commercially available alginates from standard sources, further purification is performed to further reduce fibrotic contaminants. These steps include adsorption with activated charcoal, serial filtrations to 0.1 μm, and successive alcohol precipitations. Small molecular weight fractions, that do not become stably associated with the gel matrix, are removed by ultrafiltration using a 10–17 kDa MWCO membrane. Specific protocols for the alginate purifications used in this work for mannuronate-rich and guluronate-rich alginates are available.[11] The product of these protocols is a fluffy white powder. Further characterization of these alginates is currently in progress.

### *Sheet Fabrication*

The process by which the Islet Sheet is made relies on control of the diffusion of crossing agent into soluble alginate films. Briefly, a semiporous membrane such as

0.2 μm cellulose ester filter membrane is saturated with crosslinking solution, typically 1.7% $CaCl_2$. This membrane is laid across two adjacent optically flat surfaces and a guiding shim laid atop the membrane. Sweeping an acellular alginate solution in isotonic saline over the membrane by use of a straightedge makes an alginate film. This film is destined to be the immunoprotective layers and may be of arbitrary thickness. Where this film contacts the membrane, crosslinking occurs, forming a skin of crosslinked alginate whose thickness is determined by many factors, including the chemical nature and quantity of crosslinking ion within the membrane and the viscosity of the alginate.

A soluble suspension of islets in a more viscous alginate solution in isotonic media is then applied to the center of one half of this film. A reinforcing fabric may optionally be applied to the other half. The two halves are pressed together forming a sandwich whose thickness is determined by the guiding shims. As the membranes become juxtaposed, the islet suspension is spread, displacing the uncrosslinked acellular alginate ahead. The islet core is completely covered above and below by the crosslinked skin and around the periphery by the advancing wave of acellular alginate, ensuring full lamination and complete coverage. The entire sandwich, including the semiporous membranes, is carefully slid from between the flat plates and immersed in a solution of crosslinking ions and NaCl to fully crosslink the Islet Sheet.

The fabrication process for the Islet Sheet takes less than an hour to encapsulate sufficient islets for a single patient and leaves islet viability unaffected. The insulin stimulation index in response to elevated glucose is unchanged. The *stimulation index* is the ratio of insulin produced in an hour in culture medium with 20 mM glucose relative to the insulin produced in an hour in culture medium with 2.8 mM glucose. These results indicate that the process for making thin sheets does not significantly impair islet function.

### *Alginate Permeability*

Soluble factors of unknown size may play a role in host response.[2] To demonstrate our capability to adjust permeability of the immunoprotective alginate layers we performed dialysis experiments using alginate sheets with differing compositions (in collaboration with D. Scharp, Neocrin Corp., Irvine, CA). In this example 50-micron thick sheets of 3% (w/v) alginate crosslinked with $CaCl_2$ were made using two different alginate preparations. One preparation was derived from Keltone HV alginate (further purified, from *Macrocystis pyrifera*, $F_G = 0.40$) and the other was derived from Protan XG (further purified, from *Laminaria hyperborea*, $F_G = 0.68$). These flat sheet alginate membranes were mounted within two-chamber diffusion cells. One side of each cell was filled with a protein cocktail containing vitamin $B_{12}$ (1,355 Da), myoglobin (18 kDa), albumin (67 kDa), and IgG (160 kDa) in a 0.9% NaCl solution containing 10 mM HEPES and 5 mM $CaCl_2$. The other chamber was filled with a 0.9% NaCl solution containing 10 mM HEPES and 5 mM $CaCl_2$ without protein. Following a three-day incubation at 37°C, samples were withdrawn from the buffer side and protein was determined by HPLC. A cast hydrogel membrane prepared from crosslinked polyethylene glycol is included in the chart for comparison. This type of hydrogel membrane has been shown to provide nutritional support and immunoprotection in studies using xenografted islet tissue.[12]

TABLE 1. Permeability constants of molecular weight markers through alginate membranes

| Species | B-12 | myoglobin | ovalbumin | NA | IgG |
|---|---|---|---|---|---|
| Molecular weight (Da) | 1,355 | 12,000 | 45,000 | 85,000 | 150,000 |
| PEG hydrogel | 1.30 | $6.00 \times 10^{-1}$ | | $4.00 \times 10^{-4}$ | |
| MPA alginate, $F_G = 0.40$ | $4.20 \times 10^{-1}$ | $4.00 \times 10^{-2}$ | 0.00 | | 0.00 |
| XG alginate, $F_G = 0.68$ | 1.33 | $4.50 \times 10^{-1}$ | $2.30 \times 10^{-1}$ | | $1.16 \times 10^{-1}$ |

TABLE 1 shows the permeability of three membranes to molecular species of selected weights. The results demonstrate a very broad high permeability profile for "XG" (from *L. hyperborea*, $F_G = 0.68$) and a sharp cutoff between 12 kDa and 45 kDa for the less permeable "MPA" (from *M. pyrifera*, $F_G = 0.40$). By intermediate modification of the alginate chemistry (i.e., concentration, molecular weight, and $F_G$, as well as crosslinking ion) an optimal coating can be designed which allows IgG to either pass freely or be substantially excluded.

### *Foreign Body Response to Alginate Slabs*

When sufficiently purified, alginate gels do not provoke a foreign body response as small beads less than 500 μm in diameter, regardless of the uronic acid composition.[13,14] We sought to demonstrate the bioinvisibility of alginate in the sheet configuration. There are two main differences between these settings. First, the alginate used in sheets is preferably at higher concentrations than that achievable in beads since this imparts greater strength. Second, the sheets do not move about as freely within the peritoneum, and may preferably not move at all. Early experiments investigated the response to well-known alginate compositions in a sheet format implanted intraperitoneally in BALB/c mice.

Flat slabs 250 μm thick of 3% alginate (without cells) purified from *M. pyrifera* ($F_G = 0.40$) or from *L. hyperborea* ($F_G = 0.68$), crosslinked with various $Ca^{2+}$ salts, were divided into 1 cm$^2$ sections and individually implanted without tether in the peritoneum of triplicate female BALB/c mice. Two to three weeks later the animals were euthanized and their peritonea examined for the disposition of the alginate implants. In no case was gross fibrosis evident. Microscopic examination of the recovered material revealed an accumulation of cells in defects with the sheet surface. These cells were not firmly adhered and could be removed with gentle irrigation. We have focused on the less permeable *M. pyrifera* alginates because soluble, high molecular weight factors such as IgG may play a role in immunoprotection.

### *Surface Properties*

In the study of alginate slabs in BALB/c mice already described, microscopic examination of the explanted alginate revealed an accumulation of fibroblasts in surface defects of the slabs. The cells appeared in cracks and folds of the alginate and did not appear in most cases to be responding with collagen deposition. However, their persistence in surface defects raised concern about reaction to the large surfaces required for a clinical Islet Sheet.

To further investigate this observation, subcutaneous fibrotic response studies were performed in rats using acellular sheets. In this experiment 2–250-μm-thick sheets were constructed using alginate purified from *Macrocystis pyrifera* ($F_G = 0.40$), crosslinked with 1.7% $CaCl_2$, both containing a polyester scrim to provide reinforcement for suture attachment. One sheet had no cellular material in the core, whereas the other had autoclaved baker's yeast encapsulated in the core. These sheets were separated into 1-$cm^2$ sections and implanted subcutaneously in the dorsal flank of Fischer rats.

Three weeks later a gross fibrotic response was evident in all yeast sheet implants, as manifested by a raised lump at the site of implant. Upon dissection these lumps proved to be fibrotic capsules fed by new vessels not evident on the contralateral flank. No such response was apparent at the site of implant of the acellular sheets, which were not adhered to the subcutaneous tissue.

Microscopic examination of the explanted acellular sheets showed a modest accumulation of fibroblasts at the perimeter of the sheet where the polyester reinforcement was exposed. However, these fibroblasts were unable to adhere to the surface of the sheet (see FIGURE 4). Examination of the vascularized capsules from the yeast implants demonstrated the presence of the yeast sheet within a fibrotic capsule

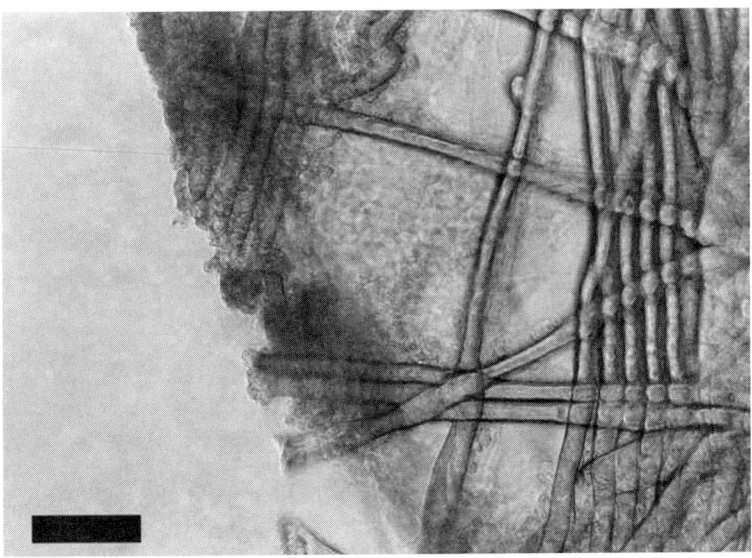

**FIGURE 4.** Micrograph of an acellular Islet Sheet recovered from a three-week subcutaneous implantation in the dorsal flank of a Fischer rat (H & E stained). There is an accumulation of fibroblasts at the edge of the sheet where the reinforcing polyester mesh was exposed when the sheet was cut into 1 cm × 1 cm sections prior to implantation. However, these fibroblasts were unable to adhere to the smooth surface of the sheet. *Bar,* 100 μm.

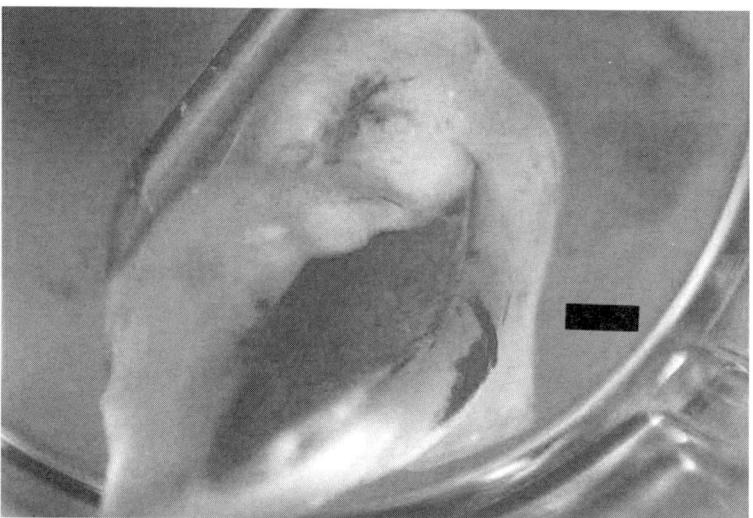

**FIGURE 5.** Photograph of sheet containing autoclaved yeast, recovered within fibrotic capsule. Sheet was implanted for three weeks subcutaneously in the dorsal flank of a Fischer rat. The surface of the sheet is not adhered to the capsule. The sheet is attached to the capsule only at the perimeter. *Bar*, 2 mm.

(see FIGURE 5). In general only the edges of these sheets were adhered to the fibrotic mass; the surfaces of the sheet did not adhere even in the context of mitogenic stimulation. The surface of the Islet Sheet is sufficiently smooth that, even in the context of aggressive fibrotic response, the capsule does not adhere.

## CANINE STUDIES

Breakthrough metabolic studies in pancreatectomized beagle dogs were initiated in September 1998. The first experiment used allogeneic islets isolated from two mongrel donors encapsulated in an Islet Sheet with a nylon mesh reinforcement (Nitex 3-325/58; Tetko, Inc. NY) made with alginate from *L. hyperborea* and a first-generation over coating process. These sheets delaminated *in vivo*, exposing the islets and nylon mesh, which proved highly fibrogenic. Metabolic parameters including C-peptide levels and insulin requirements were influenced for only a few days.

A second experiment, in late October 1998, used unreinforced alginate sheets and a process similar to that described above using partially crosslinked films. Unfortunately there was an error in preparing the solutions used to make the sheets (one of the reagents was acidic) and the islets were dead before encapsulation, a fact not discovered until after implantation. Upon explantation these unreinforced sheets rolled upon themselves and were fibrosed (see FIG. 2). Since the islets inside were dead the cause of the fibrosis is open to speculation. However, it was clear that measures were needed to keep the sheet flat.

Several rounds of *in vitro* experimentation and the mice and rat studies described above identified an acceptable sheet construction. Using *M. pyrifera* alginate and the process described above, a non-woven polyester scrim (Hollytex 3251; Ahlstrom, PA) is coencapsulated in the core of the sheet for reinforcement and to provide stable suture points. This material is at most 25 μm thick and its area is 40% occluded, minimizing the diffusion barrier and allowing the alginate gel to crosslink through. It is simultaneously robust to suture tearing (due to the non-woven characteristic) and flexible to allow conformity to the adjacent tissue. It is autoclavable and FDA-approved for blood contact (although not for implantation).

## *Experimental—Canine Studies*

In February 2000 experiments implanting these refined Islet Sheets into pancreatectomized beagle dogs began. Islets were isolated from two mongrel donors using standard collagenase digestion followed by density gradient purification. Two hundred microliters of islet tissue are recovered and washed twice in normal saline. The final pellet suspended by gentle stirring with a 16G nylon catheter in 300 μl of purified alginate from *M. pyrifera* ($F_G = 0.40$), 5% (w/v) in a buffer containing 20 mM HEPES pH 7.0, 3 mM glucose, 0.5 mM sodium citrate, and 0.9% NaCl. The suspension was drawn into a 1-cc tuberculin syringe using this catheter and used to form the core of six Islet Sheets as described above.

In a single procedure a female beagle dog was pancreatectomized and implanted with the six sheets on both sides of the omentum. Each sheet was sutured in place with single sutures at each corner. Following recovery from anesthesia the animal was fed standard chow supplemented with Viocase in the mornings and allowed to eat *ad lib*. Antibiotics were administered for two weeks following surgery to reduce the risk of sepsis. Peripheral blood samples were obtained before feeding and in the early evening from the forelimb and tested for blood glucose using a LifeScan Fast Take portable glucose meter (Johnson and Johnson, Milpitas CA). Eighty-four days later the omentum with the attached sheets was removed for analysis. Blood sampling continued for another seven days until two successive blood glucose measurements exceeded 200 mg/dL, demonstrating the underlying diabetic state of the pancreatectomized recipient. During the in-life period the dog received a single injection of 2 U insulin on day 9.

Three intravenous glucose tolerance tests (IVGTTs) were conducted before and at 30 and 60 days after pancreatectomy/implantation. In brief: 50% dextrose at a dose of 0.5 g/kg (1 mL of 50% dextrose/kg) was administered by intravenous injection over a 15-second period. From a cannula in the contralateral forelimb 1-ml blood samples were removed at −5, 0, 1, 5, 10, 20, 30, 45, 60, 90, and 120 minutes. These samples were immediately tested for blood glucose as described above. Serum from these samples was harvested and frozen for later analysis.

## *Results—Canine Studies*

The venous blood sugar measurements are shown in FIGURE 6. It is evident that the morning or fasting blood sugars were well controlled while the sheets were in

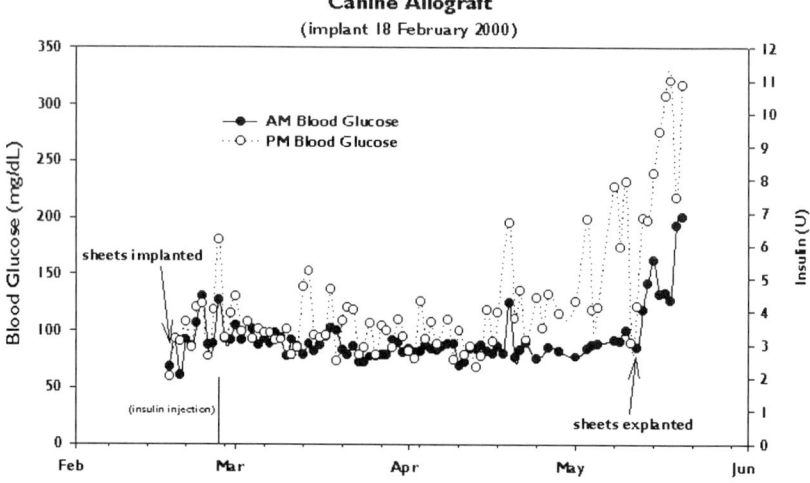

**FIGURE 6.** Peripheral blood sugars from a pancreatectomized beagle dog implanted with six Islet Sheets containing 75,000 islet equivalents sutured to the omentum. Sheet implantation was concurrent with pancreatectomy. *Closed circles*, AM blood sugars prior to feeding; *Open circles*, PM blood sugars. The dog was fed standard chow supplemented with Viocase once in the morning and allowed to eat *ad lib*. One injection of 2 U insulin was administered on Day 7. The Islet Sheets were removed at Day 84 by omentectomy. Blood sugars rose above 200 mg/dL by day seven.

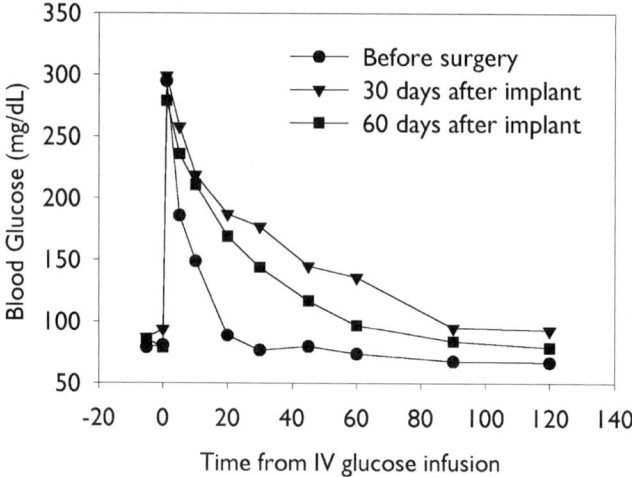

**FIGURE 7.** Blood sugars from serial intravenous glucose tolerance tests (IVGTT). 50% dextrose was administered by intravenous injection at a dose of 0.5 g/kg over a 15-second period. Blood samples were removed from a cannula in the contralateral forelimb. Although the IVGTT data 30 and 60 days after implantation with 75,000 islet equivalents in six Islet Sheets was not normal, improvement is evident between these data.

place. The afternoon or fed blood sugars were more variable, yet rarely exceeded 150 mg/dL during this period. Following explantation of the omentum and the sheets both AM and PM blood sugars rose progressively, with the AM blood sugars exceeding 200 mg/dL seven days post explant.

Blood sugar measurements from the IVGTT experiments are shown in FIGURE 7. Prior to surgery the sugars returned to normal within 30 minutes. Blood sugars returned to normal within 90 minutes of the glucose challenge 30 and 60 days following pancreatectomy and sheet implantation. The blood sugars at 60 days were lower at every measurement time compared to 30 days. Clearly glucose metabolism remains impaired, although the animal is not frankly diabetic and may be improving with time. At no time after surgery was insulin detected at levels above baseline. C-peptide analysis is pending.

The disposition of the sheets after 84 days was not encouraging. Our efforts at keeping the sheet unfolded in the peritoneal cavity were not successful. Two masses were identified in the omentum that appeared to contain all six sheets. One was a 2-cm sphere; the other was 2 cm in diameter and roughly 5 cm long. On dissection the larger mass revealed Islet Sheets, pleated and attached at the edges to a hard

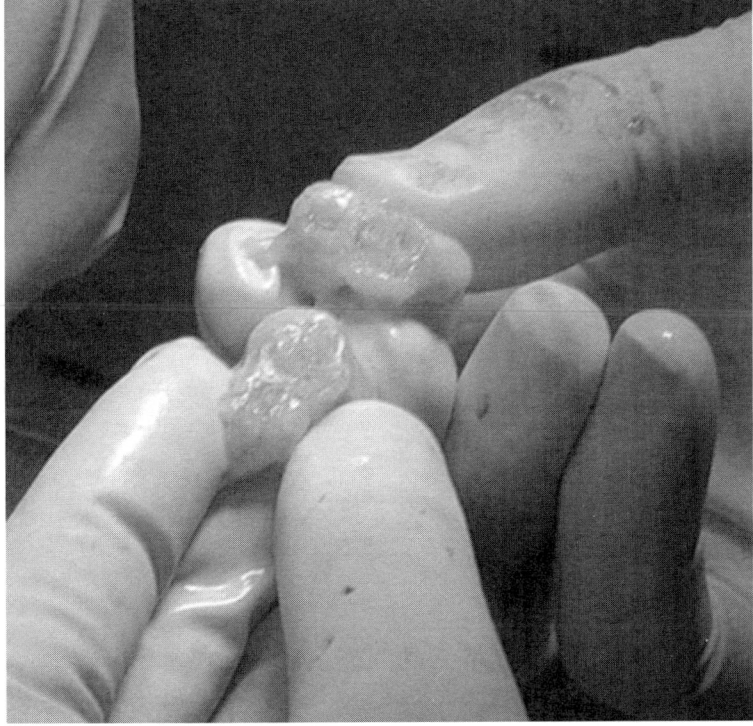

**FIGURE 8.** Photograph of the mass recovered from canine omentum implanted with six Islet Sheets 84 days earlier. The mass was cut open with scissors, exposing multiple folds of the Islet Sheets adhered at the edges to a hard capsule.

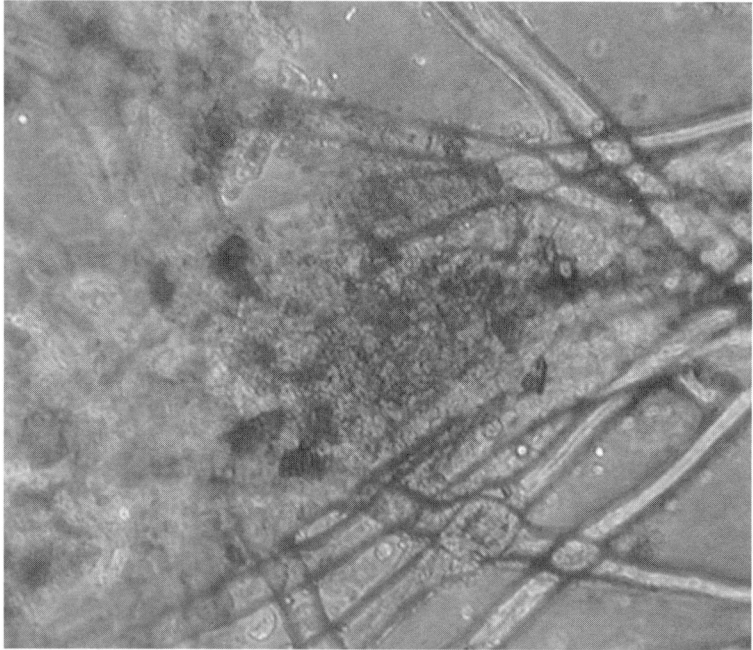

**FIGURE 9.** Wet mount of material recovered from the interior of the mass in FIGURE 8, stained with dithizone. Islets are visible above the non-woven polyester scrim coencapsulated in the Islet Sheets to provide physical strength.

fibrotic capsule (see FIGURE 8). Infiltration of the fibrotic capsules between the pleats was minimal compared to the surrounding capsule. The reinforcing polyester scrim and dithizone-positive cell clusters were identifiable in the interior (see FIGURE 9).

The histology of these masses revealed extensive striated acellular fibrils in the periphery of the capsule, occasionally punctuated by monocytes. Each fibril measured 5–7 μm across, with the entire capsule 2–3 mm thick. Fragments of polyester scrim were visible in some areas of the capsule. Alginate and insulin-positive tissue were evident in several of these inclusions. The central portions of the mass were generally missing from the sections. Rarely fragments of alginate remained on some sections. This is most likely an artifact of processing because pieces dissected from the interior of the mass stained positive for dithizone and had both alginate and polyester evident at the time of explant.

## DISCUSSION

Implantation of allogenic islets of Langerhans encapsulated in six alginate Islet Sheets measuring 3 cm × 7 cm × 250 μm onto the omentum of a pancreatectomized beagle dog maintained fasting euglycemia for 84 days. Upon sheet removal by omentectomy at 84 days, fasting and fed blood sugars steadily rose to exceed 200 mg/dL on day 91, seven days after explant. This confirms the metabolic effectiveness of the implanted immunoprotected islet tissue.

IVGTT data at 60 days was improved compared to 30 days, although still not close to normal. Presurgery the IVGTT data yields a K value of 4.24. At 30 days post surgery the K value was 0.88, improving to 1.25 at 60 days. This improvement is encouraging and may reflect the improvement seen with a similar experiment using microencapsulated islets in an omental pouch. (J. Lakey, unpublished data) One likely explanation is improvement in vascularity in the nearby tissue due to either the increased metabolic load from the implanted tissue or from the action of insulin as a growth factor. However, the robust, mostly acellular fibrotic capsule that developed around the graft during this period complicates these explanations.

The efforts to maintain sheet planarity *in vivo* were not successful. Although metabolically active, the implant elicited a strong fibrotic response and was completely encapsulated in a hard mass. On dissection this mass evidently consisted of a shell of collagen adhering to the edges of pleated Islet Sheets. As was seen with the rat implanted with encapsulated yeast, the fibrotic reaction did not adhere to the areas where the sheet remained flat but only at regions where the sheet folded on itself, likely exposing the polyester reinforcement.

Recent experiments have addressed the reaction to acellular polyester-reinforced alginate sheets attached to various organs of rats and dogs. Preliminary results indicate that sheet planarity is critical to avoidance of fibrotic response. In every instance where the sheet remained unfolded no significant fibrosis was evident at one month. Significantly all mesentery and omental implants appeared to be grossly similar to the results presented here. In several instances the sheet remained flat by attachment to a solid organ. Experiments are in progress to determine whether maintaining planarity of the sheets will support long term viability and function of islets within an Islet Sheet.

## REFERENCES

1. VAN SCHILFGAARDE, R. & P. DE VOS. 1996. Aspects of immunoprotection of islets. Transplant Proc. 28(6): 3516–3517.
2. ZEKORN, T.D., A. HORCHER, J. MELLERT, *et al.* 1996. Biocompatibility and immunology in the encapsulation of islets of Langerhans (bioartificial pancreas). Int. J. Artif. Organs 19(4): 251–257.
3. SUN, A.M., G.M. O'SHEA & M.F. GOOSEN. 1984. Injectable microencapsulated islet cells as a bioartificial pancreas. Appl. Biochem. Biotechnol. 10(99): 87–99.
4. LACY, P.E., O.D. HEGRE, A. GERASIMIDI-VAZEOU, *et al.* 1991. Maintenance of normoglycemia in diabetic mice by subcutaneous xenografts of encapsulated islets. Science 254: 1782–1784.
5. CALAFIORE, R., G. BASTA, G. LUCA, *et al.* 1999. Transplantation of pancreatic islets contained in minimal volume microcapsules in diabetic high mammalians. Ann. N.Y. Acad. Sci. 875: 219–232.
6. COLTON, C.K. 1995. Implantable biohybrid artificial organs. Cell Transplant 4(4): 415–36.
7. DE VOS, P., B. DE HAAN, G.H. WOLTERS, *et al.* 1996. Factors influencing the adequacy of microencapsulation of rat pancreatic islets. Transplantation 62(7): 888–893.

8. VAN SCHILFGAARDE, R. & P. DE VOS. 1999. Factors influencing the properties and performance of microcapsules for immunoprotection of panreatic islets. J. Mol. Med. **77**(1): 199–205.
9. XU, K., D.M. HERCULES, I. LACIK, *et al.* 1998. Atomic force microscopy used for the surface characterization of microcapsule immunoisolation devices. J. Biomed. Mater. Res. **41**(3): 461-467.
10. HILLGARTNER, M., H. ZIMMERMANN, S. MIMIETZ, *et al.* 1999. Immunoisolation of transplants by entrapment in 19F-labelled alginate gels: production, biocompatibility, stability, and long-term monitoring of functional integrity. Mat.-wiss. u. Werkstofftech **30**: 783–792.
11. Specific protocols are available at <http://www.isletmedical.com/define_methods3.htm> for mannuronate-rich alginates and <http://www.isletmedical.com/define_ methods5.htm> for guluronate-rich alginates.
12. CRUISE, G.M., O.D. HEGRE, F.V. LAMBERTI, *et al.* 1999. *In vitro* and *in vivo* performance of porcine islets encapsulated in interfacially photopolymerized poly(ethylene glycol) diacrylate membranes. Cell Transplant **8**(3): 293–306.
13. COCHRUM, K., S. JEMTRUD, & R. DORIAN. 1995. Successful xenografts in mice with microencapsulated rat and dog islets. Transplant Proc. **27**(6): 3297–3301.
14. HASSE, C., A. ZIELKE, G. KLOCK, *et al.* 1998. Amitogenic alginates: key to first clinical application of microencapsulation technology. World J. Surg. **22**(7): 659–665.

# Engineering Tolerance into Transplanted β Cell Lines

BERNARD THORENS,[a] PHILIPPE DUPRAZ,[b] AND SANDRA COTTET[a]

[a]*Institute of Pharmacology and Toxicology, University of Lausanne, 27, rue du Bugnon, 1005 Lausanne, Switzerland*

[b]*Modex Thérapeutiques, 1004 Lausanne, Switzerland*

> ABSTRACT: In this paper we explore the possibility of improving, by genetic engineering, the resistance of insulin-secreting cells to the metabolic and inflammatory stresses that are anticipated to limit their function and survival when encapsulated and transplanted in a type 1 diabetic environment. We show that transfer of the Bcl-2 antiapoptotic gene, and of genes specifically interfering with cytokine intracellular signaling pathways, greatly improves resistance of the cells to metabolic limitations and inflammatory stresses.
>
> KEYWORDS: engineering tolerance; transplanted β cell lines; genetic engineering

## INTRODUCTION

Transplantation of encapsulated β cell lines for the treatment of type 1 diabetes requires the cells to survive and function in an unnatural environment characterized by high cell density and exposure to unfavorable gradients of nutrients and oxygen. Furthermore, accumulation of inflammatory and immune cells at the surface of the encapsulation device may be triggered by the shedding of antigens from the transplanted cells into an already autoimmune environment and by the surgical procedure required to implant the device. This would then lead to a local release of cytokines which, due to their relatively small size, are expected to freely diffuse into the encapsulation device. Cytokines, in particular, Il-1β, TNFα, and INF-γ have been shown to decrease glucose-stimulated insulin secretion and induce β cell apoptosis.

To evaluate the possibility of improving the resistance of β cells to these metabolic and inflammatory stresses, we chose to work with a well-defined insulin-secreting cell line. We used the βTc-Tet cell line derived a few years ago by S. Efrat.[1] These cells can be growth-arrested, due to the presence of a tetracycline-dependent genetic switch controlling expression of the transforming SV-40 T antigen. In the presence of tetracycline, these cells stop proliferating and display a normal glucose-stimulated insulin secretory activity. Furthermore, when transplanted unencapsulated under the kidney capsule of syngeneic or allogeneic diabetic mice, they can correct hyperglycemia for several months.[1,2]

---

Address for correspondence: Bernard Thorens, Institute of Pharmacology and Toxicology, University of Lausanne, 27, rue du Bugnon, 1005 Lausanne, Switzerland. Voice: + 41-21-692-5390; fax: + 41-21-692-5355.

Bernard.Thorens@ipharm.unil.ch

We tested several genetic modifications of these βTc-Tet cells in improving their resistance to metabolic and inflammatory stress.

## EXPRESSION OF BCL-2 IMPROVES RESISTANCE TO METABOLIC STRESS

βTc-Tet cells grow relatively slowly and are therefore difficult to genetically engineer by standard transfection techniques. We therefore used recombinant lentiviruses to routinely transfer cDNAs in these cells.[3] Lentiviruses allow a very good efficiency of gene transfer into slowly or non-dividing cells.

Transfer of the Bcl-2 gene into βTc-Tet cells improved many characteristics. First, a markedly improved resistance to apoptosis, induced by non-specific activators, such as staurosporine, could be demonstrated. Importantly, there was also a considerably improved survival at high cell density and an apparent faster doubling time. These cells, referred to as CDM3D, also show improved resistance to hypoxia and to apoptosis induced by a combination of the three cytokines Il-1β, TNFα, and INF-γ. They retain their capability to be growth-arrested in the presence of tetracycline and to correct diabetic hyperglycemia when transplanted under the kidney capsule of diabetic mice.[2]

## RESISTANCE TO CYTOKINE ACTION BY TRANSFER OF PROTEINS INTERFERING WITH INTRACELLULAR SIGNALING PATHWAYS

### *The IL-1 Signaling Pathway*

The Il-1β receptor consists of a transmembrane receptor and an associated protein (IL-1R and IL-1RAcP). Binding of the cytokine to its receptor activates various intracellular pathways, in particular, activation of the NFkB and JNK pathways. One of the initial events in activation of these pathways is the association of MyD88 to the IL-1 receptor.[4] Myd88 is an adaptor protein consisting of a Toll domain that interacts with the receptor and of a death domain that interacts and activates downstream effector molecules. Overexpression of the MyD88 Toll domain or of the MyD88 protein in which a mutation of the DD domain is introduced (lpr mutation), interferes with the IL-1β signaling pathway.[4]

We, therefore, evaluated the possibility to block IL-1β action on CDM3D cells by overexpressing either the MyD88Toll or MyD88lpr proteins. We were able to demonstrate that, in the presence of either of the dominant negative forms of MyD88, we could prevent activation of NFkB, induction of iNOS gene expression, and NO production in response to IL-1β and IFN-γ or to a combination of all three cytokines. We further showed that this was accompanied by an increased resistance to apoptosis induction by the three cytokines. However, blocking the IL-1β signaling pathway did not prevent the negative effect of the cytokines on insulin secretion. Indeed, we demonstrated that the negative effect of cytokines on this β cell function could be explained by the action of IFN-γ, which induced decreased insulin gene expression, lowered the cellular insulin content, and also reduced the glucose-stimulated secretory activity of the cells.[5]

## The IFN-γ Signaling Pathway

Interferon-γ binds to a heterotetrameric receptor that transmits its intracellular signal by activating JAK kinase, which activates, by phosphorylation, the STAT1 transcription factors.[6] These dimerize and translocate to the nucleus, where they can induce gene transcription. It has been claimed that induction of this signaling pathway stimulates expression of specific suppressors of cytokine signaling proteins, in particular SOCS-1.[7] This protein acts by inhibiting signal transduction by the IFN-γ receptor, by binding to JAK, and by preventing phosphorylation of STAT1.

We, therefore, generated CDM3D cells overexpressing SOCS-1 and evaluated the resistance of these cells to the effect of IFN-γ. We were able to demonstrate a suppression of the effect of this cytokine on reducing the cellular insulin content.[8]

## The TNF-α Signaling Pathway

The TNF-α receptor is a trimeric receptor that induces apoptosis by stimulating a cascade of caspase activation. This cascade is initiated by binding of a FADD adaptor molecule to the trimeric receptor, which recruits and allows activation of FLICE/caspase 8 by proteolytic cleavage. Association of FLICE/caspase 8 with the FADD adaptor can be prevented by cellular or viral FLICE inhibitory protein (c- or v-FLIPs).[9,10]

In attempts at blocking the TNF-α intracellular pathway, we genetically engineered CDM3D cells to express v-FLIP or overexpress c-FLIP. We demonstrated that activation of caspase 8 activity by TNF-α and cycloheximide, or by a combination of all three cytokines, could be almost totally suppressed in the presence of the FLIP molecules. This was also accompanied by a markedly improved resistance to cytokine-induced apoptosis.

## CONCLUSIONS

We have demonstrated that the major cellular problems related to the use of cells in an encapsulation device for transplantation therapy of type 1 diabetes (that is, resistance to the metabolic and inflammatory challenges) can be tested systematically. This approach requires the use of an insulin-secreting cell line possessing characteristics similar to those of β cells. This means that the glucose dose dependence for insulin secretion should be similar to that of normal β cells and that the cells have the capability of controlling diabetes when transplanted into diabetic recipients. Furthermore, these cells should be amenable to genetic engineering. The βTc-Tet cells possess all of these characteristics.

Using the approach described we were able to demonstrate that resistance to hypoxia, high cell density, and cytokines could be greatly improved by the transfer of general antiapoptotic genes (Bcl-2) and by inhibitors of specific cytokine intracellular signaling pathways. Although the present studies were performed mostly under *in vitro* conditions, we have performed a number of encapsulation experiments, using mostly flat sheet technology. We were able to demonstrate that survival *in vivo* in an encapsulation device was considerably improved by Bcl-2 expression.

Similarly, we are evaluating whether blocking the cytokine signaling pathways can improve survival of the cells when transplanted in diabetic NOD mice.

Using this approach we hope to be able to define a minimal set of genes required to confer improved survival in an encapsulation device placed in an autoimmune environment and to preserve function of the encapsulated cells. Indeed, our data have shown that survival and preservation of glucose-dependent secretory function can be separately affected by cytokines, with IFN-γ having a major negative impact on insulin expression and secretion, whereas IL-1β and TNF-α may have a more critical role in induction of apoptosis without markedly affecting glucose-stimulated insulin secretion.

Finally, although the work with βTc-Tet cells may allow us to greatly improve our knowledge of the cellular requirement for survival and function in a transplanted device, the ultimate cell line to be used for transplantation therapy of type 1 diabetes should probably be of human origin.

## REFERENCES

1. EFRAT, S., D. FUSCO-DEMANE, H. LEMBERG, et al. 1995. Conditional transformation of a pancreatic β-cell line derived from transgenic mice expressing a tetracycline-regulated oncogene. Proc. Natl. Acad. Sci. USA **92:** 3576–3580.

2. DUPRAZ, P., C. RINSCH, W.F. PRALONG, et al. 1999. Lentivirus-mediated Bcl-2 expression in βTc-Tet cells improves resistance to hypoxia and cytokine-induced apoptosis while preserving *in vitro* and *in vivo* control of insulin secretion. Gene Ther. **6:** 1160–1169.

3. NALDINI, L., U. BLÖMER, P. GALLAY, et al. 1996. *In vivo* gene delivery and stable transduction of nondividing cells by a lentiviral vector. Science **272:** 263–267.

4. BURNS, K., F. MARINON, C. ESSLINGER, et al. 1998. MyD88, an adaptor protein involved in interleukin-1 signaling. J. Biol. Chem. **273:** 12203–12209.

5. DUPRAZ, P., S. COTTET, F. HAMBURGER, et al. 2000. Dominant-negative Myd88 proteins inhibit IL-1β/IFN-g-mediated induction of nuclear factor kB-dependent nitrite production and apoptosis in β cells. J. Biol. Chem. **275:** 37672–37678.

6. PESTKA, S., S.V. KOTENKO, G. MUTHUKUMARAN, et al. 1997. The interferon gamma (IFN-g) receptor: a paradigm for the multichain cytokine receptor. Cyt. Growth Fact. Rev. **8:** 189–206.

7. YASUKAWA, H., A. SASAKI & A. YOSHIMURA, 2000. Negative regulation of cyotkine signaling pathways. Ann. Rev. Immunol. **18:** 143–164.

8. COTTET, S., P. DUPRAZ, F. HAMBURGER, et al. 2001. SOCS-1 protein prevents Janus kinase/STAT-dependent inhibition of β cell insulin gene transcription and secretion in response to interferon-γ. J. Biol. Chem. **276:** 25862–25870.

9. IRMLER, M., M. THOME, M. HAHNE, et al. 1997. Inhibition of death receptor signals by cellular FLIP. Nature **388:** 190–195.

10. THOME, M., P. SCHNEIDER, K. HOFMANN, et al. 1997. Viral FLICE-inhibitory proteins (FLIPs) prevent apoptosis induced by death receptors. Nature **386:** 517–521.

# In Vitro Test of New Biomaterials for the Development of a Bioartificial Pancreas

N. LEMBERT,[a] P. PETERSEN,[b] J. WESCHE,[a] P. ZSCHOCKE,[c] A. ENDERLE,[c]
M. DOSER,[c] H. PLANCK,[c] H.D. BECKER,[b] AND H.P.T. AMMON[a]

[a]Institute of Pharmaceutical Sciences, Auf der Morgenstelle 8,
University of Tübingen, 72076 Tübingen, Germany

[b]Institute of General Surgery, Hoppe-Seyler Str. 3, University of Tübingen,
72076 Tübingen, Germany

[c]Institute of Textile and Process Engineering, Körschtalstraße 26,
73770 Denkendorf, Germany

ABSTRACT: The implantation of macroencapsulated islets has the potential to restore endogenous insulin secretion in type 1 diabetics, with no need for lifetime immunosuppression. To match the physiological fluctuations of blood glucose concentrations with appropriate insulin release, the macroencapsulation material must combine immunoprotection with optimal diffusion properties for glucose and insulin. The impact of chemical modifications of polysulphone (PSU) capillary polymers with a cutoff of 50 kD on glucose-induced insulin secretion of macroencapsulated rat islets was studied in perifusion experiments. The insulin release of free-floating islets showed the typical rapid response to glucose stimulation. Total insulin release (AUC between minute 30 and 120 of perifusion) reached $117 \pm 22$ ng/ml. Blending PSU with polyvinylpyrrolidone or sodium-dodecyl-sulfate was not suitable for islet macroencapsulation, since glucose-induced insulin release was absent or disturbed. Hydroxy-methylation ($CH_2OH$) of PSU improved the secretory behavior of macroencapsulated islets depending on the degree of PSU substitution (DS 0.8, AUC $62 \pm 15$ ng/ml; DS 1.8, $111 \pm 24$ ng/ml). In highly substituted PSU-capillaries the kinetics of glucose-induced insulin release was very similar to that observed in free-floating islets. Two consecutive glucose stimulations potentiated insulin release of free-floating islets during the second period of stimulation. Furthermore, freshly isolated macroencapsulated islets responded with more efficient insulin secretion after the initial priming. In conclusion, *in vitro* membrane screening identified highly substituted hydroxy-methylated PSU as the material of choice for islet encapsulation in a bioartificial pancreas.

KEYWORDS: new biomaterials; bioartificial pancreas

## INTRODUCTION

The transplantation of encapsulated islets has the potential to restore endogenous insulin secretion in type 1 diabetics with no need for lifetime immunosuppression.[1]

Address for correspondence: Dr. Nicolas Lembert, Institute of Pharmaceutical Sciences, Auf der Morgenstelle 8, University of Tübingen, 72076 Tübingen, Germany. Voice: + 49 7071 29 72471; fax: + 49 7071 29 2476.
nicolas.lembert@uni-tuebingen.de

It would allow early treatment after manifestation of type 1 diabetes and, thus, prevent development of secondary complications. In addition, immunoisolation may offer the use of xenogenic islets to bypass a possible shortage of human islets in the future. Immunoisolation can be achieved by encapsulation of a large number of islets in a compartment that is in close contact with blood (see FIGURE 1 A). Such a vascular device has already been tested in large animals including pancreatectomized dogs.[2–4] After implantation the fasting blood glucose concentrations were reduced to normal values and most dogs survived without exogenous insulin for several months. However, dogs never gained tight glycemic control after glucose stimulation. Restricted diffusion through the biomaterial used for macroencapsulation may have been one cause of this problem. Following macroencapsulation there was a delayed insulin secretion *in vitro*. The lagtime after glucose stimulation was more than 20 min and the risetime to reach maximal release was approximately one hour. This is approximately ten times slower than the physiological onset of insulin secretion.[5] In addition, the relatively large diffusion distance between blood and central islets in the compartment may have contributed to the blunted insulin response to glucose in dogs after implantation. Thus, pancreatectomized dogs bearing a bioartificial pancreas showed no glucose-induced insulin secretion after oral or intravenous glucose challenge.[2–4]

The project described here aims to develop a bioartificial pancreas as a vascular prothesis. To achieve tight glycemic control, the diffusion distance between blood and islets needs to be reduced and new biomaterials for macroencapsulation need to be developed with improved diffusion properties for glucose and insulin. To reduce the diffusion distance between macroencapsulated islets and blood, islets are encapsulated in narrow capillaries instead of using a large islet compartment (FIG. 1 B). These capillaries are coiled and form the inner surface of an artificial vessel. This

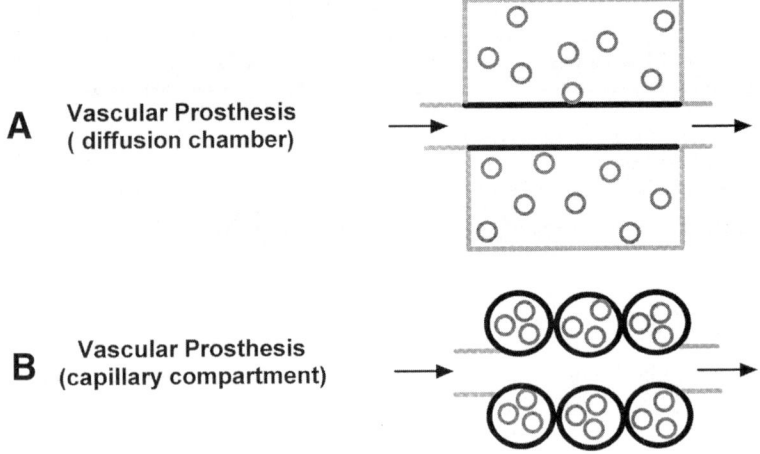

**FIGURE 1.** Different types of islet compartments in a bioartifical pancreas as vascular prothesis. ○, islets; ▬▬, membrane; ▬▬▶, blood.

type of encapsulation offers the additional advantage of islet replacement in case of functional loss since capillaries will remain accessible over a port-system placed subcutaneously.

## MATERIAL AND METHODS

Polysulphone (PSU) was chosen as starting material to produce capillaries for macroencapsulation. PSU forms stable polymers and can be chemically modified. Since native PSU is hydrophobic and adsorbs large amounts of insulin, it is not suited to macroencapsulation. It must be rendered hydrophilic, at least to some extent, to allow protein diffusion.[6] Adsorptive hydrophilization was achieved by blending PSU, dissolved in dimethylacetamide, with hydrophilic substances like sodium-dodecyl-sulfate (SDS) or polyvinylpyrrolidone (PVP). Precipitation by phase inversion yielded PSU capillaries with entrapped SDS or PVP molecules. Chemical modification was achieved by metallization of PSU, dissolved in tetrahydrofurane, with $n$-buthyllithium followed by reaction of the Li-compound with formaldehyde to produce hydroxymethylated PSU capillaries ($PSU-CH_2OH$). All capillaries tested had a molecular cutoff of 50 kD, as judged from the diffusion of IgG, polyetherglycol, or albumin.

Wistar rats (200–300 g) of both sexes with free access to food were used for islet isolation. Islets were isolated by collagenase digestion[7] and purified by hand picking. In order to identify a biomaterial with optimal diffusion properties for glucose and insulin rat islets were macroencapsulated and insulin secretion was studied in perifusion experiments. The perifusion setup consisted of a heated housing with two chambers that could be sealed by a cellulose filter. One chamber was filled with 50 free-floating islets, the other was loaded with 50 islets macroencapsulated in a PSU capillary. The chambers were perifused with glucose solution (Krebs-Ringer buffer supplemented with 20 mM Hepes and 0.5% albumin, pH 7.4), and the perifusate was collected with a fraction sampler. This equipment allows one to compare the kinetics of insulin secretion and the efficiency of glucose-induced insulin release in parallel experiments with free-floating islets and with macroencapsulted islets. The capillary under examination had a length of approximately 1 cm, an inner diameter of 0.9 mm, and a wall thickness of about 0.1 mm. All capillaries were sterilized by γ-irridation and stored in distilled water at room temperature. Before use they were incubated for 24 h at 37°C in cell culture medium containing 10% fetal calf serum to additionally saturate surface binding sites for proteins.

## RESULTS AND DISCUSSION

In perifusion experiments, freshly isolated, free-floating islets respond with a lagtime of about five minutes and a maximum of insulin release 30 min after glucose stimulation (see FIGURE 2, upper panel). After changing to substimulatory glucose concentrations insulin secretion was reduced to basal release within 30 min. The total amount of insulin release was 111 ± 22 ng/ml × 90 min. No glucose-induced insulin secretion was detected after islet macroencapsulation in PSU/SDS or PSU/PVP capillary material (FIG. 2, middle panel). With PSU/PVP capillary material, total insulin release amounts to 32 ± 11 ng/ml × 90 min. Macroencapsulation in PSU/SDS severely interfered with proper islet function. A large insulin secretion was already observed at substimulatory glucose concentrations, whereas a paradoxal decrease in insulin secretion was observed during glucose stimulation. An

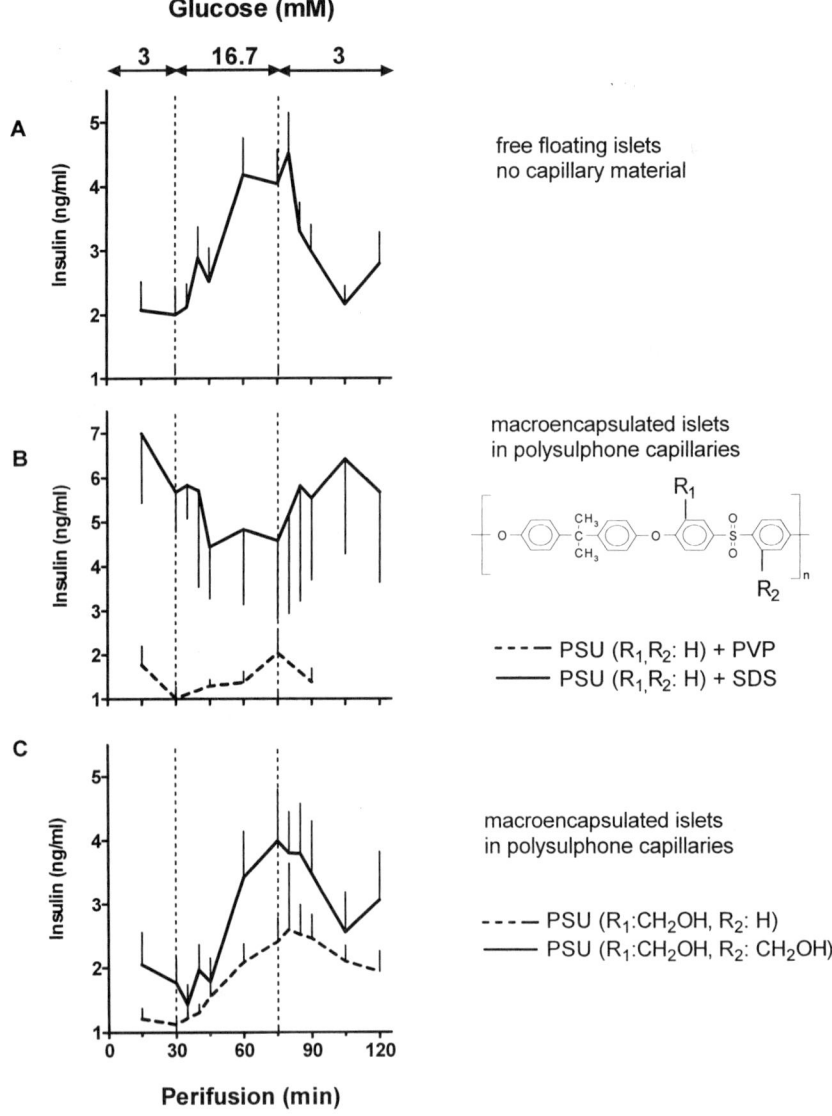

**FIGURE 2.** Effect of polysulphone modifications on glucose-induced insulin secretion in macroencapsulated rat islets.

alternative approach to improving surface hydrophilicity of polysulphone is surface modification by substitution with hydroxy-methyl groups ($CH_2OH$). A PSU capillary modified with $CH_2OH$ at a degree of substitution of approximately 0.7 is clearly more suitable for insulin diffusion than previously tested capillaries (FIG. 2, lower panel). There was a glucose-induced insulin release of about $63 \pm 15$ ng/ml × 90 min which was, however, significantly less than insulin release in control measurements. The best results were obtained by increasing the degree of PSU substitution near two. The kinetics and the efficiency ($117 \pm 24$ ng/ml × 90 min) of insulin release after macroencapsulation were almost identical compared to that observed for free-floating islets indicating that the capillary does not represent any diffusion barrier.

To further characterize the impact of macroencapsulation on islet function, insulin secretion was studied during two consecutive glucose stimulations. It is already known that insulin release in the perfused pancreas and in perfused free-floating islets increases following an initial glucose stimulation.[8] This priming depends on the production of metabolites that persist in the cytosol for some time after the first stimulation and facilitate insulin release during a second stimulation. Freshly isolated, free-floating islets respond to two consecutive glucose stimulations with a typical secretion pattern. The second stimulation is associated with an increased insulin release compared with the initial stimulation (see FIGURE 3). Like free-floating islets,

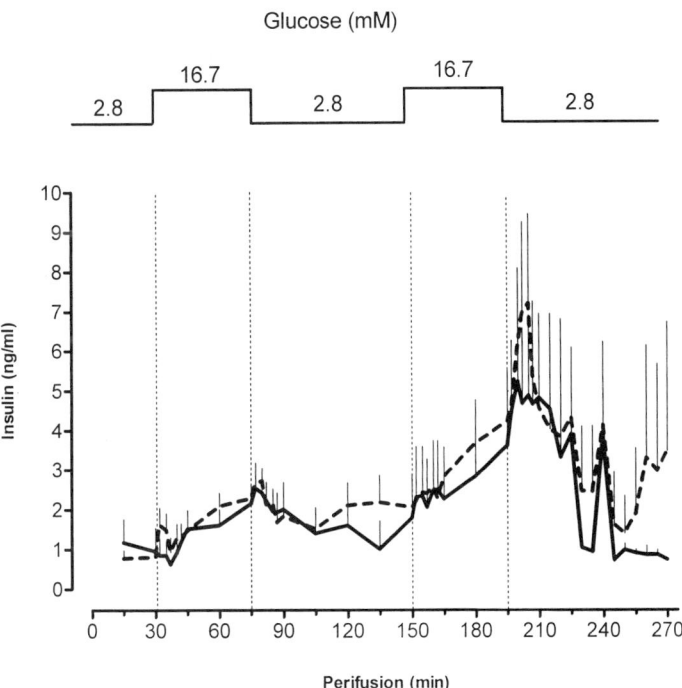

**FIGURE 3.** Priming of insulin secretion in macroencapsulated rat islets. - -, free-floating islets; ——, macroencapsulated islets.

insulin release of freshly isolated, macroencapsulated islets is stimulated by a second glucose stimulation (FIG. 3). Thus, the metabolic effect of priming is present after islet macroencapsulation.

In vitro tests of new biomaterials identified a new biomaterial with improved diffusion properties for glucose and insulin. Highly substituted hydroxy-methylated polysulphone capillary material does not alter insulin secretion kinetics following islet macroencapsulation. This material preserves proper islet function *in vitro* after an encapsulation period of two days. PSU/CH$_2$OH capillary material combines immunoisolation with optimal insulin secretion kinetics and is suitable for islet encapsulation in a vascular bioartificial pancreas.

Based on this new biomaterial a prototype of a vascular device has been developed. Since some of the critical factors responsible for restricted insulin release of previous devices are improved,[2–4] it is hoped that the new device may allow achievement of tight glycemic control after implantation. This prototype awaits a first *in vivo* test in allogenic islet transplantation in pancreatetomized pigs.

## ACKNOWLEDGMENTS

This work was supported by grants of BMBF 03N4901, Matech, Land Baden-Württemberg, and Universität Tübingen.

## REFERENCES

1. CALAFIORE, R. 1998. Actual perspectives in biohybrid artificial pancreas for the therapy of type 1, insulin dependent diabetes mellitus. Diabetes Metab. Rev. **14:** 315–324.
2. SULLIVAN, S.J., T. MAKI, K.M. BORLAND, *et al.* 1991. Biohybrid artificial pancreas: longterm implantation studies in diabetic, pancreatectomized dogs. Science **252:** 718–721.
3. MAKI, T., J.P. LOGDE, M. CARETTA, *et al.* 1993. Treatment of severe diabetes mellitus for more than one year using a vascularized hybrid artificial pancreas. Transplantation **55:** 713–718.
4. MAKI, T., I. OTSU, J.J. O'NEIL, *et al.* 1996. Treatment of diabetes by xenogenic islets without immunosuppression. Use of a vascularized bioartificial pancreas. Diabetes **45:** 342–347.
5. CALLES-ESCANDON, J. & D.C. ROBBINS. 1987. Loss of early phase of insulin release in humans impairs glucose tolerance and blunts thermic effect of glucose. Diabetes **36:** 1167–1172.
6. DIAMANTOGLOU, M. & J. VIENKEN. 1996. Strategies for the development of haemocompatible dialysis membranes. Macromol. Symp. **103:** 31–42.
7. LACY, P.E. & M. KOSTIANOVSKY. 1967. Method for the isolation of intact islets of Langerhans from the rat pancreas. Diabetes **16:** 35–39.
8. NESHER, R & E. CERASI. 1994. Signal modulation for phasic insulin release in normal and diabetic pancreatic B-cells. *In* Insulin Secretion and Pancreatic B-Cell Research. P.R. Flatt & S. Lenzen, Eds.: 411–419. Smith-Gordon.

# Newly Developed Aminopropyl-Silicate Immunoisolation Membrane for a Microcapsule-Shaped Bioartificial Pancreas

SHINJI SAKAI, TSUTOMU ONO, HIROYUKI IJIMA, AND KOEI KAWAKAMI

*Department of Materials Process Engineering, Graduate School of Engineering, Kyushu University, 6-10-1 Hakozaki, Higashi-ku, Fukuoka 812-8581, Japan*

ABSTRACT: An aminopropyl-silicate membrane, synthesized from tetramethoxysilane (TMOS) and 3-aminopropyltrimethoxysilane (APTrMOS) by the sol–gel method, was formed onto Ca-alginate gel beads via electrostatic interactions. The permeability of the membrane could be controlled easily by changing the molar ratio of both the precursors ([APTrMOS]/[TMOS]). The aminopropyl-silicate membrane prepared at a molar ratio of 2.40 rejected γ-globulin and BSA successfully, whereas it permeated ovalbumin. This result indicates that the molecular weight cutoff point of this newly developed aminopropyl-silicate membrane is approximately 60 kDa.

KEYWORDS: aminopropyl-silicate membrane; immunoisolation; bioartificial pancreas

## INTRODUCTION

Transplantation of encapsulated islets of Langerhans in a biocompatible and permselective membrane has been proposed as a method of great promise in treating insulin-dependent diabetes mellitus. The permeability of the membrane governs the success of this device. The membrane has to permeate low molecular weight substances, such as necessary nutrients, oxygen, and cellular waste products, whereas it has to exclude immune molecules, to protect the transplanted islet from host immune response. Since Lim and Sun reported the effectiveness of alginate/polylysine/alginate microcapsules in 1980,[1] many techniques and materials have been studied to develop this device. Almost all the materials used to date have been organic polymers, such as alginate,[2,3] polylysine,[1,4] cellulose,[5] protamine,[6] agarose,[7] polyethylene glycol,[8] and glycol chitosan.[9]

Sol–gel synthesized inorganic matrices are prepared from metal alkoxide precursors and the process is composed of a two-step network-forming process. The first step is hydrolysis, involving the formation of metal hydroxide intermediates. The subsequent step is a condensation of these species, resulting in a three-dimensional metal oxide network. These matrices have been widely studied for encapsulation of various biomolecules during the past decade,[10] for the following reasons: they are

---

Address for correspondence: Shinji Sakai, Department of Materials Process Engineering, Graduate School of Engineering, Kyushu University, 6-10-1 Hakozaki, Higashi-ku, Fukuoka 812-8581, Japan. Voice and fax: +81-92-642-4109.
sakai@chem_eng_kyushu-u.ac.jp

porous and the pore size is large enough to allow the diffusion of substances; the pore size can be controlled easily by changing several conditions during the sol–gel process, such as pH, aging time, and mixing procedure; and the process can take place at room temperature.

Inorganic matrices derived from the sol–gel synthesis offer several advantages over organic polymers, such as negligible swelling in solvents, chemical inertness, and hardness. However, one of the well-known shortcomings of the sol–gel synthesized matrices is their brittleness. To overcome this shortcoming, a novel method was developed: the silicate membrane was formed on the flexible alginate polymer via electrostatic interactions.

This paper deals with the permeability of the sol–gel synthesized silicate membranes from tetramethoxysilane (TMOS) [$Si(OCH_3)_4$] and 3-aminopropyltrimethoxysilane (APTrMOS) [$(CH_3O)_3Si(CH_2)_3NH_2$].

## MATERIALS AND METHODS

### Materials

Two kinds of silicon alkoxide precursors, TMOS and APTrMOS, were obtained from Tokyo Kasei Co. (Tokyo, Japan). Sodium alginate (Kelton LV) was generously donated by Kelco Co. (San Diego, USA). All the chemicals were used without further purification.

### Measurement of Permeability of Membrane

An aqueous sodium alginate solution (1.5 wt%, 200 ml) was extruded through a 22-gauge needle into an aqueous stirred 100 mM calcium chloride solution (500 ml) to prepare Ca-alginate gel beads (ca. 3.0 mm in diameter) and cured for two hours. In the case of the preparation of Ba-alginate gel beads, the sodium alginate solution was extruded into an aqueous 20 mM barium chloride solution. The resultant gel beads were suspended in distilled water. After swelling for two days in distilled water, 10 ml of the gel beads were mixed with 14 ml of $n$-hexane and kept at 4°C in an ice bath. APTrMOS (3.4 mmol, 0.60 ml) was added first and stirred for one minute with a vortex mixer, and then TMOS was added and stirred for another one minute. The quantity of TMOS was varied from 0.6 mmol (0.09 ml) to 5.4 mmol (0.80 ml). All of the sol–gel reactions were performed at 4°C. After the formation of the aminopropyl-silicate membrane, the gel beads were suspended in a stirred 0.05 wt% sodium alginate aqueous solution (100 ml) for three minutes to form an outer alginate layer via electrostatic interactions.

The membrane derived from APTrMOS alone was prepared by adding APTrMOS (1.7, 5.4, or 8.1 mmol, respectively) into a mixture of Ca-alginate gel beads and $n$-hexane and the suspension was stirred for two minutes. The membrane derived from TMOS alone was prepared by adding TMOS (67 mmol) into the mixture of Ca-alginate gel beads and $n$-hexane and the suspension was stirred for one hour.

The time-course of the diffusion of substance into the membrane-coated gel beads was measured as follows: membrane-coated gel beads (5 ml) were put into a well stirred, 0.2 M Tris buffer solution (10 ml, 37°C, pH7.4) containing one of the substances. The substances used in this study were glucose (180 Da), myoglobin (16.9 kDa), ovalbumin (45 kDa), bovine serum albumin (BSA, 67 kDa), and γ-globulin (157 kDa). Samples of 20 µl volume were taken from the solution containing gel beads. Sampling times were varied for each substance, ranging from every minute for glucose to every 0.5–4 hour for proteins, depending on the rate of diffusion of individual substrates. The initial concentrations of substances in each solution were 2 mg/ml for glucose and 1 mg/ml for proteins. The concentration of glucose was determined by an enzymatic colorimetric method (Glucose CII-Test Wako, Wako Chemical Co., Osaka, Japan). The concentrations of myoglobin, ovalbumin, BSA, and γ-globulin were determined spectrophotometrically according to Lowry's method.

The experimental data were used to calculate the effective diffusion coefficient, $D_e$, for each substance. The value was determined by the nonlinear least squares method from Equation (1),[11] which was derived under the assumptions that the concentration of solute in the solution was uniform, volume of solution was finite, and the structure inside the beads was homogeneous,

$$C_L = \frac{\alpha C_{L0}}{1+\alpha}\left\{1 + \sum_{n=1}^{\infty} \frac{6(1+\alpha)\exp(-D_e q_n^2 t/a^2)}{9 + 9\alpha + q_n^2 \alpha^2}\right\} \quad (1)$$

where $\alpha = (V/n)/(4\pi a^3 K/3)$, $q_n$ is defined by $\tan(q_n) = 3q_n/(3+\alpha q_n^2)$, $a$ is diameter of a bead, $t$ is time, $C_{L0}$ is the initial concentration of solute, $C_L$ is the concentration of solute at time $t$, $V$ is the volume of solution, and $n$ is the number of gel beads. The partition coefficient, $K$, is defined by $K = C_{GE}/C_{LE}$. $C_{LE}$ is the equilibrium concentration of substance in solution and was determined as a constant value observed for six hour. $C_{GE}$ is the substance concentration in the bead at equilibrium, obtained by mass balance using the known values of $V$, $n$, $a$, $C_{LE}$ and $C_{L0}$.

## RESULTS AND DISCUSSION

### Permeability of Membrane Derived from Either APTrMOS or TMOS

FIGURE 1 shows the equilibrium concentrations of BSA and γ-globulin in aqueous phase after the gel beads (5 ml), coated or non-coated with inorganic silicate membrane derived from TMOS alone, were incubated for 20 hours in 0.2 M Tris buffer solution (10 ml, pH7.4) at 37°C. The dotted line in FIGURE 1 ($C_{LE}/C_{L0} = 0.667$) indicates that the partition coefficient is unity; that is, both the concentrations of substance in the gel beads and the aqueous phase are the same. The concentration of each substance was well below value indicated by the dotted line. This result indicates that BSA and γ-globulin were adsorbed onto the silicate derived from TMOS alone. It is well known that such protein adsorption onto implanted materials induces a cellular adherence and a fibrotic overgrowth. These difficulties have been a cause of graft failure in a microcapsule-shaped bioartificial pancreas.[12]

FIGURE 2 shows the time-courses of the diffusion of γ-globulin from aqueous solution into the gel beads coated with aminopropyl-silicate membrane. The membrane was derived from 1.7, 5.4, or 8.1 mmol APTrMOS, respectively, per 10 ml of Ca-

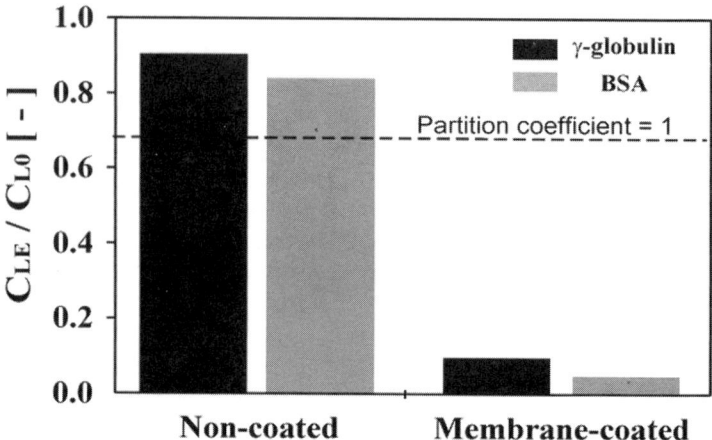

**FIGURE 1.** Equilibrium concentrations of BSA and γ-globulin after Ca-alginate gel beads (5 ml), non-coated or coated with silicate membrane derived from TMOS alone, were put into 0.2 M Tris buffer solution (10 ml, pH7.4) containing one of substances and incubated for 20 h at 37°C.

alginate gel beads. The diffusion rate of γ-globulin became somewhat slow with an increase in the amount of APTrMOS. However, the membrane permeated γ-globulin even when it was derived from 8.1 mmol APTrMOS.

*Permeability of Membrane Derived from Both APTrMOS and TMOS*

FIGURE 3 shows the time-course of γ-globulin concentration in the aqueous phase. In this experiment, three kinds of gel beads were used; non-coated Ca-alginate, Ca-alginate and Ba-alginate gel beads coated with aminopropyl-silicate membranes prepared at a ratio of [APTrMOS]/[TMOS] = 2.40. The Ca-alginate gel beads had good permeability for γ-globulin. On the other hand, the Ca-alginate gel beads coated with the aminopropyl-silicate membrane rejected γ-globulin. The Ba-alginate gel beads coated with the membrane permitted the diffusion of γ-globulin. Such a different result on the membrane-coated gel beads is probably due to a difference in a degree of electrostatic interaction between amino groups and carboxyl groups resulting from the fact that the affinity of divalent cations for alginate is $Ba^{2+} > Ca^{2+}$.[13] The core alginate gel serves as a template for the aminopropyl-silicate membrane. Therefore, the degree of electrostatic interactions could affect the structure of the membrane; that is, it would be one of the factors that affects the permeability of the membrane.

FIGURE 4 shows the effective diffusion coefficients in Eq. **(1)**, $D_e$, normalized by the molecular diffusion coefficients in pure water, $D_{water}$, against the molecular weights of the substances used in this study. This figure also shows the effect of the molar ratio of APTrMOS to TMOS during the membrane formation on the $D_e/D_{water}$ values. The effective diffusion coefficients of glucose were almost the same for four different membrane types, exhibiting about 70% of the molecular diffusion coeffi-

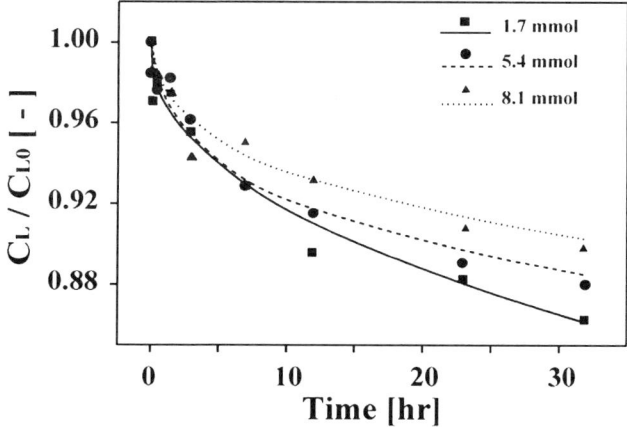

**FIGURE 2.** Time course of diffusion of γ-globulin at 37°C from 0.2 M Tris buffer solution (10 ml, pH7.4) into Ca-alginate gel beads (5 ml) coated with aminopropyl-silicate membrane derived from APTrMOS alone. The amount of APTrMOS added was varied.

cients in pure water. It follows from FIGURE 4 that the substances (excluding glucose) became more difficult to diffuse across the membrane with an increase in the molar ratio of APTrMOS to TMOS from 0.60 to 2.40. However, a further increase in the

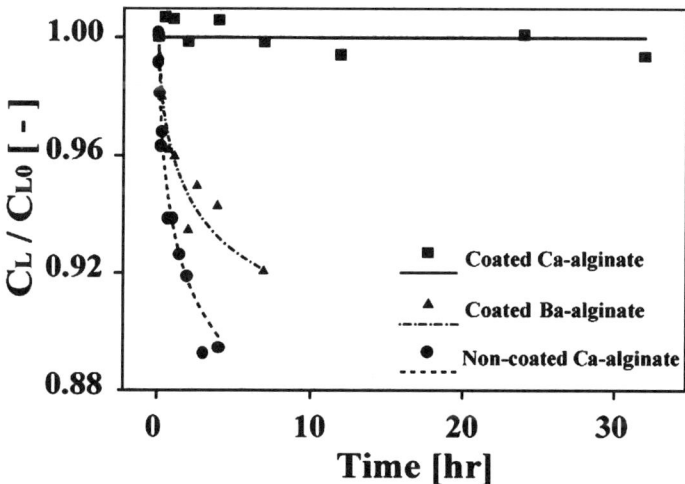

**FIGURE 3.** Time-course of diffusion of γ-globulin from 0.2 M Tris buffer solution (pH7.4) into Ca-alginate gel beads, Ca-alginate, and Ba-alginate gel beads coated with aminopropyl-silicate membrane derived from APTrMOS and TMOS. The molar ratio of APTrMOS to TMOS was 2.40.

molar ratio above 2.40 allowed these substances to permeate the membrane. In the case that the membrane was prepared at the molar ratio of 2.40, the concentrations of γ-globulin (157 kDa) and BSA (67 kDa) in the solution containing the gel beads were unchanged for 12 hours of incubation, whereas a decrease in the concentration of ovalbumin occurred. To confirm the diffusion of ovalbumin (47 kDa) through the membrane, Ca-alginate gel beads containing about 2 mg/ml ovalbumin were coated with the membrane and then suspended in 0.2 M Tris buffer solution. It was observed that ovalbumin was released into the solution through the membrane. It was, thus, estimated that the molecular weight cut-off point of this membrane was about 60 kDa.

The membranes prepared at various molar ratios of APTrMOS to TMOS showed different molecular permeabilities. This could be explained by the change of electric charge of monomer and cluster that participate in the condensation and are incorporated in the aminopropyl-silicate membrane, and by the total quantity of precursors added. The change in the electrostatic repulsion forces between these particles is expected to result in different three-dimensional membrane structures. That is, it affects the permeability of the membranes prepared at the molar ratios of 2.40, 3.60, and 5.40. For the membrane prepared at the molar ratio of 0.60, the total quantity of precursors is insufficient to form the membrane.

In order to discuss the permeability of the aminopropyl-silicate membrane in further detail, we attempted to measure the thickness of the membrane. It was found that the thickness of the membrane prepared at the molar ratio of 2.40 was about 10–20 μm in the dry state, by measurement with a scanning electron microscope.

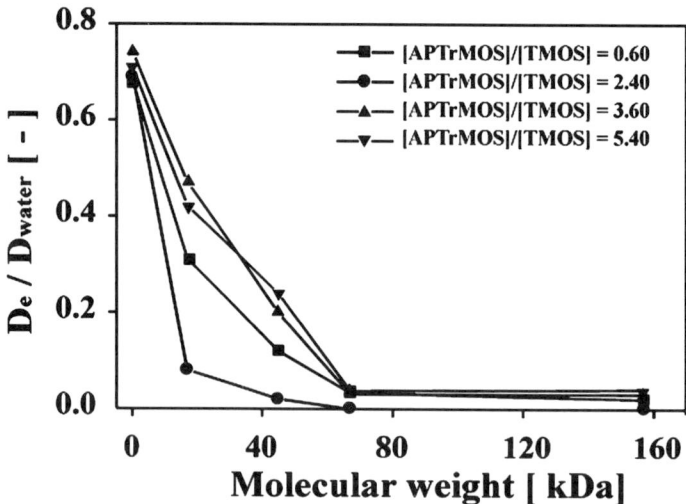

**FIGURE 4.** Relation between the ratio of $D_e$ to $D_{water}$ and molecular weight of substances (glucose, myoglobin, ovalbumin, BSA, and γ-globulin) for Ca-alginate gel beads coated with aminopropyl-silicate membranes. The molar ratio of APTrMOS to TMOS was varied.

However, at the present, we cannot determine the thickness of the membrane in a wet state because the degree of contraction during drying is unclear.

## CONCLUSION

A novel membrane composed of aminopropyl-silicate was developed for a microcapsule-shaped bioartificial pancreas. From the measurements of the diffusion rates of several substances through the membranes, it was found that the permeabilities of the membranes depend on the molar ratio of APTrMOS to TMOS. The membranes prepared from either TMOS or APTrMOS gave no effective results. With the membrane prepared at a molar ratio of [APTrMOS]/[TMOS] = 2.40, the molecular weight cut-off point of approximately 60 kDa, required for immunoisolation, was achieved.

## REFERENCES

1. LIM, F. & A.M. SUN. 1980. Microencapsulated islets as bioartificial endocrine pancreas. Science **210:** 908–910.
2. ZEKORN, T.D.C., A. HORCHER, J. MELLERT, et al. 1996. Biocompatibility and immunology in the encapsulation of islets of Langerhans (bioartificial pancreas). Int. J. Artif. Organs **19:** 251–257.
3. SIEBERS, U., A. HORCHER, R.G. BRETZEL, et al. 1997. Alginate-based microcapsules for immunoprotected islet transplantation. Ann. N.Y. Acad. Sci. **831:** 304–312.
4. SUN, Y., X. MA, D. ZHOU, et al. 1996. Normalization of diabetes in spontaneously diabetic cynomolgus monkeys by xenografts of microencapsulated porcine islets without immunosuppression. J. Clin. Invest. **98:** 1417–1422.
5. DAUTZENBERG, H., U. SCHULDT, G. GRASNICK. et al. 1999. Development of cellulose sulfate-based polyelectrolyte complex microcapsules for medical applications. Ann. N.Y. Acad. Sci. **875:** 46–63.
6. TATAKIEWICZ, K., E. SITAREK, M. SABAT & T. ORLOWSKI. 1995. Multilayer coating of islets of Langerhans: *in vitro* studies on a new method for immunoisolation. Transplant. Proc. **27:** 617.
7. IWATA, H., Y. MURAKAMI & Y. IKADA. 1999. Control of complement activities for immunoisolation. Ann. N.Y. Acad. Sci. **875:** 7–23.
8. CHEN, J.-P., I.-M. CHU, M.-Y. SHIAO. et al. 1998. Microencapsulation of islets in PEG-amine modified alginate-poly(L-lysine)-alginate microcapsules for constructing bioartificial pancreas. J. Ferment. Bioeng. **86:** 185–190.
9. SAKAI, S., T. ONO, H. IJIMA & K. KAWAKAMI. 2000. Control of molecular weight cut-off for immunoisolation by multilayering glycol chitosan-alginate polyion complex on alginate-based microcapsule. J. Microencapsul. **17:** 691–699.
10. AVNIR, D., S. BRAUN, O. LEV & M. OTTOLENGHI. 1994. Enzymes and other proteins entrapped in sol-gel materials. Chem. Mater. **6:** 1605–1614.
11. CRANK, J. 1975. The Mathematics of Diffusion. Clarendon Press, Oxford.
12. VOS, P.D., B.J.D. HAAN, G.H.J. WOLTERS. et al. 1997. Improved biocompatibility but limited graft survival after purification of alginate for microencapsulation of alginate for microencapsulation of pancreatic islets. Diabetologia **40:** 262–270.
13. GOMBOTZ, W.R. & S.F. WEE. 1998. Protein release from alginate matrices. Adv. Drug Deliv. Rev. **31:** 267–285.

# The Role of a Bioengineered Artificial Kidney in Renal Failure

WILLIAM H. FISSELL, JASON KIMBALL, SHERRILL M. MACKAY, ANGELA FUNKE, AND H. DAVID HUMES

*Departments of Internal Medicine, VA Medical Center and University of Michigan, Ann Arbor, Michigan, USA*

ABSTRACT: Renal failure continues to carry substantial burden of morbidity and mortality in both acute and chronic forms, despite advances in transplantation and dialysis. There is evidence to suggest that the kidney has metabolic, endocrine, and immune effects transcending its filtration functions, even beyond secretion of renin and erythropoietin. Our laboratory has developed experience in the tissue culture of renal parenchymal cells, and has now been able to demonstrate the metabolic activity of these cells in an extracorporeal circuit recapitulating glomerulotubular anatomy. We have observed active transport of sodium, glucose, and glutathione. We describe the design and initial preclinical testing of the bioartificial kidney, as well as future directions of our research.

KEYWORDS: bioengineering; artificial kidney; renal failure

## SCOPE OF THE PROBLEM OF RENAL FAILURE

The kidney is unique among body organs in that it is the first organ for which long-term *ex vivo* substitutive therapy has been available. Kolff's first hemodialyzer was successfully applied to a human patient with acute renal failure in 1948, and the first successful allograft transplantation was a kidney by David Humes, John Merrill, and Joseph Murray in 1951, for which a Nobel prize was awarded. Both treatments are used today. The annual mortality for patients between 40 and 60 years of age with end-stage renal disease receiving hemodialysis is 13.3%, whereas that for age-matched recipients of first cadaveric renal transplant is a mere 4%.[1] The statistics for acute renal failure are similarly grim, with overall survival unmoved from its pre-dialysis era statistic of approximately 50%.[2] Acute renal failure as a component of multiorgan dysfunction syndrome (MODS) carries an especially poor prognosis, with survival rates around 10%.[3–5] The problem is likely to continue to grow in magnitude, since the population of patients with end-stage renal disease (ESRD) in the United States has been increasing at a constant 8% per year, although the number of kidneys transplanted has risen at about only 3% per year.[6,7]

The reasons for the markedly improved prognosis of patients transplanted with allograft kidneys cannot be explained solely by the better health of patients listed for

---

Address for correspondence: H. David Humes, Department of Internal Medicine, Division of Nephrology, 3914 Taubman Center, University of Michigan Health System, Ann Arbor, MI 48109-0364, USA.

dhumes@umich.edu

transplant, since those awaiting an organ have higher mortality than those actually receiving a transplant.[7] We deduce that the intact or transplanted kidney provides function to the host that intermittent hemodialysis does not.

Hemodialysis provides clearance of small molecules in blood by diffusive flow across a semipermeable membrane, and control of volume status by bulk flow of water and solutes through that membrane. These short-term effects are sufficient to abrogate the lethal acidosis, volume overload, and uremic syndromes that accompany renal failure, but do not protect the patient from the increased mortality associated with dialysis-treated renal failure in either the acute or chronic form. Thus, the metabolic, endocrine, and immune roles of the functioning kidney are candidate mechanisms for the difference in survival noted above. The dialytic clearance of glutathione, a key tripeptide in free radical scavenging and protection against oxidant stress, the negative nitrogen balance and energy loss in the clearance of peptides and amino acids in dialysate, loss of oxidative deamination and gluconeogenesis in the tubule cell, and loss of cytokine and hormone metabolic activity by the kidney each impose substantial stress upon the dialyzed patient, and as such are appropriate targets for improved renal replacement therapy.

## RENAL CELLS AND RENAL ROLES

The kidney's functional unit, the nephron, provides for the elimination of wastes and toxins without the need for specific enzymes and transporters for each toxin. All but the large proteins and cellular elements in the blood are filtered; a system of cells reclaims specific filtered substances needed by the body, and allows all others to pass as urine. Teleologically, this allows each organism to cope with novel insults its genetic forebears may not have encountered.

Filtration is accomplished by the glomerulus, a tuft of capillaries supported by a basement membrane and specialized epithelial cells called podocytes. The renal proximal tubule, a hollow tube of cells surrounded by capillaries, receives the filtrate from the glomerulus and accomplishes the bulk of reclamation of salt, water, glucose, small proteins, amino acids, glutathione, and other substances. The tubule also accomplishes metabolic functions including excretion of acid as ammonia, hydroxylation of 25-OH-Vit $D_3$, and others.

Intermittent hemodialysis is thought to replace the filtration function of the glomerulus. Our attention is drawn to duplicating the function of the proximal tubule. The transport of solutes and water is accomplished by ATP-driven electrolyte transporters in the luminal cell membrane. Reabsorption of small proteins and peptides in the filtrate stream is accomplished by membrane-bound proteases and specific amino acid transport proteins within the luminal membrane of the tubule cell. These amino acids are either used for protein and peptide synthesis in the tubule cell, or are transported into the capillaries for transport to and use by the body. The diversity and specificity of the functions of the proximal tubule cell argue against the development of an electromechanical or polymeric substitute, and thus, a number of years ago, our research group turned its attention to the isolation and culture of renal proximal tubule cells. That research has culminated in the hollow-fiber bioreactor discussed below.

## DESIGN AND IMPLEMENTATION OF A HOLLOW-FIBER BIOREACTOR

### *Selection of Proximal Tubule Cells*

Implementation and eventual manufacture of a device based on cell therapy requires a steady and predictable supply of tissues from which cells may be isolated and cultured. Until such time as stem cells may be isolated and induced to differentiate into organ-specific cell types, cells for allotransplantation, xenotransplantation, or bioartificial organ use will need to be procured through the harvest of animal or human tissues.

Human kidneys unsuitable for cadaveric transplant have been used as a source of proximal tubule cells in our laboratory, but the potential for infectious complications looms large and mandates extensive screening and testing of each donor and each harvested kidney. There is also a limited supply of these organs since they represent a side-stream of the limited supply of organs for available for transplant. Similarly, some of the characteristics rendering them unsuitable for transplantation may adversely affect the harvest of cells from the kidneys.

There has been extensive research in xenotransplantation and bioengineering with porcine cells. Researchers developing bioartificial livers[8–18] and bioartificial pancreases[19–25] have achieved a degree of comfort with porcine cells. Pigs are commercially bred and available in large number, and have similar organ sizes to humans. There is considerable concern about the potential for zoonotic spread of viruses, particularly after the demonstration that porcine endogenous retroviruses can infect human cells.[26,27]

Although most preclinical studies have used porcine cells in preparation of clinical trials, the FDA encouraged us to carry out experiments using human cells in our bioartificial kidney to continue progress in this field. Accordingly, biocomparability studies, including metabolic, transport, and endocrine functionality have been completed between porcine and human proximal tubule cells. Human cells were obtained both from postmortem specimens as well as transplant discards. Human proximal tubule cells (HPTC) have recently been characterized in order to compare functionality between the two tissue sources. Metabolic assessment included ammonia and glutathione metabolism. Porcine proximal tubule cells (PPTC) produce $10 \pm 4$ μg ammonia/$10^6$ cells/24 hours. Ammonia production rates were pH responsive in both cell types. Glutathione metabolism in the PPTC and HPTC was 4.44 and 8.16 mmol/$10^6$ cells/hour, respectively. Glutathione metabolism was inhibited in both cell types by the addition of acivicin, a specific inhibitor of glutathione metabolism. The reabsorptive function was evaluated with glucose transport. PPTC and HPTC reabsorbed $84 \pm 15$ and $96 \pm 8$ mg of glucose/$10^6$ cells/day, respectively. Glucose transport in both cell types was inhibited by the addition of phlorizin, a specific inhibitor of glucose reabsorption. Endocrine function was assessed by 1–25 dihydroxyvitamin $D_3$ production. With the addition of parathyroid hormone, PPTC and HPTC converted $37.5 \pm 2.1$ and $48.2 \pm 5.2$ pg/$10^6$ cells/24 hours, respectively. Cytokine production was measured in both cell types. Interleukin-8 secretion was $4.7 \pm 1.7$ and $10.2$ ng/$10^6$ cells/24 hours, for PPTC and HPTC respectively, when cells were stimulated with endotoxin. These data suggest that both PPTC and HPTC are biocomparable with respect to transport, metabolic, and endocrine functions in cell culture.

## Isolation and Culture of Proximal Tubule Cells

Our laboratory developed experience in the isolation and culture of porcine proximal tubule cells until we could reproducibly harvest cells and maintain them stably in culture.[28,29] In brief, Yorkshire breed pigs were sacrificed at four to six weeks of age and their kidneys harvested. The renal cortices were dissected, minced, digested with collagenase, and the resulting mixture was separated on a Percoll density gradient. Renal proximal tubule fragments were isolated and grown in a serum-free, hormonally derived medium. After third passage and reaching confluence on 100-mm culture dishes, cells were mobilized with trypsin into a suspension and seeded into polysulfone single hollow-fiber bioreactors (Fresenius AG BadHamburg, Germany, or Minntech, Inc., Minneapolis, MN, USA) for *in vitro* assessment of cell viability and metabolic activity.

## Characterization of a Single Hollow-Fiber Bioreactor

Cellular attachment, stability, and confluence on the interior lumen of the bioreactor is of paramount importance. To promote attachment of the cells, the luminal surface of the polysulfone membrane was coated with ProNectin-L (Protein Polymer, San Diego, CA, USA). ProNectin-L is a synthetic protein sharing the intercellular attachment domains of laminin, a protein found in the renal glomerular and tubular basement membrane.[30] Laminin and collagen type IV, key components of the tubular basement membrane, also provide an effective biomatrix for cell attachment and growth. After seeding of the hollow fiber with tubule cells, the hollow fibers were perfused with culture media. Because newly seeded cells need time to attach, perfusion was initially performed via diffusion from the exterior through the polysulfone membrane, and after time for attachment, convective flow through the interior of the fiber was initiated. A graduated increase in flow (and, thus, shear forces) was used to condition the cells and minimize cellular detachment. Studies demonstrated that confluence was reached in seven to ten days. After fourteen days in culture the hollow fiber bioreactors were assessed for cellular confluency and viability. Light microscopy of fixed sections showed evidence of a confluent monolayer formed on the inside of the hollow fibers.[31]

Experiments were undertaken to verify the confluency of the monolayer of cultured cells. $C^{14}$-labelled inulin, a compound freely filtered by the glomerulus and by dialysis membranes, but not absorbed nor secreted by the tubule, was perfused through the lumen of the bioreactor. The amount of radioactivity in the luminal fluid and in the extraluminal fluid were compared, to verify minimal insulin transport across the monolayer, with less than two percent leak across the monolayer.[32]

## Transport and Metabolic Characteristics of Hollow-Fiber Bioreactors

Because initial experiments using the single hollow-fiber model were promising, the design was scaled up to use commercially available polysulfone hollow fiber dialysis cartridges from the manufacturers of the single hollow fibers. Single hollow-fiber measurements of transport and metabolic activity were repeated with 97 cm$^2$ and 0.4 m$^2$ surface area cartridges.

Vectorial transport of sodium and water across the monolayers was assessed by perfusion of the lumen and the extraluminal space (ECS) with calibrated flows of culture media and measurement of timed collections of media from each flow. The bioreactor was tested to see if transport could be increased by creating an oncotic driving force across the monolayer, and if that increase could be abrogated by ouabain, a specific inhibitor of Na$^+$/K$^+$ ATPase, the enzyme responsible for the bulk of sodium transport across the luminal surface of the cell, which suggested that the transport was an active process, rather than passive flow governed by Starling forces across a semipermeable membrane. To increase the oncotic pressure, bovine serum albumin (BSA) was added to the ECS perfusate, and then ouabain was also added to the ECS perfusate. The data are summarized in TABLE 1. As expected, the transport was active and mediated by sodium–potassium ATPase.[31]

We further explored the metabolic characteristics of the cultured proximal tubule cells. We examined the transport of glucose, bicarbonate, and glutathione and expressed the data in terms of fractional reabsorption accomplished by the bioreactor, now termed the renal tubule assist device, or RAD. For each of the molecules listed, fractional excretion was measured in the absence and presence of a known inhibitor of an enzyme essential for the reabsorption. In the case of glucose, the compound phlorizin was used; for bicarbonate, a carbonic anhydrase inhibitor, acetazolamide, was used; for glutathione, an inhibitor of γ-glutamyltranspeptidase,

TABLE 1. Fluid transport[a]

| Ouabain Experiments | Absolute Reabsorption (ml/30 min) | Inulin Leak (percent) |
|---|---|---|
| Baseline | 1.05 ± 0.40 | 3.25 ± 0.21 |
| Albumin | 4.87 ± 0.66 | 3.10 ± 0.21 |
| Albumin and ouabain | 1.73 ± 0.43 | 2.98 ± 0.19 |

[a]Adapted from Reference 31.

TABLE 2. Solute transport[a]

| Molecule | Condition | Fractional Reabsorption (percent) |
|---|---|---|
| Glucose | baseline | 25.0 ± 1.2 |
|  | phlorizin | 9.2 ± 0.7 |
| Bicarbonate | baseline | 21.9 ± 1.8 |
|  | acetazolamide | 4.1 ± 0.5 |
| Glutathione | baseline | 44 ± 2 |
|  | acivicin | 25 ± 4 |

[a]Adapted from Reference 31.

TABLE 3. Effect of porcine cytokines on human monocytes

**Stimulation with Porcine TNF-α**

| | Control | Human TNF-α (ng/ml) | | | | Porcine TNF-α (ng/ml) | | | |
|---|---|---|---|---|---|---|---|---|---|
| | | 0.05 | 0.5 | 5 | 50 | 0.05 | 0.5 | 5 | 50 |
| IL-8 ng/$10^6$ cells | 29 ± 16 | 27 ± 17 | 33 ± 19 | 35 ± 16 | 38 ± 16 | 46 ± 22 | 105 ± 48 | 153 ± 51** | 157 ± 47** |

**Stimulation with Lipopolysaccharide 1 μg/ml**

| | Control | Human IL-10 (ng/ml) | | | | Porcine IL-10 (ng/ml) | | | |
|---|---|---|---|---|---|---|---|---|---|
| | | 0.05 | 0.5 | 5 | 50 | 0.05 | 0.5 | 5 | 50 |
| IL-8 ng/$10^6$ cells | 91 ± 20 | 113 ± 33 | 119 ± 35 | 103 ± 29 | 59 ± 17* | 118 ± 35 | 104 ± 29 | 69 ± 21 | 30 ± 9* |
| TNF-α ng/$10^6$ cells | 1.49 ± 0.60 | 1.46 ± 0.59 | 1.34 ± 0.68 | 0.83 ± 0.48** | 0.23 ± 0.90** | 1.52 ± 0.88 | 1.16 ± 0.71* | 0.30 ± 0.10** | 0.14 ± 0.46** |

*$p < 0.05$. **$p < 0.01$ by paired Student's $t$-test compared with baseline controls.

acivicin, was used. The data are summarized in TABLE 2. In each case, there was evidence of active transport and specific inhibition.[31]

The synthesis and secretion of ammonia into the tubule is essential for renal excretion of an acid load, since it buffers secreted protons. Proximal tubule cells are able to upregulate their ammoniagenesis in response to a decline in pH, and the proximal tubule cells in the bioreactor demonstrated a stepwise increase in ammonia production with changes in pH.[31]

The experiments detailed above were performed with porcine tubule cells. However, our laboratory has demonstrated similar results in culture, attachment, and activity with human proximal tubule cells from cadaveric organs. The final selection of cell type for use in a renal tubule device rests, not only on supply and safety of cells, but also on the ability of xenotransplanted cells to participate in the homeostasis of the host. The bioequivalence of large proteins and signalling molecules from pigs and humans is not well established in the literature to date. Our laboratory undertook a series of experiments to explore this issue. Human monocytes were isolated from healthy controls by standard methods.[33] Human and porcine TNF-α were used to stimulate monocyte production of IL-8 *in vitro*. Similarly, porcine IL-10 was used to attenuate monocyte secretion of TNF-α and IL-8 response to lipopolysaccharide stimulation. The results of our experiments are summarized in TABLE 3.[34]

This demonstration of response of human monocytes to porcine-derived cytokines is encouraging for xenotransplantation research. Of special interest is the finding that porcine IL-10 seems to be able to blunt inflammatory cytokine release from human monocytes.

The field of xenotransplantation, we must note, although a promising area of research, is challenged by much more than the aforementioned issue of bioequivalence of signals between organ and host. Detailed understandings of interactions between MHC-incompatible organs, the immune cells they harbor, and the host, as well as of zoonotic transmission in both directions are necessary before xenotransplantation research can move from laboratory to clinic.[35,36]

The above data suggest that our laboratory has successfully isolated and cultured renal proximal tubule cells, established stable confluent monolayers within hollow fiber bioreactors, and scaled the initial construct to a level approximating the number of proximal tubule cells in a single kidney. We termed the large-scale bioreactor the renal assist device, or RAD.

## *EX VIVO* AND PRECLINICAL CHARACTERIZATION OF THE RENAL ASSIST DEVICE

### *Experimental Model*

Following the demonstration of *in vitro* metabolic activity, we sought to determine if the metabolic and transport functions we observed in the RAD could be observed in an *ex vivo* system. Nephrectomized uremic mongrel dogs were placed on a modified continuous venovenous hemofiltration (CVVH) circuit. In an analogue to the glomerular/tubule relationship seen in the kidney, ultrafiltrate from a conventional hollow-fiber dialyzer (Fresenius AG Bad Hamburg, Germany, Model F-40) was directed to the luminal space of the RAD, and a portion of the posthemofilter

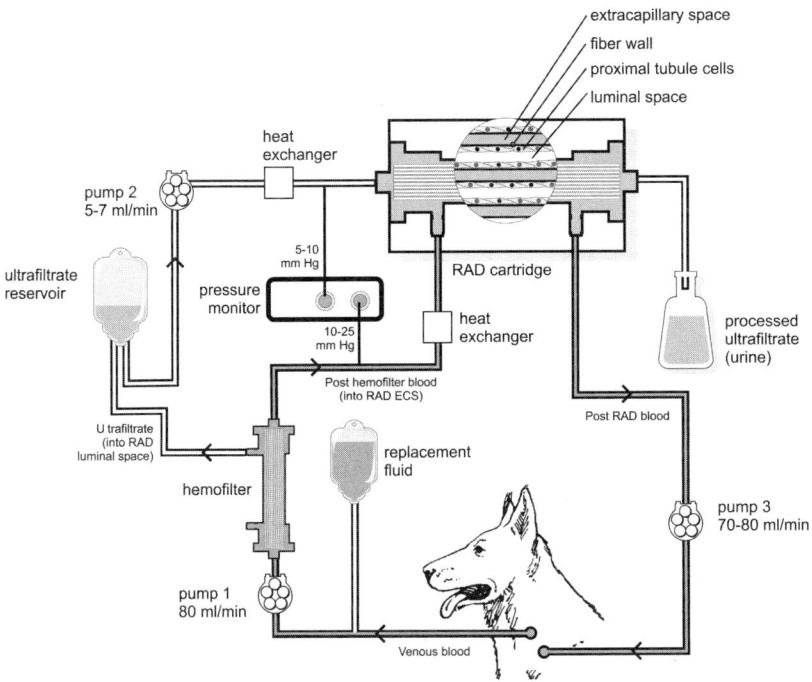

**FIGURE 1.** Extracorporeal hemoperfusion circuit.

blood was directed to the extracapillary space of the RAD. Roller pumps were used to dictate the flow rates of blood and ultrafiltrate to the RAD, as illustrated in FIGURE 1. The proximal tubule is responsible for reabsorption of approximately 50% of gloneulus ultrafiltrate, and adjustment of the flow rates and pressures in the RAD allowed us to mimic that reabsorption rate in our extracorporeal perfusion circuit. A series of experiments with RADs seeded with proximal tubules and equivalent hollow-fiber cartridges without cells were conducted. To quantify cell viability, cell counts were performed on the urine leaving the RAD hourly during the RAD treatment. After removal from the circuit at the conclusion of the experiment, RAD cartridges were assessed for cell viability and confluence immediately and after return to *in vitro* perfusion with culture media. We examined the ultrafiltrate entering (tubular fluid) and leaving (urine) the RAD for evidence of vectorial transport and secretion by the cells. Plasma levels of electrolytes, Vitamin $D_3$, and glutathione were measured before nephrectomy, before RAD treatment, and after RAD treatment.

### Cell Viability and Confluence

Urine cell counts obtained during the treatment revealed low levels of detachment during the first hour of treatment, and little or no detachment thereafter.[37] Histologic sections revealed persistence of the monolayer. Inulin leak rates increased from 5.8% ± 0.9% before the experiment to 10.0% ± 0.9% after the experiment, but after

14 days of culture had improved to 6.1% ± 0.6%, suggesting that the cells were able to replicate and reline the interior of the lumen.

### Transport Functions of the RAD

We chose to measure the homeostatic properties of the RAD not only by assessing serum concentrations of biologically important compounds, but also by quantifying vectorial transport from the ultrafiltrate to the bloodstream. The ratio of concentrations between tubular fluid leaving the RAD and ultrafiltrate entering the RAD (TF/UF) is a convenient expression of vectorial transport, as it quantifies extraction of a compound from the ultrafiltrate stream. Sodium and water are transported isoosmotically by the proximal tubule in the kidney and in the RAD. TF/UF ratios for sodium were approximately 1.00 in our circuit, as expected.[37] Fractional excretion of sodium did reflect active transport across the RAD, which was measured at 66.5% ± 2.0% in RADs with tubule cells and 52.5% ± 1.4% in sham-treated controls.[37] TF/UF ratios were calculated for the sodium, potassium, chloride, bicarbonate, BUN, creatinine, glucose, and glutathione, and are shown in TABLE 4.[37]

We assessed two other measures of tubule cell metabolism: ammoniagenesis and serum 1–25 dihydroxy-Vitamin $D_3$ levels in RAD-treated and sham-treated animals. Total ammonia excretion was assessed by collection of tubular fluid from the RAD. Excretion of ammonia was measured at –1.38 ± 1.2 μmol/h in sham-treated animals, and at 41 ± 19.9 μmol/h, ($p < 0.02$) in treated animals, with peak levels exceeding 90 μmol/h in animals treated for 20–24 hours.[37]

Serum 1–25 dihydroxy-Vitamin $D_3$ levels in animals treated with the RAD were also significantly different from levels in sham-treated controls, with levels decreasing by 4.0 pmol/ml over the course of a sham treatment, compared with an increase of 5.8 pmol/ml in RAD-treated animals.[37]

We have evidence that cell therapy with proximal tubule cells in our RAD bioreactor, in both *in vitro* and *ex vivo* models can reproduce many of the key functions of the renal proximal tubule. Furthermore, in large mammal models, we have demonstrated significant endocrinologic and metabolic activity reflected in serum

TABLE 4. Tubular fluid/ultrafiltrate ratios (TF/UF)[a]

| Molecule | Sham Treated | RAD Treated | $p$ |
|---|---|---|---|
| sodium | 1.01 ± 0.01 | 1.00 ± 0.01 | NS |
| potassium | 1.00 ± 0.02 | 0.94 ± 0.02 | $p < 0.001$ |
| chloride | 1.01 ± 0.01 | 1.00 ± 0.01 | NS |
| bicarbonate | 0.98 ± 0.01 | 0.96 ± 0.01 | $p < 0.05$ |
| BUN | 1.00 ± 0.01 | 0.99 ± 0.01 | NS |
| creatinine | 1.00 ± 0.01 | 0.99 ± 0.01 | NS |
| glucose | 0.98 ± 0.01 | 0.88 ± 0.04 | $p < 0.01$ |
| glutathione | 0.99 ± 0.07 | 0.52 ± 0.06 | $p < 0.001$ |

[a]Adapted from Reference 37.

chemistries of the treated animal. We then directed our attention to answering one of the initial questions posed: can functioning proximal tubule cells protect against the increased mortality seen when acute renal failure complicates other illness?

## Role of the RAD in Animal Models in Sepsis

Charles Natanson and others at the National Institutes of Health have developed and refined a large animal model of septic shock, using lipopolysaccharide infusions to trigger the proinflammatory cascade that characterizes the sepsis syndrome.[38] We adapted that model to healthy and to bilaterally nephrectomized mongrel dogs to simulate acute renal failure. Of note, even healthy dogs subject to the stress of lipopolysaccharide infusions displayed evidence of oliguric renal failure. Preliminary data suggest that some of the clinical markers of septic shock, such as hypotension, as well as serum levels of cytokines, such as IL-10, are different between dogs treated with the RAD and treated with sham controls. Further exploration is underway in defining our model.

## CLINICAL TRIALS OF THE RAD

The accumulation of several years' experience with the RAD in large animal models, as well as the encouraging data from our models of septic shock have brought us to clinical trials in human patients. The FDA has given approval to proceed to a PhaseI/II clinical trial of the RAD containing human rather than porcine cells. We plan to enroll ten patients during the first half of 2001. Our inclusion criteria are designed to enroll patients with acute tubular necrosis already receiving continuous renal replacement therapy, with APACHE-III predicted mortalities between 50% and 90%. We eagerly look forward to ushering in a new era of treatment for patients with acute and chronic renal failure.

### REFERENCES

1. WOLFE, R., V. ASHBY, E. MILFORD, *et al.* 1999. Comparison of mortality in all patients on dialysis, patients on dialysis awaiting transplantation, and recipients of a first cadaveric transplant. N. Engl. J. Med. **341:** 1725–1730.
2. ALKHUNAIZI, A.M. & R.W. SCHRIER. 1996. Management of acute renal failure: new perspectives. AJKD **28:** 315–328.
3. BONE, R.C., C.J. FISCHER, T.P. CLEMMER, *et al.* 1987. A controlled clinical trial of high-dose methylprednisolone in the treatment of severe sepsis and septic shock. N. Engl. J. Med. **317**(11): 653–658.
4. DAVIES, M.G. & P.-O. HAGEN. 1997. Systemic inflammatory response syndrome. Br. J. Surg. **84**(7): 920–935.
5. GROENEVELD, A., D. TRAN, J. VAN DER MEULEN, *et al.* 1991. Acute renal failure in the medical intensive care unit: predisposing, complicating factors and outcome. Nephron **59:** 602–610.
6. HARAHARAN, S., C. JOHNSON, B. BRESNAHAN, *et al.* 2000. Improved graft survival after renal transplantation in the United States, 1988 to 1996. N. Engl. J. Med. **342:** 605–612.
7. NEILSON, E., A. HULL, J. WISH, *et al.* 1997. The ad hoc committee report on estimating the future workforce and training requirements for nephrology. J. Am. Soc. Nephrol. **8**(5 Suppl. 9): S1–S4.

8. OHSHIMA, N., K. YANAGI & H. MIYOSHI. 1999. Development of a packed-bed type bioartificial liver: tissue engineering approach. Transplant. Proc. **31:** 2016–2017.
9. BUSSE, B. & J. GERLACH. 1999. Bioreactors for hybrid liver support: historical aspects and novel designs. Ann. N.Y. Acad. Sci. **875:** 326–339.
10. DIXIT, V. & G. GITNICK. 1998. The bioartificial liver: state-of-the-art. Eur. J. Surg. Suppl. **582:** 71–76.
11. NARUE, K., I. NAGASHIMA, Y. SAKAI, et al. 1998. Efficacy of a bioreactor filled with porcine hepatocytes immobilized on nonwoven fabric for *ex vivo* direct hemoperfusion treatment of liver failure in dogs. Artificial Organs **22:** 1031–1037.
12. NAKA, S., K. TAKESHITA, T. YAMAMOTO, et al. 1999. Bioartificial liver support system using porcine hepatocytes entrapped in a three-dimensional hollow fiber module with collagen gel: an evaluation in the swine acute liver failure model. Artificial Organs **23:** 822–828.
13. MCLAUGHLIN, B., C. TOSONE, L. CUSTER, et al. 1999. Overview of extracorporeal liver support systems and clinical results. Ann. N.Y. Acad. Sci. **875:** 310–325.
14. PATZER, J., G. MAZARIEGOS, R. LOPEZ, et al. 1999. Novel bioartificial liver support system: preclinical evaluation. Ann. N.Y. Acad. Sci. **875:** 340–352.
15. ROGER, V., P. BALLADUR, J. HONIGER, et al. 1998. Internal bioartificial liver with xenogeneic hepatocytes prevents death from acute liver failure: an experimental study. Ann. Surg. **228:** 1–7.
16. IWATA, H., T. SAJIKI, H. MAEDA, et al. 1999. *In vitro* evaluation of metabolic functions of a bioartificial liver. ASAIO J. **45:** 299–306.
17. WATANABE, F., C. MULLON, W. HEWITT, et al. 1997. Clinical experience with a bioartificial liver in the treatment of severe liver failure. a phase I clinical trial. Ann. Surg. **225:** 484–491.
18. WATANABE, F., C. SHACKLETON, S. COHEN, et al. 1997. Treatment of acetaminophen-induced fulminant hepatic failure with a bioartificial liver. Transplant. Proc. **29:** 487–488.
19. HAYASHI, H., K. INOUE, T. AUNG, et al. 1996. Long survival of xenografted bioartificial pancreas with a mesh-reinforced polyvinyl alcohol hydrogel bag employing a b-cell line (min6). Transplant. Proc. **28:** 1428–1429.
20. DELAUNAY, C., S. DARQUY, J. HONIGER, et al. 1998. Glucose-insulin kinetics of a bioartificial pancreas made of an an69 hydrogel hollow fiber containing porcine islets and implanted in diabetic mice. Artificial Organs **22:** 291–299.
21. CALAFIORE, R., G. BASTA, L. OSTICIOLI, et al. 1996. Coherent microcapsules for pancreatic islet transplantation: a new approach for bioartificial pancreas. Transplant. Proc. **28:** 812–813.
22. OHGAWARA, H., S. HIROTANI, J. MIYAZAKI, et al. 1998. Membrane immunoisolation of a diffusion chamber for bioartificial pancreas. Artificial Organs **22:** 788–794.
23. OBERHOLZER, J., F. TRIPONEZ, J. LOU, et al. 1999. Clinical islet transplantation: a review. Ann. N.Y. Acad. Sci. **875:** 189–199.
24. HUNTER, S., Y. WANG, C. WEINER, et al. 1997. Encapsulated beta-islet cells as a bioartificial pancreas to treat insulin-dependent diabetes during pregnancy. Am. J. Obstet. Gynecol. **177:** 746–752.
25. HUNTER, S., Y. WANG & V. RODGERS. 1999. Bioartificial pancreas use in diabetic pregnancy. ASAIO J. **45:** 13–17.
26. MARTIN, U., V. KIESSIG, J. BLUSCH, et al. 1998. Expression of pig endogenous retrovirus by primary porcine endothelial cells and infection of human cells. Lancet **352:** 692–694.
27. PATIENCE, C., Y. TAKEUCHI & R. WEISS. 1997. Infection of human cells by an endogenous retrovirus of pigs. Nat. Med. **3:** 282–286.
28. HUMES, H. & D. CIESLINSKI. 1992. Interaction between growth factors and retinoic acid in the induction of kidney tubulogenesis in tissue culture. Exp. Cell Res. **201:** 8–15.
29. HUMES, H., J. KRAUSS & D. CIESLINSKI, et al. 1996. Tubulogenesis from isolated single cells of adult mammalian kidney: clonal analysis with a recombinant retrovirus. Am. J. Physiol. **271:** F42–49.

30. OGAWA, S., Z. OTA, K. SHIKATA, et al. 1999. High-resolution ultrastructural comparison of renal glomerular and tubular basement membranes. Am. J. Nephrol. **19:** 686–693.
31. HUMES, H., S. MACKAY, A. FUNKE, et al. 1999. Tissue engineering of a bioartificial renal tubule assist device: *in vitro* transport and metabolic characteristics. Kidney Int. **55:** 2502–2514.
32. MACKAY, S., A. FUNKE, et al. 1998. Tissue engineering of a bioartificial renal tubule. ASAIO J. **44:** 179–183.
33. BOYUM, A. 1998. Isolation of mononuclear cells and granulocytes from human blood. Scand. J. Clin. Lab. Invest. **21:** 77.
34. KIMBALL, J., A. FUNKE, D. BUFFINGTON, et al. 2000. Effect of porcine cytokines on human peripheral blood mononuclear cells. Abstract. J. Am. Soc. Nephrol. **11:** 665A.
35. COZZI, E., S. MASROOR, B. SOIN, et al. 2000. Progress in xenotransplantation. Clin. Nephrol. **53:** 13–18.
36. GODDARD, M., J. FOWERAKER & J. WALLWORK. 2000. Xenotransplantation-2000. J. Clin. Pathol. **53:** 44–48.
37. HUMES, H., D. BUFFINGTON, S. MACKAY, et al. 1999. Replacement of renal function in uremic animals with a tissue-engineered kidney. Nat. Biotech. **17:** 451–455.
38. NATANSON, C., P. ELCHENHOLZ, R. DANNER, et al. 1989. Endotoxin and tumor necrosis factor challenges in dogs simulate the cardiovascular profile of human septic shock. J. Exp. Med. **169:** 823–832.

# Derivation of Pharmacokinetics Equations for Quantitative Evaluation of Bioartificial Liver Functions

Y.-G. PARK, H. IWATA, AND Y. IKADA

*Institute for Frontier Medical Sciences, Kyoto University, Kyoto, Japan*

ABSTRACT: A bioartificial liver (BAL) is an extracorporeal medical device incorporating living hepatocytes in a cartridge. A variety of BALs have been developed and new devices are being introduced. Some of them have been clinically applied and from the results obtained they are claimed to be useful devices for assisting the liver functions of patients. However, there is still uncertainty as to their efficacy and their limitations are not clear. It is important to establish methods to quantitatively evaluate the metabolic and synthetic functions of BAL. In this paper, we derive simple equations for the quantitative evaluation of BAL functions on the basis of pharmacokinetics. Pharmacokinetics was originally developed to understand the processes of absorption, distribution, and elimination of administered drugs. Metabolic functions of the natural liver have been analyzed using pharmacokinetics and values of the useful parameters, clearance ($CL$) and intrinsic clearance ($CL_{int}$), have been reported. The metabolic functions of the BAL expressed using values of CL and CLint are easily compared with those of the normal human liver. We believe that our method provides a useful basis for estimating the clinical effectiveness of BAL.

KEYWORDS: pharmacokinetics; quantitative evaluation; bioartificial liver; *in vitro* circulating system

## INTRODUCTION

Bioartificial livers (BALs) are extracorporeal medical devices that incorporate living hepatocytes in a cartridge. They have been developed to assist the liver functions of patients with severe liver failure. Several research groups[1–4] have started clinical applications of their BAL devices. For example, the group at Cedars-Sinai medical center in Los Angeles has demonstrated the safety of their BAL[1] and Circe biomedical group has started multicenter trials to collect the data required to show the efficacy of their BAL. However, the multiplicity of liver functions is so great that it is still unknown what functions BAL should support in the treatment of patients with severe liver failure. Furthermore, there have been few studies to establish methods for quantitative evaluation of BAL functions. The authors believe that it is important to establish methods for quantitatively evaluating the metabolic and

Address for correspondence: H. Iwata, 53 Kawahara-cho, Shogoin, Sakyo-ku, Kyoto 606-8507, Japan. Voice: +81-75-751-4119; fax: +81-75-751-4144.
iwata@frontier.kyoto-u.ac.jp

synthetic functions of BAL in order to compare the functions of BAL with each other, and with those of the normal human liver.

In this paper we derive pharmacokinetics equations that can evaluate the concentration decreases in drugs loaded to the *in vitro* circuit and the concentration increases in the substances produced by BAL. Pharmacokinetics provides a basis for the studies on drug absorption, distribution, and elimination, and also for the dynamics of these processes.[5] The authors believe that it also provides a suitable basis for the quantitative evaluation of BAL functions.

## EQUATIONS FOR FUNCTIONAL EVALUATION OF BAL

### Basic Equations

Some BAL systems contain, not only a BAL cartridge, but also a plasmapheresis cartridge and/or a charcoal cartridge. The functions of BAL systems are modified by these appendices, although they are mainly determined by the BAL cartridge. However, difficulties in the quantitative functional evaluation of the BAL cartridge itself are encountered in such BAL systems. An *in vitro* circuit that is used for the evaluation of the BAL cartridge functions should be set up as simply as possible, as shown in FIGURE 1. The circuit consists of a BAL cartridge, an oxygenator, and a reservoir connected by tubes.

In this study, pharmacokinetics equations that describe the concentration changes in the drug are derived using the well-stirred model.[5] In this model, instantaneous, complete mixing is assumed to occur within the BAL cartridge. A drug is loaded into the reservoir by a bolus ($D$) at time zero, followed by continuous infusion at a constant rate ($R$). The drug exists in various forms, such as in a free state or bond to plasma proteins and blood cells. Unless otherwise stated, a concentration is defined by the total amount of the drug in any form in a unit volume of the perfusate. The drug is brought into the BAL cartridge by the perfusate at the concentration $C_1$ in the reservoir, and a fraction of the drug is metabolized by the hepatocytes in the BAL cartridge and then the perfusate leaves it with a reduced drug concentration $C_2$.

Clearance ($CL$) is the most important parameter in pharmacokinetics and is defined as the volume of the inflow to the BAL cartridge from which the drug would be entirely removed in unit time. Thus, the rate of drug metabolism in BAL is expressed by:

$$R_m = CLC_1 \tag{1}$$

The changes in drug amounts in the reservoir and the BAL cartridge, respectively, can be expressed by the following differential equations:

$$\frac{dX_1}{dt} = -QC_1 + QC_2 + R \tag{2}$$

$$\frac{dX_2}{dt} = -QC_2 + QC_1 - CLC_1, \tag{3}$$

where $Q$ is the circulating rate of the perfusate, $X_1$ and $X_2$ are the drug amounts in the reservoir and the BAL cartridge, respectively. The drug concentrations in the

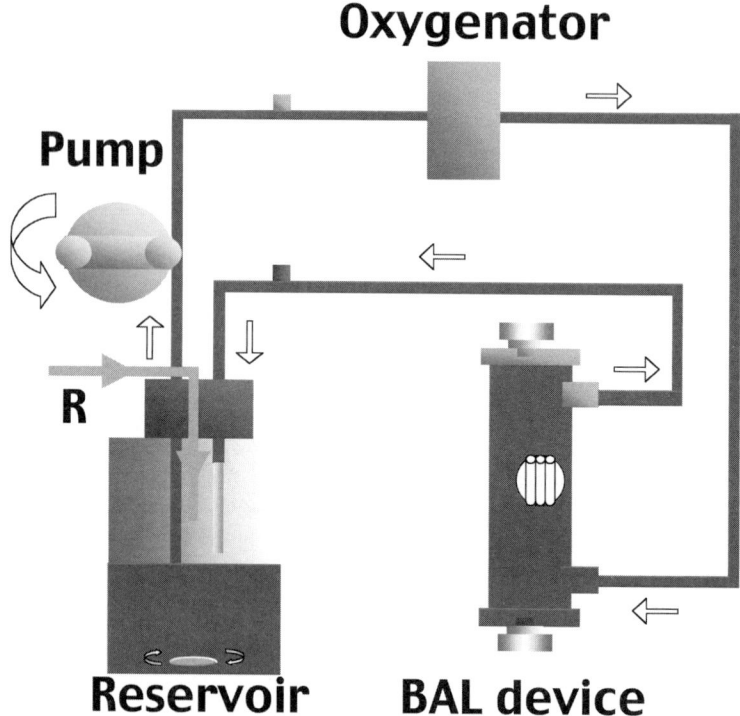

**FIGURE 1.** Schematic representation of the *in vitro* circulating system employed for bioartificial liver functional analyses. The perfusate is assumed to be composed of culture medium, plasma, and blood cells and is well mixed in the reservoir.

reservoir, the oxygenator, and the tubes from the reservoir to the BAL can be assumed to be the same as $C_1$. Equation (2) can be rewritten as:

$$V_1 \frac{dC_1}{dt} = -QC_1 + QC_2 + R, \tag{4}$$

where $V_1$ is the total volume of the reservoir, the oxygenator, and the tubes. When the well-stirred model is employed, the drug concentration in the BAL cartridge is assumed to be homogeneous and to be the same as that of the outflow, $C_2$. Equation (3) can be rewritten:

$$V_2 \frac{dC_2}{dt} = -QC_2 + QC_1 - CLC_1, \tag{5}$$

where $V_2$ is the total volume of the BAL cartridge and the tubes from the BAL to the reservoir. However, it rarely corresponds to the real volume since some drugs might adsorb on the large surface of hollow fibers, and some of the inner space of the BAL cartridge is occupied by hepatocytes. The former effect increases the $V_2$ value, whereas the latter reduces it. In addition, drugs binding to hepatocytes also introduce uncertainty in the value of $V_2$. It is not realistic to determine its value geometrically from the experimental setup. Thus, this value should be determined from the pharmacokinetics analyses of a drug-loading test.

The initial conditions at time zero for $C_1$ and $C_2$, which are used to solve the two simultaneous differential Equations **(4)** and **(5)**, are assumed to be:

$$C_1\big|_{t=0} = \frac{D}{V_1}, \quad C_2\big|_{t=0} = 0, \tag{6}$$

where $D$ is the amount of the drug loaded by the bolus injection at time zero.

Solving Equations **(4)** and **(5)** under the initial conditions **(6)** yields:

$$C_1 = \frac{QR}{V_1 V_2 \alpha \beta} + \frac{(D\alpha - R)(Q - \alpha V_2)}{V_1 V_2 \alpha (\beta - \alpha)} e^{-\alpha t} + \frac{(D\beta - R)(Q - \beta V_2)}{V_1 V_2 \beta (\alpha - \beta)} e^{-\beta t} \tag{7}$$

$$C_2 = \frac{(Q - CL)R}{V_1 V_2 \alpha \beta} + \frac{(D\alpha - R)(Q - CL)}{V_1 V_2 \alpha (\beta - \alpha)} e^{-\alpha t} + \frac{(D\beta - R)(Q - CL)}{V_1 V_2 \beta (\alpha - \beta)} e^{-\beta t}. \tag{8}$$

Here, $\alpha$ and $\beta$ are given by:

$$\alpha = \frac{1}{2}\left[\left(\frac{Q}{V_1} + \frac{Q}{V_2}\right) + \left\{\left(\frac{Q}{V_1} + \frac{Q}{V_2}\right)^2 - \frac{4CLQ}{V_1 V_2}\right\}^{1/2}\right] \tag{9}$$

$$\beta = \frac{1}{2}\left[\left(\frac{Q}{V_1} + \frac{Q}{V_2}\right) - \left\{\left(\frac{Q}{V_1} + \frac{Q}{V_2}\right)^2 - \frac{4CLQ}{V_1 V_2}\right\}^{1/2}\right] \tag{10}$$

These equations can be simplified for each experimental setup.

## *Bolus-Loading Test*

The bolus administration is a simple method for drug-loaded tests. In this method, the constant infusion rate, $R$, is zero in the above equations. The decrease in the drug concentration in the reservoir is given by the sum of the two exponential terms as expressed by Eq. **(7)** under $R = 0$. The term $e^{-\alpha t}$, which is mainly determined by dilution of the drugs in the BAL cartridge, approaches zero more rapidly than does the term $e^{-\beta t}$. Hence, when the concentration $C_1$ is plotted against the perfusion time ($t$) on a semilogarithmic scale, the initial fall is rapid, followed by a slower decline. After a certain time interval, the term $e^{-\alpha t}$ becomes virtually zero, and thus, the extrapolated line is expressed by:

$$\underline{C}_1 = \frac{D(Q - \beta V_2)}{V_1 V_2 (\alpha - \beta)} e^{-\beta t} = B e^{-\beta}. \tag{11}$$

Subtracting $\underline{C}_1$ from $C_1$ yields:

$$C_1 - \underline{C}_1 = \frac{D(Q - \alpha V_2)}{V_1 V_2 (\beta - \alpha)} e^{-\alpha t} = A e^{-\alpha t}. \tag{12}$$

Equation **(12)** expresses the initial rapid fall. The values of $\alpha$ and $\beta$, and $A$ and $B$ can be determined from the slope and the zero-time intercept of the linear fitting semilogarithmic plots of Eqs. **(11)** and **(12)** with the experimental data. The relationships between a set of parameters, $\alpha$ and $\beta$, and $A$ and $B$, with another set of parameters, $V_1$, $V_2$, and $CL$, are given by:

$$A + B = \frac{D}{V_1} \tag{13}$$

$$\alpha + \beta = \frac{Q}{V_1} + \frac{Q}{V_2} \tag{14}$$

$$\alpha\beta = \frac{CLQ}{V_1 V_2} \tag{15}$$

$$\frac{A}{\alpha} + \frac{B}{\beta} = \frac{D}{CL}. \tag{16}$$

The $CL$ value can be determined from Eq. (16) using the values of $\alpha$ and $\beta$, and $A$ and $B$, and the amount of the drug loaded ($D$). The value of $V_2$ that can be obtained from Eq. (14) or Eq. (15) will give information about the interaction between the drug and the BAL cartridge.

It is tedious to estimate the $CL$ value from the values of the parameters, $A$, $B$, $\alpha$, and $\beta$ that are determined by applying Eqs. (11) and (12) to the observations. If attention is paid to the fact that integration of $C_1$ with time gives the total area under the concentration–time curve ($AUC$),[5] the $CL$ value can be more easily estimated. The left side of Eq. (16) is derived by integration of Eq. (7), with the assistance of Eqs. (11) and (12), from time zero to infinite time. Thus, $AUC$ is expressed by:

$$AUC = \frac{A}{\alpha} + \frac{B}{\beta}. \tag{17}$$

Equations (16) and (17) give:

$$CL = \frac{D}{AUC}. \tag{18}$$

A value for $AUC$ can be easily obtained by the trapezoidal rule from the observations. The $CL$ value can be estimated using Eq. (18) from the values of $D$ and $AUC$. This is the simplest method to determine the $CL$ value. However, it can be more accurately determined, and other valuable information can be obtained at the same time, by using Eqs. (7), (14), (15), and (16) as discussed above.

### *Constant Infusion Test*

When a drug solution is infused into the reservoir at a constant rate $R$, without bolus administration, the drug concentration in the perfusate continues to increase until a plateau is reached. After that, the input rate equals the clear rate, so that a simple equation is derived.

$$R = CLC_1\big|_{t = \infty}, \tag{19}$$

where $C_1\big|_{t = \infty}$ is the concentration at the infinite infusion time. This can also be derived from Eqs. (4) and (5). After the stationary-state condition is achieved,

$$0 = -QC_1\big|_{t = \infty} + QC_2\big|_{t = \infty} + R \tag{20}$$

$$0 = -QC_2\big|_{t = \infty} + QC_1\big|_{t = \infty} - CLC_1\big|_{t = \infty}. \tag{21}$$

Appropriate rearrangements give

$$R = CLC_1\big|_{t=\infty} \tag{22}$$

$$R = \frac{C_2\big|_{t=\infty}}{\dfrac{1}{CL} - \dfrac{1}{Q}} \tag{23}$$

The $CL$ value can be simply evaluated by using Eq. (22), from the plateau level of the drug concentration in the reservoir.

Since the drug is removed during passage through the BAL cartridge, it provides a measurable concentration gradient between the inlet and the outlet of the BAL cartridge. The relationship between the $CL$ value and the trans-BAL drug concentration difference can be derived from Eqs. (21) and (22) as follows:

$$C_1\big|_{t=\infty} - C_2\big|_{t=\infty} = \frac{R}{Q} = \frac{CLC_1\big|_{t=\infty}}{Q} \tag{24}$$

Thus, the $CL$ value can also be evaluated using this relationship.

The evaluation methods described above are simple, but the experiment is time consuming, since there can be long delay between the start of the infusion and the establishment of the plateau concentration. The concentration change exhibits biexponential disposition characteristics expressed by Eq. (7), in which $D$ should be taken as zero for the constant infusion test without the bolus administration. The halflives of the second and third terms of Eq. (7) are given by:

$$t_{\alpha_{1/2}} = \frac{0.693}{\alpha} \tag{25}$$

$$t_{\beta_{1/2}} = \frac{0.693}{\beta}. \tag{26}$$

Theoretically, a plateau is only reached when a drug solution has been infused for an infinite number of halflives. It takes four halflives to reach 94% of the plateau. It is desirable to exclude this time-consuming step for the $CL$ determination.

Since $\beta$ is assumed to be smaller than $\alpha$, the rate-limiting step is caused by the third term of the right side of Eq. (7). The long tail of the concentration increase can be removed by an initial bolus injection:

$$D = \frac{R}{\beta}. \tag{27}$$

Equation (7) becomes

$$C_1 = \frac{QR}{V_1 V_2 \alpha \beta} - R\frac{\left(\dfrac{Q}{V_2} - \alpha\right)}{V_1 \alpha \beta} e^{-\alpha t} = \frac{R}{CL} - R\frac{\left(\dfrac{Q}{V_2} - \alpha\right)}{V_1 \alpha \beta} e^{-\alpha t} \tag{28}$$

The plateau concentration ($C_1\big|_{t=\infty} = R/CL$) is nearly attained after 4 $t_{\alpha_{1/2}}$ by combination of the bolus administration $R/\beta$, and the constant infusion $R$. However, there is a self contradiction in this method for the determination of the $CL$ value, since the $CL$ value should be known beforehand in order to calculate the $\beta$ value. This method can only be applied to confirm a $CL$ value obtained by other methods.

## Intrinsic Clearance

The perfusate flow rate influences the clearance of the loaded drug, because the perfusate delivers the drug to the BAL cartridge in which it is cleared.[5] Binding of the drug to plasma proteins and blood cells determines whether the drug will cross the membrane or not. The extent of this binding determines how much of the drug is available in a form that can be cleared. Thus, the metabolic capacity of the BAL system setup, as shown in FIGURE 1 is a function of the intrinsic metabolic capacity of the BAL system, the perfusate flow rate, and the binding of drug to plasma proteins and blood cells. The *CL* value, which can be evaluated by the methods described above, only reflects the metabolic capacity of the BAL system under a certain experimental condition. Intrinsic clearance ($CL_{int}$), which can represent the intrinsic metabolic capacity of the BAL cartridge, should be introduced. This is useful as a quantitative comparison of the metabolic functions of the BAL cartridge with those of human liver or the BAL cartridges of other groups.

The intrinsic clearance ($CL_{int}$) relates the metabolic rate of a drug to its unbound concentration at the enzyme site. In this paper, we adopted the well-stirred model in which instantaneous, complete mixing is assumed to occur within the BAL cartridge. The equations derived under this model represent simple, and predictably significant features of $CL_{int}$. Rowland et al.[6] reported that the well-stirred model is suitable for predicting the *in vivo* phamacokinetics behavior of loaded lidocaine, which has been frequently employed to evaluate the detoxification ability of the human liver and BAL. The removal rate of a drug from the perfusate $R_m$ is expressed by

$$R_m = CL_{int} f_{uB} C_2, \qquad (29)$$

where $f_{uB}$ is defined as the concentration of unbound drug in plasma divided by concentration of drug in perfusate.

The removal rate of a drug from the perfusate is also expressed by Eq. (1). Thus:

$$CLC_1 = CL_{int} f_{uB} C_2. \qquad (30)$$

Under the stationary-state condition, the relationship of $C_1$ and $C_2$ is given by Eq. (21). From Eqs. (21) and (30), the clearance *CL* is expressed using the intrinsic clearance ($CL_{int}$) and the perfusate flow rate ($Q$) as

$$CL = \frac{Q CL_{int} f_{uB}}{Q + CL_{int} f_{uB}}. \qquad (31)$$

Equation (31) predicts that the *CL* increases with the increasing flow rate of the perfusate and approaches a plateau at the infinite flow rate, that is, $CL_{int} f_{uB}$.

## Bolus Loading of a Large Amount of a Drug

The galactose-loading test has been clinically used for patients with hepatic failure to determine the functional liver mass.[7] It has also been adopted to evaluate the metabolic function of BALs.[8,9] The concentration of galactose, administered by bolus *in vivo*, declines exponentially with time only in a low concentration range (less than 200 μg/ml).[10] The galactose *CL* value can be estimated in a manner similar to the methods mentioned above under such circumstances. However, the enzymatic method, which has been conventionally used in clinical tests to determine galactose concentrations, is not sensitive enough to determine such low concentrations. Galactose pharmacokinetics in a high concentration range have been clinically studied and the galactose elimination capacity (GEC) instead of the $CL$ has been used to express the functional liver mass remaining in patients for more than 30 years. The galactose elimination capacity is defined by[11]

$$\text{GEC} = -(V_1 + V_2)\frac{d[G]}{dt}, \quad (32)$$

where [G] is the galactose concentration. This can be related to the pharmacokinetics parameters used above as follows. The galactose concentration change after bolus loading can also be expressed by Eqs. (4) and (5). When the well-stirred model is employed, Eq. (5) can be rewritten using Eq. (30):

$$V_2\frac{dC_2}{dt} = -QC_2 + QC_1 - CL_{\text{int}}f_{uB}C_2 \quad (33)$$

Since phosphorylation of galactose to galactose-1-phosphate is involved as a rate-determining process in the elimination of the loaded galactose,[11] the galactose metabolic velocity can be assumed to obey the simple kinetics of enzymatic reactions (Michaelis-Menten kinetics).[12] The rate of metabolism is expressed by

$$R_g = \frac{V_{\max}C_2 f_{uB}}{K_m + C_2 f_{uB}}. \quad (34)$$

Consequently,

$$CL_{\text{int}} = \frac{V_{\max}}{K_m + C_2 f_{uB}}, \quad (35)$$

where $V_{\max}$ is the maximum elimination rate and $K_m$ is the Michaelis-Menten constant. Since the galactose concentration is much higher than the reported $K_m$ value[13] in most of the galactose loading tests for BAL functional evaluations, the enzyme site is saturated with galactose. Equation (36) can be simplified to

$$CL_{\text{int}} = \frac{V_{\max}}{C_2 f_{uB}}. \quad (36)$$

Thus, addition of Eq. (2) to (33) without constant infusion ($R = 0$) gives:

$$V_1\frac{dC_1}{dt} + V_2\frac{dC_2}{dt} = -V_{\max}. \quad (37)$$

Since galactose elimination is not rapid, the difference between $C_1$ and $C_2$ is small. As a result, Eq. (37) can be simplified to

$$(V_1 + V_2)\frac{dC_1}{dt} = \frac{d(\text{Galactose amount})}{dt} = -\text{GEC} = -V_{\max}. \quad (38)$$

Integrating Eq. (38) from the time of the drug administration to time $t$ provides

$$C_1 - C_1\big|_{t=0} = \frac{-tV_{\max}}{V_1 + V_2} = \frac{-t\text{GEC}}{V_1 + V_2}. \quad (39)$$

Thus, the value of GEC can be determined from the slope of the linear plot of $C_1$ against the perfusion time using Eq. (39).

## Synthesis

The liver performs crucial functions to produce various bioactive substances, such as blood coagulation factors. Their syntheses by a BAL cartridge are beneficial to patients with severe liver failure. Changes in $C_1$ and $C_2$ of a bioactive substance in the reservoir and the BAL cartridge, respectively, are as follows:

$$V_1 \frac{dC_1}{dt} = -QC_1 + QC_2 \tag{40}$$

$$V_2 \frac{dC_2}{dt} = -QC_2 + QC_1 + R_p, \tag{41}$$

where $R_p$ is a synthesis rate of the bioactive substance by the BAL cartridge. The initial conditions at time zero for $C_1$ and $C_2$, which will be used to solve the two simultaneous differential equations, are

$$C_1\big|_{t=0} = 0, \quad C_2\big|_{t=0} = 0. \tag{42}$$

Solving Eqs. (40) and (41) under these conditions yields

$$C_1 = \frac{RV_1 V_2}{Q(V_1 + V_2)^2}\left(e^{-\left(\frac{Q}{V_1} + \frac{Q}{V_2}\right)t} - 1\right) + \frac{Rt}{V_1 + V_2} \tag{43}$$

$$C_2 = \frac{RV_1^2}{Q(V_1 + V_2)^2}\left(1 - e^{-\left(\frac{Q}{V_1} + \frac{Q}{V_2}\right)t}\right) + \frac{Rt}{V_1 + V_2}. \tag{44}$$

After a transient period, $C_1$ linearly increases with time. The slope of the linearly increased part gives $R/(V_1 + V_2)$ and the intercept of the extrapolation of the linear part to the time axis gives $V_1 V_2/Q(V_1 + V_2)$. Values of $Q$ and $V_1$ are determined from the experimental setup. However, some uncertainty might be introduced in determining the value of $V_2$ when produced substance is adsorbed on the large surface of the BAL cartridge. Thus, we recommend that $R$ and $V_2$ are determined from the slope and the intercept of the time axis.

## DISCUSSION

Several research groups have carried out drug-loading tests on BALs to evaluate their functions. Each group analyzed the results of loading using its own method and presented the BAL functions in a unique form. Therefore, the reported values do not allow us to compare the BAL metabolic abilities with each other. In addition, it is difficult to predict from the reported values the proportion of the metabolic capacity of the normal human liver that can be replaced by their BAL. We proposed that the detoxification abilities of a BAL cartridge are expressed using $CL$ and $CL_{int}$, and GEC. These values can be directly compared with the reported $CL$ and $CL_{int}$, and GEC values of the normal human liver.

In the following, the authors discuss the methods reported by other groups and attempt to relate their parameters with $CL$ or $CL_{int}$. Ohshima et al.[14] took the permeation process through a membrane into consideration and derived three equations

$$V_1 \frac{dC_1}{dt} = -QC_1 + QC_{21} + R \tag{45}$$

$$V_{21} \frac{dC_{21}}{dt} = -QC_{21} + QC_1 - KA(C_{21} - C_{22}) \tag{46}$$

$$V_{22} \frac{dC_{22}}{dt} = KA(C_{21} - C_{22}) - K_s N_0 \upsilon C_{22} V_{22}, \tag{47}$$

where the subscripts 1, 21, and 22 represent the reservoir, the shell space, and the inner space separated by a membrane, respectively, $K$ is the overall mass transfer coefficient, $A$ is the surface contact area of the membrane, $N_0$ is the initial number of living hepatocytes, $K_s$ is the metabolic reaction rate constant, and $\upsilon$ is the ratio of living hepatocytes to the whole cell population.

There are many variations in BAL systems. They can be classified into two groups from the standpoint of how to expose hepatocytes to patient blood or plasma. It is not necessary to take the permeations step into consideration in the systems where the hepatocytes are directly exposed to patient blood or plasma.[8,15] In such systems, it is not necessary to assume differences in concentrations between the shell space and the inner space. Equations (45) and (46) are reduced to

$$V_1 \frac{dC_1}{dt} = -QC_1 + QC_2 + R \tag{48}$$

$$V_2 \frac{dC_2}{dt} = -QC_2 + QC_1 - K_s N_0 \upsilon C_2 V_{22}, \tag{49}$$

where $V_2$ is the total volume, $V_{21} + V_{22}$, of the BAL cartridge and $C_2$ is the drug concentration in the BAL cartridge. From a comparison of Eqs. (2) and (33) with Eqs. (48) and (49), the coefficient of the third term of the left side of Eq. (49), $K_s N_0 \upsilon V_{22} K_t$ appears to be equivalent to $CL_{int} f_{uB}$.

In other systems,[3,16] hepatocytes are exposed to patient blood or plasma through a semipermeable membrane. A BAL cartridge should be designed in which toxin permeation through the membrane is not a rate-limiting step. There should be no difficulty in finding a highly permeable membrane, since a variety of membranes have been developed for various medical devices. When the permeation rates of toxins through a membrane are higher than the toxin metabolic rate by BAL, the quasiequilibrium of the toxin concentration between the blood side and the hepatocyte existing side is established, and thus, toxin distribution through the membrane can be simply expressed using $C_{21}$ and the partition coefficient $K_t$, instead of $KA(C_{21} - C_{22})$. Equations (45), (46), and (47) can be simplified to

$$V_1 \frac{dC_1}{dt} = -QC_1 + QC_{21} + R \tag{50}$$

$$(V_{21} + K_t V_{22}) \frac{dC_{21}}{dt} = -QC_{21} + QC_1 - K_s N_0 \upsilon V_{22} K_t C_{21}. \tag{51}$$

From a comparison of Eqs. (4) and (33) with Eqs. (50) and (51), the coefficient of the third term of the left side of Eq. (51) $K_s N_0 \upsilon V_{22} K_t$ appears to be equivalent to the $CL_{int} f_{uB}$, and the term $(V_{21} + K_t V_{22})$ can be replaced by the apparent volume $V_2$.

Although the Ohshima's expression apparently gives a deeper insight into the meaning of $CL_{int}f_{uB}$, each parameter cannot be separately determined from the analysis of the detoxification behavior of BAL. Furthermore, the detoxification ability of BAL as a cartridge, that is expressed by $CL$ or $CL_{int}$, but not that of each cell and living cell number, is important in determining the clinical efficacy of the BAL. Equations (**4**) and (**5**) are sufficient to assess the detoxification ability of a BAL cartridge.

Nyberg *et al.*[17] carried out pharmacokinetics studies for quantitative estimation of their BAL functions. They employed a single compartment model to analyze the concentration decay curves after lidocaine loading. Their experimental data were well reproduced by the single compartment model, but it has several disadvantages. (1) In most drug-loaded tests, the semilogarithmic plot of the drug concentration with time does not give a single straight line. (2) It is difficult to relate the parameters used in the single compartment model to those used to express the experimental set-up for an *in vitro* closed circuit. (3) Although the elimination rate of the loaded drug depends on the perfusate flow rate as discussed above in relation to $CL_{int}$; however, the single compartment does not take this into consideration. All these disadvantages come from the implicit assumption included in the single compartment model, where the perfusing rate is assumed to be so high, or the drug metabolic rate is assumed to be so slow, and thus the difference in the drug concentration between the inflow and the outflow of the BAL is negligible.

Pharmacokinetics was originally developed to understand the processes of absorption, distribution, and elimination of administered drugs. They can also provide various useful concepts to quantitatively evaluate the metabolic capacities of BAL. In this study, we derived the equations on the basis of pharmacokinetics to quantitatively evaluate the metabolic functions of BAL. These can be easily expressed using $CL$ and $CL_{int}$ and compared with those of the normal human liver. The authors believe that the method reported in this paper gives a useful basis for estimating the clinical efficacy of BAL.

## ACKNOWLEDGMENT

This work was supported by Grant JSPS-RFTF 96I 00204 from the Japan Society for the Promotion of Science.

## REFERENCES

1. KAMOHARA, Y., J. ROZGA & A.A. DEMETRIOU. 1998. Artificial liver: review and Cedars-Sinai experience. Hepatobiliary Pancreat. Surg. **5**(3): 273–852.
2. BUSSE, B. & J.C. GERLACH. 1999. Bioreactors for hybrid liver support: historical aspects and novel designs. Ann. N.Y. Acad. Sci. **875**: 326–339.
3. SUSSMAN, N.L., G.T. GISLASON & J.H. KELLY. 1994. Extracorporeal liver support: application to fulminant hepatic failure. J. Clin. Gastroenterol. **18**(4): 320–324.
4. RIORDAN, S.M. & R. WILLIAMS. 2000. Acute liver failure: targeted artificial and hepatocyte-based support of liver regeneration and reversal of multiorgan failure. J. Hepatol. **32**(1 Suppl): 63–76.
5. ROWLAND, M. & T.N. TOZER. 1989. Clinical Pharmacokinetics: Concepts and Applications. 101–193. Lea & Febiger, Philadelphia.

6. PANG, K.S. & M. ROWLAND. 1977. Hepatic clearance of drugs. II. Experimental evidence for acceptance of the well-stirred model over the parallel tube model using lidocaine in the perfused rat liver in situ preparation. J. Pharmacokinet. Biopharm. **5**(6): 655–680.
7. FABBRI, A., G. BIANCHI, E. MOTTA, et al. 1996. The galactose elimination capacity test: a study of the technique based on the analysis of 868 measurements. Am. J. Gastroenterol. **91:** 991–996.
8. GERLACH, J.C., J. ENCKE, O. HOLE, et al. 1994. Bioreactor for a larger scale hepatocyte in vitro perfusion. Transplantation **58**(9): 984–988.
9. FLENDRIG, L.M., J.W. LA-SOE, G.G. JORNING, et al. 1997. In vitro evaluation of a novel bioreactor based on an integral oxygenator and a spirally wound nonwoven polyester matrix for hepatocyte culture as small aggregates. J. Hepatol. **26**(6): 1379–1392.
10. HU, O.Y., T.M. HU & H.S. TANG. 1995. Determination of galactose in human blood by high-performance liquid chromatography: comparison with an enzymatic method and application to the pharmacokinetic study of galactose in patients with liver dysfunction. J. Pharm. Sci. **84**(2): 231–235.
11. FRIEDMAN, L.S., P. MARTIN & S.J. MUNOZ. 1996. Liver function tests and the objective evaluation of the patient with liver disease. In Hepatology. A Textbook of Liver Disease, 3rd edit. D. Zakin & T.D. Boyer, Eds.: 805–806. W.B. Saunders Company, Philadelphia.
12. KEIDING, S., S. JOHANSEN, K. WINKLER, et al. 1976. Michaelis-Menten kinetics of galactose elimination by the isolated perfused pig liver. Am. J. Physiol. **230:** 1302–1313.
13. KEIDING, S., S. JOHANSEN & K. WINKLER. 1982. Hepatic galactose elimination kinetics in the intact pig. Scand. J. Clin. Lab. Invest. **42:** 253–259.
14. OHSHIMA, N., M. SHIOTA, H. KUSANO, et al. 1994. Kinetic analyses of the performance of a hybrid-type artificial liver support system utilizing isolated hepatocytes. Mater. Sci. Engin. C1 **79:** 8515.
15. HASEGAWA, H., M. SHIMADA, T. GION, et al. 1999. Modulation of immunologic reactions between cultured porcine hepatocytes and human sera. ASAIO J. **45**(5): 392–396.
16. IWATA, H., T. SAJIKI, H. MAEDA, et al. 1999. In vitro evaluation of metabolic functions of a bioartificial liver. ASAIO J. **45**(4): 299–306.
17. NYBERG, S.L., H.J. MANN, R.P. REMMEL, et al. 1993. Pharmacokinetic analysis verifies P450 function during in vitro and in vivo application of a bioartificial liver. ASAIO J. **39:** M252–M256.

# Development of a Hybrid Liver Support System

I.M. SAUER, N. OBERMEYER, D. KARDASSIS,
T. THERUVATH, AND J.C. GERLACH

*Medizinische Fakultät der Humboldt Universität zu Berlin, Berlin, Germany*

ABSTRACT: Hybrid liver systems are being developed as temporary extracorporeal liver support therapy. The overview given here emphasizes the development of both hepatocyte culture models for bioreactors and of systems for clinical therapy. *In vitro* studies demonstrate long term external metabolic function in isolated primary hepatocytes within bioreactors. These systems are capable of supporting essential liver functions. Animal experiments verify the possibility of upscaling bioreactors for clinical treatment. However, since there is no reliable animal model for investigating the treatment of acute liver failure, the promising results obtained from these studies have limited relevance to human beings. The small number of clinical studies performed thus far are not sufficient to enable any conclusions concerning improvements in the therapy of acute liver failure. Although important progress has been made in the development of these systems, multiple hepatocyte culture models and bioreactor constructions are being discussed in the literature, indicating competition in this field of medical research. For the use of hepatocytes and sinusoidal endothelial cells in coculture, a bioreactor has been designed. The construction is based on capillaries for hepatocyte aggregate immobilization. Four separate capillary membrane systems, each permitting a different function, are woven in order to create a three-dimensional network. Cells are perfused via independent capillary membrane compartments. Decentralized oxygen supply and carbon dioxide removal with low gradients is possible. The parallel use of identical units enables easy upscaling. Initial studies on the use of discarded organs that are unsuitable for transplantation as a source for primary human liver cells seem to be promising.[1]

KEYWORDS: hybrid liver support system; bioreactor

## INTRODUCTION

Recent developments in biotechnology have enabled the clinical use of temporary extracorporeal hybrid liver support. Contrary to implantable hepatocyte systems[2] for therapy of chronic liver diseases, the authors have focused on extracorporeal liver support systems (LSS) for temporary extracorporeal therapy[3] in acute liver failure (ALF). In publications concerning biotechnology-based therapy systems for acute liver failure, various terms are used to describe these systems. We believe that these should distinguish between:

Address for correspondence: Dr. med. Igor M. Sauer, Charité, Campus Virchow-Klinikum, Medizinische Fakultät der Humboldt Universität zu Berlin, Klinik für Allgemein, Viszeral- und Transplantationschirurgie, Augustenburger Platz 1, D-13353 Berlin, Germany. Voice: +49-30-450-559002; fax: +49-30-450-552900.
igor.sauer@charite.de   <www.charite.de/avt>

*(a)* systems with additional non-biological components as therapeutic tools (e.g., charcoal columns and resin adsorbers), and

*(b)* systems based on biological components.

Demetriou *et al.* introduced the term "bioartificial liver" to describe the combination of liver cells in a system with an additional artificial detoxification component in the same circuit as the liver cells.[4] The term "cartridge" was used for the apparatus, containing hepatocytes, cultivated on microcarriers. The term "hybrid system" was applied by Chang *et al.*, in 1988, for therapeutic devices using biological tissue,[5] whereas Pappas used the term "hybrid liver" to describe liver cells cultivated in a bioreactor, and employed in extracorporeal perfusion systems.[6] Since tissue engineering aims to implement systems that support liver functions (including artificial detoxification), we use the term "hybrid liver" to describe combined systems. The term "cartridge" is employed for devices using liver cells in conventional culture techniques and the term "bioreactor" is used for systems employing liver cells forming liver tissue structures.

In developing an LSS two complementary basic approaches have been followed:

1. In order to reverse the deteriorating course of patients with acute liver failure and progressive hepatic coma, biochemical and physiological activity provided by liver cells is thought to be necessary.

2. Efforts are necessary to stabilize and maintain the cellular functions of primary liver cells. Consequently one of the biggest challenges of bioengineering and tissue engineering is to mimic the physiologic conditions and the optimization of the cellular microenvironment.

For both approaches, the clinical logistics, and the possibility of upscaling the device, need to be considered. As soon as the need for treatment arises, a long period of preparation may not be acceptable due to potentially dramatic progression of the disease and its complications.

All considerations are driven by the fact that our knowledge of the mechanisms of the disease and associated complications (namely progressive encephalopathy, hyperdynamic cardiovascular insufficiency, renal failure, and increased risk of infection) is limited. The success of orthotopic liver transplantation proves that biologic treatments are effective, whereas no benefit concerning survival has been shown for otherwise highly effective artificial detoxification methods. It is the aim of hybrid liver support to fill the gap between these two therapeutic concepts.

One of the most important questions concerning efficiency relates to the dimension of the appropriate cell mass. Although clinical and experimental studies of partial hepatectomy showed the possibility of survival after reduction of the liver mass to one-fifth, the cell mass necessary for LSS is not known. Transfer of the data concerning hepatectomy are too optimistic since the patient with ALF already presents dramatic disturbances in metabolic state compared to the compensated state of a patient with partial hepatectomy due to liver metastasis. Furthermore, the reduction in mass transfer of a LSS compared to the native liver should be mitigated by an efficient and biochemically active cell mass. Attempts at compromising between demands of bioengineering and cell physiology, as well as clinical and logistic requests during our own work are described.

## CONSIDERATIONS FOR THE DEVELOPMENT OF THE CULTURE MODEL

Conventional culture techniques lead to a remarkable alteration in the environmental conditions of liver cells in comparison to their *in vivo* situation.[7] Electron microscopy investigations have demonstrated that major differences in the ultrastructure of hepatocytes can be observed, when cultured in monolayer technique. The endocytosis of the junctional complexes with secondary effects on the orientation of the cytoskeleton and cell organelles are important findings.[8] If a culture model were able to support high cell densities,[9] as well as a free three-dimensional cell rearrangement, a more physiological microenvironment of hepatocytes could be established. Cell-to-cell aggregation[10] would enable the reconstruction of junctional complexes, as well as reorientation of the cytoskeleton and cell organelles *in vitro*. Furthermore, a liver tissue–like formation of parenchymal and non-parenchymal cells is thought to support cellular orientation and differentiated function. A culture technique in which the various cell populations can reorganize themselves into three-dimensional structures may result in a hepatocyte microenvironment more akin to the physiological situation along the liver sinusoids.

Most conventional culture models present important differences in mass exchange features, compared to the liver. They rely on diffusion for substrate exchange, whereas hepatocytes *in vivo* operate under continuous perfusion conditions. Furthermore the natural zonation within a liver lobulus results in gradients of oxygen, carbon dioxide and metabolites, and various metabolic functions can be identified along the liver sinusoids. In conventional culture models, gradients and vectors for metabolite transfer are often greatly distorted when compared with the *in vivo* situation. A culture technique that allows the cells to operate under more physiological conditions, for example, convection with low metabolite gradients, may result in a cell microenvironment more closely related to the situation in the liver sinusoids.

## BACKGROUND OF THE HYBRID LIVER DEVELOPMENT

In order to use primary hepatocytes for LSS with high cell mass (approximately half or one-third of the liver mass of an adult human), techniques for large scale cell isolation have been developed.[11–14] Liver cell immobilization is an important factor in the maintenance of differentiated hepatocyte function *in vitro*.[15] In addition, the immobilization technique appears to be problematic when several hundred grams of liver cells are to be cultivated. Furthermore, a module (bioreactor) is necessary in order to introduce a large cell mass into an extracorporeal circuit for therapeutic use. Monolayer cultivation of hepatocytes allows a cell density of $3 \times 10^5$ cells per cm$^2$. Scale up of monolayer cultures for 500 grams of cells would call for an adhesion surface of about 100 m$^2$. The monolayer technique seems to be inappropriate both for techniques of well-distributed cell seeding and for construction of modules ready for extracorporeal perfusion.[16] The surface can be enlarged using microcarriers. By using microcarriers, a cell density of $10^6$ cells per ml bioreactor volume can be achieved (depending on the microcarrier volume). In contrast, by high density immobilization between capillary membranes, more than $10^7$ cells can be used per milliliter bioreactor volume. For a cell mass of $10^{10}$ hepatocytes, considered a minimum for clinical application, this results in a construction of a 10-liter reactor for microcarrier culture and a 1-liter reactor for high cell density immobilization. Cell-to-cell aggregate formation,[17] leading to cell immobilization, allows the reduction of artificial substrates and reduces the total volume of the culture model.

From a clinical point of view it is important to decrease the volume of the culture model in order to reduce patients' extracorporeal plasma compartment. Unfortunately the spontaneous aggregation of the cells induces new problems. Special nutrition and oxygenation of larger cellular clusters must be guaranteed. The deconstruction of the vascular system of the liver during enzymatic dissociation calls for alternative solutions to enable sufficient mass exchange and oxygenation. Artificial flat sheet or hollow-fiber membranes, may act as substrate to immobilize cell aggregates.[18] In addition to cell immobilization,[19] the arrangement of membranes included in a bioreactor construction is able to define the size of the cellular aggregates.

Shape, chemical structure and permeability are all important membrane properties. Control of permeability make it possible to distinguish between hydrophilic and hydrophobic membranes. Hydrophilic membranes can be used, for example, for metabolite/plasma exchange and hydrophobic membranes for cell oxygenation.[20]

Numerous approaches are possible in the design of a bioreactor incorporating liver cells for plasma perfusion. Concerning the culture technique and bioreactor design we aimed to meet the following requirements:

- The ability to scale up for clinical application resembling a natural model of liver lobules and liver lobes.

- Reorganization of the isolated liver cell populations into three-dimensional structures.

- The attainment of suitable microenvironmental conditions leading to physiological gradients of plasma and oxygen compared to the liver sinusoids.

- The development of culture techniques enabling coculture of all liver cell populations.

## DEVELOPMENT OF A NOVEL BIOREACTOR

There are some disadvantages using conventional dialysis cartridges for seeding the cells and for extracorporeal perfusion. For example, oxygenation of the cells is possible only by external oxygenation of the circulating fluids. In the absence of hemoglobin, a very high flow rate is necessary to meet the demands of upscaled cell masses. Furthermore, any interruption of circulation will lead to hypoxia. Conventional dialysis cartridges only allow a reduced ultrafiltration rate from the inner-capillary space (ICS) to the outer-capillary space (OCS). Depending on the cartridge length and pressure gradients, zones of filtration from the ICS to OCS can be found at the inflow side of the cartridge. At the outflow side the flow direction is reversed. The result is a convection of fluids in the cell compartment only in a range of centimeters, compared to a maximum of 500 μm within the liver sinusoids. In addition, perfusion of the open ended, single bundle, hollow-fiber device allows a substantial part of the circulating fluid to be shunted without contact with the OCS.

In order to overcome these handicaps and to meet the demands of liver cells, a bioreactor was designed (see FIGURE 1). The system consists of interwoven hollow fiber membranes, creating a three-dimensional framework over which self-assembling hepatocyte aggregates are distributed. The more complex design requires the following explanatory notes: the bioreactor may be considered as three separate parallel hollow-fiber bundles. Two sets of hydrophilic, high NMWCO (about 300,000) hollow-fiber membranes are incorporated into the bioreactor. By closing one end of each set, plasma entering the reactor via one set must enter the extracapillary space before leaving the reactor, via the second set of membranes. An alternative way to enable high mass exchange would be through the cross flow plasma perfusion of the two capillary systems in the counter direction, by using both bundles. The third set of hollow fibers is made of hydrophobic membranes that are used for supply of oxygen and surplus $CO_2$ removal. A proprietary technique for combining these three sets of hollow-fiber membranes results in a complex extracapillary framework. The periphery of the bioreactor is sealed by polyurethane potting. This produces a central region in which the hepatocytes are distributed upon the membrane framework. The extracapillary space is, therefore, perfused with plasma (or culture medium) while gas exchange occurs by diffusion across the hydrophobic membranes. The framework allows a close localization of inflow-, outflow- and oxygenation-membranes. Due to the size of hollow fibers, distances of 400–800 μm are produced in the extracapillary space. Therefore, a multitude of repetitive units for perfusion and oxygenation are formed. The bioreactor design allows further independent capillary systems to be added. Additional functions could be integrated into the module. For example, the incorporation of dialysis membranes or the use of adsorbents are both feasible. The use of water-impermeable capillaries as a heat exchanger might also permit cryopreservation of cells within the reactor.

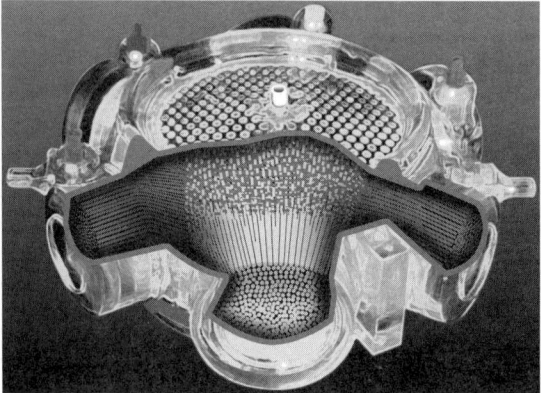

**FIGURE 1.** Bioreactor construction with three independent capillary membrane systems that create a three-dimensional artificial framework for adhesion, aggregation, and reorganization of tissue structures. One capillary system enables oxygen supply.

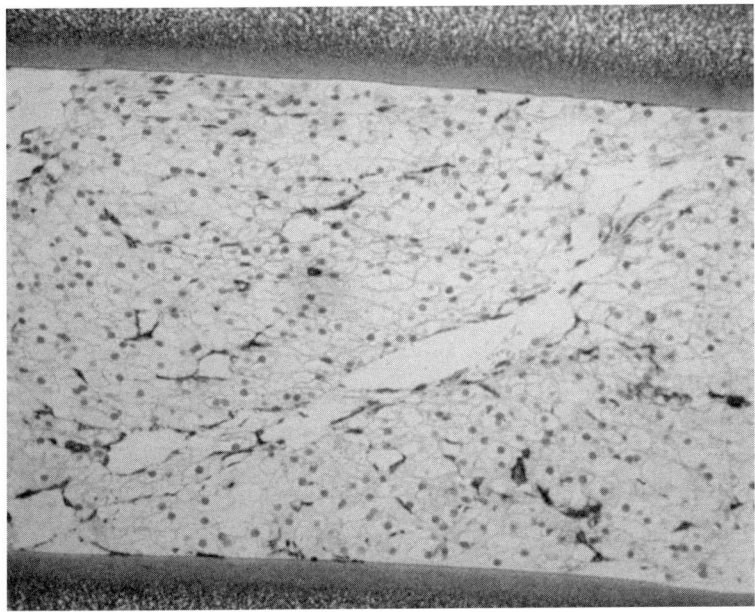

**FIGURE 2.** Cell reoganization by coculture of parenchymal and non-parenchymal cells between the capillaries (light microscopy).

In this bioreactor (FIG. 1) liver cell populations immobilize to aggregates, produce their own biomatrix and reform liver tissue-like structures between the capillaries (see FIGURE 2). The smallest repetitive unit resembles the liver lobulus. Within the cellular aggregates, liver sinusoidal structures are reformed. In actual size, the bioreactor contains up to 600 grams, thereby maintaining the cell mass of a human liver lobe.

## INVESTIGATIONS USING THE NEW BIOREACTOR

The biochemical activity of primary porcine liver cell cultures within the bioreactor was followed for up to eight weeks. Twenty-five cultures with an initial liver cell mass of 210 g to 680 g (representing $1.2$–$4.0 \times 10^{10}$ cells) were evaluated (see FIGURE 3). Enzyme release (lactatedehydrogenase, asparaginaminotransferase, and glutamatdehydrogenase), albumin release, urea formation, carbohydrate metabolism (glucose, galactose, and sorbitol), amino acid metabolism, lignocaine uptake, and monoethylglycinxylidid formation have been investigated. The examinations included the response of the cultures to various substrate dosages and feed rates. The data showed a highly reproducible time course, with an initial enzyme release peak during the first 48–72 hours, accompanied by a temporary disturbance in nitrogen metabolism. This initial phase was followed by a period of stable metabolic function for up to three weeks. After three weeks, differentiated hepatocyte functions began

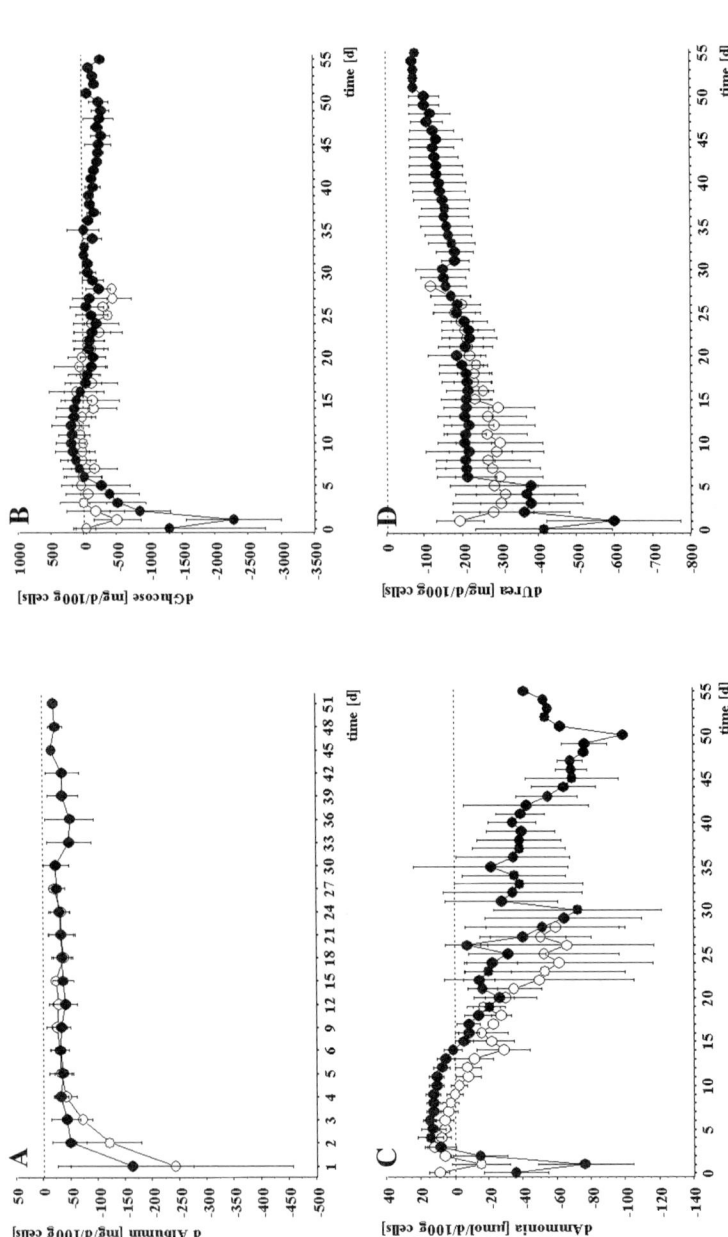

**FIGURE 3.** Twenty-five stand-by cultures with 150 g–400 g cells: net-balances of the parameters (**A**) albumin, (**B**) glucose, (**C**) ammonia, and (**D**) urea depending on various fresh-media flow-rates (*white*, media supply day 0–end, 1.2 l/d; *black*, day 0–1, 4.8 l/d, day 2–5, 2.4 l/d, day 6–end, 1.2 l/d—positive values, substrate uptake; negative values, substrate release).

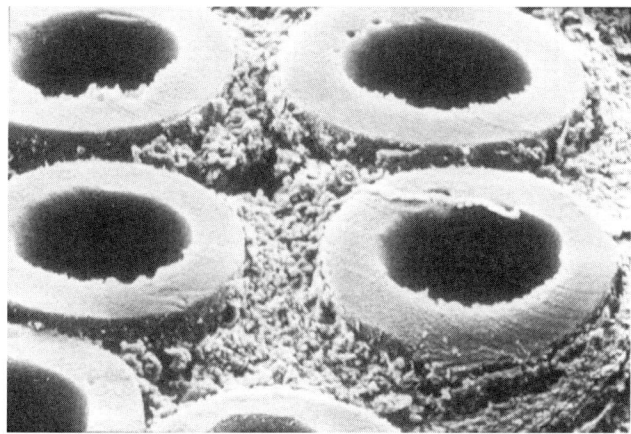

**FIGURE 4.** Three-dimensional structure of reactor showing capillaries and liver cells (TEM).

to decrease gradually. At the end of the culture periods, the bioreactor housings were opened and biopsies of the cellular aggregates were taken for morphologic studies. Freshly isolated pig hepatocytes form a tissue-like structure in the culture model. Scanning electron microscopy shows that hepatocytes spontaneously form aggregates in a three-dimensional structure between and on the surface of artificial capillaries (see FIGURE 4). Transmission electron microscopy reveals that even after seven weeks of *in vitro* perfusion the cell ultrastructure remains similar to that of the parenchyma *in vivo*. Golgi complexes, active membrane processes, reorganization of cell junctions, and bile canaliculi-like intercellular spaces were observed.

The results of the studies indicate that primary hepatocyte cultures can be maintained over a period of several weeks *in vitro* and that they reorganize themselves to give tissue-like structures within the artificial system. The cells spontaneously form aggregates on and between the capillaries and reorganize into a three-dimensional array. Rebuilt cell junctions and the reconstitution of bile canaliculi-like structures were demonstrated in all reactors under investigation. Even after seven weeks of perfusion, the cells display a relatively intact ultrastructure. Cell organelles that depend on intact cytoskeleton, such as the endoplasmatic reticulum and the Golgi apparatus, are well maintained.

## DEVELOPMENT OF A PERFUSION SYSTEM FOR EXTRACORPOREAL HYBRID LIVER SUPPORT

For the therapeutic use of liver cell cultures for temporary extracorporeal hybrid liver support, a perfusion system complying with clinical standards had to be developed. Consideration of technical problems due to direct hemoperfusion of the bioreactor resulted in the introduction of a continuous plasma separation unit between the patient and the bioreactor circuit. Due to plasma separation before bioreactor perfusion, the following features can be supported:

- Perfusion of the cell cultures is enabled in contrast to a diffusion.
- Platelet aggregation within the bioreactor can be avoided leading to a prolongation of the life cycle of the device.
- Direct cellular immunological interactions between the patient's specific and non-specific immunocompetent cells and the heterologous cell cultures can be avoided.
- The running of an extracorporeal blood circuit and a parallel bioreactor circuit allows an easy connection and disconnection of the two circuits without producing stasis in either circuit (reduction of technical complications).

Animal experiments were performed in order to develop a system for plasma perfusion,[21,22] and to enable[23–25] first clinical applications of the bioreactor. The extracorporeal liver system[26] was used in a phase I study on eight patients listed for highly urgent liver transplantation. All applications (7–46 h) could be performed as successful bridging to transplantation and survival rate after two years was 100%. In response to the discussion on PERV transmission from pig cells to patients, we are now focussing on the clinical application of primary human liver cells, isolated from discarded transplantation organs. By November 2000, three patients with acute liver failure were treated with four bioreactors containing human liver cells. All patients have undergone liver transplantation successfully.

## DISCUSSION

Preliminary clinical trials for various concepts of hybrid liver support systems and bioartificial liver devices have been performed during the last decade. The knowledge of possible side effects has therefore increased, but it remains difficult to evaluate clinical efficacy since larger controlled trials are difficult to conduct and a multicenter approach is necessary to treat an appropriate number and wide sample of patients. In addition relatively little information about biochemical functions of liver cell cultures used during clinical applications has been published. This is particularly important, insomuch as the biological feature of these devices is outlined in their concept. Furthermore, the description of adaptation of metabolic activity in the pathophysiologic state of acute liver failure may provide information on pathomechanisms of the disease. Naturally, future work in this field is of high interest.

A prerequisite for sufficient extracorporeal hybrid liver support is a cell culture system that presents features close to physiologic liver functions. For this approach, within our own model, it was thought that the reconstruction of some features of liver architecture within the reactors contributes to the long term stability of hepatocytes. The interwoven capillaries provide a three-dimensional artificial framework as a macroenvironment for cell reorganization. Since expression of differentiated cell functions in tissue culture is strongly affected by cell density,[27,28] the microenvironment of hepatocytes in the presented culture model may partly result from cell contacts promoted by dense packing. In the actual model, a cultivation of a cell mass up to 600 g is possible. This could be compared to a single lobe of the liver. The multicapillary fluid distribution within the device maintains the function of the medium and small size vessels of the liver. Perfusion channels in the intercapillary space reach the dimension and shape of sinusoidal structures. The rearrangement of parenchymal and non-parenchymal liver cells in these structures was a finding that was interpreted as a prerequisite for maintenance of biochemical activity for a period of several weeks.

The morphology of the surviving cells appears to be well preserved but amounts of non-surviving cells could also be detected. This phenomenon could be due to a suboptimal bioreactor design: the diameter of the capillaries used is relatively large in comparison to the size of the hepatocytes and the liver sinusoids. Consequently, the distances between the packed capillaries are, depending on the localization of the cells, in some cases increased by a factor of 2–5. These technical problems could be improved in the future by using specially adapted capillaries and weaving techniques.

Initial clinical experience in experimental transplantation surgery[29] provides information that the cell mass of a liver lobe should be sufficient to support patients in acute liver failure. The developed bioreactor in its actual size incorporates 300–600 gram of cells, a value that can be compared to that of the liver lobe. However, it is unlikely, that this quantity of *in vitro* culture enables qualitative and quantitative organ functions equivalent to that of the same cell mass in a liver lobe. Furthermore, the mass exchange between the patient and the device is not comparable to the physiologic blood supply of the liver. Clinical investigations need to show whether a sufficient clinical function can be enabled by simply adjusting the cell mass, or if a radical redevelopment of the liver support devices is necessary.

The biological approach to liver support with primary cells has its general technical limitations. Foremost is the gradual loss of cell metabolism with time in culture. A significant amount of work needs to be done to enable a halflife of liver cells *in vitro* comparable to that of liver cells *in vivo*. Halflife of biochemical activity of the cells influences the logistics of hybrid liver support. To avoid further critical damage of the cells, a cryopreservation step to facilitate distribution and handling of the devices was excluded from the novel concept, presented herein. The crossover from organ to culture and from *in vitro* culture to therapeutic use are critical points for metabolic adaptation. Another problem that may influence the logistics of clinical application of primary hepatocytes is their need for time for recovery after the trauma of cell isolation. This may also be relevant after the trauma of thawing and reoxygenation in case of using frozen cells. An initial metabolic disorder[30] following cell isolation was observed. This normalizes after the reorganization of the cells to liver tissue-like structures inside the bioreactor. During this process of 24–48 hours, cell function is impaired. Considering the time required after cell isolation and the halflife of cell function *in vitro*, a time window for possible clinical applications of bioreactors may be defined. A further finding from our own investigations was that detection of viability of the initial cell suspension does not enable a prediction of biochemical activity. Therefore, a critical evaluation of every single cell culture before its clinical use is indicated. These considerations result in a standby cultivation of liver cells, to enable on-demand availability of biochemically active devices and to allow screening of the pretreatment biochemical activity. From clinical and practical points of view, the concept of centralized cell culture laboratories and on-demand distribution of the devices to different clinics needs to be evaluated. The vulnerability of function of primary liver cell cultures asks for sophisticated physiologic support during all periods of device handling. Whether the high demands concerning logistics will be accepted, depends on the proof of clinical benefits. The problems due to the limited lifespan of primary liver cells and the control of possible transmission of infectious diseases or immunological risks bring permanent liver cells of human origin into the center of interest. Our initial results on employing discarded transplant organs as an ethically desired cell source are promising. However, the enormous research efforts required in the past to prolong the maintenance of differentiated cellular functions of primary liver cells suggest that research remains. Unsolved problems of long term *in vitro* hepatocyte cultivation will also affect the work on natural or artificially immortalized cell lines, as well as the developments in hepatic stem cell cultivation.

## REFERENCES

1. RUNGE, D., G.K. MICHALOPOULOS, S.C. STROM & D.M. RUNGE. 2000. Recent advances in human hepatocyte culture systems. Biochem. Biophys. Res. Commun. **274**(1): 1–3.
2. CHANG, T.M.S. 1987. Applications of artificial cells in medicine and biotechnology. Biomat. Art. Cells Art. Organs **15**: 1–20.
3. GERLACH, J., R. ZIEMER & P. NEUHAUS. 1996. Fulminant liver failure: relevance of extracorporeal hybrid liver support systems. Int. J. Art. Org. **19**: 7–13.
4. DEMETRIOU, A.A., J. WHITING, S.M. LEVENSON, *et al.* 1986. New method of hepatocyte transplantation and extracorporal liver support. Ann. Surg. **204**: 259–271.
5. CHANG, T.M.S. 1988. The role of biotechnology in bioartificial or hybrid artificial cells and organs. Biomater. Artif. Cells Artif. Organs **16**: 5–6.
6. PAPPAS, S.C. 1988. Fulminant hepatic failure and the need for artificial liver support. Mayo Clin. Proc. **63**: 198–200.
7. REID, L.M. & D.M. JEFFERSON. 1984 . Culturing hepatocytes and other differentiated cells. Hepatology 4(3): 548–559.
8. BERRY, M.N., A.M. EDWARDS & G.J. BARRIT. 1991. Isolated hepatocytes preparation, properties and applications. *In* Laboratory Techniques in Biochemistry and Molecular Biology. R.H. Burdon & P.H. van Knippenberg, Eds. Elsevier, Amsterdam, Netherlands.
9. CLAYTON, D.F., A.L. HARRELSON & J.E. DARNELL. 1985. Dependence of liver-specific transcription on tissue organisation. Mol. Cell Biol. **5**: 2623–2632.
10. KOIDE, N., K. SAKAGUCCI & Y. KOIDE. 1990. Formation of multicellular spheroids composed of adult rat hepatocytes in dishes with positive charged surfaces and under other nonadherent environments. Exp. Cell Res. **186**: 227–235.
11. GERLACH, J., J. BROMBACHER, J.M. COURTNEY & P. NEUHAUS. 1993. Nonenzymatic versus enzymatic hepatocyte isolation from pig livers for larger scale investigations of liver cell perfusion systems. Int. J. Art. Org. **16**: 677–681.
12. GERLACH, J., K. KLÖPPEL, M.R. SCHÖN, *et al.* 1993. Comparison of pig hepatocyte isolation using intraoperative perfusion without warm ischemia and isolation of cells from abattoir organs after warm ischemia. Art. Org. **17**: 950–953.
13. GERLACH, J., J. BROMBACHER, K. KLÖPPEL, *et al.* 1994. Comparison of four methods for mass hepatocyte isolation from pig and human livers. Transplantation **57**: 1318–1322.
14. GERLACH, J., J. BROMBACHER, M. SMITH & P. NEUHAUS. 1996. High yield hepatocyte isolation from pig livers for investigation of hybrid liver support systems: Influence of collagenase concentration and body weight. J. Surg. Res. **62**: 85–89.
15. GERLACH, J., J. VIENKEN, P. WALKER & K. AFFELT. 1990. Computer aided time-lapse video analysis of hepatocyte morphology during adhesion to cellulose membranes. Int. J. Art. Org. **13**: 365–369.

16. GERLACH, J., H.H. SCHAUWECKER, K. KLÖPPEL, et al. 1989. Use of hepatocytes in adhesion and suspension cultures for liver support bioreactors. Int. J. Art. Org. **12:** 788–793.
17. GERLACH, J., K. KLÖPPEL, C. MÜLLER, et al. 1993. Hepatocyte aggregate culture technique for bioreactors in hybrid liver support systems. Int. J. Art. Org. **16**(12): 843–846.
18. GERLACH, J., P. STOLL, N. SCHNOY & E.S. BÜCHERL. 1990. Membranes as substrates for hepatocyte adhesion in liver support bioreactors. Int. J. Art. Org. **13:** 436–441.
19. GERLACH, J., P. STOLL, N. SCHNOY & P. NEUHAUS. 1996. Comparison of hollow fibre membranes for hepatocyte immobilisation in bioreactors. Int. J. Art. Org. **19:** 610–616.
20. GERLACH, J., K. KLÖPPEL, P. STOLL, et al. 1990. Gas supply across membranes in bioreactors for hepatocyte culture. Art. Org. **14:** 328–333.
21. GERLACH, J., T. TROST, C.J. RYAN, et al. 1994. Hybrid liver support system in a short term application on hepatectomized pigs. Int. J. Art. Org. **17:** 549–553.
22. GERLACH, J., A. JÖRRES, O. TROST, et al. 1993. Side effects of hybrid liver support therapy: TNF-$\alpha$ liberation in pigs, associated with extracorporeal bioreactors. Int. J. Art. Org. **16:** 604–608.
23. JANKE, J., J. GERLACH, D. KARDASSIS, et al. 1997. Effect of a hybrid liver support system on cardiopulmonary function in healty pigs. Int. J. Artif. Org. **20:** 570–576.
24. GLEISNER, M., R. BORNEMANN, R. STEMEROWICZ, et al. 1997. Immunisolation of hybrid liver support systems by semipermeable membranes. Int. J. Artif. Org. **20:** 644–649.
25. BORNEMANN, R., M.D. SMITH & J. GERLACH. 1996. Consideration of potential immunological problems in the application of xenogenic hybrid liver support. Int. J. Art. Org. **19:** 655–663.
26. GERLACH, J. 1996. Development of a hybrid liver support system—a review. Int. J. Art. Org. **19:** 645–655.
27. CLAYTON, D.F., A.L. HARRELSON & J.E. DARNELL. 1985. Dependence of liver-specific transcription on tissue organisation. Mol. Cell Biol. **5:** 2623–2632.
28. YUASA, C., Y. TOMITA, K. SHONO, et al. 1993. Importance of cell aggregation for expression of liver functions and regeneration demonstrated with primary cultured hepatocytes. J. Cell. Phys. **156:** 522–530.
29. GUBERNATIS, G., R. PICHLMAYR, J. KEMNITZ & K. GRATZ. 1991. Auxiliary partial orthotopic liver transplantation for fulminant hepatic failure: first successful case report. World J. Surg. **15:** 660–666.
30. GERLACH, J., M. FUCHS, M. SMITH, et al. 1996. Is a clinical application of hybrid liver support systems limited by an initial disorder in cellular amino acid and keto acid metabolism, rather than by later gradual loss of primary hepatocyte function? Transplantation **62:** 224–228.

# Advances in Bioartificial Liver Assist Devices

JOHN F. PATZER II

*Departments of Surgery and Chemical Engineering,
Thomas E. Starzl Transplantation Institute,
McGowen Center for Artificial Organ Development,
University of Pittsburgh, Pittsburgh, Pennsylvania, USA*

ABSTRACT: Rapid advances in development of bioartificial liver assist devices (BLADs) are exciting clinical interest in the application of BLAD technology for support of patients with acute liver failure. Four devices (Circe Biomedical HepatAssist®, Vitagen ELAD™, Gerlach BELS, and Excorp Medical BLSS) that rely on hepatocytes cultured in hollow-fiber membrane technology are currently in various stages of clinical evaluation. Several alternative approaches for culture and perfusion of hepatocytes have been evaluated in preclinical, large animal models of liver failure, or at a laboratory scale. Engineering design issues with respect to xenotransplantation, BLAD perfusion, hepatocyte functionality and culture maintenance, and ultimate distribution of a BLAD to a clinical site are delineated.

KEYWORDS: bioartificial liver assist device; acute liver failure; hepatocyte

## INTRODUCTION

Development of efficacious bioartificial liver assist devices (BLADs) for the treatment of acute liver failure, either fulminant or acute decompensation on chronic liver failure, remains one of the most elusive biomedical engineering endeavors. One reason for this is that hepatocytes (liver cells) have proven one of the most difficult mammalian cells to maintain in culture. The necessary knowledge and ability to maintain functional hepatocytes in long term, three-dimensional culture systems has only been developed in the past decade or so. A second, equally important, reason is that the "engineering" requirements for a BLAD are not well defined. A listing of various artificial organ technologies, together with times to coma or death in the absence of intervention and engineering design concepts, is provided in TABLE 1. The minimal intervention requirement for an artificial organ technology is based on the time to coma or death without intervention. In contrast to other artificial organ technologies, where the engineering need is fairly well understood or identifiable, engineering requirements for a BLAD are yet to be developed. Despite the lack of a well-defined engineering problem, great progress is being made in the development of BLADs.

Address for correspondence: John F. Patzer II, Departments of Surgery and Chemical Engineering, 1249 Benedum Hall, University of Pittsburgh, Pittsburgh, PA 15261, USA. Voice: 412-624-9819; fax: 412-624-9639.
patzer+@pitt.edu

TABLE 1. Artificial organ technologies

| Organ | Time Frame | Problem | Intervention Requirement | Technology |
|---|---|---|---|---|
| heart | minutes | pump | continuous | LVAD |
| lung | minutes | mass transfer | continuous | ECMO |
| pancreas | hours to days | insulin/glucagon | intermittent, hours | IIT |
| kidney | days | mass transfer | intermittent, days | hemodialysis |
| liver | days | ? | intermittent(?) continuous(?) | best care |

NOTE: LVAD, left ventricular assist device; ECMO, extracorporeal membrane oxygenation; IIT, intensive insulin therapy.

From a biomedical engineering viewpoint, the healthy liver is a complex biochemical reactor that has several functions: oxidative *detoxification* (primarily through the cytochrome P450 enzyme system); *biotransformation* (e.g., urea synthesis, gluconuridation, and sulfation); *excretion* (through the bile system); protein and macromolecule *synthesis*; intermediate *metabolism* (gluconeogenesis, fatty acid, and amino acid); and immune and hormonal system *modulation*. Detoxification and biotransformation are primary housekeeping functions performed by the liver that alter potential toxins for elimination through renal or bile mechanisms. Excretion through the bile is also one of the primary housekeeping roles of the liver. Synthesis, metabolism, and modulation are important homeostasis maintenance functions that are provided by the liver.

The sequences in the cascading loss of liver function associated with liver failure are largely unknown in clinical cases because patients tend to present with liver failure well after the initial liver injury has occurred. However, from studies with animal models of acute liver failure,[1] the likely progression results from an overload of an hepatotoxin, such as acetaminophen, that sequentially saturates available detoxification routes, leading to loss of further detoxification ability. The buildup of toxin intermediates is associated with endotoxin and cytokine production and, ultimately, interruption of other cellular processes and cell death. Patients presenting with acute liver failure often have little or no detectable levels of known primary hepatotoxins or their major metabolites, yet liver failure and liver necrosis are progressing. This leads to the speculation that once the primary detoxification routes have been disabled, low concentrations of secondary toxins, such as endotoxin and cytokines, are capable of sustaining progressive cell necrosis.[2] There is also a possibility that the putative toxins are highly bound to albumin with little free concentration to detect.

Many therapeutic approaches to liver failure have been tried.[2] Treatment modalities directed toward detoxification that are currently in clinical trials[3–6] may have potential to abrogate the course of liver failure if the intervention is made early enough. Plasma exchange therapies,[7,8] which should provide detoxification as well as homeostasis functions, have had limited success.

## BLAD APPROACHES

BLAD therapy is based upon the premise that a patient with progressing acute liver failure can benefit from the combination of active detoxification, intermediate metabolism, and possibly macromolecule synthesis and excretion capability that can only be provided by liver cells (hepatocytes). A perceived advantage of using hepatocytes is that they can replace necessary biochemical function for the patient without the need to identify the particular biochemical pathways out of numerous possibilities that have been compromised by liver failure. TABLE 2 provides a partial listing of BLADs that are in clinical evaluations, have been evaluated preclinically in large animal models of liver failure, or are under development.

### *Devices in Clinical Evaluation*

The first generation of BLADs that are in clinical evaluation are all based on the use of hollow-fiber cartridges housing hepatocytes cultured in the extraluminal space of the hollow fibers. The Circe Biomedical HepatAssist® device[9–12] uses cryopreserved primary porcine hepatocytes that have been seeded onto collagen-coated dextran beads prior to placement in the bioreactor. The Vitagen ELAD™ device[13–15] uses the C3A derivative of the HepG2 human hepatocyte cell line that have been seeded and grown to confluence within the extraluminal space. The BELS device, developed by Gerlach *et al.*,[16,17] uses either primary human hepatocytes (if available) or primary porcine hepatocytes embedded in a collagen matrix in the extraluminal space of a unique tripartite arrangement of hollow fibers. The Excorp Medical BLSS device[18–20] uses a high-density culture of primary porcine hepatocytes. The Circe Biomedical HepatAssist is currently in a Phase II/III randomized, multicenter clinical efficacy evaluation. The other three are in various stages of a Phase I/II clinical safety/efficacy evaluation.

With the exception of the Excorp Medical BLSS, which perfuses whole blood directly through the luminal space of the hollow-fiber cartridge, the other three approaches use some means of plasma separation to create a plasma stream that perfuses the luminal space in the bioreactor. All four devices use an oxygenator placed before the bioreactors to raise the available oxygen levels in the perfusing stream. The HepatAssist also uses a charcoal column prior to the bioreactor to help remove any putative toxins prior to reaching the hepatocytes. The BELS has three different hollow fibers woven in an interlocking pattern. One set is used for patient plasma, another set for hepatocyte nutrient media, and the third set for direct oxygen flow. All four systems rely on diffusion of all species, including oxygen, from the perfusate stream across the fiber membrane to the hepatocytes for detoxification and other metabolic hepatocyte functions.

### *Devices in Large Animal Evaluations*

Several alternative device configurations have advanced to the stage of large animal, preclinical evaluations. Flendrig *et al.*[21–23] have developed a novel approach that directly perfuses patient plasma in an axial flow path over and/or through a nonwoven polyester fabric that has been seeded with primary porcine hepatocytes. This approach allows more active convective transport of plasma constituents to the hepatocytes than is possible by diffusive means alone. Additional oxygenation and

TABLE 2. Comparison of BLAD approaches

| Status/Device | Plasma Separator | | | Bioreactor | | | | | |
|---|---|---|---|---|---|---|---|---|---|
| | Membrane | MW Cutoff, kD | Clinical Perfusate | Cell Type | Amount, g | Membrane | MW Cutoff, kD | Cell Matrix |
| *Clinical Trials* | | | | | | | | |
| HepatAssist® [9-12] | centrifuge | 5,000 | plasma | porcine | 50-100 | cellulose acetate | 5,000 | dextran beads |
| ELAD™ [13-15] | cellulose acetate | 120 | plasma | C3A line | 800 | cellulose acetate | 120 | none |
| BELS [16,17] | polysulphone | 400 | plasma | porcine/human | 500 | polysulfone | 400 | collagen |
| BLSS [18-20] | none | | blood | porcine | 100 | cellulose acetate | 100 | none |
| *Preclinical Trials* | | | | | | | | |
| Flendrig et al. [21-23] | centrifuge | 5,000 | plasma | porcine | 200 | none | | polyester |
| Funatsu et al. [24-26] | ? | ? | plasma | porcine | 200-600 | none | | polyurethane foam |
| Kodama et al. [27,28] | polysulfone | 5,000 | plasma | porcine | 50 | polysulfone | 5,000 | collagen |
| Cerra et al. [29-31] | none | | blood | porcine | 30-50 | cellulose acetate | 100 | collagen |
| *Development* | | | | | | | | |
| Sakai & Naruse et al. [32-34] | | | blood | porcine | 200 | none | | polyester |
| Iwata & Sajiki et al. [35,36] | | | plasma[a] | porcine | 30-50 | cellulose acetate | 70 | none |
| Miyoshi & Ohshima et al. [37-39] | | | plasma[a] | rat | 0.7 | | | polyvinyl formal resin |
| Toner et al. [48-50] | | | plasma[a] | | | | | microchannels |

[a] These systems have used media as the perfusate in publications to date, indicating potential use of plasma in the clinical setting. However, the use of blood as a clinical perfusate is possible as these systems move to larger scale evaluation.

carbon dioxide elimination capacity is provided through a network of hydrophobic polypropylene fibers that span the bioreactor. Preclinical evaluation of the system has demonstrated improved survival time in a pig liver ischemia model.[21]

Funatsu et al.[24–26] have also developed an approach that uses direct plasma perfusion through channels cored in an highly porous polyurethane foam structure that has been seeded with primary porcine hepatocytes. Species transport from the plasma to the hepatocytes is diffusive, but without the additional diffusion resistance represented by the fiber membrane in hollow-fiber–based devices. The system has shown large reduction in ammonia levels when used with a canine ischemia model of liver failure.[24]

Kodama et al.[27,28] have developed a system using primary porcine hepatocytes that is similar to the Excorp Medical BLSS.[18–20] The primary differences lie in the use of microporous polysulfone hollow-fiber membranes in the hepatocyte bioreactor and perfusion of plasma through the bioreactor. The system has shown some efficacy in support of an ischemic pig liver failure model.[27]

Cerra et al.[29–31] demonstrated increased survival times in a canine D-galactosamine model of liver failure[31] when supported with a BLAD with inverted configuration from the normal hollow-fiber cartridge: primary porcine hepatocytes housed in the luminal space of a hollow-fiber cartridge with blood flow through the extraluminal space. An additional media flow through the luminal space provides hepatocyte nutrients and a mechanism for excretion separate from return to the patient for excretion.

### *Approaches Under Development*

Sakai and Naruse et al.[32–34] have been working with primary porcine hepatocytes seeded into a nonwoven polyester matrix, similar to that of Flendrig et al.[21–23] In contrast to the Flendrig approach, however, Sakai and Naruse form a cylindrical shell of the matrix and then force blood flow from the outside of the shell to the interior of the shell in a radial crossflow reactor. They rely upon an external oxygenator to provide all oxygen requirements for the hepatocytes. Blood is forced convectively across the hepatocytes, limiting the diffusive mass transport that might be present with channeling in the axial flow path of the Flendrig approach. Although the system has been used successfully in support of an ischemic pig model of liver failure,[33] no mention has been made of the possible hemolytic effects of the flow configuration and the potential immunological problems that would be confronted with human blood. Iwata and Sajiki et al.[35,36] have published some excellent hepatocyte metabolic kinetics and reactor visualization work with primary porcine hepatocytes in a system similar to that of Cerra et al.[29–31] The work validates and extends many of the results observed by Cerra et al. and provides a standard for reaction engineering investigations into hepatocyte-based bioreactors. In the early stages of development, it is not clear whether the developers intend to flow blood or plasma through the extraluminal space in the cartridge.

Miyoshi and Ohshima et al.[37–39] have been working with hepatocyte culture systems in a microporous polyvinyl formal resin material. Cubes of the material are seeded with primary rat hepatocytes and placed in a packed-bed axial flow column. Studies have shown long term maintenance of protein synthesis and metabolic function. Further development will require use of an hepatocyte source suitable for clinical use.

Several researchers[40–47] have proposed the use of hepatocyte encapsulation in creation of a BLAD. The encapsulating material serves several functions: immunoisolation, protection of the hepatocyte from shear forces, and an anchorage medium required for the anchorage-dependent hepatocytes to maintain functionality. Encapsulated hepatocytes could then be placed in a packed bed reactor or a fluidized bed reactor. A major advantage perceived for such BLAD systems based on encapsulated hepatocytes is improved mass transport from the perfusing plasma or blood to the hepatocytes.

Toner et al.[48–50] have been studying the effects of hepatocyte cell coculture with fibroblasts in two-dimensional micropatterned systems. They indicate that the long term metabolic maintenance of such systems may be better than that observed with hepatocyte culture alone. Although in the early stages of development, it is possible to imagine a plasma-perfused BLAD based upon stacks of thin-film micropatterned coculture layers.

## BLAD DESIGN ISSUES

Numerous design issues confront the developers of BLAD systems. Some of the more important issues are noted in TABLE 3. Early consideration of all of the issues will improve the probability that any particular approach will reach the stage of clinical evaluations.

### Xenotransplantation

The vast majority of the devices and approaches listed in TABLE 2 use primary porcine hepatocytes. This choice is based upon an extreme shortage of preferable human hepatocytes, the general loss of hepatocyte-specific functions associated with

TABLE 3. Design issues in BLAD development

- Xenotransplantation
  - Infectious diseases (PERV)
  - Immunologic response
- Perfusion
  - Whole blood vs plasma
  - Intermittent vs continuous
  - Dose (number of cells)
- Function
  - Detoxification, excretion, synthesis
  - Kinetics (bioreactor configuration dependence)
  - Long term culture
  - Reactor modeling
- Distribution

hepatocyte cell lines, the similarity of function between porcine and human hepatocytes, and the general availability of porcine hepatocytes. However, the choice of primary porcine hepatocytes has associated risks that need to be considered. In the United States, use of primary porcine hepatocytes places BLADs into full xenotransplantation regulation by the Food and Drug Administration (FDA). Animals that provide hepatocytes must come from herds managed according to the draft xenotransplantation guidelines.[51]

Early BLAD development focused on the immunoisolation issues in xenotransplantation.[52–55] This issue has two sides. The first is potential development of porcine immune responses in patients post perfusion with a BLAD. The second is protection of the porcine hepatocytes from the potentially adverse effects of human immune response during a perfusion. Mitigation of this potential problem has been primarily through the use of membranes that have nominal molecular weight diffusive transmission cutoffs of around 100 kD. Such membranes permit the passage of albumin-sized proteins (60–80 kD) while rejecting human immunoglobulins (about 2,500 kD). The notable exception to this is the Circe Biomedical HepatAssist, which uses microporous membranes that permit passage of species up to 5,000 kD. The only study with humans,[55] involving the HepatAssist, indicated no sustained humoral immune response after six-hour perfusions with the device. Although limited in scope, this study provides some support that systems without immunoisolation membranes may not have a perceived immunological response problem.

However, the seminal work by Patience et al.[56] on active infection of a human cell line by porcine endogenous retrovirus (PERV) changed forever the focus of the xenotransplantation issue from immune response protection to potential opportunistic disease transmission. Discussions of the wisdom of whether human tissue or bodily fluids should be exposed directly to porcine tissue has limited the progression of porcine–human xenotransplantation.[57] Whether the membranes that are used for immunological protection in BLADs are sufficient protection from PERV transmission has become a very important research issue in BLAD development.[58,59] In the only clinical study published to date,[60] no infective transmission of PERV was detected with the HepatAssist. Although the study is encouraging for BLAD development, patient exposure was limited. An active plan to assess the potential of PERV transmission will need to be a major component of any clinical evaluation of a BLAD device.

## BLAD Perfusion

A BLAD can be perfused either directly by whole blood or by a plasma stream as depicted in FIGURE 1. Advantages to whole blood perfusion in comparison to plasma perfusion include one less processing step in the system, greater oxygen-carrying capacity of the perfusing stream, and higher initial diffusive gradient driving force because plasma circuits generally contain a reservoir for flow and pressure balance that dilutes the plasma stream. A primary advantage of plasma perfusion is the ability to decouple the bioreactor flows and maintenance from the patient, thus isolating potential problems with patient blood access from the system.

The primary disadvantage of whole blood perfusion is clot formation in the lumen of the hollow fibers leading to loss of a fiber to blood flow and eventual unacceptably high pressure drops through the device to maintain flow rates. In this

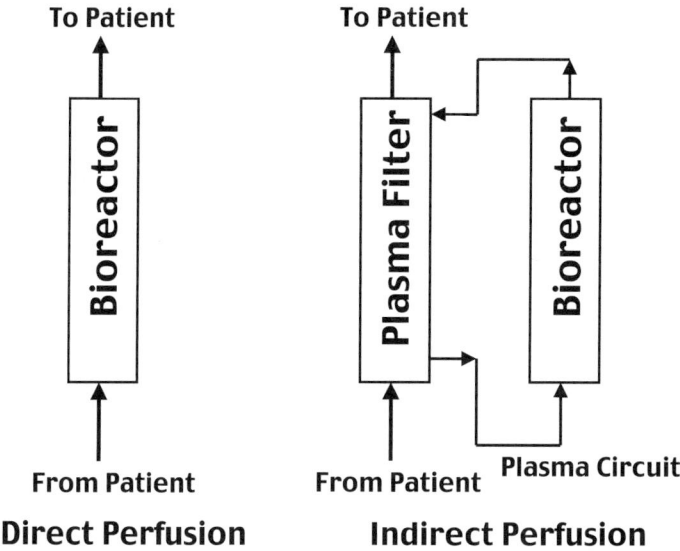

**FIGURE 1.** BLAD perfusion options.

scenario, a very expensive bioreactor is lost. With plasma perfusion provided by a plasma filter, the same progression leads to the loss of a relatively inexpensive plasma filter cartridge that can be replaced while protecting the bioreactor. Improved understanding of the coagulopathy issues surrounding patients with liver failure will improve both whole blood and plasma perfusion systems.

An associated issue is whether clinical perfusion should be continuous or intermittent, or whether it matters. Of the four devices in clinical evaluations, the ELAD and BELS provide continuous perfusion while the HepatAssist uses six-hour perfusion periods and BLSS uses 12-hour perfusion periods. Proponents of continuous perfusion note that the liver is a continuously perfused organ *in vivo* and that provision of continuous liver support to patients with liver failure is, therefore, only reasonable. As noted in TABLE 1, however, whether continuous perfusion is required is moot. Both diabetes (artificial pancreas) and renal failure (artificial kidney), with a time course of days, are treatable with intermittent therapy. (This is not to say that continuous intervention for diabetes and renal failure is not desirable. Indeed, great efforts are under way to develop continuous intervention therapies. However, the disease state is treatable with intermittent therapy.) Given a similar time course for acute liver failure, intermittent therapy may be suitable for either bridging to transplant or reversing the course of the acute episode of liver failure.

Continuous versus intermittent perfusion has an impact on BLAD design from several perspectives. The most important is patient tolerance for the perfusion. Patients with acute liver failure tend to be hemodynamically unstable. Initiation of an extracorporeal perfusion must be closely monitored for any changes in hemodynamic status. Problems with or ease of maintenance of patient physiologic and hemodynamic status with long term perfusion is largely unknown at this time. A second issue is maintenance of patient coagualopathy parameters over long periods, previously discussed. The third issue is maintenance of bioreactor functionality in long term perfusion. Not much information is available about pre- and postperfusion hepatocyte viability and bioreactor performance. Development of such information is requisite for adequately addressing the feasibility of long term or continuous perfusion.

Included with perfusion as a BLAD design issue is the question of how many grams of liver cells are required for a clinically acceptable BLAD. Estimates range from 100 g for the HepatAssist and BLSS, to 500 g for the BELS, to 800 g for the ELAD. The 500 g estimate is based upon surgical observations that patients with 70% liver resections (leaving approximately 30% of an initial 1,500 g liver mass) generally have good prognosis for survival whereas those with greater than 70% resections have poor prognosis. Although this observation is relevant to establishing an upper bound on the requisite hepatocyte mass in BLADs, the relevancy to establishing a lower bound is moot. The real issue is to determine what constitutes a reasonable therapeutic dose of BLAD support for a patient with acute liver failure. Quantification of therapeutic dose involves whole blood versus plasma perfusion, intermittent versus continuous perfusion, perfusion rates, and mass transfer limitations in the bioreactor, as well as the mass of liver cells used. An important first step in this debate would be an analysis of the time course changes in measurable (blood chemistry) patient parameters as a function of whole blood versus plasma perfusion. The hemodialysis literature provides suitable models for such an analysis.

## *BLAD Function*

The vast majority of hepatocyte function literature deals with rat hepatocytes maintained in monolayer culture. Rat hepatocytes are known to have different metabolic pathways than human and porcine hepatocytes[61] and are unacceptable for use in a BLAD for xenotransplantation reasons. Also, maintenance of differentiated function in long term (days) monolayer culture is problematic at best, even with manipulations of extracellular matrix factors and/or media composition.[62–67] Additionally, although proposals have been made[68] little agreement exists with respect to appropriate metabolic function measures for BLADS. As a result, little information is available in the literature that permits *a priori* estimation of hepatocyte metabolic function in any particular reactor design.

Several factors complicate the development of knowledge about "intrinsic" hepatocyte metabolic kinetics and function that can be used in *a priori* design of new bioreactor configurations. First is the well-known fact that hepatocytes are inducible; that is, hepatocytes respond to increased concentrations of a stimulant by producing more enzyme to process the stimulant. Second, experimental observations indicate that the apparent intrinsic kinetics are likely a function of cell density,[69] even in the absence of external mass transport limitations. A third is that hepatocytes tend to lose their differentiated function with extended times in culture.[35–36]

Several groups are working on development of reaction engineering descriptions of BLAD bioreactors. Catapano *et al.*[70–72] have used basic reaction engineering concepts to delineate the need for better kinetic understanding of hepatocyte-based bioreactors. Gaylor *et al.*[69,73] have examined the issue of hepatocyte oxygen requirements and developed techniques for measuring metabolic oxygen demand. Application of conventional reaction engineering modeling[74,75] to hepatocyte oxygen consumption in a hollow-fiber reactor[73] has produced a conundrum, however. The conclusion drawn from the modeling effort, that primary hepatocytes will experience large regions of anoxia and, therefore, cell death, is contrary to the practical experience of the four BLADs in clinical evaluations and contrary to at least one published photograph of healthy hepatocytes in a region extending far beyond the fiber wall.[27] The answer to the conundrum appears to lie in the acknowledged observation that intrinsic hepatocyte kinetics are modulated by cell density. The problem from the modeling analysis lies, not with the modeling, but with the far reaching conclusion on hollow fiber-based bioreactors in general, based upon insufficient knowledge about kinetics.

Clearly, understanding and being able to adequately model hepatocyte function *a priori* in the development of new bioreactor configurations is crucial to developing improved bioreactor designs for improved BLAD systems. Realization of this goal requires BLAD researchers to more clearly identify and characterize their systems with respect to hepatocyte culture density, perfusion parameters, mass transfer resistances, and metabolic performance within the context of a reasonably detailed reaction engineering model.

## *BLAD Distribution*

Distribution of the BLAD to the site of need is an important issue in BLAD development that should be considered as early as possible in the development cycle. The HepatAssist is distributed as cryopreserved hepatocytes with associated microcarrier beads and bioreactor. When need arises at a site, a trained team will thaw the hepatocytes, allow them to attach to the microcarrier beads, and then infuse them into the bioreactor. This strategy allows rapid response when a patient with acute liver failure presents at a clinical site. The ELAD is maintained in culture at a central site and then shipped by express courier to a clinical site when an appropriate patient with acute liver failure presents. Depending upon when the patient presents, a delay of up to 24 hours is possible before initiating treatment. The BELS and BLSS have not yet disclosed distribution plans.

Assuming that initiation of BLAD therapy for acute liver failure should commence within 12–36 hours from patient presentation in a clinical setting, the distribution issue is not so much rapid response as an assurance that a fully functional bioreactor be delivered to the clinic. Hepatocyte cryopreservation has been shown to successfully meet this criterion.[11] Kodama *et al.*[76] have shown reasonable recovery of collagen-embedded hepatocyte functionality after several days' maintenance at 4°C in University of Wisconsin organ preservation solution. They suggest that this may prove a practical method for shipping BLAD bioreactors to sites of need.

## ACKNOWLEDGMENT

This work was funded in part by Excorp Medical, Inc., Oakdale, MN, USA.

## REFERENCES

1. NEWSOME, P.N., J.N. PLEVRIS, L.J. NELSON & P.C. HAYES. 2000. Animal models of fulminant hepatic failure: a critical evaluation. Liver Transplant. **6:** 21–31.
2. HUGHES, R.D. & R. WILLIAMS. 1996. Use of bioartificial and artificial liver support devices. Seminars in Liver Disease **16:** 435–444.
3. STANGE, J., S.R. MITZNER, T. RISLER, et al. 1999. Molecular adsorbent recycling system (MARS): clinical results of a new membrane-based blood purification system for bioartificial liver support. Artif. Organs **23:** 319–330.
4. STANGE, J. & S. MITZNER. 1996. A carrier-mediated transport of toxins in a hybrid membrane. Safety barrier between a patients blood and a bioartificial liver. Int. J. Artif. Organs **19:** 677–691.
5. ELLIS, A.J., R.D. HUGHES, D. NICHOLL, et al. 1999. Temporary extracorporeal liver support for severe acute alcoholic hepatitis using the BioLogic-DT. Int. J. Artif. Organs **22:** 27–34.
6. HUGHES, R.D., A. PUCKNELL, D. ROUTLEY, et al. 1994. Evaluation of the BioLogic-DT sorbent-suspension dialyser in patients with fulminant hepatic failure. Int. J. Artif. Organs **17:** 657–662.
7. KAMOHARA, Y., H. FUJIOKA, S. EGUCHI, et al. 2000. Comparative study of bioartificial liver support and plasma exchange for treatment of pigs with fulminant hepatic failure. Artif. Organs **24:** 265–270.
8. IWAI, H., M. NAGAKI, T. NAITO, et al. 1998. Removal of endotoxin and cytokines by plasma exchange in patients with acute hepatic failure. Crit. Care Med. **26:** 873–876.
9. DETRY, O., N. ARKADOPOULOS, P. TING, et al. 1999. Clinical use of a bioartificial liver in the treatment of acetaminophen-induced fulminant hepatic failure. Am. Surg. **65:** 934–938.
10. CHEN, S.C., C. MULLON, E. KAHAKU, et al. 1997. Treatment of severe liver failure with a bioartificial liver. Ann. N.Y. Acad. Sci. **831:** 350–360.
11. WATANABE, F.D., C.J. MULLON, W.R. HEWITT, et al. 1997. Clinical experience with a bioartificial liver in the treatment of severe liver failure. A phase I clinical trial. Ann. Surg. **225:** 484–491.
12. CHEN, S.C., W.R. HEWITT, F.D. WATANABE, et al. 1996. Clinical experience with a porcine hepatocyte-based liver support system. Int. J. Artif. Organs **19:** 664–669.
13. SUSSMAN, N.L. & J.H. KELLY. 1997. Extracorporeal liver support: cell-based therapy for the failing liver. Am. J. Kidney Dis. **30**(5 Suppl. 4): S66–71.
14. ELLIS, A.J., R.D. HUGHES, J.A. WENDON, et al. 1996. Pilot-controlled trial of the extracorporeal liver assist device in acute liver failure. Hepatology **24:** 1446–1451.
15. SUSSMAN, N.L., G.T. GISLASON & J.H. KELLY. 1994. Extracorporeal liver support application to fulminant hepatic failure. J. Clin. Gastroenterol. **18:** 320–324.
16. GERLACH, J.C. 1997. Long-term liver cell cultures in bioreactors and possible application for liver support. Cell Biol. Toxicol. **13:** 349–355.
17. GERLACH, J.C., P. LEMMENS, M. SCHON, et al. 1997. Experimental evaluation of a hybrid liver support system. Transplant. Proc. **29:** 852.
18. PATZER II, J.F., G.V. MAZARIEGOS, R. LOPEZ, et al. 1999. Novel bioartificial liver support system: preclinical evaluation. Ann. N.Y. Acad. Sci. **875:** 340–352.
19. MAZARIEGOS, G.V., J.F. PATZER II, R.C. LOPEZ, et al. 2001. First clinical use of a novel bioartificial liver support system (BLSS). Am J. Transplant. Submitted.
20. MAZARIEGOS, G.V., D.J. KRAMER, R.C. LOPEZ, et al. 2001. Safety observations in the phase I clinical evaluation of the Excorp Medical BLSS after the first four patients. ASAIO J. In press.
21. FLENDRIG, L.M., F. CALISE, E. DI FLORIO, et al. 1999. Significantly improved survival time in pigs with complete liver ischemia treated with a novel bioartificial liver. Int. J. Artif. Organs **22:** 701–709.
22. FLENDRIG, L.M., R.A. CHAMULEAU, M.A. MAAS, et al. 1999. Evaluation of a novel bioartificial liver in rats with complete liver ischemia: treatment efficacy and species-specific alpha-GST detection to monitor hepatocyte viability. J. Hepatol. **30:** 311–320.

23. FLENDRIG, L.M., D. SOMMEIJER, N.C. LADIGES, et al. 1998. Commercially available media for flushing extracorporeal bioartificial liver systems prior to connection to the patient's circulation: an in vitro comparative study in two and three dimensional porcine hepatocyte cultures. Int. J. Artif. Organs **21:** 467–472.
24. GION, T., S. MITSUO, K. SHIRABE, et al. 1999. Evaluation of a hybrid artificial liver using a polyurethane foam packed-bed culture system in dogs. J. Surg. Res. **82:** 131–136.
25. NAKAZAWA, K., H. IJIMA, M. KANEKO, et al. 1999. Development of a hybrid artificial liver support system and its application to hepatic failure animals. *In* Tissue Engineering for Therapeutic Use 3. K. Ikada & T. Okano, Eds. Elsevier Science.
26. IJIMA, H., T. MATSUSHITA, K. NAKAZAWA, et al. 1998. Hepatocyte spheroids in polyurethane foams: functional analysis and application for a hybrid artificial liver. Tissue Engin. **4:** 213–226.
27. NAKA, S., K. TAKESHITA, T. YAMAMOTO, et al. 1999. Bioartificial liver support system using porcine hepatocytes entrapped in a three-dimensional hollow fiber module with collagen gel: an evaluation in the swine acute liver failure model. Artif. Organs **23:** 822–828.
28. SUZUKI, M., K. TAKESHITA, T. YAMAMOTO, et al. 1997. Hepatocytes entrapped in collagen gel following 14 days of storage at 4 degrees C: preservation of hybrid artificial liver. Artif. Organs **21:** 99–106.
29. SIELAFF, T.D., S.L. NYBERG, M.D. ROLLINS, et al. 1997. Characterization of the three-compartment gel-entrapment porcine hepatocyte bioartificial liver. Cell Biol. Toxicol. **13:** 357–364.
30. SIELAFF, T.D., M.Y. HU, B. AMIOT, et al. 1995. Gel-entrapment bioartificial liver therapy in galactosamine hepatitis. J. Surg. Res. **59:** 179–184.
31. SIELAFF, T.D., M.Y. HU, M.D. ROLLINS, et al. 1995. An anesthetized model of lethal canine galactosamine fulminant hepatic failure. Hepatology **21:** 796–804.
32. SAKAI, Y., K. NARUSE, I. NAGASHIMA, et al. 1999. A new bioartificial liver using porcine hepatocyte spheroids in high-cell-density suspension perfusion culture: in vitro performance in synthesized culture medium and in 100% human plasma. Cell Transplant. **8:** 531–541.
33. NARUSE, K., I. NAGASHIMA, Y. SAKAI, et al. 1998. Efficacy of a bioreactor filled with porcine hepatocytes immobilized on nonwoven fabric for *ex vivo* direct hemoperfusion treatment of liver failure in pigs. Artif. Organs **22:** 1031–1037.
34. NARUSE, K., Y. SAKAI, I. NAGASHIMA, et al. 1996. Comparisons of porcine hepatocyte spheroids and single hepatocytes in the non-woven fabric bioartificial liver module. Int. J. Artif. Organs **9:** 605–609.
35. SAJIKI, T., H. IWATA, H.J. PAEK, et al. 2000. Morphologic studies of hepatocytes entrapped in hollow fibers of a bioartificial liver. ASAIO J. **46:** 49–55.
36. IWATA, H., T. SAJIKI, H. MAEDA, et al. 1999. *In vitro* evaluation of metabolic functions of a bioartificial liver. ASAIO J. **45:** 299–306.
37. YANAGI, K., H. MIYOSHI & N. OHSHIMA. 1998. Improvement of metabolic performance of hepatocytes cultured *in vitro* in a packed-bed reactor for use as a bioartificial liver. ASAIO J. **44:** M436–440.
38. MIYOSHI, H., K. OOKAWA & N. OHSHIMA. 1998. Hepatocyte culture utilizing porous polyvinyl formal resin maintains long-term stable albumin secretion activity. J. Biomat. Sci. Polym. Edit. **9:** 227–237.
39. OHSHIMA, N., K. YANAGI & H. MIYOSHI. 1997. Packed-bed type reactor to attain high density culture of hepatocytes for use as a bioartificial liver. Artif. Organs **21:** 1169–1176.
40. WONG, H. & T.M. CHANG. 1991. A novel two step procedure for immobilizing living cells in microcapsules for improving xenograft survival. Biomat. Artif. Cells Immobil. Biotechnol. **19:** 687–697.
41. CHANG, T.M. 1992. Hybrid artificial cells: microencapsulation of living cells. ASAIO J. **38:** 128–130.
42. CHANG, T.M. 1992. Artificial liver support based on artificial cells with emphasis on encapsulated hepatocytes. Artif. Organs **16:** 71–74.

43. DIXIT, V. 1994. Development of a bioartificial liver using isolated hepatocytes. Artif. Organs **18:** 371–384.
44. DIXIT, V. & G. GITNICK. 1996. Artificial liver support: state of the art. Scand. J. Gastroenterol. Suppl. **220:** 101–114.
45. STANGE, J. & S. MITZNER. 1996. Hepatocyte encapsulation--initial intentions and new aspects for its use in bioartificial liver support. Int. J. Artif. Organs **19:** 45–48.
46. SELDEN, C., A. SHARIAT, P. MCCLOSKEY, et al. 1999. Three-dimensional *in vitro* cell culture leads to a marked upregulation of cell function in human hepatocyte cell lines—an important tool for the development of a bioartificial liver machine. Ann. N.Y. Acad. Sci. **875:** 353–363.
47. LEGALLAIS, C., E. DORÉ & P. PAULLIER. 2000. Design of a fluidized bed bioartificial liver. Artif. Organs **24:** 519–525.
48. GREGORY, P.G., C.K. CONNOLLY, M. TONER & S.J. Sullivan. 2000. In vitro characterization of porcine hepatocyte function. Cell Transplant. **9:** 1–10.
49. LEDEZMA, G.A., A. FOLCH, S.N. BHATIA, et al. 1999. Numerical model of fluid flow and oxygen transport in a radial-flow microchannel containing hepatocytes. J. Biomech. Engin. **121:** 58–64.
50. BHATIA, S.N., U.J. BALIS, M.L. YARMUSH & M. TONER. 1998. Microfabrication of hepatocyte/fibroblast co-cultures: role of homotypic cell interactions. Biotech. Prog. **14:** 378–387.
51. FOOD AND DRUG ADMINISTRATION. 2000. Center for Biologics Evaluation and Research: Draft PHS guideline on infectious disease issues in xenotransplantation. Food and Drug Administration. <http://www.fda.gov/cber/guidelines.htm>.
52. BORNEMANN, R., M.D. SMITH & J.C. GERLACH. 1996. Consideration of potential immunological problems in the application of xenogenic hybrid liver support. Int. J. Artif. Organs **19:** 655–663.
53. TE VELDE, A.A., L.M. FLENDRIG, N.C. LADIGES & R.A. CHAMULEAU. 1997. Possible immunological problems of bioartificial liver support. Int. J. Artif. Organs **20:** 418–421.
54. GLEISSNER M, R BORNEMANN, R STEMEROWICZ, et al. 1997. Immunoisolation of hybrid liver support systems by semipermeable membranes. Int. J. Artif. Organs **20:** 644–649.
55. BAQUERIZO, A., A. MHOYAN, M. KEARNS-JONKER, et al. 1999. Characterization of human xenoreactive antibodies in liver failure patients exposed to pig hepatocytes after bioartificial liver treatment: an *ex vivo* model of pig to human xenotransplantation. Transplantation **67:** 5–18.
56. PATIENCE, C., Y. TAKEUCHI & R.A. WEISS. 1997. Infection of human cells by an endogenous retrovirus of pig. Nat. Med. **33:** 282–286.
57. FIANE, A.E., T.E. MOLLNES & M. DEGRE. 2000. Pig endogenous retrovirus—a threat to clinical xenotransplantation? APMIS **108:** 241–250.
58. FALASCA, E., U. BACCARANI, C. PIPAN, et al. 2000. Is PERV transfer across hollow fiber membranes relevant to bioartificial liver model? Transplantation **69:** 1755.
59. NYBERG, S.L., J.R. HIBBS, J.A. HARDIN, et al. 1999. Transfer of porcine endogenous retrovirus across hollow fiber membranes: significance to a bioartificial liver. Transplantation **67:** 1251–1255.
60. PITKIN, Z. & C. MULLON. Evidence of absence of porcine endogenous retrovirus (PERV) infection in patients treated with a bioartificial liver support system. Artif. Organs **23:** 829–833.
61. DONATO, M.T., J.V. CASTELL & M.J. GOMEZ-LECHON. 1999. Characterization of drug metabolizing activities in pig hepatocytes for use in bioartificial liver devices: comparison with other hepatic cellular models. J. Hepatol. **31:** 542–549.
62. LANDRY, J., D. BERNIER, C. OUELLET, et al. 1985. Speroidal aggregate culture of rat liver cells: histotypic reorganization, biomatrix deposition, and maintenance of functional activities. J. Cell Biol. **101:** 914–923.
63. SHINJI, T., N. KOIDE & T. TSUJI. 1988. Glycosaminoglycans partially substitute for proteoglycans in spheroid formation of adult rat hepatocytes in primary culture. Cell Struct. Func. **13:** 179–188.

64. TONG, J.Z., S. SARRAZIN, D. CASSIO, et al. 1994. Application of spheroid culture to human hepatocytes and maintenance of their differentiation. Biol. Cell **81:** 77–81.
65. SUN, J., L. WANG, M.A. WARING, et al. 1997. Simple and reliable methods to assess hepatocyte viability in bioartificial liver support system matrices. Artif. Organs **21:** 408–413.
66. BLOCK, G.D., J. LOCKER, W.C. BOWEN, et al. 1996. Population expansion, clonal growth, and specific differentiation patterns in primary cultures of hepatocytes induced by HGF/SF, EGF and TGF alpha in a chemically defined (HGM) medium. J. Cell Biol. **132:** 1133–1149.
67. KOEBE, H.G., M. WICK, U. CRAMER, et al. 1994. Collagen gel immobilisation provides a suitable cell matrix for long term human hepatocyte cultures in hybrid reactors. Int. J. Artif. Organs **17:** 95–106.
68. KARDASSIS, D., B. BUSSE, A. BESSELING, et al. 1999. Enzyme release in hybrid liver support systems: marker for quality prior to clinical application. Transplant. Proc. **31:** 668–669.
69. SMITH, M.D., A.D. SMIRTHWAITE, D.E. CAIRNS, et al. 1996. Techniques for measurement of oxygen consumption rates of hepatocytes during attachment and post-attachment. Int. J. Artif. Organs **19:** 36–44.
70. CATAPANO, G. & L. DE BARTOLO. 1996. Importance of the kinetic characterization of liver cell metabolic reactions to the design of hybrid liver support devices. Int. J. Artif. Organs **19:** 670–676.
71. CATAPANO, G. 1996. Mass transfer limitations to the performance of membrane bioartificial liver support devices. Int. J. Artif. Organs **19:** 18–35.
72. CATAPANO, G., L. DE BARTOLO, C.P. LOMBARDI & E. DRIOLI. 1996. The effect of oxygen transport resistances on the viability and functions of isolated rat hepatocytes. Int. J. Artif. Organs **19:** 61–71.
73. PIRET, J.M. & C.L. COONEY. 1991. Model of oxygen transport limitations in hollow fiber bioreactors. Biotech. Bioeng. **37:** 80–92.
74. BROTHERTON, J.D. & P.C. CHAU. 1996. Modeling of axial-flow hollow fiber cell culture bioreactors. Biotech. Prog. **12:** 575–590.
75. HAY, P.D., A.R. VEITCH, M.D. SMITH, et al. 2000. Oxygen transfer in a diffusion-limited hollow fiber bioartificial liver. Artif. Organs **24:** 278–288.
76. SUZUKI, M., K. TAKESHITA, T. YAMAMOTO, et al. 1997. Hepatocytes entrapped in collagen gel following 14 days of storage at 4 degrees C: preservation of hybrid artificial liver. Artif. Organs **21:** 99–106.

# Effect of Flow Configuration and Membrane Characteristics on Membrane Fouling in a Novel Multicoaxial Hollow-Fiber Bioartificial Liver

JEFFREY M. MACDONALD,[a] STEPHEN P. WOLFE,[a]
INDRAJIT ROY-CHOWDHURY,[b] HIROSHI KUBOTA,[c] AND LOLA M. REID[c]

[a]*Department of Biomedical Engineering, University of North Carolina School of Medicine, Chapel Hill, North Carolina, USA*

[b]*Department of Biological Sciences, Duke University Medical Center, Durham, North Carolina, USA*

[c]*Department of Cellular and Molecular Physiology, Program in Molecular Biology and Biotechnology, University of North Carolina School of Medicine, Chapel Hill, North Carolina, USA*

ABSTRACT: A novel "multicoaxial hollow fiber bioreactor" has been developed consisting of four concentric tubes, the two innermost tubes are called hollow fibers. Bioartificial livers are created by culturing liver progenitors in the space between the two innermost hollow fibers and with culture media contained in the two compartments (intracapillary and extracapillary) sandwiching the cell compartment. The outermost compartment is used for gas exchange. A hydrodynamic model has recently been established to predict the optimum hydraulic permeability and bioreactor operational parameters to create the physicochemical environment found in the liver acinus.[1] However, perfusion with serum-free hormonally-defined media and inoculation of cells introduces membrane fouling into the equation, and this parameter must be incorporated into the model. Using commercially available semipermeable hollow fibers (1 mm [0.65 µm pores] and 3 mm [0.1 µm pores] outer diameters [o.d]), the primary cause of resistance is the middle hollow fiber. Preliminary studies using bioreactors inoculated with isolated rat hepatocytes and perfused with serum-containing culture media demonstrated that the middle hollow fiber is the primary site of fouling, and this fouling ultimately causes cell mortality by blocking the transfer of nutrients. Experiments were performed to determine the best commercially available middle hollow fiber for construction of bioreactors and two 3-mm outer-diameter middle hollow fibers were compared: polypropylene and polysulfone, with 0.2 µm and 0.1 µm pore sizes, respectively. Dead-ended and cross flow configurations were compared for their effectiveness at reducing membrane fouling in the middle hollow fiber by determining the change in resistance with time. The results demonstrate that the 0.2-µm pore size polypropylene hollow fiber is the best choice for construction of the multicoaxial hollow-fiber bioreactor, and that cross flow results in two orders of magnitude lower resistance than dead-ended flow after 36 h.

Address for correspondence: Lola M. Reid, Department of Biomedical Engineering, Program in Molecular Biology and Biotechnology, University of North Carolina School of Medicine, Chapel Hill, NC 27599-7038, USA.

KEYWORDS: multicoaxial bioreactor; membrane fouling; polysulfone; polypropylene; hollow fiber; cross flow; dead-ended flow

## INTRODUCTION

A novel multicoaxial hollow-fiber bioreactor has been developed[1] to permit expansion and differentiation of human hepatic progenitors into normal human liver tissue and, thus, the establishment of a human bioartificial liver.[2] The bioreactor is composed of two innermost coaxial semipermeable hollow fibers. Cells are cultured in the space between two fibers (1-mm outer diameter [o.d.] and 2-mm inner diameter [i.d.]) with culture media contained in the two compartments sandwiching the cell compartment. Integral oxygenation occurs in the outermost (aeration) compartment created by a third coaxial outer silicone tube and the polycarbonate housing. Orientation of the four compartments is shown in FIGURE 1A. The outermost media stream in the extracapillary compartment (ECC) is oxygenated via the aeration compartment, and peripheral-to-central blood flow is mimicked by radial flow from the ECC to the innermost compartment, or intracapillary compartment (ICC).[1] A hydrodynamic model based on Darcy's law was recently developed to determine the optimum hydraulic permeability and bioreactor operational parameters to create the physicochemical environment found in the liver acinus.[1] With the use of serum-free hormonally defined media and cells, the membranes foul and the hydraulic permeability decreases, as defined by some function.

The rate of membrane fouling depends on membrane characteristics and the flow configuration, decreasing from dead-ended to cross flow configurations. Dead-ended and cross flow configuration are perpendicular and parallel, respectively, to the plane of the membrane, therefore, the former has a more rapid rate of membrane adsorption of components from the media.[3] The cross flow configuration generates a shear force that scrubs the membrane surface of adsorbed molecules. Furthermore, the molecular and physical characteristics of the membrane affect the rate of fouling.[3] For example, polysulfone is typically used for cell culture filtration, because media components do not adsorb as well in comparison to other polymers, such as polypropylene.[3] Smaller pore size results in increased fouling rates.[3] Therefore, "membrane-fouling" experiments were performed using 3-mm o.d. polypropylene and polysulfone hollow fibers with 0.2-µm and 0.1-µm pore size, respectively. Dead-ended and cross flow configurations, were compared by monitoring the change in resistance between bioreactors constructed from the two different hollow fibers. To demonstrate that membrane-fouling of the middle hollow fiber causes the death of the cells, a viability study was performed using isolated rat hepatocytes inoculated into bioreactors constructed with 3-mm o.d. polysulfone middle hollow fibers (0.1 µm pore size). One bioreactor was perfused directly in the cell compartment containing the hepatocytes with serum-containing culture media (FIG. 1B) and the other had a cross flow configuration, but the transmembrane pressure was relatively small and the middle fiber became clogged, halting radial flow (FIG. 1D).

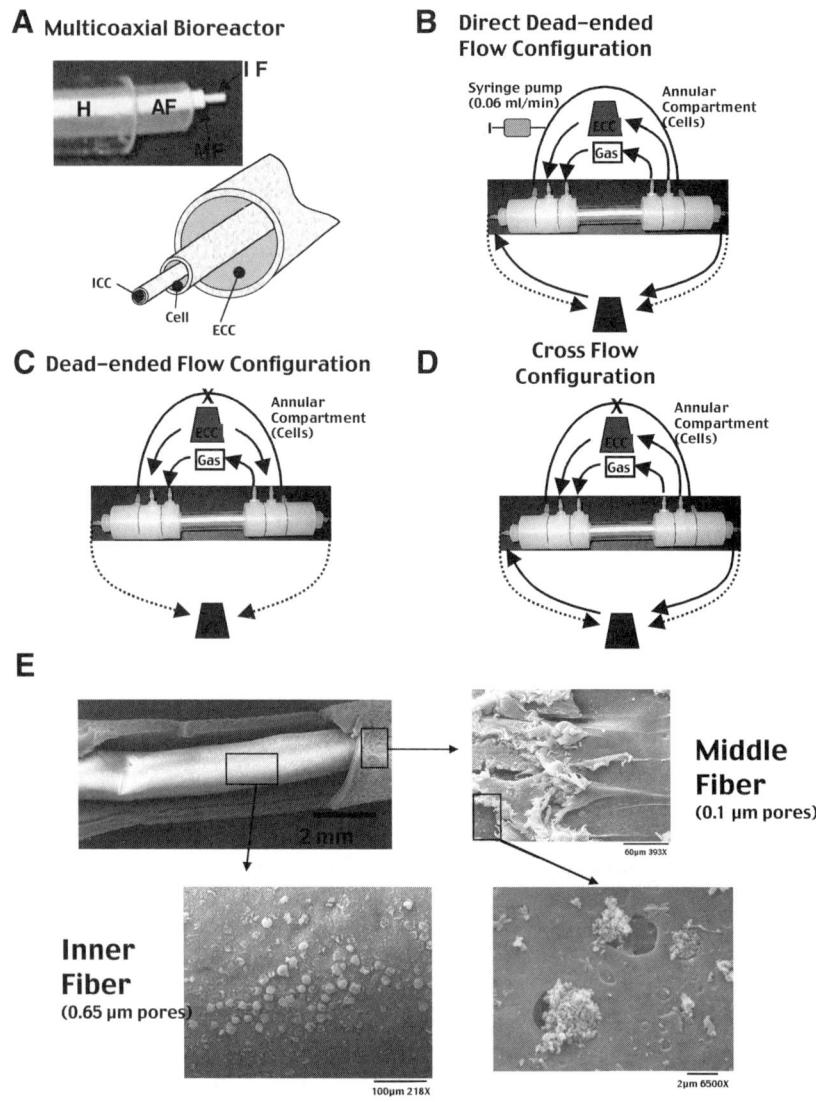

**FIGURE 1.** A picture and schematic representation showing the three concentric tubes, housing, and three major compartments of the multicoaxial bioreactor (**A**). The bioreactor loop for the radial perfusion and hepatocyte viability study (**B**) and dead-ended (**C**) and cross flow (**D**) configurations used in the membrane fouling study. The SEMs of the coaxial fibers after the hepatocyte viability study using the direct dead-ended flow configuration shown in **B** (**E**). ABBREVIATIONS: H, housing; AF, aeration tube; MF, middle hollow fiber; IF, inner hollow fiber; ICC, intracapillary compartment; ECC, extracapillary compartment. Note: in **B–D**, the ECC and ICC reservoirs are on the top and bottom, respectively, of the flow diagram.

## METHODS

Materials for the construction of bioreactors were polysulfone hollow fibers, polypropylene hollow fibers, Silastic™ tubing and silicone glue, 10-mm NMR tubes, 1-inch diameter polypropylene rod, 0.394 inch by 0.079 inch viton O-rings, and medical-grade polyurethane purchased from AG/Technology (Needham, MA), Akzo Nobel (Wuppertal, Germany), Dow Corning (Midland, MI), Wilmad/Lab Glass (Buena, NJ), Piedmont Plastics Inc. (Raleigh, NC), Apple Rubber Products (Lancaster, NY), and Caschem Inc. (Bayonne, NJ), respectively. The 1–60 rpm variable pump, Pharmed™ tubing, polypropylene barbed fittings, plastic tubing clamps, and Teflon needle valves were purchased from Cole Parmer (Chicago IL). The pressure monitoring apparatus was constructed using 0 to 5 psi pressure sensors, a pressure calibrator, and TDS210 oscilloscope purchased from Sensym Inc., (Milpitas, CA), Crystal Engineering Inc. (San Luis Obispo, CA), and Tektronix (Beaverton, OR), respectively. Details of the pressure monitoring system are described elsewhere by Wolfe and others.[1]

Construction of bioreactors and quality assurance were performed as described by Wolfe and others.[1] Two sets of bioreactor experiments were performed: isolated rat hepatocyte viability and membrane fouling studies. RPMI 1640 (calcium concentration less than 0.5 mM) was used for both hepatocyte and membrane-fouling studies, but the former contained 10% fetal calf serum and the latter contained a serum-free medium supplemented with four major components (0.1% BSA-fatty acid free, 5 µg/ml insulin, 10 µg/ml transferrin, and 10 µg/ml HDL]. To both recipes, penicillin and streptomycin were added, and the medium was filtered to 0.2 µm. The tubing and glassware used to construct the bioreactor loops were autoclaved prior to use. Experimental setup of the bioreactor loop is shown in FIGURE 1 B–D for direct dead-end, dead-end, and cross flow configurations, respectively. The bioreactor loops were maintained at 37°C in a Wedco incubator (Silver Spring, MD).

### Isolated Rat Hepatocyte Viability Studies

Rat hepatocytes were isolated using the procedure of Seglen.[4] To obtain a crude enrichment for the smaller, less dense hepatocytes, the mixture of isolated hepatocytes was suspended in 20 ml of RPMI 1640 with 10% fetal calf serum, penicillin, and streptomycin and permitted to settle at unit gravity on ice for 8 min. The supernatant was obtained and centrifuged for 1 min at 75 rpm to remove the majority of dead cells. The pellet was used for the viability study. The bioreactors were inoculated with $4 \times 10^6$ hepatocytes. MacDonald and others[5] describe the inoculation procedure: in brief, the hepatocytes were introduced into the cell compartment via the cell inoculation ports by reversing the pump attached to the ICC and clamping off all ports leading from the ECC similar to the bioreactor loop configuration shown in FIGURE 1 B. Two flow configurations were tested for their efficacy at maintaining viability and after one day in the bioreactors, the hepatocytes were removed and the viability was determined by trypan blue exclusion assay. The two flow configurations are shown in FIGURE 1 B and D. They consist of direct dead-ended flow to the cell compartment (FIG. 1 B) with cross-flow in the ECC and ICC but with no pressure gradient, thus no radial flow (FIG. 1 D). After inoculation the bioreactor was maintained at 37°C without perfusion for 0.5 to 1.0 h, at which point the pumps were activated.

## Membrane-Fouling Studies

The optimum hydraulic permeability, $k$, for the middle hollow fiber was determined using a model based on Darcy's Law, $v = -k\nabla P/\mu$, where $v$ is velocity, $P$ is pressure, and $\mu$ is viscosity of the fluid.[16] The model does not account for fouling and cell attachment, both of which decrease $k$. Therefore, the two commercially available hollow fibers and flow configurations were investigated.

Bioreactors were constructed as described elsewhere[1] except the inner fiber was deleted, and the cell ports were blocked with silicone glue. Intraluminal ($P_i$) and extraluminal ($P_e$) pressures were measured with a pressure monitoring system described elsewhere[1] and gauge hydrostatic pressures values were noted at 0, 0.5, 1, 2, 4, 8, 12, 24, 36, and 48 h. The two flow configurations are shown in FIGURE 1C and D. Radial flow rates ($Q_r$) were calculated by measuring the total volume accumulation in the waste reservoir (FIG. 1C and D) per time interval. The radial flow rate and pressure data were used to calculate the total resistance ($R_{Tot}$), which is the reciprocal of hydraulic permeability, as shown by Equation (1).[6]

$$R_{Tot} = \frac{2\pi L \Delta P}{Q_r \mu \ln\left(\frac{r_{o2}}{r_{i2}}\right)}, \qquad (1)$$

where, $\Delta P = P_e - P_i$, $R_{Tot} = 1/k$, and $K = k/\mu$. $L$ is the length of the middle hollow fiber, $K$ is the conductivity of the middle hollow fiber, and $r_{i2}$ and $r_{o2}$ are the inner and outer radii for the middle hollow fiber, respectively.

## SEM Studies

Bioreactors were fixed by slow injection via 20 cc syringe of fixative (2.5% glutaraldehyde and 2% paraformaldehyde, 157 mM phosphate buffered saline) across the middle fibers and flowing out through the ICC ports. Fibers were extricated from the bioreactors using a bandsaw, and the fibers were dehydrated in serial dilution from fixative to 100% ethanol. The samples were critical point dried using a Hummer X critical point dryer (Anatech LTD., Alexandria, VA), mounted on SEM stubs, coated with a gold:palladium (40:60) alloy using a sputter coater (Bal-tec Products Inc., Middlebury, CT), and attached to the SEM. A Cambridge S200 SEM (Cambridge, England) was used to obtain the images.

## RESULTS

The results from the hepatocyte studies found that after 24 h hepatocytes survived using direct dead-ended flow configuration as shown in FIGURE 1B, and died with no radial perfusion directed from the ECC to ICC. The SEMs in FIGURE 1E are the outside of the inner and outer fibers in the bioreactor with no radial perfusion but a cross flow configuration (FIG. 1C). The bottom left SEM (FIG. 1E) shows that hepatocytes are attached to the inner fiber and the bottom right SEM (FIG. 1E) shows that cell-derived and medium-derived components are clogging pores on the outer membrane. It was concluded that the relatively low hydraulic permeability of the middle hollow fiber was the primary cause of stopping radial flow and likely due

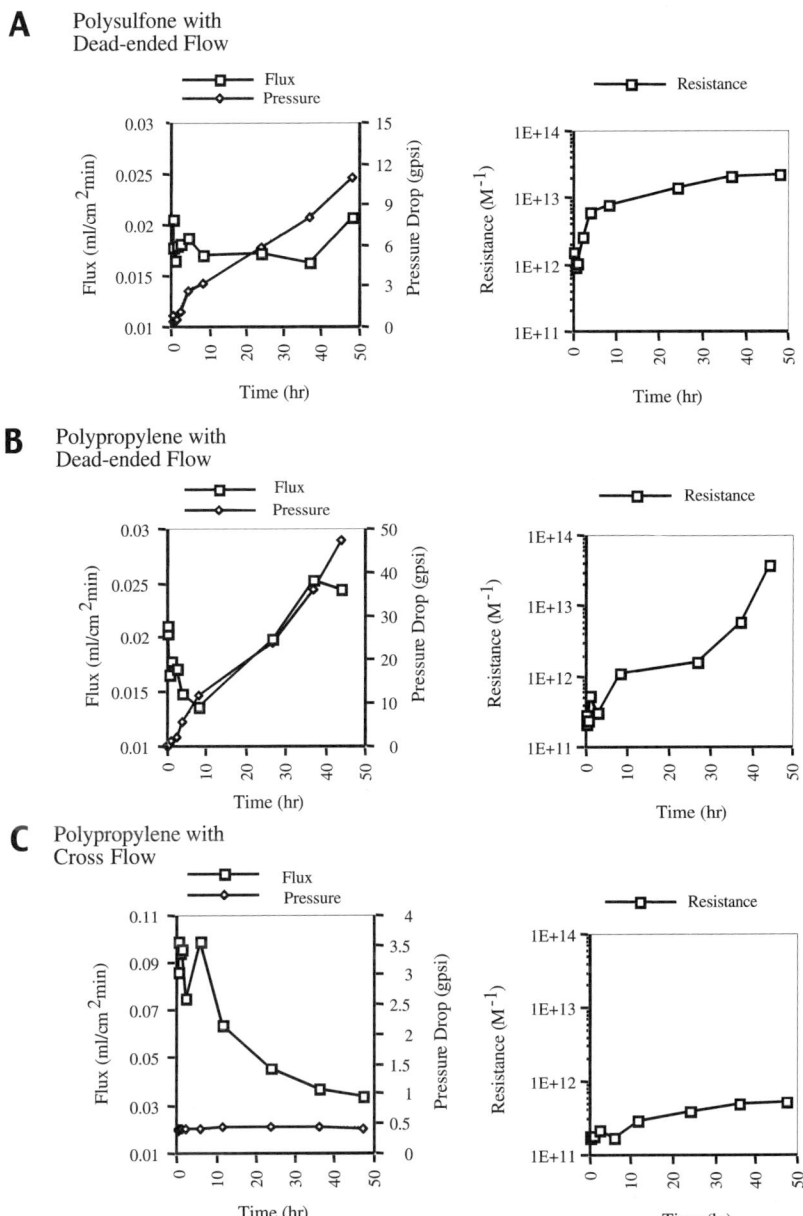

**FIGURE 2.** The results of the membrane-fouling experiment between the two hollow fibers and dead-ended and cross flow configurations (**A–C**). The time course on the left plots pressure and flux; those on the right plot resistance.

to membrane fouling. To test this hypothesis, membrane-fouling studies were performed with bioreactors made only using the middle hollow fiber and not the inner hollow fiber in order to simplify analysis. The membrane-fouling studies showed that larger pore size had greater flux per unit pressure (compare FIGURE 2A and B), and the dead-ended flow configuration (FIG. 1C) caused far more fouling than the cross-flow configuration, as shown by the increase in resistance (compare FIG. 2B and C). In typical fouling studies, the pressure is kept constant and radial flow is measured to yield a rate of fouling, defined by resistance Eq. (**1**), for a given filtration rate.[3,7–10] The goal of this experiment was to obtain a constant radial flow rate, since this is the most important mass transfer parameter for satisfying the

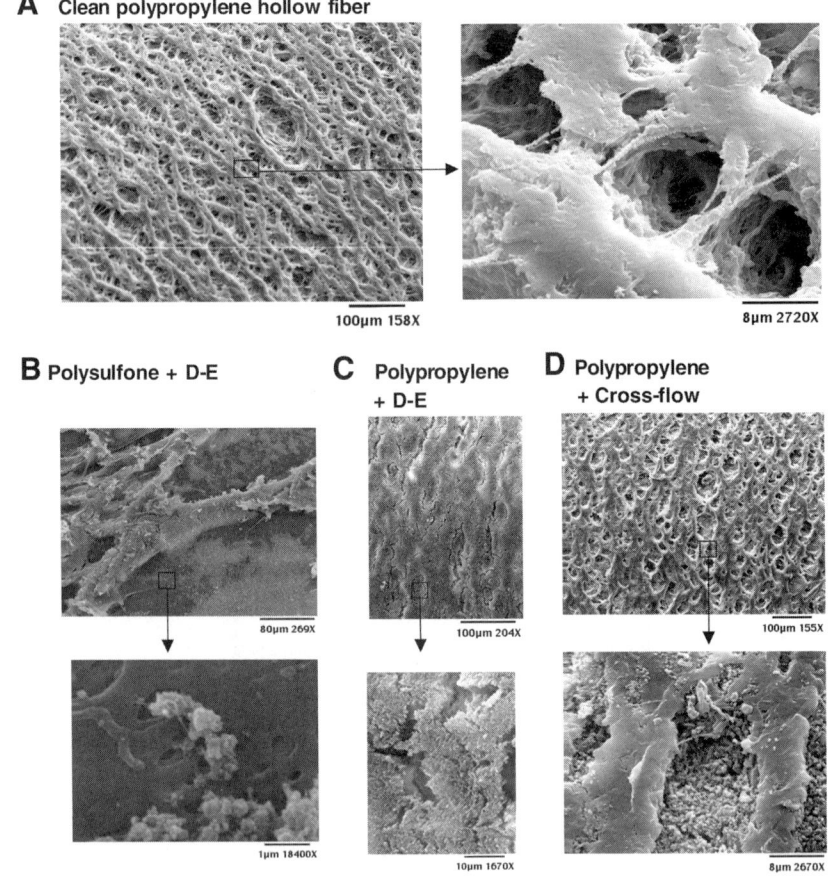

**FIGURE 3.** SEMs of the clean polypropylene middle hollow fiber (**A**), and the middle hollow fiber after each of the three experiments: polysulfone with direct dead-ended flow and cross flow (**B**), polypropylene with dead-ended flow (**C**), and polypropylene with cross flow (**D**).

oxygen demands of the cell culture.[11] The elevated pressure in the ECC associated with maintaining a given radial flow rate was shown not to significantly transmit to the cell compartment,[1] thus, the high pressures associated with long term dead-ended flow filtration were investigated.

In the dead-ended flow experiments the flux was maintained nearly constant as illustrated by the left graph of both pressure and flux shown in FIGURE 2A, demonstrating relatively constant flux with increasing pressure. The graphs on the right in FIGURE 2A and B show the resulting rate of membrane fouling as related by resistance Eq. (1). The fouling with the dead-ended flow configuration using the polypropylene fiber was so extensive that all radial flow ceased, and the hollow fiber collapsed at 44 h due to excessive pressure in the ECC (FIG. 2B). However, with the cross flow configuration, the axial flow rates in the ICC and ECC were constant, and thus the pressures were relatively constant and flux decreased, ultimately reaching a steady-state radial flow rate by two days (left graph, FIG. 2C). Cross flow also resulted in relatively minor membrane fouling as supported by the two orders of magnitude difference in total resistance by two days (compare right graphs in FIG. 2B and C).

Medium-derived components can be seen in SEM photos clogging a 0.1-μm pore on the outside of the polysulfone hollow fiber (see FIGURE 3B). The SEMs demonstrate the enormous amount of material forming a "cake" on the polypropylene hollow fiber with the dead-ended configuration (FIG. 3C) as compared to the cross flow configuration (FIG. 3D) and a clean hollow fiber (FIG. 3A). Therefore, the polypropylene hollow fiber using cross flow configuration resulted in far longer retention of the initial hydraulic permeability values.

## DISCUSSION

Before cells can be established in bioreactors and with retention of viability, a physical analysis of the bioreactor must be performed to optimize mass transfer during operation. Previous studies have shown that isolated rat hepatocytes die within a few hours in a similar coaxial hollow fiber bioreactor without radial perfusion,[5] and studies with extant commercially available bioreactors indicate survival for relatively short periods of time (less than a week) and no growth,[12] such as those presently in clinical trials.[13,14] The study shown in FIGURE 1 demonstrates that fouling of the middle fiber ultimately will stop radial flow and cause hepatocytes to die. Therefore, we compared two commercially available hollow fibers and flow configurations to determine which is best for liver culture.

We found the polypropylene (0.2-μm pore size) hollow fiber resisted fouling the best with a cross flow configuration. The flux time course from the cross flow configuration (FIG. 2C) was consistent with other membrane-fouling studies in hollow-fiber bioreactors,[3,15] where there is an initial exponential decrease due to fouling, followed by a plateau over which flux remains relatively constant. In this study, a plateau was reached by 48 h (FIG. 2C). An experimental protocol should be employed whereby the conditioning phase should be used to establish steady-state flux values before inoculating the bioreactor with cells. Therefore, based on FIGURE 2C, the starting point for axial flow rate and resulting pressure in the ECC should be an order of magnitude greater and conditioned with serum-free hormonally defined medium for

12–24 h to establish a relatively stable radial flux before cells are inoculated. This exponential phase is also characterized by a decrease in the filtrate of key culture components essential for cell survival, such as oncotic agents like albumin or growth factors like insulin (unpublished results).[1] Therefore, media should be changed prior to inoculation of cells to achieved desired oncotic and hormonal concentrations.

The difference between the two flow configurations depicted in FIGURE 1B and C is illustrated by comparing the two SEMs shown in FIGURE 3B and C. "Cake" is the term used for the material formed on membrane surfaces due to adsorption of components from the perfusate and is clearly shown in the SEM with dead-ended flow (FIG. 3B) but not cross flow (FIG. 3C). The cake acts like a second membrane, but with much less permeability.[16] Adsorption of proteins in the culture media such as, albumin, is enhanced by concentration polarization, which is the reversible build-up of dissolved or suspended solute in the solution phase near the membrane–solution interface. The build-up is due to a balance between the convective drag toward and through the membrane resulting from the radial flux.[3] Hydrophobic and solvation effects between the solute and membrane surface are significant factors with polypropylene material.[16] The SEMs in FIGURE 3B and C demonstrate the effectiveness of cross flow in reducing cake formation and ultimately maintaining relatively constant radial flow rates. Furthermore, outgassing, or the movement of gases from solution to gas phase, can occur due to the drop in pressure and the potential decrease in gas solubility at the surface due to concentration polarization.[1] Small bubbles were observed on the middle fiber surface of the cake during dead-ended flow but not with cross flow.

These results indicate that cross flow should be used for maintaining radial flux in the multicoaxial bioreactor. Furthermore, hollow fibers with a larger pore size is indicated. Previous studies have shown that commercially available 3-mm o.d. and 2-mm i.d. hollow fibers are nearly two orders of magnitude less permeable than needed to maintain values of radial flux at acceptable pressures for providing oxygen mass transfer requirements of cultured liver cells.[1] The final parameter in establishing this bioartificial liver is the culturing of liver cells, which will greatly reduce hydraulic permeability of the membranes and the cell compartment. Novel membranes are presently being investigated to obtain an optimal hydraulic permeability that can be easily changed, depending on future *in vivo* experimental findings.[17]

## ACKNOWLEDGMENTS

Funding for these studies derived from NIH (1-R01 DK52851; L.M. Reid), an NRSA fellowship (1-F32-DK09713; J.M. MacDonald), a Sponsored Research Grant from Renaissance Cell Technologies Inc. (L.M. Reid), and the Johns Hopkins Center for Alternatives to Animal Testing (J.M. MacDonald and L.M. Reid). We thank Dr. YiWei Rong from the Advance Cell and Tissue Engineering Facility for the isolated rat hepatocytes and Dr. Robert Bagnell from the Microscopy Services Laboratory for technical support with the SEMs, both are at the University of North Carolina at Chapel Hill.

## REFERENCES

1. WOLFE, S., E. HSU, L.M. REID & J.M. MACDONALD. 2001. A novel multi-coaxial hollow fiber bioreactor for adherent cell types. Part 1: hydrodynamic studies. Biotech. Bioeng. In press.
2. XU, A., T. LUNTZ, J.M. MACDONALD, et al. 2000. Liver stem cells and lineage biology. *In* Principles of Tissue Engineering. R. Lanza, R. Langer & J. Vacanti, Eds. Academic Press, San Diego.
3. BELFORT, G., R. DAVIS & A. ZYDNEY. 1994. The behavior of suspensions and macromolecular solutions in crossflow microfiltration. J. Mem. Sci. **96:** 1–58.
4. SEGLEN, P.O. 1973. Preparation of rat liver cells. II. Effects of ions and chelators on tissue dispersion. Exp. Cell Res. **76**(1): 25–30.
5. MACDONALD, J.M., M. GRILLO, O. SCHMIDLIN, et al. 1998. NMR spectroscopy and MRI investigation of a potential bioartificial liver. NMR Biomed. **11:** 55–66.
6. TRACEY, E. & R. DAVIS. 1994. Protein fouling of track-etched polycarbonate microfiltration membranes. J. Coll. Inter. Sci. **167:** 104–116.
7. DORP, E., D. SCHNEDITZ & M. MOSER. 1991. The measurement of blood density to investigate protein deposition at the blood/hollow fiber membrane interface during ultrafiltration. Inter. J. Art. Org. **14:** 424–429.
8. GUELL, C. & R.H. DAVIS. 1996. Membrane fouling during microfiltration of protein mixtures. J. Mem. Sci. **119:** 269–284.
9. KELLY, S.T. & A.L. ZYDNEY. 1995. Mechanisms for BSA fouling during microfiltration. J. Mem. Sci. **107:** 115–127.
10. OPONG, W.S. & A.L. ZYDNEY. 1991. Hydraulic permeability of protein layers deposited during ultrafiltration. J. Coll. Inter. Sci. **142:** 41–60.
11. CIMA, L.G., H.W. BLANCH & C.R. WILKE. 1990. A theoretical and experimental evaluation of a novel radial-flow hollow fiber reactor for mammalian cell culture. Bioproc. Eng. **5:** 19–30.
12. MACDONALD, J.M., J.P. GRIFFIN, H. KUBOTA, et al. 1999. Bioartificial livers. *In* Cell Encapsulation Technology and Therapeutics. W. Kuhtreiber, R.P. Lanza & W.L. Chick, Eds. Birkhauser, Boston.
13. CUSTER, L. & C.J. MULLON. 1998. Oxygen delivery to and use by primary porcine hepatocytes in the HepatAssist 2000 system for extracorporeal treatment of patients in end-stage liver failure. Adv. Exp. Med. Biol. **454:** 261–271.
14. NAIK, S., H.A. SANTANGINI, D.M. TRENKLER, et al. 1997. Functional recovery of porcine hepatocytes after hypothermic or cryogenic preservation for liver support systems. Cell Transplant. **6:** 447–454.
15. CONRAD, P.B. & S.S. LEE. 1998. Two-phase bioconversion product recovery by microfiltration I. Steady state studies. Biotech. Bioeng. **57:** 631–641.
16. MEAGHER, L., C. KLAUBER & R.M. PASHLEY. 1996. The influence of surface forces on the fouling of polypropylene microfiltration membranes. Coll. Surf. A: Physicochem. Eng. Asp. **106:** 63–81.
17. GUPTA, B.S. 1998. Medical textile structures: an overview. Med. Plast. Biomat. **5:** 16–30.

# Evaluating the Performance of a Hybrid Artificial Liver Support System With a Recoverable Hepatic Failure Rat Model

HIROYUKI IJIMA, AYAKO NOGUCHI, TAKEYUKI KATSUNO, TSUTOMU ONO, KOHJI NAKAZAWA, KAZUMORI FUNATSU, AND KOEI KAWAKAMI

*Department of Chemical Engineering, Faculty of Engineering, Graduate School of Engineering, Kyusyu University, 6-10-1 Hakozaki, Higashi-ku, Fukuoka 812-8581, Japan*

ABSTRACT: To evaluate the performance of an artificial liver, we created a recoverable hepatic failure rat model. This involves a 30–60 minute warm ischemia, via clamping, of one-third of the liver with a partial (two-thirds) hepatectomy. Variations on this method provide for the possibility of several modes of hepatic failure. Survival time of the rats was prolonged (35%) by applying our hybrid artificial liver. However, the extracorporeal circulation is a considerable burden to the rat. Therefore, we need to apply the hybrid artificial liver intermittently and repeatedly.

KEYWORDS: hybrid artificial liver; support system; hepatic failure; rat model

## INTRODUCTION

Generally, liver transplantation is the only method that can be used to save patients suffering from fulminant hepatic failure, particularly acute in chronic hepatic failure patients. However, we are not able to provide liver transplantation to the majority of the patients due to a donor shortage.[1-3] Therefore, development of a hybrid artificial liver is required.[4] There is no method for evaluating the performance of an artificial liver, except via animal experimentation. However, there are many problems with these techniques, including cost and reliability of the data. Eguchi[5] and Suh et al.[6] have created a fulminant hepatic failure rat model in which partial hepatectomy (68%) is combined with induction of right liver lobe necrosis. They reported that liver mass, PCNA, hepatocyte growth factor (HGF), and HGF receptor c-met levels increased as a result of using their hybrid artificial liver. They also concluded that their artificial liver can induce regeneration of host liver. However, they were not able to evaluate the recovery ratio by using this model. On the other hand, there is no animal model that can evaluate liver regeneration and recovery of the animal except drug-induced hepatic failure animals.

In the study reported in this paper, we created a novel hepatic failure rat model that has enabled us to evaluate the performance of a hybrid artificial liver, including

Address for correspondence: Dr. Hiroyuki Ijima, Associate Professor, Department of Chemical Engineering, Faculty of Engineering, Graduate School of Engineering, Kyushu University 6-10-1 Hakozaki, Higashi-ku, Fukuoka 812-8581, Japan. Voice/fax: +81-92-642-4114.
ijima@apex.chem-eng.kyushu-u.ac.jp

liver regeneration induction ability. Furthermore, we have developed an extracorporeal circulation system for applying the artificial liver to rats without anesthesia. Thus, we have been able to establish an evaluation method for artificial liver by using these techniques. The methods are reproducible, reduce cost, are simple to operate, and fast in terms of the evaluation of artificial liver.

## MATERIALS AND METHODS

Adult male Wistar rats (7–8 weeks old, approximately 250 g) were used in this study. This experiment was reviewed by the Ethics Committee on Animal Experiments in Kyushu University and was carried out under the control of the Guideline for Animal Experiments at Kyushu University.

### *Hepatic Failure Rat Model*

The two anterior liver lobes (2/3 liver) were removed using a standard partial hepatectomy method. Subsequently the remaining liver lobes (1/3) experienced 30–60 minutes of warm ischemia by clamping the hepatic artery and portal vein, as is shown in FIGURE 1. After this period, the clamp was released and the rat was used in our study.

### *Hybrid Artificial Liver Support System*

*Hybrid Artificial Liver Module*

A multicapillary polyurethane foam packed-bed type artificial liver module[7] was used in this study. This module consisted of cylindrical PUF block that had many capillaries in a triangular arrangement for uniform medium flow. Hepatocytes were isolated from a rat using a two-step collagenase perfusion method.[8] The isolated hepatocytes ($7 \times 10^7$ cells) were inoculated[7] to the artificial liver module at a density of $1 \times 10^7$ cells/ml and cultured for one day. The culture medium was exchanged four hours after inoculation.

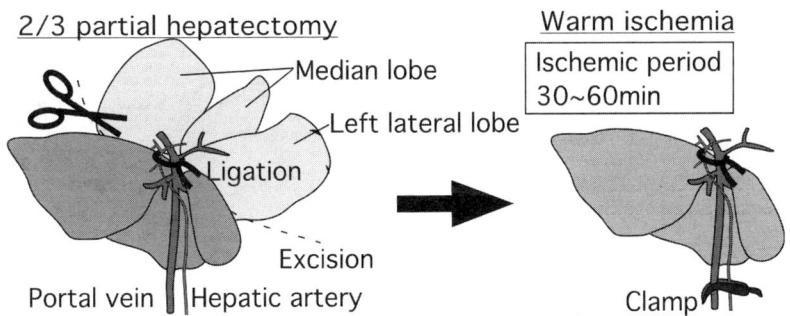

**FIGURE 1.** Hepatic failure rat model.

*Rat Extracorporeal Circulation*

We placed the access points to draw and return blood for extracorporeal circulation on the carotid artery and jugular vein of a recipient rat (dorsal incision on the neck).[9] After connecting an extracorporeal circulation line, hepatic failure was induced by the operation described above. The hybrid artificial liver support system was composed of a rat extracorporeal circulation line and a module side plasma circulation line, with these lines connected via a plasma separator as shown in FIGURE 2. The total volume in the extracorporeal circulation line including a plasma separator was approximately 1.5 ml.

*Prevention of Blood Clotting*

Before using a hybrid artificial liver support system, both circulation lines were filled with 100 U-heparin/ml isotonic sodium chloride solution to prevent blood clotting in the lines. The solution was then exchanged to normal rat plasma supplemented with 10 U/ml heparin. Furthermore, 50 U heparin (1,000 U/ml) was injected to a recipient rat via carotid artery before inducing hepatic failure.

*Treatment Protocol*

The efficiency of an artificial liver was evaluated by comparing the survival period of two different groups; a hybrid artificial liver treatment group (AL group) to which was applied a hybrid artificial liver support system, and a control group that was connected to the system without hepatocytes. Blood (0.3 ml) was obtained as a sample and injected with 0.5–1.0 ml transfusion mixture, composed of normal rat plasma and 5% glucose solution mixture at the same volume via an extracorporeal blood circulation line every 0.5 hours during extracorporeal circulation.

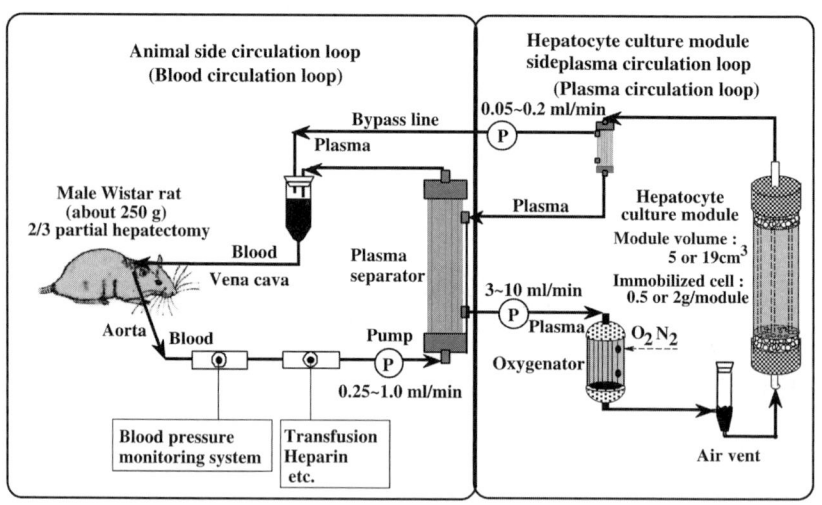

**FIGURE 2.** Hybrid artificial liver support system.

## RESULTS AND DISCUSSIONS

### Hepatic Failure Rat Model

FIGURE 3 shows the relation between warm ischemic period and survival ratio of rats. The relation is linear during the period from 30 to 60 minutes of ischemia. From the result, we were easily able to control the degree of hepatic failure in rats by changing the warm ischemic period. When we applied the relation to non-ischemic rats, the survival ratio reached 140%. This result indicates that there is an ischemic threshold period to load irreversible damage to the liver.

### Artificial Liver Support

When we applied an artificial liver support system with 0.5 g hepatocytes to the 50-minute warm ischemic hepatic failure rat model for the entire period, the survival times of the control group and the AL group were 84 ± 42 minutes ($n = 4$) and 115 ± 15 minutes ($n = 5$), respectively. We consider our hybrid artificial liver support system to be effective for the treatment of the hepatic failure rat. However, the ammonia concentration in blood rapidly increased during three hours, extracorporeal circulation in both cases, as is shown in FIGURE 4A.

Damage of extracorporeal circulation to normal rat was evaluated. At the result, the degree of damage was not significantly changed at flow rates between 0.25 and 1.0 ml/minute. Therefore, we attempted to evaluate the performance of ammonia metabolism activity of our hybrid artificial liver support system for two hours' circulation at 1.0 ml/minute with 2 g of hepatocytes immobilized in the module (FIG. 4B). By applying this hybrid artificial liver support system, ammonia was well metabolized. However, the concentration in blood line is twice that in plasma of hybrid artificial liver module side. This was caused by the insufficient mass transfer. In future, we need to establish an improved protocol to use a hybrid artificial liver for clinical treatment. The treatment period and performance required (hepatocyte mass)[10] will be major topics of study.

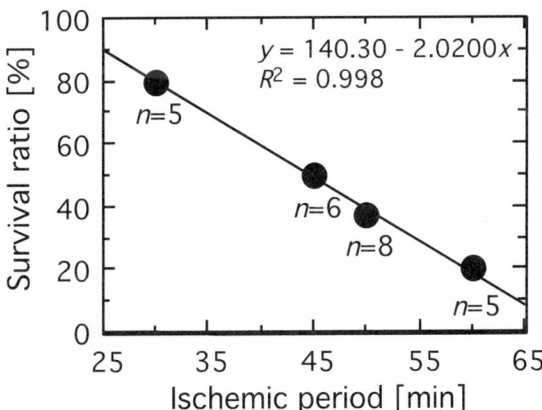

**FIGURE 3.** Relation between warm ischemic period and survival ratio of rats: $n$ denotes the number of rats in this study.

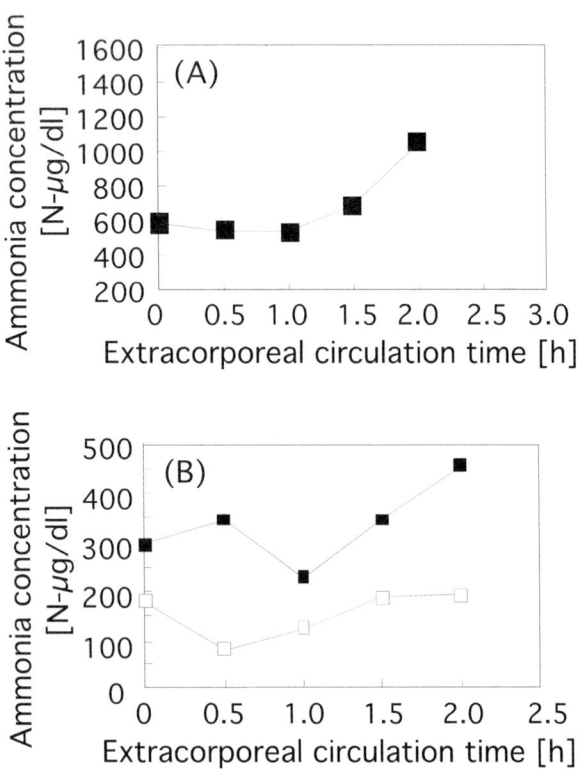

**FIGURE 4.** Ammonia concentration during the extracorporeal circulation. Immobilized hepatocytes in (**A**) and (**B**) are 0.5 g and 2 g, respectively. Ammonia concentration in blood line (■) and in module side plasma line (□).

## CONCLUSIONS

The authors offer the following conclusions based on this concise experimental design:
1. We have created a fulminant hepatic failure rat model in which the severity of hepatic failure can be controlled by changing the warm ischemic period.
2. Our hybrid artificial liver support system improved survivability relative to the control group, although plasma ammonia levels continued to rise.

## ACKNOWLEDGMENT

This work was supported in part by a Grant-in-Aid for Encouragement of Young Scientists (A): 11750694 from the Ministry of Education, Science, Sports and Culture of Japan.

## REFERENCES

1. IJIMA, H., K. NAKAZAWA & K. FUNATSU. 1998. Development of a hybrid artificial liver. Organ Biol. **5:** 35–40.
2. SCHRAA, E.O., R.L. MARQUET & J.N.M. IJZERMANS. 1999. The fourth barrier. Curr. Med. Res. Opin. **15:** 327–338.
3. SIM, K.H., A. MARINOV & G.A. LEVY. 1999. Can. J. Gastroenterol. **13:** 311–318.
4. IJIMA, H., K. NAKAZAWA, S. KOYAMA, et al. 2000. Development of a hybrid artificial liver support system and preclinical animal experiments. J. Artif. Organs **3:** 112–116.
5. EGUCHI, S., H. LILJA, W.R. HEWITT, et al. 1997. Loss and recovery of liver regeneration in rats with fulminant hepatic failure. J. Surg. Res. **72:** 112–122.
6. SUH, K.S., H. LILJA, Y. KAMOHARA, et al. 1999. Bioartificial liver treatment in rats with fulminant hepatic failure efect on DNA-binding activity of liver-enriched and growth-associated transcription factors. J. Surg. Res. **85:** 243–250.
7. IJIMA, H., T. MATSUSHITA & K. FUNATSU. 1994. Development of a hybrid artificial liver using multi capillary PUF/spheroid packed bed. Jpn. J. Artif. Organs **23:** 463–468.
8. SEGLEN, P.O. 1976. Preparation of isolated rat liver cells. In Methods in Cell Biology, Vol. 13. D.M. Prescott, Ed.: 29–83. Academic Press, New York.
9. IJIMA, H., T. MATSUSHITA, M. TAGA, et al. 1994. Establishment of a rat extracorporeal circulation system to estimate the performance of a hybrid artificial liver. In Animal Cell Technology: Basic & Applied Aspect, Vol. 6. T. Kobayashi, et al., Eds.: 395–399. Kluwer Academic Publishers, Netherlands.
10. IJIMA, H., K. NAKAZAWA, M. KANEKO, et al. 2000. Conditions required for a hybrid artificial liver support system using a PUF/hepatocyte-spheroid packed-bed module and its use in dogs with liver failure. Int. J. Artif. Organs **23:** 446–453.

# Development of a Coculture Model of Encapsulated Cells

LAURENCE CANAPLE,[a] NATHALIE NURDIN,[b] NELA ANGELOVA,[b] DAVID HUNKELER,[b] AND BÉATRICE DESVERGNE[a]

[a]*Institute of Animal Biology, University of Lausanne, CH-1015 Lausanne, Switzerland*

[b]*Laboratory of Polyelectrolytes and BioMacromolecules, EPFL, CH-1015 Lausanne, Switzerland*

ABSTRACT: In the whole animal, metabolic regulations are set by reciprocal interactions between various organs, via the blood circulation. At present, analyses of such interactions require numerous and uneasily controlled *in vivo* experiments. In a search for an alternative to *in vivo* experiments, our work aims at developing a coculture system in which different cell types are isolated in polymer capsules and grown in a common environment. The signals exchanged between cells from various origins are, thus, reproducing the *in vivo* intertissular communications. With this perspective, we evaluated a new encapsulation system as an artificial housing for liver cells on the one hand and adipocytes on the other hand. Murine hepatocytes were encapsulated with specially designed multicomponent capsules formed by polyelectrolyte complexation between sodium alginate, cellulose sulphate and poly(methylene-co-guanidine) hydrochloride, of which the permeability has been characterized. We demonstrated the absence of cytotoxicity and the excellent biocompatibility of these capsules towards primary culture of murine hepatocytes. Encapsulated hepatocytes retain their specific functions—transaminase activity, urea synthesis, and protein secretion—during the first four days of culture in minimum medium. Mature adipocytes, isolated from mouse epidydimal fat, were embedded in alginate beads. Measurement of protein secretion shows an identical profile between free and embedded adipocytes. We finally assessed the properties of encapsulated hepatocytes, cryopreserved over a periods of up to four months. The perspective of using encapsulated cells in coculture are discussed, since this system may represent a promising tool for fundamental research, such as analyses of drug metabolism, intercellular regulations, and metabolic pathways, as well as for the establishment of a tissue bank for storage and supply of murine hepatocytes.

KEYWORDS: coculture model; encapsulated cells; cryopreservation; metabolic signals

## INTRODUCTION

### *From* In Vivo *to* In Vitro *Analyses of Metabolic Regulation*

Homeostasis refers to the ability of an organism to maintain constant vital parameters, such as blood pressure, blood composition, energy balance, and hydration

Address for Correspondence: Béatrice Desvergne, Bâtiment de Biologie, Faculté des Sciences, CH-1015 Lausanne, Switzerland. Voice: 41 21 692 41 40; fax: 41 21 692 41 15.
beatrice.desvergne@iba.unil.ch

level. It requires that each organ—and within it, each cell—adjusts its program according to the information it gains from the systemic environment; that is, mainly from the blood, which carries informative molecules. Understanding how a tissue or a cell modifies its functional status in response to a given stimulus is well known in a classical cell culture system, which combines ease of manipulation with cell-specific responses. However, few models are available at present for understanding regulatory networks at the molecular level. Primary cultures in monolayer are simple and amenable to molecular studies but cannot be considered for crosstalk analysis. *In vivo* models of metabolic studies have provided a wealth of information, and the generation of mice that are functionally deleted for one gene has renewed the interest for such studies. However, the interpretation of mice phenotype at the molecular level, in basal condition and upon challenges, remains complex and often hypothetical. The need for *in vitro* tools has prompted the development of coculture methods. In one type of application, cell–cell interactions are direct and provide a structural organization, reminiscent of that of an organ, in which different cell types create a matrix that participates in organ-specific function maintenance. Closer to our interest are the cocultures in cell well inserts that allow free diffusion but no direct physical contact between two cell types. In this assay, one cell type is grown on the bottom plastic surface of the well and the second cell type resides on the membrane of the insert suspended in the well. It was first used to demonstrate the phenomenon of induction in early developmental processes. More recently, this device was used to analyze muscle/fat cell lines in coculture.[1] The limitations of this model are that interactions between no more than two tissues can be analyzed at one time. Thus, the development of a coculture system combining several cell types could be used to understand intercellular communication mechanisms and could also be a substitute for numerous preliminary experiments conducted in animals. Ideally, such a system should allow (1) free diffusion and access to the various cell types of any secreted molecules that may act as a signal; (2) the possibility of retrieving each cell type without contamination by the others, in order to analyze the cell-specific change in the gene transcription program; and (3) ease of manipulation and of production of the corresponding materials and cells for experimental reliability.

## *Cell Encapsulation as a Method for Compartmentation*

Encapsulation is presently being developed as a tool for immunoisolating cells to be transplanted into the human body in order to replace a deficient organ or deliver a therapeutic agent. The therapeutic potential of encapsulated cells is promising for treating patients who suffer from tissue loss, neurodegenerative disorders, diabetes, severe liver failure, and others diseases due to specific deficiencies. With this goal for clinical application, Chang has proposed an encapsulation system in which cells are retained in a semipermeable membrane that both protects them from damages by the host immune system and maintains their survival and metabolic functions by allowing the bidirectional diffusion of oxygen, nutrients, and cellular products.[2] Numerous studies have, indeed, demonstrated the efficiency of capsules such as alginate-poly (L-lysine) composite capsules to immunoisolate hepatocytes in xenograft attempts.[3–7] Because the properties described above are reminiscent of those required for cell compartmentation in a coculture system, we decided to assess the possibility of applying this new encapsulation technology to cocultures of various

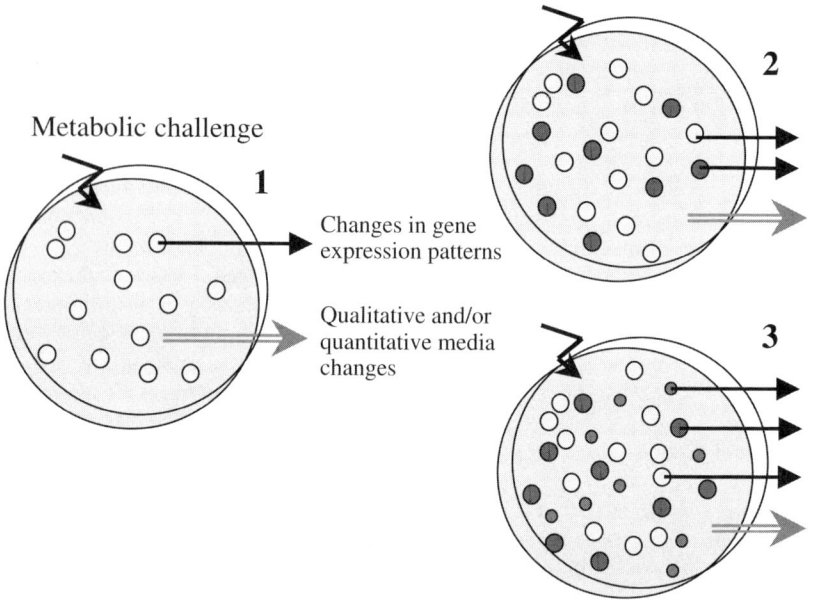

**FIGURE 1.** Schematic view of the coculture of encapsulated cells as a tool for analyzing tissue crosstalk and coordination upon metabolic challenge. In this system, a given metabolic challenge, such as a hormonal signal (insulin, glucocorticoids, etc.) or a modification of glucose availability, is expected to provoke different changes measured in the culture medium or at the level of gene expression, in the absence (*1*) or the presence of one (*2*) or two (*3*) other cell types.

cell types. Cells obtained from various tissues would be enclosed in a polymer capsule whose permeability allows adequate exchange of soluble molecules with the media. Allowing capsules containing various cells to be cultivated in a common environment, while not being in direct contact with each other, will reproduce the long-range crosstalk and coordination between the tissues, as it occurs *in vivo* via the vascular system (see FIGURE 1). Moreover, encapsulation has been proven to protect the cells from injury that can occur upon cryopreservation, during handling and in freezing/thawing steps.[8–11]

### *Control of Energy Metabolism: an Example of the Biological Relevance of the Coculture Approach*

Three organs have a main impact on lipid metabolism. The liver determines the metabolic fate of fatty acids, directing the fatty acids either to the esterification into triglycerides or to the oxidation pathway. On one hand the esterification pathway leads to the secretion into the bloodstream of the triglyceride excess in form of the very low density lipoproteins that are mainly taken up by the adipose tissue for triglyceride storage. On the other hand, when the plasma fatty acid levels are high, the oxidative pathway leads to the production and the secretion of ketone bodies, which serve as fuel for brain, muscles, and kidneys. In contrast, the adipose tissue is the site of the fatty acid synthesis and storage as triglycerides. Beside accumulating triglycerides, one crucial physiological function of the adipose tissue is to release in a highly controlled manner fatty acids into the bloodstream. Finally, the muscles are important consumers of fatty acids as an energy source, when the glucose level is low. The biological question on which we focus our research concerns the regulatory events that control lipid metabolism and that are taking place between liver, fat tissue, and muscle. According to the glucose availability, lipid concentration, and the hormonal environment, each of these tissues needs permanently to adjust its decision about utilization, storage or secretion of lipids and/or signal molecules. Disruption of the coordination between these three tissues with respect to lipid metabolism is believed to explain, at least in part, diabetes mellitus type II, often associated with obesity, which is a complex metabolic disorder involving both glucose and lipid metabolism pathways.[12]

At the molecular level, the nuclear receptors called peroxisome proliferator-activated receptors (PPARs) are ligand-activated transcription factors that modulate many aspect of energy metabolism.[13] They are activated by various compounds, among which the fibrate hypolipidemic drugs as well as mono and polyunsaturated fatty acids are important representatives. Three different PPAR isotypes have been identified ($\alpha$, $\beta/\delta$, and $\gamma$). PPAR$\alpha$ is highly expressed in the liver and its target genes comprise those encoding key enzymes in peroxisomal and mitochondrial fatty acid $\beta$-oxidation. The upregulation of the PPAR$\alpha$ gene by glucocorticoids also suggests that PPAR$\alpha$ plays an important role in regulating the catabolism of fatty acids mobilized during energy-demanding physiological situations, such as fasting. In contrast, PPAR$\gamma$ is predominantly expressed in the adipose tissue and its target genes are involved in all critical steps of lipid accumulation. Moreover, PPAR$\gamma$ directly participates in the adipose differentiation program. Thus, the nature of the PPAR ligands, the preferential expression of PPAR$\alpha$ in hepatocytes and that of PPAR$\gamma$ in adipocytes, and the identification of the main PPAR targeted pathways identify PPARs as a key regulator of lipid metabolism. Interestingly, thiazolidinediones (TZD) are high-affinity ligands for PPAR$\gamma$. They are antidiabetic agents that reduce hyperglycemia observed in diabetes mellitus type II, by improving the insulin sensitivity of several target tissues, including adipose tissue, liver, heart, and muscles. This reinforces the hypothesis that the alteration of lipid metabolism importantly contributes to the mechanism of the diabetes mellitus type II and that PPARs are likely to be involved in the signalling between liver and adipose tissue that coordinate and maintain energy homeostasis.

The important question that remains unsolved is the nature of the signals between the liver, the adipose tissue, and the muscles. There are several candidate signals, among which are the free fatty acids themselves, which can be envisioned as messenger molecules between adipose and other tissues. Adipose tissue also secretes the hormone-like substances TNF$\alpha$ and leptin. TNF$\alpha$ has a strong antiadipogenic action whereas secretion of leptin results in a complex modulation of insulin secretion and action, in addition to a role in regulating food intake. Two other substances recently identified, resistin[14] and FIAF,[15] are secreted by the adipose tissue and might also be of interest (see FIGURE 2). The difficulty of proving this concept comes from the complexity of the *in vivo* situation. We believe that our coculture system will provide the tools for an understanding of molecular signalling between these tissues.

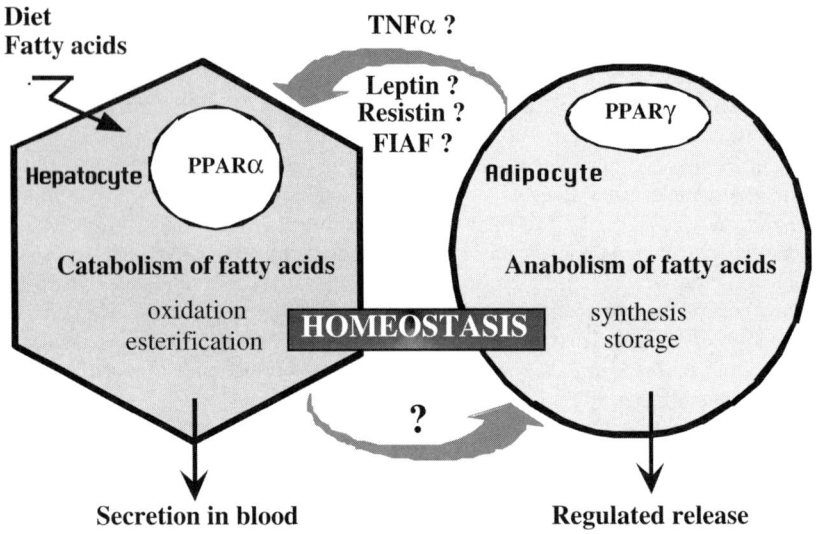

**FIGURE 2.** Homeostasis in lipid metabolism, and more generally in energy metabolism requires crosstalk between liver and adipocyte (see the text for further details).

Because of their central role in metabolic regulations, we first analyzed the survival and the functionality of encapsulated hepatocytes (liver cells) and adipocytes (fat cells). In addition, we also performed studies of cell using encapsulation as a means to optimize cell recovery after cryopreservation.

## MATERIALS AND METHODS

Murine hepatocytes were isolated, encapsulated, and cultured as described in detail elsewhere by the authors.[16]

Murine adipocytes were prepared from white epididymal fat pads after tissue dissociation with collagenase digestion, filtration through 150-μm nylon membrane, and centrifugation (5 min, 300 rpm). Adipocytes were then encapsulated in 1.5-mm alginate beads prepared by dropping 0.6% w/v alginate solution containing adipocytes into a 1.1% $CaCl_2$ solution buffered with 10 mM HEPES, 20 mM fructose. Free and encapsulated adipocytes were cultured in minimum DMEM medium (Life Technologies) supplemented with streptomycin/penicillin (100 μg/ml each) at 37°C. Total secreted proteins released in the medium both by free and encapsulated adipocytes during the first days of culture were quantified by a Bradford dye-binding assays (Bio-Rad Laboratories).

Encapsulated cells were cryopreserved in Cryotube vials (Nunc) containing serum-free media with 10% DMSO. The freezing steps consist of 30 minutes at 4°C, two hours at −20°C, 24 hours at −80°C, and final storage in a liquid nitrogen tank. Thawing was performed by a quick immersion at 37°C. Capsules were then washed three times and cultured in minimum medium. (For additional details, see REF. 16).

## EXPERIMENTAL DATA

### General Properties of the Biocapsules

Previously, various approaches utilizing different principles of capsule formation, such as alginate poly(L-lysine),[17,18] alginate–propylene glycol alginate–human serum albumin,[19] polyacrylonitrile–sodium methallyl-sulphonate,[20] hydroxyethyl methacrylate–methyl methacrylate copolymer,[21] or cellulose sulphate–polydimethyldiallylammonium chloride hydrogels[22] were developed and showed a great potential for cell encapsulation. For our purpose of constructing a coculture system, we were interested in identifying a suitable non-toxic polymer chemistry for the encapsulation of various cells, and in producing mechanically stable microcapsules with controllable permeability. For that purpose, we used a new system based on polyelectrolyte complexation between sodium alginate, cellulose sulphate, and poly(methylene-co-guanidine) hydrochloride.[23–25]

We first evaluated the biocompatibility of several capsule components. For that purpose, we used primary culture of hepatocytes from mouse liver, on the one hand, and primary culture of murine mature adipocytes from white epididymal fat, on the other hand, and assessed the cytotoxicity of polymers in solution at various concentrations. On the basis of our observations, reported in Canaple et al.,[16] anionic solutions composed of high viscosity Keltone alginate and cellulose sulphate were retained as the main components of the capsules.

We next established that the ratio of 0.6% alginate Keltone HV/0.6% cellulose sulphate provided capsules with satisfactory mechanical properties. To further the encapsulation process, an outer membrane was formed by dropping these cell-containing capsules in a $CaCl_2$/PMCG solution. The duration of the exposure to the PMCG solution determines the membrane thickness and, thus, the permeability properties of the capsule. We set up conditions such that this permeability was compatible with a free diffusion of the soluble molecules between the encapsulated cells and the medium. In the final protocol, described in detail elsewhere,[16,26] hepatocytes were encapsulated in 1.5-mm diameter capsules with a 90-μm-thick membrane.

In order to be able to use a differential means to retrieve hepatocyte- versus adipocyte-containing capsules, adipocytes were encapsulated in 1.5-mm alginate beads, with no outer membrane. Indeed, capsules containing different cell types can be mixed in a single culture dish and a simple and reliable method for differential sorting of these capsules needs to be devised. In this first approach, adipocyte cell extraction can be obtained via decomplexation of alginate beads by sodium citrate. This will not affect the membrane-covered beads, for which a mechanical stress can be applied in order to retrieve the cells. During this procedure, cell survival is not necessarily required, as many biological markers can be measured on total cell extract or following specific extraction methods (e.g., RNA preparation).

As shown in TABLE 1, the molar mass cutoff for both beads and capsules is sufficiently high to allow the free passage of most of the biological molecules of potential interest.

### Functional Consequences of Cell Encapsulation

The suitability of these systems was evaluated with respect to the survival and the specific functions of adipocytes and hepatocytes. The process of encapsulation

TABLE 1. Permeability properties of beads and capsules used for adipocyte and hepatocyte encapsulation

| | Molar Mass Cut-off Evaluation | |
|---|---|---|
| | Using polymer ingress detection by size exclusion chromatography | Using protein ingress/egress detection by electrophoresis and coomassie blue staining |
| Beads 1.5-mm diameter | 110–200 kDa | 150–220 kDa |
| Capsules 1.5-mm diameter 90-μm-thick membrane | 80–90 kDa | 116–150 kDa |

did not alter cell survival, as assessed by trypan blue staining and cytological observations. Cellular damage was measured by the release of the cytosolic liver enzyme glutamic oxaloacetic transaminase, whose release from encapsulated hepatocytes was prolonged compared to non-encapsulated cells, maintained in primary culture. However, the functional properties of the hepatocytes were not altered, as demonstrated by the comparable activities of encapsulated and non-encapsulated cells in albumin and urea production, at least during the first four days of culture in serum-free Williams' E medium (see TABLE 2 and FIGURE 3A). Thus, we demonstrated that the encapsulation does not adversely affect specific functions of hepatocytes, as compared to classic primary cultures.

The functional characterization of mature adipocytes in alginate beads was more difficult because of the rather low metabolic activities of the adipocytes in culture. Nevertheless, we tested their ability to secrete proteins during the first days of culture

TABLE 2. *In vitro* functional activities of free and encapsulated hepatocytes cultured in serum-free Williams' E medium

| Days of Culture | GOT Secretion (U/ml/million cells) | | Urea/Ammonia Secretion (μg/million cells) | | Albumin Secretion |
|---|---|---|---|---|---|
| | Non-Encapsulated Hepatocytes | Encapsulated Hepatocytes | Non-Encapsulated Hepatocytes | Encapsulated Hepatocytes | Non-Encapsulated Hepatocytes |
| 1 | 32.2 ± 9.7 | 33.3 ± 9.6 | 11 ± 2.2 | 11.6 ± 4.7 | Days of Culture 1 2 3 4 |
| 2 | 15.2 ± 8.0 | 24.4 ± 9.9 | 3.4 ± 1.3 | 7 ± 1.7 | [blot bands] |
| 3 | 3.1 ± 1.1 | 10.1 ± 1.4 | 1.5 ± 1.0 | 8.2 ± 1.8 | Encapsulated Hepatocytes |
| 4 | 0.6 ± 0.6 | 11.3 ± 5.9 | 2.6 ± 1.8 | 5.8 ± 3.7 | |
| 5 | 1.5 ± nd | 5.5 ± nd | 4.9 ± nd | 14 ± nd | Days of Culture 1 2 3 4 |
| 6 | 1.6 ± 3.9 | 8.7 ± 2.2 | 2.8 ± 2.8 | 14.3 ± 2.1 | [blot bands] |

NOTE: The values are means ± SD of three independent experiments in duplicate or triplicate. For albumin secretion, the data shown are representative of all experiments performed.

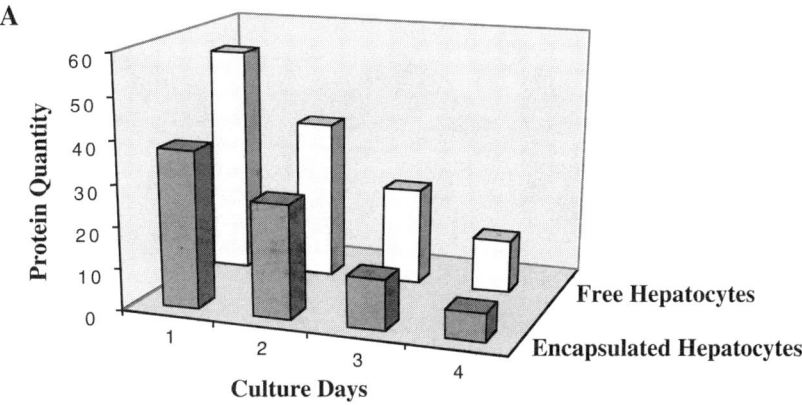

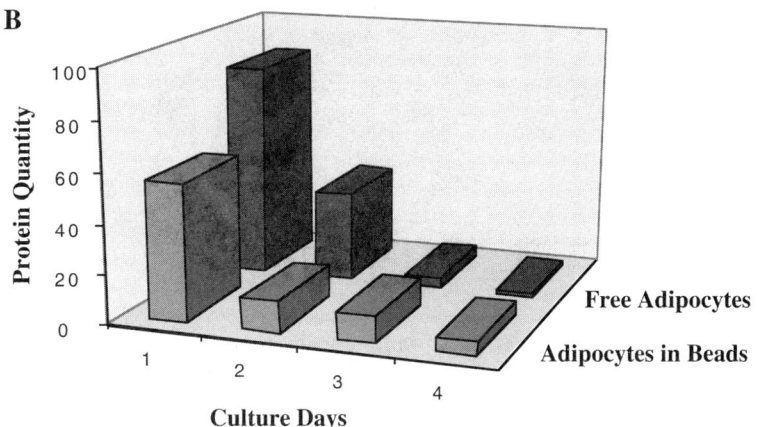

**FIGURE 3.** (**A**) Comparison of total protein secretion by hepatocytes encapsulated and in monolayer culture. Protein quantity is expressed as µg/ml per $10^6$ cells. (**B**) Comparison of total protein secretion by adipocytes in beads or free in the culture dish. Protein quantity is expressed as µg/ml. In all cases, cells were cultured in serum-free minimal medium to avoid interference with protein secretion measurement.

in minimum DMEM medium (FIG. 3 B). Protein amounts were generally lower for encapsulated cells compared to free cells as evaluated by the Bradford assays. Nevertheless, all experiments performed suggested that adipocytes in beads maintained their protein secretion and this activity is comparable to that observed for their nonencapsulated counterparts.

### *Cryopreservation: Preliminary Experiments*

Preliminary experiments were initiated on the suitability of our encapsulation system for cryopreservation of cells. Our first observations showed that the freezing and

## Cryopreservation of Encapsulated Hepatocytes

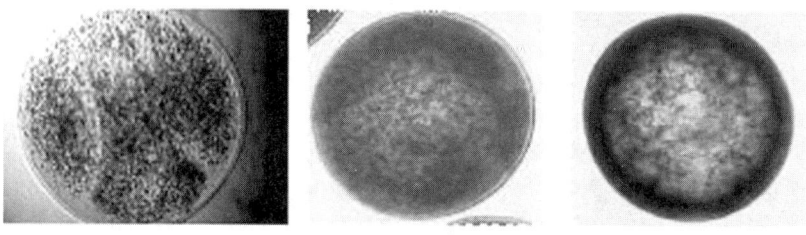

## Cryopreservation of Adipocytes in Bead

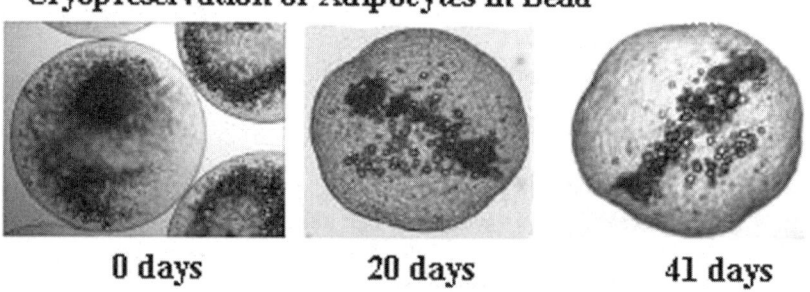

0 days          20 days          41 days

**FIGURE 4.** Morphology analysis of capsules and beads after various time periods of preservation in liquid nitrogen.

thawing processes do not distort the capsules containing hepatocytes; the capsules were spherical without apparent alteration. Only a small fraction of capsules were broken due to handling. Comparatively, the beads containing adipocytes treated in the same freeze–thaw conditions were deformed and showed a great fragility towards handling, indicating that the outer membrane plays an important role in the maintenance of the capsule structure (see FIGURE 4). We then evaluated the viability and the

**TABLE 3. Total protein secretion by encapsulated hepatocytes cryopreserved during one or two months in comparison to freshly encapsulated hepatocytes.**

| | Total Protein Secretion by Encapsulated Hepatocytes ($\mu$g/ml/$10^6$ cells) | | |
|---|---|---|---|
| | Cryopreservation Days | | |
| Days of Culture | 0 | 30 | 60 |
| 1 | 52.4 ± 9.5 | 59.7 ± 23 | 81.9 ± 4.0 |
| 2 | 30.3 ± 5.3 | 28.4 ± 1.5 | 35.8 ± 0.1 |
| 3 | 12.0 ± 9.6 | 13.0 ± 3.7 | 23.6 ± 0.9 |
| 4 | 10.2 ± 11.3 | 9.6 ± 3.2 | 12.4 ± 2.7 |

NOTE: The values are means ± SD of three independent experiments.

secretory functions of encapsulated hepatocytes after various cryopreservation times in liquid nitrogen. The cell viability as assessed by trypan blue exclusion was barely affected by the cryopreservation step, with a loss not exceeding 15% of the initial viability from seven days to 60 days of cryopreservation. In addition, as seen in TABLE 3, no significant difference in the protein secretion profile was observed between cryopreserved encapsulated hepatocytes after thawing and classical primary hepatocyte culture. Albumin secretion was also found to be similar for both freshly encapsulated hepatocytes and cryopreserved hepatocytes. All these data suggest that encapsulation allows the murine hepatocytes to overcome the cryopreservation procedure without significant loss of their viability and of their functions.

## DISCUSSION

Our previous reports on murine hepatocyte encapsulation, combined with the new experimental observations presented herein concerning adipocyte encapsulation, have identified a polymer combination that is biocompatible for these two murine cell types. We obtained mechanically stable capsules with controlled permeability. We demonstrated that the encapsulation of hepatocytes and adipocytes does not alter their functional characteristics, as compared to those obtained in classic primary cultures. Finally we have made a first evaluation of an easy and reliable method for hepatocyte cryopreservation. Several practical applications can now be generated from the establishment of our coculture model of encapsulated cells.

First, and as detailed in the introduction, it represents a handy and simplified *in vitro* tool for understanding reciprocal interactions between organs. Information can already be gained by analyzing the change in the gene expression profile of a given cell type, depending on the presence or absence of another cell type, and/or depending on a given hormone-like substance, such as TNFα, leptin, FIAF, or resistin. The identification of soluble signals that are responsible for crosstalk can be searched for either by high throughput techniques such as proteomics, applied to the culture medium obtained from various culture conditions. Other classical methods such as media fractionation could also be used. As discussed above, validation of our coculture model of encapsulated cells will first be centered on the mechanisms of lipid metabolism regulation and provide insights into possible molecular determinants of metabolic disorders affecting energy balance, such as obesity or diabetes. With that particular aim in view, muscle cells and pancreatic islets are the next candidates for this culture system of encapsulated cells. The use of null-mutant mice and/or transgenic mice as a source of genetically variant tissues is also of great interest in a search for the molecular relays of the metabolic pathways.

Other perspectives are particularly important in toxicology. Our model can be envisioned as extremely useful for assessing the beneficial and detrimental effects of new drugs on a given metabolic pathway, implicating several organs, rather than on a given tissue. For example, assessing the action of a drug on any cell type *in vitro* could be performed in presence of encapsulated hepatocytes, thus taking into account the liver-dependent modification of the drug.

Finally, cell encapsulation offers a simple tool for the cryopreservation of cells and more particularly hepatocytes, which are currently used in toxicology as well as in fundamental research. Preliminary results suggest that encapsulation may protect liver cells from the adverse effects of cryopreservation. Efforts now have to be undertaken to cryopreserve other tissue than hepatocytes (i.e., adipocytes and muscle cells).

## ACKNOWLEDGMENT

We thank Walter Wahli for critical reading of the manuscript. The work done in the authors' laboratory was supported by UNIL-EPFL Funds and the Etat de Vaud.

## REFERENCES

1. DODSON, M.V., J.L. VIERCK, K.L. HOSSNER, et al. 1997. The development and utility of a defined muscle and fat co-culture system. Tissue Cell **29**: 517–524.
2. CHANG, T. 1964. Semipermeable microcapsules. Science **146**: 524–525.
3. BRUNI, S. & T.M. CHANG. 1989. Hepatocytes immobilised by microencapsulation in artificial cells: effects on hyperbilirubinemia in Gunn rats. Biomater. Artif. Cells Artif. Organs **17**: 403–411.
4. CAI, Z.H., Z.Q. SHI, M. SHERMAN & A.M. SUN. 1989. Development and evaluation of a system of microencapsulation of primary rat hepatocytes. Hepatology **10**: 855–860.
5. DIXIT, V., R. DARVASI, M. ARTHUR, et al. 1990. Restoration of liver function in Gunn rats without immunosuppression using transplanted microencapsulated hepatocytes. Hepatology **12**: 1342–1349.
6. DIXIT, V., M. ARTHUR & G. GITNICK. 1993. A morphological and functional evaluation of transplanted isolated encapsulated hepatocytes following long-term transplantation in Gunn rats. Biomater. Artif. Cells Immobilization Biotechnol. **21**: 119–133
7. GOMEZ, N., P. BALLADUR, Y. CALMUS, et al. 1997. Evidence for survival and metabolic activity of encapsulated xenogeneic hepatocytes transplanted without immunosuppression in Gunn rats. Transplantation **63**: 1718-1723.
8. GROUT, B., J. MORRIS & M. MCLELLAN. 1990. Cryopreservation and the maintenance of cell lines. Trends Biotechnol. **8**: 293-297.
9. KARLSSON, J.O. & M. TONER. 1996. Long-term storage of tissues by cryopreservation: critical issues. Biomaterials **17**: 243-256.
10. DIXIT, V., R. DARVASI, M. ARTHUR, et al. 1993. Cryopreserved microencapsulated hepatocytes—transplantation studies in Gunn rats. Transplantation **55**: 616–622.
11. GUYOMARD, C., L. RIALLAND, B. FREMOND, et al. 1996. Influence of alginate gel entrapment and cryopreservation on survival and xenobiotic metabolism capacity of rat hepatocytes. Toxicol. Appl. Pharmacol. **141**: 349–356.
12. FERRANNINI, E. 1998. Insulin resistance versus insulin deficiency in non-insulin-dependent diabetes mellitus: problems and prospects. Endocr. Rev. **19**: 477–490.
13. DESVERGNE, B. & W. WAHLI. 1999. Peroxisome proliferator-activated receptors: nuclear control of metabolism. Endocrine Rev. **20**: 649–688.
14. STEPPAN, C.M., S.T. BAILEY, S. BHAT, et al. 2001. The hormone resistin links obesity to diabetes. Nature **409**: 307–312.
15. KERSTEN, S., S. MANDARD, N.S. TAN, et al. 2000. Characterization of the fasting-induced adipose factor FIAF, a novel peroxisome proliferator-activated receptor target gene. J. Biol. Chem. **275**: 28488-28493.
16. CANAPLE, L., N. NURDIN, N. ANGELOVA, et al. 2001. Maintenance of primary murine hepatocyte functions in multicomponent polymer capsules—*in vitro* cryopreservation studies. J. Hepatol. **34**: 11–18.
17. SUN, A.M., Z. CAI, Z. SHI, et al. 1987. Microencapsulated hepatocytes: an *in vitro* and *in vivo* study. Biomater. Artif. Cells Artif. Organs **15**: 483–496.
18. WONG, H. & T. M. CHANG. 1988. The viability and regeneration of artificial cell microencapsulated rat hepatocyte xenograft transplants in mice. Biomater. Artif. Cells Artif. Organs **16**: 731–739.

19. JOLY, A., J.F. DESJARDINS, B. FREMOND, et al. 1997. Survival, proliferation, and functions of porcine hepatocytes encapsulated in coated alginate beads: a step toward a reliable bioartificial liver. Transplantation **63**: 795–803.
20. HONIGER, J., P. BALLADUR, P. MARIANI, et al. 1995. Permeability and biocompatibility of a new hydrogel used for encapsulation of hepatocytes. Biomaterials **16**: 753–759.
21. CROOKS, C.A., J.A. DOUGLAS, R.L. BROUGHTON & M.V. SEFTON. 1990. Microencapsulation of mammalian cells in a HEMA-MMA copolymer: effects on capsule morphology and permeability. J. Biomed. Mater. Res. **24**: 1241–1262.
22. STANGE, J., S. MITZNER, H. DAUTZENBERG, et al. 1993. Prolonged biochemical and morphological stability of encapsulated liver cells—a new method. Biomater. Artif. Cells Immobilization Biotechnol. **21**: 343–352.
23. WANG, T., I. LACIK, M. BRISSOVA, et al. 1997. An encapsulation system for the immunoisolation of pancreatic islets. Nat. Biotechnol. **15**: 358–362.
24. BARTKOWIAK, A., L. CANAPLE, I. CEAUSOGLU, et al. 1999. New multicomponent capsules for immunoisolation. Ann. N.Y. Acad. Sci. **875**: 135–145.
25. LACIK, I., M. BRISSOVA, A.V. ANILKUMAR, et al. 1998. New capsule with tailored properties for the encapsulation of living cells. J. Biomed. Mater. Res. **39**: 52–60.
26. NURDIN, N., L. CANAPLE, A. BARTKOWIAK, et al. 2000. Capsule permeability via polymer and protein ingress/egress. J. Appl. Polym. Sci. **75**: 1165–1175.

# Present Status of Modified Hemoglobin as Blood Substitutes and Oral Therapy for End Stage Renal Failure Using Artificial Cells Containing Genetically Engineered Cells

THOMAS MING SWI CHANG

*Faculty of Medicine, McGill University, Montreal, Quebec, Canada*

> ABSTRACT: Artificial cell or bioencapsulation has been developed for use in bioartificial organs, drug delivery, blood substitutes, and other areas. Recent rapid advances in modified hemoglobin blood substitutes have resulted in advance stages of Phase III clinical trials. Another area of use is in oral therapy, using artificial cells microencapsulated with genetically engineered cells for use in end stage renal failure and other conditions.
>
> KEYWORDS: modified hemoglobin; blood substitutes; oral therapy; end state renal therapy; artificial cells; genetically engineered cells

## INTRODUCTION

The first reports on artificial cells including bioencapsulation were published as early as 1964.[1] Our early research shows the feasibility of artificial cells in biotechnology including blood substitutes, enzyme technology, cell encapsulation, drug delivery, biosorbents, and other applications[1–3] (see FIGURE 1). Interest in this approach increased only in early 1980 following the explosive international interest in all areas of biotechnology at about that time. This has resulted in progress in the use of artificial cells in biotechnology, especially in bioencapsulation.[4–7] Artificial cells are prepared in different configurations depending on the area of application. Thus, in bioencapsulation of enzymes or drugs they are usually in the form of microcapsules or nanocapsules, whereas for cell or tissue encapsulation they are usually in the form of larger macrocapsules. For blood substitutes they are usually in the form of nanocapsules or even smaller in the form of crosslinked polyhemoglobin. The basic principle is based on the ability of artificial cells to isolate the contents from the external environment, but the same type allows permeant material to diffuse rapidly into the microcapsules (FIG. 1). Hormone and reaction products can readily diffuse out of the artificial cells.

Two of the recent rapidly advancing areas are found in modified hemoglobin as blood substitutes and oral therapy, using artificial cells that are microencapsulated

---

Address for correspondence: Thomas Ming Swi Chang, O.C.,M.D.,C.M.,Ph.D.,FRCP(C), Director, Artificial Cells & Organs Research Centre, Professor of Physiology, Medicine & Biomedical Engineering, Faculty of Medicine, McGill University, Montreal, Quebec, Canada H3G 1Y6

artcell@med.mcgill.ca  <www.artcell.mcgill.ca>

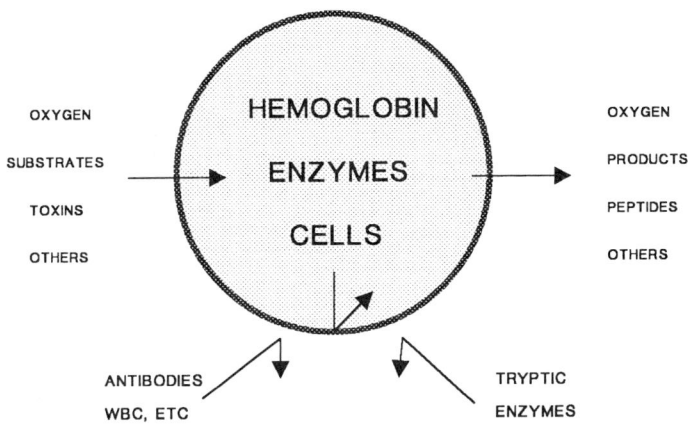

**FIGURE 1.** Basic principle of artificial cells or bioencapsulation.[1-3]

and genetically engineered cells for end stage kidney failure and other conditions. Concerns of HIV in donor blood has stimulated the development of blood substitutes based on modified hemoglobin.[8,9] These can be stored at 4°C, or room temperature, for more than one year. They have no blood group antigen and can be used as universal donor. They can also be sterilized to remove and inactivate infectious agents like HIV and hepatitis viruses. In the case of end stage kidney failure, dialysis is an established and effective method of treatment. However, most patients prefer oral therapy rather than dialysis. Furthermore, 85% of the world's uremic population (half a million/year) died because they could not afford dialysis. If they were all treated and maintained alive, the total number of patients would plateau at 7–8 million. Thus, there is some urgency in finding a solution to this problem.

## MODIFIED HEMOGLOBIN AS BLOOD SUBSTITUTES

### Polyhemoglobin

Inside red blood cells, hemoglobin is a tetramer of with a 2,3-GPD pocket. When infused, the tetramer breaks down into toxic dimers. Our research shows that bifunctional agents can be used to crosslink hemoglobin to prevent its breakdown.[1-3] We first used sebacyl chloride to crosslink hemoglobin into polyhemoglobin.[1-3] The reaction is as follows:

$$Cl(CH_2)_8Cl + HBNH_2 = HB(CH_2)_8HB$$
$$\text{sebacyl chloride} \quad \text{hemoglobin} \quad \text{crosslinked polyhemoglobin}$$

We then used another bifunctional agent, glutaraldehyde, to crosslink hemoglobin and a rbc enzyme, catalase, into soluble polyhemoglobin.[10] The reaction is as follows:

$$H\text{-}CO\text{-}(CH_2)_3\text{-}CO\text{-}H + HBNH_2 = HB\text{-}NH\text{-}CO\text{-}(CH_2)_3\text{-}CO\text{-}NH\text{-}HB$$
$$\text{glutaraldehyde} \quad \text{hemoglobin} \quad \text{cross-linked polyhemoglobin}$$

This glutaraldehyde crosslinked polyhemglobin approach has been developed by a number of groups[8,9] to its present state, suitable for clinical use, as described below.

### Glutaraldehyde Crosslinked Human Pyridoxalated Polyhemoglobin (Polyheme) in Clinical Trial

Gould et al. from Northfield have reported their clinical trial using glutaraldehyde polymerized pyridoxalated human polyhemoglobin with the following characteristics.[11,12] They removed most of the single crosslinked tetrameric hemoglobin (less than 1% remaining), leaving more than 99% of hemoglobin in the form of polyhemoglobin. Each unit (500 ml) contains 50 g of the polymerized hemoglobin in lactated Ringer's solution. It has a $P_{50}$ of 28–30 mmHg, its halflife in the circulation after infusion is 24 hours, and its shelf life is more than one year. Their Phase I clinical trial shows that infusion of 500 ml did not produce any gastrointestinal smooth muscle spasm or vasoconstriction nor any effects on the kidney or other organs. In their Phase II clinical trial in trauma surgery,[12] 44 trauma patients, aged 19–75, with an injury severity score (ISS) of 21 ± 10 were randomized to received red cells ($n$ = 23) or up to six units of PolyHeme ($n$ = 21) after trauma and during emergent operations. After six units of PolyHeme, any further transfusion needed would be given as allogeneic blood. Thus, 12 patients received 6 U, 3 patients received 4 U, 1 patient received 3 U, 2 patients received 2 U, and 1 patient received 1 U of PolyHeme. There was no significant difference between the control group using RBC and the experimental group using polyhemoglobin with respect to any adverse events. There were no vasoactive properties, renal dysfunction, fever, or other measurements of organ functions. The authors followed the total hemoglobin as: Total (Hb) = RBC (Hb) + Poly (Hb). They showed that each 500 ml of PolyHeme (50 g Hb) raises the Poly (Hb) of the plasma about 1 g/dl. In the experimental group, at the end of infusion, Total (Hb) was 9.0 ± 2.0 g/dl with 5.8 ± 2.8 g/dl from red blood cells and 3.9 ± 1.3 g/dl from the infused Poly (Hb). The authors calculated this to represent the replacement of greater than 40% of the Total circulating (Hb) by PolyHeme. They also found that PolyHeme with a circulation halflife of 24 hours was able to significantly decrease the need for blood transfusion during the first 24 hours. They updated their clinical trial in the FDA workshop on blood substitutes in the fall of 1999. The number of recipients (and amount) receiving polyhemoglobin were: 7 (14–20 units), 19 (10 units), 27 (6–9 units), 31 (3–5 units), and 67 (1–2 units). Infusion of PolyHeme maintains adequate total (Hb) even in those with RBC (Hb) of less than 3 g/dl. It is safe during rapid, massive infusion to the amount of 20 units studied. These authors' data show that this approach very significantly decreases the mortality of trauma patients with less than 3 g/dl total red blood cell hemoglobin when compared to historical controls.

### Glutaraldehyde Crosslinked Bovine Polyhemoglobin

Biopure has developed glutaraldehyde crosslinked polyhemoglobin using bovine hemoglobin instead of human hemoglobin and their investigators have described this in some detail elsewhere.[13,14] Bovine hemoglobin is available in large amounts; furthermore, unlike human hemoglobin, even without 2–3 DPG or its analogue, pyridoxal-phosphate, bovine hemoglobin has much higher $P_{50}$ than human hemoglobin. This polyhemoglobin preparation contains less than 5% of crosslinked tetrameric hemoglobin. Each unit (500 ml) contains 6–7 g of hemoglobin in lactated Ringer's solution with a $P_{50}$ of 38 mmHg and halflife in the circulation of 24 hours. One of the most surprising findings is that its shelf life at room temperature is more than two years. LaMuraglia et al.[14] recently reported their Phase II single blind, multicenter trial in infrarenal aortic aneurysm surgery. Seventy-two patients were randomized to receive blood substitute ($n = 48$) or allogenic red blood cells ($n = 24$) at the time of the first transfusion decision. Those randomized to the blood substitute group received 60 g of polyhemoglobin for the initial transfusion and had the option to receive three further doses of 30 g each within 96 hours. After this, allogenic red blood cells were given for any further requirements in the 28 days following randomization. The two groups were comparable for all baseline characteristics. All patients in the control group required allogenic red blood cell transfusion. Among those in the blood substitute group, 27% did not require allogenic red blood cell transfusion in the 28-day period. Antibody levels of IgE to bovine hemoglobin were not induced in any of the patients in this study. There was a transient 15% increase in blood pressure, but the cardiac index and pulmonary pressures were not affected. The transfusions were well tolerated and there was no significant differences in complications, morbidity, or mortality rates between the two groups. Phase III clinical trials in humans are now in progress. Very recently these researchers reported, in the *New England Journal of Medicine*, the use of this product in a patient with acute hemolytic anemia.[15] Hemolysis was so severe that the hemoglobin level was less than 4 g/dl despite standard treatment plus daily infusion of 8 units of donor blood. Infusion of their polyhemoglobin in the amounts of 5, 3, and 3 units, a total of 11 units over 7 days, was able to maintain the total hemoglobin level at 5.5 g/dl. The patient eventually recovered and was discharged. The FDA has approved a glutaraldehyde polymerized bovine hemoglobin product from this group for routine use in veterinary medicine.

### *o-Raffinose Crosslinked Human Polyhemoglobin*

Another polyhemoglobin is based on the use of *o*-raffinose to crosslink human hemoglobin.[16] Hemosol has developed this in the form of Hemolink: each unit of 500 ml contains 50 g of Hemolink in Ringer's lactate solution with a $P_{50}$ of 34 mmHg and containing $33 \pm 10\%$ of crosslinked tetrameric hemoglobin. Its halflife in the circulation is 18–20 hours. The report of this by Adamson and Moore[16] and at the 1999 Fall FDA workshop on blood substitutes show that their Phase I clinical trial, with dose escalation study from 0.025 g/kg to 0.6 g/kg, was safe in humans with no renal or other systems effects. At the highest dose in unanesthetized volunteers, they reported small increases in blood pressure and transient GI effects. The small effects on blood pressure and GI effects are not observed in anesthetized surgical patients. Hemosol has carried out Phase II clinical trials in orthopedic surgery, where intraoperative, autologous blood is used, and blood substitutes are given when needed. They have also carried out Phase II clinical trials in cardiovascular surgery using their blood substitutes for perioperative transfusion requirements. They have recently announced the completion of their Phase III clinical trials in coronary artery bypass surgery in Canada and the United Kingdom and are applying for regulatory approval.[17]

### Tetrameric Crosslinked Hemoglobin

Hemoglobin can also be crosslinked intramolecularly to form a single crosslinked tetrameric hemoglobin.[18] This was developed by Baxter and studied in multicenter clinical trials.[18] Higher doses of crosslinked tetrameric hemoglobin can result in increase in vasoactivity and, in unanesthetized patients, GI side effects such as oesophageal spasm.[18] They have used a diaspirin crosslinked hemgolobin (DCLHb) for smaller volume replacement. The results of Baxter's Phase III clinical trials have led them to discontinue this approach and to develop a second-generation recombinant human hemoglobin as discussed below.

### Recombinant Human Hemoglobin

Hoffman et al.[19] prepared recombinant tetrameric human hemoglobin from genetically engineered *E coli*. Somatogen has developed this for several clinical trials.[20] Using tetrameric hemoglobin, they reported vasoactivity and, in unanesthetized patients, GI effects as discussed above. They are, therefore, developing a second generation recombinant human hemoglobin[21] in which they modify the nitric oxide binding site of the recombinant hemoglobin molecule. They have successfully produced recombinant human hemoglobin that no longer exhibits vasoactivity in animal studies.[21] Somatogen has joined Baxter to develop this new generation recombinant human hemoglogin for clinical trails.

### Conjugated Hemoglobin

Hemoglobin can be crosslinked to polymer to form insoluble conjugated hemoglobin.[1-3] This has been extended by Wong and others to form soluble conjugated hemoglobin by crosslinking individual hemoglobin molecule to a soluble polymer.[8] Hemoglobin conjugated to polyoxyethylene has been developed by Ajinomoto, who has now joined with Apex Bioscience, USA to carry out clinical trials.[22] They have completed Phase I clinical trials using doses of up to 7 grams/patient without reporting any significant toxicity. They are studying the use of this in Phase II clinical trials, especially in septic shock with increase in nitric oxide levels, and have demonstrated its efficacy in maintaining blood pressure and removal of nitric oxide.[22] Enzon Inc. has used polyethylene glycol (PEG) to crosslink to bovine hemoglobin and showed in Phase 1a clinical trials that this is well tolerated.[8] They have carried out Phase 1b clinical trials to evaluate the safety of PEG hemoglobin as an adjuvant to radiation therapy in human cancer patients to oxygenate hypoxic tumor tissue and thereby increase their sensitivity to radiation therapy.[8]

### Comparison of the Modified Hemoglobins

As far as oxygen dissociation is concerned, all of the modified hemoglobins mentioned above have the required properties, and are comparable or better than native hemoglobin. The major difference is that polyhemoglobin and conjugated hemoglobin do not cause vasoconstriction and, therefore, can deliver oxygen more effectively to the well-perfused tissues. Intramolecularly crosslinked single Hb molecules and the first generation recombinant single hemoglobin, as discussed, cause vasoconstriction. Vasoconstriction results in a decreased perfusion of the tissues. Therefore, even though the modified hemoglobins have good oxygen release characteristics, vasoconstriction results in a decrease in their ability to deliver oxygen to the less-well-perfused tissues. Modified hemoglobins are prepared from ultrapure hemoglobin and, therefore, do not contain the red blood cell enzyme systems of those described in the next two sections.

### *Polyhemoglobin-Superoxide Dismutase Catalase in Ischemia Reperfusion*

Reperfusion with oxygen-carrying fluids, such as blood substitutes, to ischemic tissues as in stroke, myocardial infarction, organs transplantation, severe sustained hemorrhagic shock, and other conditions can result in the release of superoxide, oxygen radicals, and other reactions leading to tissue injuries. D'Agnillo and Chang crosslinked trace amounts of catalase and superoxide dismutase (SOD) to hemoglobin (Hb) to form polyHb-SOD-catalase.[23] Compared to polyHb, polyHb-SOD-catalase removes significantly more oxygen radicals and peroxides and stabilizes the crosslinked hemoglobin, resulting in decreased oxidative iron and heme release. In the reperfusion of ischemic rat intestine, polyHb-SOD-catalase also significantly reduces the increase in oxygen radicals, as measured by an increase in 3,4 dihydroxybenzoate, when compared to polyHb.[8]

### *Encapsulated Hemoglobin as a Third Generation Modified Hemoglobin*

Molecularly modified hemoglobins in the form of crosslinked hemoglobin or recombinant hemoglobin as described above are simpler and, therefore, the first modified hemoglobins in clinical trials. However, these are not covered by a membrane and need to be ultrapure to avoid adverse reactions. Furthermore, the circulation halflife is rather short, 24 hours. As a result, Chang's original idea of a more complete artificial RBC[1,3] is now being developed as third generation blood substitutes. Submicron lipid membrane microencapsulated hemoglobin[24] is being explored, especially by the group of Tsuchida in Japan[25] and Rudolph in the USA.[26] The U.S. group has modified the surface properties to result in a circulation halflife of about 50 hours.[27] Chang and Yu are developing a new system based on

TABLE 1. Changes in the plasma concentrations of potassium, phosphate, magnesium, sodium, chloride, uric acid, cholesterol, and billirubin after 24 hours of contact *in vitro* with artificial cell encapsulated genetically engineered *E. coli* DH5 cells[33]

| Metabolites | Concentration at 0 Hours | Concentration at 24 Hours |
|---|---|---|
| Potassium | $5.80 \pm 0.40$ mEq/l | $3.50 \pm 0.03$ mEq/l ($p < 0.001$) |
| Phosphate | $2.20 \pm 0.9$ mg/dl | $1.49 \pm 0.03$ mg/dl ($p < 0.005$) |
| Magnesium | $0.90 \pm 0.04$ mg/dl | $0.66 \pm 0.09$ mg/dl ($p < 0.005$) |
| Sodium | $172 \pm 11.00$ mEq/l | $129 \pm 6.12$ mEq/l ($p < 0.001$) |
| Chloride | $137 \pm 6.60$ mEq/l | $107 \pm 2.00$ mEq/l ($p < 0.005$) |
| Uric acid | $84.80 \pm 3.40$ mg/dl | $8.80 \pm 3.12$ mg/dl ($p < 0.001$) |
| Cholesterol | $1.86 \pm 0.10$ mmol/l | $1.37 \pm 0.06$ mmol/l ($p < 0.005$) |

biodegradable polymer and nanotechnology, resulting in polylactide membrane hemoglobin nanocapsules of less than 150 nanometers in diameter.[28,29] Unlike lipid, polylactide is readily converted to water and carbon dioxide in the body and, therefore, does not accumulate in the reticuloendothelial system. They are smaller in diameter than the lipid vesicles and contain negligible amounts of lipids and, thus, have less saturating effects on the reticuloendothelial systems when large amounts are infused. We have included superoxide dismutase, catalase, carbonic anhydrase, and multienzyme systems to prevent the accumulation of methemoglobin.[29]

## ORALLY ADMINISTERED ARTIFICIAL CELLS CONTAINING GENETICALLY ENGINEERED CELLS FOR END STAGE KIDNEY FAILURE

### In Vitro *Removal of Urea, Ammonia, Uric Acid, Creatinine, Bilirubin, Cholesterol, Potassium, Phosphate, Sodium and Chloride*

Advances in molecular biology have resulted in the availability of nonpathogenic genetically engineered microorganisms that can effectively use uremic metabolites for cell growth. We have, therefore, studied the oral use of microencapsulated genetically engineered nonpathogenic *E. coli* DH5 cells containing *Klebsiella aerogenes* urease gene in renal failure rats.[30,31] We reported that $40.00 \pm 8.60$ g of encapsulated *E. coli* DH5 can remove 40 grams of urea (100 mg/dl in 40 liters), as compared to 1,212 g of microcapsulated urease-zirconium-phosphate.[31] *E. coli* DH5 cells in culture grow to many times their original number and reach a plateau after about 12 hours.[32] This rapid growth requires ions and other metabolites in addition to a nitrogen source. Our most recent *in vitro* studies using uremic rat plasma show that there are significant decreases in potassium, phosphate, sodium, chloride, cholesterol, uric acid, and creatinine.[33] The removal of uric acid was so high that we had to add a higher concentration of uric acid into the uremic plasma to carry out the studies.

### *Oral Administration in End Stage Renal Failure Rats to Remove Uremic Metabolites*

When given orally, the microcapsules containing the *E. coli* DH5 cells pass through the intestine and use uremic metabolites for their rapid growth. The microcapsules containing the microorganisms with the uremic metabolites are then excreted in the stool and there is no retention in the body.[34] We reported elsewhere daily oral administration of log phase microencapsulated genetically engineered *E. coli* DH5 cells to partially nephrectomized renal failure rats with a urea level of $52.08 \pm 2.06$ mg/dl. This resulted in lowering and maintaining at the normal range of $9.10 \pm 0.71$ mg/dl during the 21-day treatment period.[31] The blood ammonia level also decreased significantly. A return to high urea levels was observed when the treatment was stopped, showing that there was no significant retention of *E. coli* DH5 cells in the intestine. Calculations based on the results from this study showed that in a 70-kg patient with the same degree of renal failure as in the partially nephrectomized rats, we would only need to give 4 grams of *E. coli* DH5 cells orally each day. The most recent studies in uremic rats showed a reduction of uric acid, creatinine, potassium and phosphate.[35,36]

Daily oral administration of encapsulated *E. coli* DH5 cells for 21 days was started 31 days after partial nephrectomy in uremic rats. In the group of uremic rats that received control microcapsules containing no *E. coli* DH 5 cells, 25% died in the first 46 days after partial nephrectomy, 50% died after 54 days, and 75% died after 67 days.[37] The uremic rats that received daily oral microcapsulated *E. coli* DH 5 cells all survived during the 21 days of the treatment period.[37] After stopping oral administration 50% of the animals died by day 81, equivalent to 29 days after stopping treatment.[37]

In addition, we carried out a very severe test of the potential toxicity that might occur if some encapsulated cells leak during their passage through the intestinal tract. We gave another group of renal failure rats the same daily oral doses of *E. coli* DH5 cells, but all in the free form, for the same 21-day period. The results showed that even if all the *E. coli* DH5 cells were to have leaked, there was no adverse effect on the growth or survival of the renal failure rats.[37] Even though free *E. coli* DH5 cells are not toxic when given orally, it does not mean that they should be given orally in the free form.[34] When free *E. coli* DH5 cells were used, some of them were retained in the intestine.[34] Repeated large doses of these bacteria in the free form would result in their taking over the normal intestinal flora. Urea removal is based on the use of urea as a nitrogen source by the encapsulated *E. coli* DH5 cells, which are then excreted in the stool with its nitrogen content.[34] If the *E. coli* DH5 cells stay in the intestine, the urea–nitrogen is not excreted and is recycled in the body. Indeed, attempts in the past to lower urea levels by manipulating the intestinal flora[38] involved the retention of bacteria in the intestine. With the retention of the microorganisms in the intestine, the nitrogen source from the urea also stays with the microorganisms and is therefore retained in the body and recycled.[34]

### *Summary of the* in Vivo *Results*

Using encapsulated DH5 cells orally avoids the need for dialysis treatments to remove waste metabolites. Yet, of the uremic metabolites tested (e.g., urea, creatinine, uric acid, potassium, phosphate, and sodium) they are all lowered to within normal levels. Since the exact uremic toxin is not yet known, we can only follow the effectiveness by the survival and growth of the animals. In this respect, untreated uremic control animals died during the study period of 21 days, whereas treated animal continued to survive. Although untreated uremic control animals did not grow and lost weight, treated animals continued to grow at about the same rate as normal animals.[37] It is difficult to observe in detail in rats whether they are completely symptom free. However, they are at least growing and surviving. These are uremic rats that still have some ability to excrete water and electrolytes. In more advanced stages of uremia, this ability is greatly compromised and additional methods, such as oral administration of osmotic materials, are required to remove fluids.

### *Potential Uses for the Oral Administration of Artificial Cells Containing Nonpathogenic Genetically Engineered Cells*

The results show much potential for the oral administration of artificial cells containing nonpathogenic genetically engineered cells in end stage renal failure. In earlier stages of end stage renal failure, before fluid retention, this oral approach can be used by itself. In later stages, when there is fluid retention, the oral approach can be combined with an oral osmotic agent like mannitol, but in a much smaller amount, to remove about one liter of fluid per day. There have been recent demonstrations that daily dialysis prevents large fluctuations in the systemic waste metabolites, but this requires daily treatment. Here the oral approach could be used as in combination with standard dialysis to prevent large fluctuations in the systemic waste metabolites. The rapid and efficient removal of uric acid may result in other possible applications in hyperuricemia, such as in gout and in chemotherapy.

## ACKNOWLEDGMENTS

The support of the Canadian Institutes for Health Research (previously Medical Research Council of Canada), the "Virage" Centre of Excellence in Biotechnology from the Quebec Ministry and the Bayer-Canadian Blood Agency-Hema Quebec Research and Development Funds (previously Bayer-Canadian Red Cross) are all gratefully acknowledged.

## REFERENCES

1. CHANG, T.M.S. 1964. Semipermeable microcapsules. Science **146**(3643): 524.
2. CHANG, T.M.S, F.C. MACINTOSH & S.G. MASON. 1966. Semipermeable aqueous microcapsules: I. Preparation and properties. Can. J. Physiol. Pharmacol. **44**: 115–128.
3. CHANG T.M.S. 1972. Artificial cells. Monograph. Charles C Thomas, Springfield.
4. LIM, F. & A.M. SUN. 1980. Microencapsulated islets as bioartificial endocrine pancreas. Science **210**: 908–909.
5. KUHREIBEZ, W.M., P.P. LAUZA & W.L. CUICKS, Eds. 1999. Cell Encapsulation Technology and Therapy. Birkhauser, Boston.
6. HUNKELER, D., A. PROKOP, A.D. CHERRINGTON, *et al.* Eds. 1999. Bioartificial Organs II: Technology, Medicine and Material. Ann. N.Y. Acad. Sci. **875**: 271–279.
7. CHANG, T.M.S. 2000. Artificial cell biotechnology in medical applications. J. Blood Purification **18**: 91–96.
8. CHANG, T.M.S. 1997. Blood Substitutes: Principles, Methods, Products and Clinical Trials. Vol. 1. Karger, Basel.
9. CHANG, T.M.S. 2000. Red blood cell substitutes—best practice & research. Clin. Hæmatol. **13**(4): 651–668.
10. CHANG, T.M.S. 1971. Stabilization of enzyme by microencapsulation with a concentrated protein solution or by crosslinking with glutaraldehyde. Biochem. Biophys. Res. Com. **44**: 1531–1533.
11. GOULD, S.A., L.R. SEHGAL, H.L. SEHGAL, *et al.* 1998. The clinical development of human polymerized hemoglobin: *In* Blood Substitutes: Principles, Methods, Products and Clinical Trials, Vol. 2. T.M.S. Chang, Ed.: 12–28. Karger, Basel.
12. GOULD, S.A., E.E. MOORE, D.B. HOYT, *et al.* 1998 The first randomized trial of human polymerized hemoglobin as a blood substitute in acute trauma and emergent surgery. J. Am. Coll. Surg. **187**: 113–120.
13. PEARCE, L.B. & M.S. GAWRYL. 1998. Overview of preclinical and clinical efficacy of Biopure's HBOCs. *In* Blood Substitutes: Principles, Methods, Products and Clinical Trials, Vol 2. T.M.S. Chang Ed. 82–98. Karger, Basel.
14. LAMURAGLIA, *et al.* 2000. The reduction of the allogenic transfusion requirement in aortic surgery with a hemoglobin-based solution. J. Vasc. Surg. **31**(2): 243–256.
15. MULLON, J., *et al.* 2000. Transfusions of polymerized bovine hemoglobin in a patient with severe autoimmune hemolytic anemia. N. Engl. J. Med. **342**: 1638–1643.

16. ADAMSON, J.G. & C. MOORE. T.M. Hemolink, an *o*-Raffinose crosslinked hemoglobin-based oxygen carrier. *In* Blood Substitutes: Principles, Methods, Products and Clinical Trials, vol. 2. T.M.S. Chang Ed.: 62–79. Karger, Basel.
17. HEMOSOL INC. 2000. Release, September 20, 2000.
18. NELSON, D.J. 1998. Blood and HemAssistTM (DCLHb): potentially a complementary therapeutic team. *In* Blood Substitutes: Principles, Methods, Products and Clinical Trials, Vol 2. T.M.S. Chang, Ed.: 39–57. Karger, Basel.
19. HOFFMAN, S.J., D.L. LOOKER, J.M. ROEHRICH, *et al.* 1990. Expression of fully functional tetrameric human hemoglobin in *Escherichia coli.* Proc. Natl. Acad. Sci. USA **87**: 8521–8525.
20. FREYTAG, J.W. & D. TEMPLETON. 1997. OptroTM (recombinant human hemoglobin): a therapeutic for the delivery of oxygen and the restoration of blood volume in the treatment of acute blood loss in trauma and surgery. *In* Red Cell Substitutes: Basic Principles and Clinical Application. A.S. Rudolph, R. Rabinovici & G.Z. Feuerstein, Eds.: 325–334. Marcel Dekker, New York.
21. DOHERTY, D.H., M.P. DOYLE, S.R. CURRY, *et al.* 1998. Rate of reaction with nitric oxide determines the hypertensive effect of cell-free hemoglobin. Nature Biotechnol. **16**: 672–676.
22. DEANGELO, J. 1999. Nitric oxide scavengers in the treatment of shock associated with systemic inflammatory response syndrome. Exp. Opin. Pharmacother. **1**: 19–29.
23. D'AGNILLO, F. & T.M.S. CHANG. 1998. Polyhemoglobin-superoxide dismutase catalase as a blood substitute with antioxidant properties. Nature Biotechnol. **16**(7): 667–671.
24. DJORDJEVICH, L. & I.F. MILLER. 1980. Synthetic erythrocytes from lipid encapsulated hemoglobin. Exp. Hematol. **8**: 584.
25. TSUCHIDA, E., Ed. 1998. Blood Substitutes: Present and Future Perspectives. Elsevier, Amsterdam.
26. RUDOLPH, A.S., R. RABINOVICI & G.Z. FEUERSTEIN, Eds. 1997. Rbc Substitutes. Marcel Dekker, New York.
27. PHILIPS, W.T., R.W. KLPPER, V.D. AWASTHI, *et al.* 1999. Polyethylene glyco-modified liposome-encapsulated hemoglobin: a long circulating red cell substitute. J. Pharm. Exp. Therapeut. **288**: 665–670.
28. YU, W.P. & T.M.S. CHANG. 1996. Submicron polymer membrane hemoglobin nanocapsules as potential blood substitutes: preparation and characterization. Artif. Cells Blood Subst. Immob. Biotechnol. **24**:169–184.
29. CHANG, T.M.S. & W.P. YU. Nanoencapsulation of hemoglobin and rbc enzymes based on nanotechnology and biodegradable polymer. *In* Blood Substitutes: Principles, Methods, Products and Clinical Trials, Vol. 2, T.M.S. Chang, Ed.: 216–231. Karger, Basel.
30. Chang, T.M.S. & S. Prakash. 1998. Therapeutic uses of microencapsulated genetically engineered cells. Molecular Medicine Today **4**: 221–227.
31. PRAKASH, S. & T.M.S. CHANG. 1996. Microencapsulated genetically engineered live *E. coli* DH5 cells administered orally to maintain normal plasma urea level in uremic rats. Nature Med. **2**(8): 883–887.
32. PRAKASH, S. & T.M.S. CHANG. 1999. Growth kinetics of genetically engineered *E. coli* DH5 cells in artificial cell apa membrane microcapsules: preliminary report. Artif. Cells Blood Subst. Immob. Biotechnol. **27**(3): 291–301.
33. Prakash, S. & T.M.S. Chang. 1999. Artificial cell microcapsules containing genetically engineered *E. coli* DH5 cells for *in vitro* lowering of plasma potassium, phosphate, magnesium, sodium, chloride, uric acid, cholesterol, and creatinine: a preliminary report. Artif. Cells Blood Subst. Immob. Biotechnol. **28**(5,6): 475–482
34. CHANG, T.M.S. 1997. Live *E. coli* cells to treatment uremia: replies to letters to the editor. Nature Med. **3**: 2,3.
35. PRAKASH, S. & T.M.S. CHANG. 2000. Lowering of uric acid *in vitro* and *in vivo* by artificial cell microcapsulated genetically engineered *E. coli* DH 5 cells. Int. J. Artif. Organs **23**: 429–435.
36. PRAKASH, S. & T.M.S. CHANG. 2000. Artificial cells microencapsulated genetically engineered *E. coli* DH5 cells for the lowering of plasma creatinine *in vitro* and *in vivo*. Artif. Cells Blood Subst. Immob. Biotechnol. **28**(5): 397–408.

37. PRAKASH, S. & T.M.S. CHANG. 1998. Growth and survival of renal failure rats that received oral microencapsulated genetically engineered *E. coli* DH5 cells for urea removal. Artif. Cells Blood Subst. Immob. Biotechnol. **26**: 35–51.
38. WRONG, O.M., C.J. EDMONDS & V.S. CHADWICK, Eds. 1981. The Large Intestine. MTP Press, Lancaster.

# β Cell Replacement for the Treatment of Diabetes

JOSÉ OBERHOLZER, CHRISTIAN TOSO, FRÉDÉRIC RIS, PASCAL BUCHER, FRÉDÉRIC TRIPONEZ, ALP DEMIRAG, JINNING LOU, AND PHILIPPE MOREL

*Division of Surgical Research, Department of Surgery, University Hospital, Geneva 14, Switzerland*

> ABSTRACT: The replacement of insulin-producing β cells by islet transplantation can efficiently reverse diabetes. The recent improvements in clinical results were made possible by transplanting higher islet masses and through the introduction of new immunosuppressive protocols that avoid diabetogenicity. The need for alternatives to continuous immunosuppression, and an unlimited source of glucose-sensitive, insulin-secreting tissue, is emerging. In this review we discuss the various key steps in islet transplantation and offer perspectives for future developments in the replacement of insulin-producing β cells for the treatment of type I diabetes.
>
> KEYWORDS: diabetes; islet isolation; islet transplantation; β cell; bioartificial pancreas

## INTRODUCTION

Diabetes is the most frequent endocrine disease in industrialized countries. The juvenile form of diabetes, also known as type I diabetes, hits previously healthy children or adolescents and marks their entire life by a chronic disease for which only palliation can be offered. Since the beginning of attempts to treat this devastating disease, the replacement of destroyed endocrine tissue was seen as the unique path to a cure:

"On December 20th, 1893, my surgical colleague, Mr. Harsant, placed the patient under chloroform, while I extracted the pancreas with strict aseptic precautions from a freshly-slaughtered sheep, so that by the time the patient was anesthetized the pancreas was at hand, and three pieces each of the size of a brazil nut had been grafted into the subcutaneous tissues of the breast and abdomen, and the operation completed within twenty minutes of the death of the sheep."[1] Although the first *islet transplantation* was performed more than 100 years ago, the past 20 years have seen accelerated development and improved understanding.

Although the islet transplantation concept was initially thought to be simple, its widespread clinical applicability was hampered by a variety of technical and biological obstacles (see FIGURE 1). Since then, many groups have worked closely together and made many contributions that allow this promising therapy to enter into clinical

Address for correspondence: Dr. J. Oberholzer, Division of Surgical Research, Department of Surgery, University Hospital, Rue Micheli-du-Crest 24, 1211 Genève 14, Switzerland. Voice: 41 22 372 33 11; fax: 41 22 372 77 55.
celtrans@cmu.unige.ch

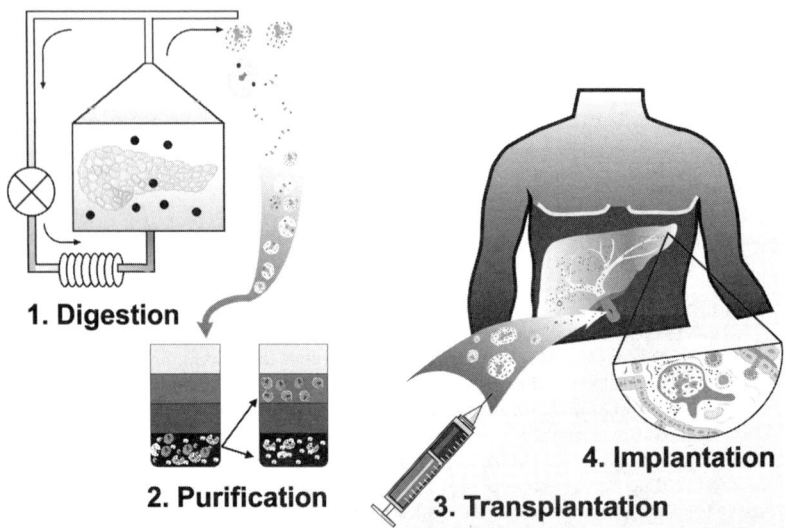

**FIGURE 1.** The concept of islet transplantation and its limitation. Following the injection of an enzyme solution (collagenase) into the main pancreatic duct, the pancreas is digested within a temperature-controlled chamber (*digestion*). The primary limitation is the specific activity of the collagenase that can vary from batch to batch, but also from the characteristic of the pancreas of an individual donor. The tissue suspension is purified by a density gradient. The endocrine islets have a lower density than the exocrine tissue and are separated by the gradient (*purification*). According to the donor conditions the density can vary and the difference in density between the endocrine and exocrine tissue may become too small for an efficient purification. Under local anesthesia and radiological control, the purified islets are injected into the main portal vein (*transplantation*). The islet will engraft into the small portal veins (*implantation*). A variety of immunological and non-immunological factors can hamper appropriate engraftment in the ectopic environment of the portal system.

reality. Since the last breakthrough in this field, the successful clinical trials for islet transplantation in non-uremic type I diabetic patients by the Edmonton group,[2] much attention has been given to the treatment of diabetes by islet transplantation. Although islet transplantation is now widely accepted, the need for alternatives to immunosuppression and an unlimited source of glucose-sensitive, insulin-secreting tissue is emerging. In this review we discuss the various key steps in islet transplantation and offer perspectives for future developments in the replacement of insulin-producing β cells for the treatment of type I diabetes.

## ISLET ISOLATION—STILL NECESSARY

During the 1970s, the pioneering work by Lacy involving the development of islet isolation[3] and islet transplantation in rats[4] was rapidly applied in large animal models,[5,6] and consequently in humans.[7,8] In the small animal models, two mice (total body weight 50 g) can be transplanted with islets from one rat (body weight 300 g); however, clinical therapy demands more efficient islet usage. For example, the results obtained by the Edmonton group[2,9] required a minimum of two pancreata per patient to achieve insulin independence. Specifically, the serious human organ shortage demands more efficient islet isolation procedures, permitting a transplant for one person from each donor. Such statistics are rarely, at present, attainable in clinical practice. Some centers have been reported to use as many as six to nine pancreata for one islet transplantation.[10] Nonetheless, most hospitals tend to use, if possible, an islet graft from one excellent isolation procedure. In our own series at the University Hospital of Geneva, insulin independence, following allogeneic islet transplantation in type I diabetic patients, was achieved for three patients with an islet preparation from a single pancreas, and in four patients with islets from two pancreata. Under optimal conditions, every third to fifth islet isolation can deliver a single pancreas islet graft. Furthermore, the enormous variability of donor factors and organ procurement-related variables reduce the potential number of clinical islet transplants.[11] Factors affecting the success of islet isolation have been extensively studied.[12,13] Although donor factors are largely fixed, and can be influenced only by adequate donor selection (donor above age of 20 years, high body mass index, no cardiac arrest, no severe hypotension, no or low vasoactive medication, and short intensive care stay), the procurement technique has a major impact on the outcome of islet isolation and a short (less than 20 min) secondary ischemia time is of crucial importance.[14] An improved selection of the donors and refined procurement parameters may decrease variability and improve human islet isolation yields. A more homogeneous population of harvested pancreata may also facilitate the appreciation of new technical modifications on the isolation process.

The development of an automated digestion and purification procedure for islet isolation by C. Ricordi[15] was a breakthrough in this field, allowing reproducible clinical application. Nonetheless, the large variability in collagenase activity adds another uncertainty to the isolation procedure.[16] Purified enzyme blends such as Liberase® (Boeringer-Mannheim) are sought, with lower batch to batch variability.[17,18] Moreover, in contrast to most crude collagenase blends, Liberase has no endotoxin contamination,[19] which improves primary function and engraftment of islet grafts.[20] However, despite initial convincing results and a less aggressive digestion allowing the isolation of more intact islets, lots with low enzymatic activity remain a problem.

Lakey *et al.* have shown that effective intraductal delivery of the enzyme collagenase into the pancreas is crucial to the subsequent ability to isolate viable islets. Most clinical islet transplant centers load the enzyme into the pancreas by retrograde injection using a syringe following cannulation of the pancreatic duct. The Edmonton group has shown an alternative approach, perfusing the pancreas via the pancreatic duct with collagenase solution using a recirculating perfusion device system. This controlled perfusion via the pancreatic duct allows the effective delivery of the enzyme, achieving maximal distension to all regions of the pancreas and leading to an increased recovery of the islets.[21]

The purification procedure of the digest has been the focus of intense research.[22–27] Although a large variety of continuous and discontinuous density gradients have been tested, the tradeoff between purity and islet loss remains unresolved due to the limiting factor of density gradients; namely, the minimal difference of density between islets and exocrine tissue. The purification of islets by magnetic beads linked to islet-specific antibodies is an interesting concept, but it has not gained acceptance for the large scale purification of human islets.[28] Thus far, purification by fluorescence-activated cell sorting has failed by lacking the means to specifically label the islets by a fluorescent dye. Recently, the group of Lille has identified a non-toxic zinc-sensitive fluorescent probe able to selectively label labile zinc in viable β cells and to exhibit excitation and emission wavelengths in the visible spectrum, making this technique exploitable by a cell sorter.[29] This more specific approach may allow us to better purify the pancreatic digest in future.

Evidently, as long as the islet isolation procedure remains unreliable, thereby rendering islet yields irreproducible among the various reporting laboratories, clinical islet transplantation will be restricted to some experienced centers. The islet isolation technique is of fundamental importance, since a good islet isolation is the *conditio sine qua non* of successful islet transplantation. Before the islet isolation process is better standardized or *in vitro* expansion of islet tissue is made clinically available, the setup of organizational improvements is the only way to address the technical difficulties in islet isolation and organ shortage in the perspective of allotransplantation. Regional organization of networks for islet transplantation is an efficient and valid modality to implement islet transplantation and make it available for large groups of diabetic patients. Such networks allow pancreas procurement, recipient recruitment, transplantation procedure, and followup in each individual center of a region, with islet isolation performed in one single laboratory. In Europe, the Swiss-French GRAGIL consortium (Groupe de Recherche Rhin Rhône Alpes Genève pour la transplantation d'Ilots de Langerhans) was implemented in 1999. It regroups the University Hospitals of Besançon, Geneva, Grenoble, Lyon, and Strasbourg and was recently enlarged to Dijon and Marseille, thus covering about one fourth of France,[30] with islet isolation performed at the core facilities at the University of Geneva. Similar to the GRAGIL group, another network is in the process of being created in England—the Diabetes UK Islet Transplantation Consortium (Diabetes UKITC)—made up of medical researchers interested and/or involved in islet cell research in the U.K. Plans are already in place to develop facilities for islet transplantation at the University Hospitals of Leicester, the King's College Hospital in London, the Royal Free Hospital in London, Worcestershire Acute Hospital NHS Trust, the Southmead Hospital in Bristol, the Addenbrooke's Hospital in Cambridge, and the John Radcliffe Hospital in Oxford. In the USA, the government has recognized the necessity of creating networks for islet transplantation with core facilities. In a Congressional Report on NIH Implementation of the Recommendations of the Congressionally Directed Diabetes Research Working Group it was proposed to establish regional islet cell centers with core laboratory facilities that can isolate and characterize human islet cells according to good manufacturing practice (GMP) guidelines.[31]

The National Center for Research Resources (NCRR), together with the National Institute of Diabetes and Digestive and Kidney Diseases (NIDDK), and the Juvenile Diabetes Research Foundation International (JDRFI), in January 2001, invited applications from institutions to establish Islet Cell Resources (ICRs) for the isolation, purification, and characterization of human pancreatic islet cells for transplantation into diabetic patients. Establishment of up to six ICRs in a wide geographic distribution across the United States is planned. These centers will be responsible for the procurement of whole pancreata, isolation and quality control of islet cell preparations, and distribution of islets for approved research or clinical protocols. They will also perform research and development to improve isolation techniques, cellular viability and function, and shipping procedures.[32]

## THE UNLIMITED ISLET SUPPLY—FACT OR FICTION

The demand for pancreatic islet transplantation significantly exceeds the current supply in human tissue. For instance, in Switzerland there are 30,000 patients with type I diabetes, where under optimal conditions only 30 islet transplantations per year could be performed. In light of the recent fear of transmission of zoonosis by xenotransplantation,[33] reproduction of human tissue by genetic engineering appears to offer an alternative. A human beta cell line could represent an unlimited supply in insulin-producing cells. One of the major obstacles of the procedure is that adult human β cells are difficult to sustain in culture and do not grow spontaneously.

Several groups in the USA and in Europe are intending to create a β cell line by introducing specific genes into adult human β cells to make them grow.[34,35] The main obstacle is to preserve the specific characteristics of the β cells during proliferation, namely, their capacity to produce insulin according to the glucose level *in vitro* and *in vivo*. Recently, NES2Y, a proliferating human insulin-secreting cell line, has been derived from a patient with persistent hyperinsulinemic hypoglycemia of infancy (nesidioblastosis) by the group of Docherty *et al.* at the University of Aberdeen.[36] This disease is characterized by unregulated insulin release despite profound hypoglycemia. Islet cells from patients with nesidioblastosis proliferate spontaneously *in vitro*. NES2Y cells, like β cells isolated from the patient of origin, lack functional ATP-sensitive potassium channels (KATP) and also carry a defect in the insulin gene-regulatory transcription factor PDX1. To repair these defects NES2Y cells were triple transfected with cDNAs encoding the two components of the K(ATP) channel and PDX1.[37] These engineered β cells seem to have an appropriate glucose-responsive insulin release.[38] Additional studies are required to evaluate if these cells will regulate glycemia in a physiological manner in humans. In addition, evidence is required that NES2Y cells and their derivatives are truly immortalized and will not undergo senescence after a certain number of passages.

The use of pancreatic ductal cell precursors is also a potential alternative for creating a cell line. The research group from Lille (France) described that, under specific culture conditions, some cells from the pancreatic duct have the ability to differentiate into insulin-producing cells.[39–41]

Zulewski *et al.* described a new type of pluripotent stem stell within islets. These nestin-positive cells are able to differentiate into cells that express liver and exocrine pancreas markers, such as alpha-fetoprotein and pancreatic amylase, and display a ductal/endocrine phenotype with expression of CK19, neural-specific cell adhesion molecule, insulin, glucagon, and the pancreas/duodenum specific homeodomain transcription factor, PDX-1.[42] Both approaches, the differentiation of pancreas-specific endocrine tissue from either ductal cells or nestin-positive stem cells, are of particular interest for clinical application. Ductal cells or nestin-positive stem cells isolated from pancreatic biopsies could be expanded *ex vivo* and transplanted into the donor/recipient.

Embryonic stem cells display the ability to differentiate in culture into a variety of cell lineages. Recently, a Spanish group at the University of Alicante successfully produced a human insulin-secreting cell derived from mouse embryonic stem cells that normalizes blood glucose when transplanted into diabetic mice.[43] Apart from ethical considerations, the use of human embryonic stem cells has various legal and political limitations. For instance, in France any experiments involving embryonic cells are forbidden. In contrast, the United Kingdom has a legal framework for the use of such embryonic stem cells. However, eight out of the 15 European Union countries have no legal provision concerning this issue.[44] Thus, the field of embryonic stem cells remains highly controversial.

## ISLET AUTOTRANSPLANTATION—
## THE IMPORTANCE OF ISLET INTEGRITY

Autotransplantation may be restricted to a small group of patients undergoing extensive pancreatectomy for benign disease. Nonetheless its clinical application has not only prevented postoperative diabetes in some patients,[45–48] but has additionally brought to light the pathophysiology of islet transplantation. Having to deal neither with allo- nor with autoimmunity, autologous islet transplantation allows for studying non-immunological factors involved in islet transplantation. As shown in FIGURE 2, islet autografts can experience an initial dysfunction and over time can lose the capacity to maintain normoglycemia.

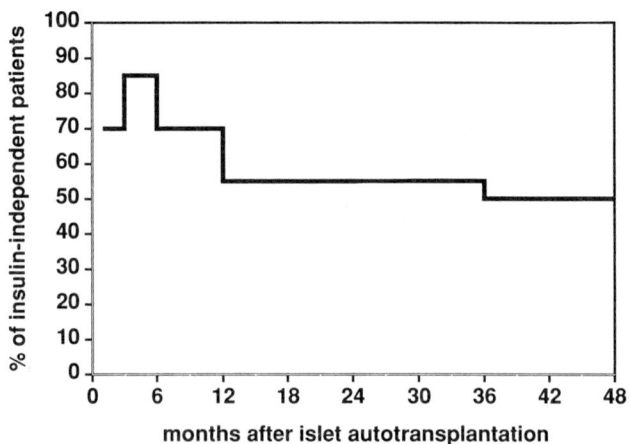

**FIGURE 2.** Actuarial insulin independence after pancreatectomy and autologous islet transplantation in a series of thirteen patients at the University of Geneva. Two patients became immediately insulin-dependant because of an insufficient islet mass isolated from a very fibrotic pancreas. Two patients required insulin therapy during the first two months after the procedure, but subsequently became insulin independent. Four patients lost insulin independence over time, three of whom had recurrent alcohol abuse.

In rodents, the survival of transplanted β cells has been shown to be prolonged by the presence of islet endocrine non-β-cells within the graft. The mechanisms underlying this effect have not yet been elucidated, but they may involve metabolic interactions of the endocrine non-β-cells.[49] The glucose-induced insulin release depends not only on the insulin-containing beta cells, but also on their interactions with other types of endocrine cells within the islet. Human beta cells express functional glucagon receptors that can generate synergistic signals for glucose-induced insulin secretion.[50] Therefore, a change of islet cell composition may affect insulin release. It has been shown that during the isolation procedure, the islet integument can be damaged[51,52] with consecutive injury or loss of islet cells.[53] Since alpha cells are mainly distributed in the islet periphery, they are more easily lost or injured during the isolation procedure.

Isolated islets transplanted to the intrahepatic portal system may lack protective mechanisms that are present in the normal pancreas. We have recently described that alpha-1 proteinase inhibitor is expressed on human islet microvascular endothelial cells.[54] Alpha-1 proteinase inhibitor blocks trypsin activity and inhibits transendothelial leukocyte migration.[55] Transplanted islets are probably revascularized by endothelial cells coming from the vascular bed of the recipient site[56] not expressing the physiological characteristics of islet endothelial cells.

Despite of these biological constraints, there is sufficient clinical evidence to validate the islet transplantation concept. The data from autologous islet transplantation suggest that the transplantation of isolated β cells may not restore physiologically normoglycemia. This can only be verified when a human β cell line is available.

## ISLET ALLOTRANSPLANTATION IN UREMIC TYPE I DIABETIC PATIENTS—TOO LATE, TOO DIFFICULT?

Thus far, islet allotransplantation has been prescribed mostly for type I diabetic patients with a functional solid organ graft, or for patients on the waiting list for an organ transplantation. This group of worst-case diabetic patients has a long history of unstable diabetes and presents all chronic diabetic complications. These patients require immunosuppression to prevent rejection of the transplanted organ (mostly a kidney graft because of end-stage diabetic nephropathy), and the islet graft does not present a relevant additional risk.

To date, more than 400 islet allotransplantations have been reported to the International Islet Transplantation Registry in Giessen (ITR). Islet transplantation in type I diabetic patients with end-stage kidney failure has had some important (see FIGURE 3), although still unreliable, success.[47,57–60] Data from our group showed that, with improved islet isolation techniques, the rate of primary islet function can be increased from 55%[61] to 100%[47] (see FIGURE 4). However, the applied immunosuppression, including a combination of steroids and high dose calcineurin inhibitors (either cyclosporine or tacrolimus), did not prevent consistently rejection or recurrence of autoimmune diabetes. In addition, the combination of steroids and calcineurin inhibitors induced a marked insulin resistance and direct beta-cell toxicity. Although in whole-pancreas transplantation this insulin-resistance can be counterbalanced by a sufficient islet mass transplanted, the islet mass in an islet graft is often inappropriate to overcome the increased metabolic demand induced by the

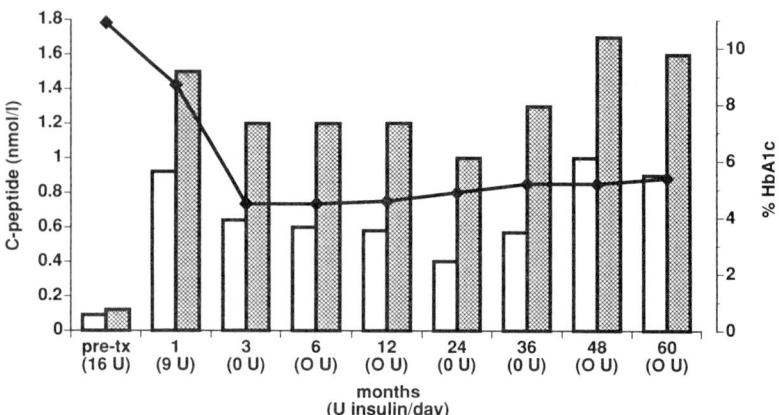

**FIGURE 3.** Metabolic follow up after successful islet allotransplantation in a 36-year-old patient with type I diabetes having received a kidney graft nine years previously. Two months following islet transplantation exogenous insulin therapy could be stopped. The patient has remained insulin independent for five years. Basal and stimulated C-peptide levels are within normal ranges. Without any dietary restriction, HbA1c is normal. The patient is under standard immunosuppression with cyclosporine, mycophenolate, and steroids. ▨, C-peptide (stimulated); ☐, C-peptide (basal); ◆, HbA1c%.

diabetogenic immunosuppression. Although only few patients became insulin independent with this conventional immunosuppression, the restoration of an endogenous insulin-production stabilized glucose homeostasis reduced hypoglycemic events,[62] normalized glycosylated hemoglobin,[47] and had potentially a beneficial effect on long term diabetic complications.[63]

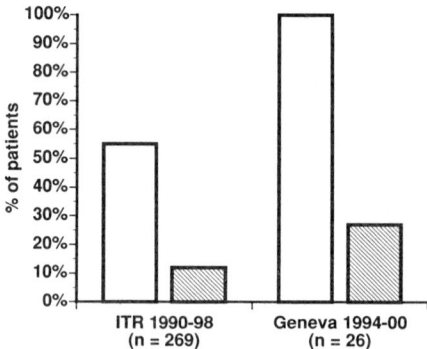

**FIGURE 4.** Comparison of the results of islet allotranplantation as reported to the International Islet Registry (ITR) and at the University of Geneva. A basal C-peptide above 0.3 nmol/l (0.9 ng/ml) indicates ongoing graft function. ☐, C-peptide > 0.3 nmol/l, two months after transplantation; ▨, insulin independence.

## ISLET ALLOTRANSPLANTATION ALONE IN NON-UREMIC TYPE I DIABETIC PATIENTS

Recently, the Edmonton group reported on a series of successful islet allografts in non-uremic type I diabetic patients (patients with normal kidney function and, thus, not requiring a kidney transplantation) using a steroid-free immunosuppressive regimen and repeated islet injections until transplantation of a sufficient islet mass so as to achieve insulin independence.[2,9] This remarkable breakthrough in the field of islet transplantation raises several questions on the reasons for the previous frequent graft failures. The amount of islets injected and engrafting thereafter are of utmost importance. In the Edmonton series, at least 9,000 islet equivalents per kilogram of body weight of the recipient were needed to achieve insulin independence. Therefore, a patient with a body weight of 70 kg would require at least 630,000 islet equivalents to achieve insulin independence. Grossly, this number corresponds to 50% of the islet content of a normal pancreas. In previous series, most patients received a lower islet mass. In our series at the University of Geneva, we transplanted a mean of 6,000 islet equivalents per kilogram body weight, giving one explanation why insulin independence was only achieved in 7 of 26 islet allotransplantations (unpublished data). With improved islet isolation techniques, 9,000 islet equivalents per kilogram body weight could be isolated from a single pancreas. However, patients with a high body weight still require more than one donor. Thus, strategies are required to lower the islet mass needed to achieve insulin independence in order to make islet transplantation accessible to more patients.

Combining immunosuppression with sirolimus and low dose tacrolimus, without steroids, is also one of the keys for the success of the Edmonton trial. The previous series of islet transplantation used a combination of high doses of calcineurin inhibitors and steroids, which is diabetogenic, as described previously. In contrast to a standard immunosuppression, this regimen has almost no diabetic side effects. Moreover, considering the relative low acute insulin response to intravenous glucose, and the excellent metabolic results described in the Edmonton series,[9] the question can be raised as to whether sirolimus may increase the effect of insulin.

When balancing the risk and benefit of islet transplantation in non-uremic patients, we must consider some rare complications that occurred in the patients grafted in Edmonton.[9] In addition to the risks of injection (bleeding and partial transitory thrombosis), some patients showed increased cholesterol and decreased kidney function. During long term followup, some patients also experienced postislet transplant diabetes (three out of twelve). Thus, as long as long term immunosuppression is required, it seems important to restrict islet transplantation only to patients with unstable diabetes at risk for severe hypoglycemia and long term complications. This particular category of patients will benefit by a better glucose regulation achieved after islet transplantation, even if low doses of exogenous insulin and life-long immunosuppression may be needed.

## FUTURE PERSPECTIVES—IMMUNE TOLERANCE OR IMMUNOPROTECTIVE DEVICES?

The main hurdles to the widespread use of islet transplantation are the insufficient number of appropriate donors and the need for immunosuppression to prevent rejection of the graft and recurrence of the eventually underlying autoimmune disease. Although new sources of cells and tissue may be found in the near future, as discussed above, to date all immunosuppressive regiments inevitably exhibit side effects, such as an increased incidence of infection and cancer.

To avoid immunosuppression, induction of immune tolerance or immunoisolation (e.g., encapsulation) have been proposed to protect the graft from the assaults of the host's immune system.[64,65] Immune tolerance has been reviewed extensively by others.[66–69] Three principal approaches for induction of immunological tolerance towards an allo- or xenogeneic graft are under investigation, namely hematopoietic chimerism, lymphocyte depletion, and costimulation blockade.[70] Although all of these principles have been applied successfully in non-human primates, clinical data in humans are still lacking.

A number of immunoisolation systems have been developed during the past decades. Three major types of immunoisolation have been studied by different groups: perfusion shunt devices anastomosed to the vascular system,[71] diffusion chambers or macrocapsules, and microcapsules. However, the clinical application of these devices is hindered, in many cases, by problems such as fragility, limited surface area, and, in the case of perfused vascular devices, the surgery required for implantation and shunt connection with risks of hemorrhage, thrombosis, embolism, and infection, and the relatively high diffusion resistance inherent in the plastic membrane.[72] Immunoisolation barriers, such as microcapsules bypass these problems and provide additional options for the method and site of implantation. Specifically, Sun, in 1980 provided the first evidence that encapsulated islets could regulate blood glucose in rats.[64] By isolating rat islets and encapsulating these in water soluble polymeric capsules with a semipermeable membrane, the ingress of nutrients and egress of cellular debris could be controlled while protecting the graft (an islet cluster containing insulin-secreting β cells) from the host's immune system. These capsules, based on naturally occurring polysaccharides and polyaminoacids, have been shown to regulate blood glucose for periods exceeding six months.[73] The results have recently been extended to spontaneously diabetic cynomogulus monkeys providing the first "large" animal (Sun's monkeys weighed 2–3 kgs) evidence of discordant xenograft function,[74] although these data remain to be duplicated.

The transplantation of microencapsulated islets has been exposed to several biomechanical limitations. Among these, the optimal site for transplantation remains to be defined. Thus far, the size and mechanical properties of most available microcapsules restricted the choice of the implantation site to the peritoneal cavity. Most researches were concentrated on the peritoneal site for implantation of encapsulated islets.[75,76] However, this site is, for several reasons, inappropriate for encapsulated cell therapy. The peritoneal cavity has a low blood supply, oxygenation tension, and concentration in essentials minerals, thus hampering the viability of the graft.[75] The release of hormones, like insulin, from the peritoneal cavity to the blood stream has a delayed and reduced kinetic compared to hormones released in the portal vein.[77]

Furthermore, peritoneal macrophages have a high cytotoxicity against encapsulated islets.[78] Most clinical islet transplantations have been performed intraportally (184 from 200 islet allografts from 1990 to 1997). The International Islet Registry reports significantly more c-peptide positive cases (at least 0.5 ng/ml) one year after transplantation in the portal vein than in any other site (36% vs. 13%, $p < 0.05$).[61] The intraportal location has a high oxygenation and nutriment supply, thanks to its double vascularization. Moreover, the liver is the main target organ for insulin. A preliminary study has demonstrated the feasibility of intraportal injections of empty microcapsules in the portal vein of the rat, with the portal pressure returning to basal level within two hours after injection.[79] Recently, we have extended these experiments to a large animal model. Intraportal injection of 10,000 microcapsules (with a diameter of 400 µm) per kilogram body weight was well tolerated in pigs without any alteration in liver function over a period of three months.[80] Additional studies are required to evaluate the function of encapsulated islets transplanted into various sites in large animals, before encapsulated islet transplantation can enter clinical reality.

In summary, the clinical data obtained thus far have validated the islet transplantation concept. The authors recommend that research in clinical islet transplantation continues to focus auto- and allotransplantation, providing a limited number of worst-case patients the chance to alleviate the burdens of an unstable diabetes, or even cure an onset diabetes, and accumulating data sufficient to scale up the technology to a larger population. Specifically, the medicoscientific community needs to enhance the investigations in finding an unlimited β cell supply and to develop strategies to overcome the need for continuous immunosuppression.

## ACKNOWLEDGMENTS

Research work performed at the University of Geneva in the fields reviewed was supported by the Swiss National Science Foundation Grants No. 32-061873.00 (to Ph. Morel and J. Oberholzer) and No. 4046-058685 (to Ph. Morel and J. Oberholzer) and the Foundation Carlos et Elsie de Reuter (to Ph. Morel), the Geneva Diabetes Foundation (to Ph. Morel and J. Oberholzer), the Swiss Committee of Technology and Innovation (to Ph. Morel, D. Hunkeler and J. Oberholzer), as well as by the Juvenile Diabetes Foundation (to B. Thorens, D. Trono, Ph. Halban, P. Aebischer, and Ph. Morel).

## REFERENCES

1. WILLIAMS, P.W. 1894. Notes on diabetes treated with grafts of sheep's pancreas. Br. Med. J. **2:** 1303.
2. SHAPIRO, A.M., J.R. LAKEY, E.A. RYAN, et al. 2000. Islet transplantation in seven patients with type 1 diabetes mellitus using a glucocorticoid-free immunosuppressive regimen. N. Engl. J. Med. **343:** 230–238.
3. LACY, P.E. & M. KOSTIANOVSKY. 1967. Method for the isolation of intact islets of Langerhans from the rat pancreas. Diabetes **16:** 35–39.
4. BALLINGER, W.F. & P.E. LACY. 1972. Transplantation of intact pancreatic islets in rats. Surgery **72:** 175–186.

5. MIRKOVITCH, V. & M. CAMPICHE. 1976. Successful intrasplenic autotransplantation of pancreatic tissue in totally pancreatectomised dogs. Transplantation **21:** 265–269.
6. LORENZ, D., R. REDING, J. PETERMANN, *et al.* 1976. Transplantation of isolated islets of Langerhans into the liver of diabetic dogs. Zentralbl. Chir. **101:** 1359–1368.
7. NAJARIAN, J.S., D.E. SUTHERLAND, A.J. MATAS, *et al.* 1977. Human islet transplantation: a preliminary report. Transplant. Proc. **9:** 233–236.
8. SUTHERLAND, D.E., A.J. MATAS, F.C. GOETZ & J.S. NAJARIAN. 1980. Transplantation of dispersed pancreatic islet tissue in humans: autografts and allografts. Diabetes **29**(Suppl. 1): 31–44.
9. RYAN, E.A., J.R. LAKEY, R.V. RAJOTTE, *et al.* 2001. Clinical outcomes and insulin secretion after islet transplantation with the Edmonton protocol. Diabetes **50:** 710–719.
10. KEYMEULEN, B., Z. LING, F. GORUS, *et al.* 1998. Implantation of standardized beta-cell grafts in a liver segment of IDDM patients: graft and recipient characteristics in two cases of insulin-independence under maintenance immunosuppression for prior kidney graft. Diabetologia **41:** 452–459.
11. BRANDHORST, D., H. BRANDHORST, M. BRENDEL & R.G. BRETZEL. 1998. Problems of islet isolation from the human and porcine pancreas for islet transplantation into men. Zentralbl. Chir. **123:** 814–822.
12. BENHAMOU, P.Y., P.C. WATT, Y. MULLEN, *et al.* 1994. Human islet isolation in 104 consecutive cases. Factors affecting isolation success. Transplantation **57:** 1804–1810.
13. TOSO, C., J. OBERHOLZER, F. RIS, *et al.* 2001. Factors affecting human islet of Langerhans isolation yields. Transplant. Proc. In press.
14. BRANDHORST, D., H. BRANDHORST, B.J. HERING, *et al.* 1995. Islet isolation from the pancreas of large mammals and humans: 10 years of experience. Exp. Clin. Endocrinol. Diabetes **103**(Suppl. 2): 3–14.
15. RICORDI, C., P.E. LACY, E.H. FINKE, *et al.* 1988. Automated method for isolation of human pancreatic islets. Diabetes **37:** 413–420.
16. JOHNSON, P.R., S.A. WHITE & N.J. LONDON. 1996. Collagenase and human islet isolation. Cell Transplant. **5:** 437–452.
17. LINETSKY, E., R. BOTTINO, R. LEHMANN, *et al.* 1997. Improved human islet isolation using a new enzyme blend, liberase. Diabetes **46:** 1120–1123.
18. OLACK, B.J., C.J. SWANSON, T.K. HOWARD & T. MOHANAKUMAR. 1999. Improved method for the isolation and purification of human islets of langerhans using Liberase enzyme blend. Hum. Immunol. **60:** 1303–1309.
19. JAHR, H., G. PFEIFFER, B.J. HERING, *et al.* 1999. Endotoxin-mediated activation of cytokine production in human PBMCs by collagenase and Ficoll. J. Mol. Med. **77:** 118–120.
20. ECKHARDT, T., H. JAHR, K. FEDERLIN & R.G. BRETZEL. 1999. Endotoxin impairs the engraftment of rat islets transplanted beneath the kidney capsule of C57BL/6-mice. J. Mol. Med. **77:** 123–125.
21. LAKEY, J.R., G.L. WARNOCK, A.M. SHAPIRO, *et al.* 1999. Intraductal collagenase delivery into the human pancreas using syringe loading or controlled perfusion. Cell Transplant. **8:** 285–292.
22. ALEJANDRO, R., S. STRASSER, P.F. ZUCKER & D.H. MINTZ. 1990. Isolation of pancreatic islets from dogs. Semiautomated purification on albumin gradients. Transplantation **50:** 207–210.
23. BEHBOO, R., P.B. CARROLL, F. UKAH, *et al.* 1994. One-hour of hypothermic incubation in Euro-Collins improves islet purification. Transplant. Proc. **26:** 645.
24. SOON-SHIONG, P., R. HEINTZ, T. FUJIOKA, *et al.* 1990. Utilization of anti-acinar cell monoclonal antibodies in the purification of rat and canine islets. Horm. Metab. Res. Suppl. **25:** 45–50.
25. SAMEJIMA, T., K. YAMAGUCHI, H. IWATA, *et al.* 1998. Gelatin density gradient for isolation of islets of Langerhans. Cell Transplant. **7:** 37–45.
26. LAKEY, J.R., T.J. CAVANAGH & M.A. ZIEGER. 1998. A prospective comparison of discontinuous EuroFicoll and EuroDextran gradients for islet purification. Cell Transplant. **7:** 479–487.

27. LONDON, N.J., S.M. SWIFT & H.A. CLAYTON. 1998. Isolation, culture and functional evaluation of islets of Langerhans. Diabetes Metab. **24:** 200–207.
28. NANDIGALA, P., T.H. CHEN, C. YANG, et al. 1997. Immunomagnetic isolation of islets from the rat pancreas. Biotechnol. Prog. **13:** 844–848.
29. LUKOWIAK, B., B. VANDEWALLE, R. RIACHY, et al. 2001. Identification and purification of functional human beta-cells by a new specific zinc-fluorescent probe. J. Histochem. Cytochem. **49:** 519–528.
30. BENHAMOU, P.Y., J. OBERHOLZER, C. TOSO, et al. 2001. Human islet transplantation network for the treatment of type 1 diabetes: first (1999–2000) data from the Swiss-French GRAGIL consortium. Diabetologia. **44:** 859–864.
31. <http://www.niddk.nih.gov/federal/dwg/DRWGREP2.htm>
32. <http://grants.nih.gov/grants/guide/rfa-files/RFA-RR-01-002.html>
33. BACH, F.H. & H.V. FINEBERG. 1998. Call for moratorium on xenotransplants. Nature **391:** 326.
34. SALMON, P., J. OBERHOLZER, T. OCCHIODORO, et al. 2000. Reversible immortalization of human primary cells by lentivector-mediated transfer of specific genes. Mol. Ther. **2:** 404–414.
35. DUFAYET DE LA TOUR, D., T. HALVORSEN, C. DEMETERCO, et al. 2001. Beta-cell differentiation from a human pancreatic cell line *in vitro* and *in vivo*. Mol. Endocrinol. **15:** 476–483.
36. MACFARLANE, W.M., H. CRAGG, H.M. DOCHERTY, et al. 1997. Impaired expression of transcription factor IUF1 in a pancreatic beta-cell line derived from a patient with persistent hyperinsulinaemic hypoglycaemia of infancy (nesidioblastosis). FEBS Lett. **413:** 304–308.
37. MACFARLANE, W.M., R.E. O'BRIEN, P.D. BARNES, et al. 2000. Sulfonylurea receptor 1 and Kir6.2 expression in the novel human insulin-secreting cell line NES2Y. Diabetes **49:** 953–960.
38. MACFARLANE, W.M., R.M. SHEPHERD, K.E. COSGROVE, et al. 2000. Glucose modulation of insulin mRNA levels is dependent on transcription factor PDX-1 and occurs independently of changes in intracellular $Ca^{2+}$. Diabetes **49:** 418–423.
39. GMYR, V., J. KERR-CONTE, S. BELAICH, et al. 2000. Adult human cytokeratin 19-positive cells reexpress insulin promoter factor 1 *in vitro*: further evidence for pluripotent pancreatic stem cells in humans. Diabetes **49:** 1671–1680.
40. KERR-CONTE, J., F. PATTOU, M. LECOMTE-HOUCKE, et al. 1996. Ductal cyst formation in collagen-embedded adult human islet preparations. A means to the reproduction of nesidioblastosis *in vitro*. Diabetes **45:** 1108–1114.
41. GMYR, V., J. KERR-CONTE, B. VANDEWALLE, et al. 2001. Human pancreatic ductal cells: large-scale isolation and expansion. Cell Transplant. **10:** 109–121.
42. ZULEWSKI, H., E.J. ABRAHAM, M.J. GERLACH, et al. 2001. Multipotential nestin-positive stem cells isolated from adult pancreatic islets differentiate *ex vivo* into pancreatic endocrine, exocrine, and hepatic phenotypes. Diabetes **50:** 521–533.
43. SORIA, B., E. ROCHE, G. BERNA, et al. 2000. Insulin-secreting cells derived from embryonic stem cells normalize glycemia in streptozotocin-induced diabetic mice. Diabetes **49:** 157–162.
44. LENOIR, N. 2000. Europe confronts the embryonic stem cell research challenge. Science **287:** 1425–1427.
45. WAHOFF, D.C., B.E. PAPALOIS, J.S. NAJARIAN, et al. 1995. Autologous islet transplantation to prevent diabetes after pancreatic resection. Ann. Surg. **222:** 562–575; discussion 75–79.
46. ROBERTSON, G.S., A.R. DENNISON, P.R. JOHNSON & N.J. LONDON. 1998. A review of pancreatic islet autotransplantation. Hepatogastroenterology **45:** 226–235.
47. OBERHOLZER, J., F. TRIPONEZ, R. MAGE, et al. 2000. Human islet transplantation: lessons from 13 autologous and 13 allogeneic transplantations. Transplantation **69:** 1115–1123.
48. WHITE, S.A., J.E. DAVIES, C. POLLARD, et al. 2001. Pancreas resection and islet autotransplantation for end-stage chronic pancreatitis. Ann. Surg. **233:** 423–431.

49. PIPELEERS, D.G., M. PIPELEERS-MARICHAL, B. VANBRABANDT & S. DUYS. 1991. Transplantation of purified islet cells in diabetic rats. II. Immunogenicity of allografted islet beta-cells. Diabetes **40:** 920–930.
50. HUYPENS, P., Z. LING, D. PIPELEERS & F. SCHUIT. 2000. Glucagon receptors on human islet cells contribute to glucose competence of insulin release. Diabetologia **43:** 1012–1019.
51. WANG, R.N., S. PARASKEVAS & L. ROSENBERG. 1999. Characterization of integrin expression in islets isolated from hamster, canine, porcine, and human pancreas. J. Histochem. Cytochem. **47:** 499–506.
52. WANG, R.N. & L. ROSENBERG. 1999. Maintenance of beta-cell function and survival following islet isolation requires re-establishment of the islet-matrix relationship. J. Endocrinol. **163:** 181–190.
53. BERTUZZI, F., C. BERRA, C. SOCCI, et al. 1995. Glucagon improves insulin secretion from pig islets *in vitro*. J. Endocrinol. **147:** 87–93.
54. LOU, J., F. TRIPONEZ, J. OBERHOLZER, et al. 1999. Expression of alpha-1 proteinase inhibitor in human islet microvascular endothelial cells. Diabetes **48:** 1773–1778.
55. CEPINSKAS, G., R. NOSEWORTHY & P.R. KVIETYS. 1997. Transendothelial neutrophil migration. Role of neutrophil-derived proteases and relationship to transendothelial protein movement. Circ. Res. **81:** 618–626.
56. VAJKOCZY, P., A.M. OLOFSSON, H.A. LEHR, et al. 1995. Histogenesis and ultrastructure of pancreatic islet graft microvasculature. Evidence for graft revascularization by endothelial cells of host origin. Am. J. Pathol. **146:** 1397–1405.
57. SECCHI, A., C. SOCCI, P. MAFFI, et al. 1997. Islet transplantation in IDDM patients. Diabetologia **40:** 225–231.
58. BRETZEL, R.G., D. BRANDHORST, H. BRANDHORST, et al. 1999. Improved survival of intraportal pancreatic islet cell allografts in patients with type-1 diabetes mellitus by refined peritransplant management. J. Mol. Med. **77:** 140–143.
59. WARNOCK, G.L., N.M. KNETEMAN, E.A. RYAN, et al. 1992. Long-term follow-up after transplantation of insulin-producing pancreatic islets into patients with type 1 (insulin-dependent) diabetes mellitus. Diabetologia **35:** 89–95.
60. ALEJANDRO, R., R. LEHMANN, C. RICORDI, et al. 1997. Long-term function (6 years) of islet allografts in type 1 diabetes. Diabetes **46:** 1983–1989.
61. BRENDEL, M.D., B. HERING, A.O. SCHULTZ & R.G. BRETZEL. 1999. International islet transplant registry. Newsletter 8, Justus-Liebig-University of Giessen.
62. MEYER, C., B.J. HERING, R. GROSSMANN, et al. 1998. Improved glucose counterregulation and autonomic symptoms after intraportal islet transplants alone in patients with long-standing type I diabetes mellitus. Transplantation **66:** 233–240.
63. LUZI, L., G. PERSEGHIN, M.D. BRENDEL, et al. 2001. Metabolic effects of restoring partial beta-cell function after islet allotransplantation in type 1 diabetic patients. Diabetes **50:** 277–282.
64. LIM, F. & A.M. SUN. 1980. Microencapsulated islets as bioartificial endocrine pancreas. Science **210:** 908–910.
65. MULLEN, Y., M. MARUYAMA & C.V. SMITH. 2000. Current progress and perspectives in immunoisolated islet transplantation. J. Hepatobiliary Pancreat. Surg. **7:** 347–357.
66. SACHS, D.H. 1999. Immunologic tolerance to organ transplants. J. Gastrointest. Surg. **3:** 105–110.
67. CALNE, R.Y. 2000. Prope tolerance: a step in the search for tolerance in the clinic. World J. Surg. **24:** 793–796.
68. WEKERLE, T. & M. SYKES. 2001. Mixed chimerism and transplantation tolerance. Annu. Rev. Med. **52:** 353–370.
69. BLUESTONE, J.A., J.B. MATTHEWS & A.M. KRENSKY. 2000. The immune tolerance network: the "Holy Grail" comes to the clinic. J. Am. Soc. Nephrol. **11:** 2141–2146.
70. KNECHTLE, S.J. 2000. Knowledge about transplantation tolerance gained in primates. Curr. Opin. Immunol. **12:** 552–556.
71. PETRUZZO, P., L. PIBIRI, M.A. DE GIUDICI, et al. 1991. Xenotransplantation of microencapsulated pancreatic islets contained in a vascular prosthesis: preliminary results. Transpl. Int. **4:** 200–204.

72. LANZA, R.P. & W.L. CHICK. 1997. Experimental pancreatic islet cell xenotransplantation. *In* Xenotransplantation. D.K.C. Cooper, E. Kemp, J.L. Platt & D.J.G. White, Eds.: 534–544. Springer, Berlin.
73. O'SHEA, G.M., M.F. GOOSEN & A.M. SUN. 1984. Prolonged survival of transplanted islets of Langerhans encapsulated in a biocompatible membrane. Biochim. Biophys. Acta **804:** 133–136.
74. SUN, Y., X. MA, D. ZHOU, *et al.* 1996. Normalization of diabetes in spontaneously diabetic cynomologus monkeys by xenografts of microencapsulated porcine islets without immunosuppression. J. Clin. Invest. **98:** 1417–1422.
75. DE VOS, P., J.F. VAN STRAATEN, A.G. NIEUWENHUIZEN, *et al.* 1999. Why do microencapsulated islet grafts fail in the absence of fibrotic overgrowth? Diabetes **48:** 1381–1388.
76. LANZA, R.P., D.M. ECKER, W.M. KUHTREIBER, *et al.* 1999. Transplantation of islets using microencapsulation: studies in diabetic rodents and dogs. J. Mol. Med. **77:** 206–210.
77. DE VOS, P., D. VEGTER, B.J. DE HAAN, *et al.* 1996. Kinetics of intraperitoneally infused insulin in rats. Functional implications for the bioartificial pancreas. Diabetes **45:** 1102–1107.
78. KESSLER, L., C. JESSER, Y. LOMBARD, *et al.* 1996. Cytotoxicity of peritoneal murine macrophages against encapsulated pancreatic rat islets: *in vivo* and *in vitro* studies. J. Leukoc. Biol. **60:** 729–736.
79. LEBLOND, F.A., G. SIMARD, N. HENLEY, *et al.* 1999. Studies on smaller (approximately 315 microM) microcapsules: IV. Feasibility and safety of intrahepatic implantations of small alginate poly-L-lysine microcapsules. Cell Transplant. **8:** 327–337.
80. TOSO, C., J. OBERHOLZER, I. CEAUSOGLU, *et al.* 2001. Intraportal injections of 400 µm multicomponent microcapsules in a large animal model. Submittted.

# Standards and Guidelines for Biopolymers in Tissue-Engineered Medical Products

## ASTM Alginate and Chitosan Standard Guides

MICHAEL DORNISH,[a] DAVID KAPLAN,[b] AND ØYVIND SKAUGRUD[a]

[a]*Pronova Biomedical a.s, Gaustadalléen 21, N-0349 Oslo, Norway*

[b]*Division of Mechanics and Materials Sciences, CDRH, FDA, Rockville, Maryland, USA*

ABSTRACT: The American Society for Testing and Materials (ASTM) is making a concerted effort to establish standards and guidelines for the entire field of tissue-engineered medical products (TEMPS). Safety, consistency, and functionality of biomaterials used as matrices, scaffolds, and immobilizing agents in TEMPS are a concern. Therefore, the ASTM has established a number of task groups to produce standards and guidelines for such biomaterials. Alginate is a naturally occurring biomaterial used for immobilizing living cells to form an artificial organ, such as encapsulated pancreatic islets. In order to aid in successful clinical applications and to help expedite regulatory approval, the alginate used must be fully documented. The ASTM alginate guide gives information on selection of testing methodologies and safety criteria. Critical parameters such as monomer content, molecular weight, and viscosity, in addition to more general parameters, such as dry matter content, heavy metal content, bioburden, and endotoxin content are described in the ASTM document. In a like manner, the characterization parameters for chitosan, a bioadhesive polycationic polysaccharide, are described in a separate guide. For chitosan, the degree of deacetylation is of critical importance. Control of protein content and, hence, potential for hypersensitivity, endotoxin content, and total bioburden are important in chitosan preparations for TEMPS. Together these two guides represent part of the effort on behalf of the ASTM and other interested parties to ensure quality and standardization in TEMPS.

KEYWORDS: ASTM; tissue-engineered medical products; TEMPS; alginate; chitosan; standardization

## INTRODUCTION

The biomedical and pharmaceutical industries are continually searching for functional materials in their development of improved devices and drug delivery systems. Alginate and chitosan have shown an interesting potential for use as scaffolds in tissue-engineered medical products,[1,2] as drug-containing materials for depot delivery,[3,4] and as an encapsulating matrix for immobilization of living cells.[5] However, in order to ensure the functionality of these biopolymers in an application they must be fully

---

Address for correspondence: Michael Dornish, Pronova Biomedical a.s, Gaustadalléen 21, N-0349 Oslo, Norway. Voice: +47-22958650; fax: +47-22696470.
mdornish@pronova.no

TABLE 1. Biomedical and pharmaceutical applications of ultrapure alginate

| Matrices and Scaffolds | Directed Drug Delivery | Artificial Organs |
|---|---|---|
| Bone regeneration<br>Maruyama, et al.[14];<br>Kenley et al.[15] | Endostatin-producing cells<br>Reed et al.[20];<br>Joki et al.[21] | Artificial pancreas<br>Lim[27];<br>Sun et al.[28] |
| Nerve regeneration<br>Suzuki et al.[16] | Parkinson's disease<br>Emerich, et al.[22] | Artificial liver<br>Wong[29];<br>Sun et al.[30] |
| Bulking agent<br>Atala, et al.[17];<br>Diamond[13];<br>Gentile[18] | Hormones and growth<br>Chang et al.[23];<br>Peirone et al.[24];<br>Stockley et al.[25] | Artificial kidney<br>Chang[31] |
| Soft tissue implant<br>Brunstedt, et al.[19] | CNS<br>Chen[26] | |

characterized. There is, therefore, a need for guidance in the characterization and testing of these materials in order to ensure uniformity and from batch to batch.

Commodity alginates are well known to the biomedical and pharmaceutical industry for their traditional uses in the treatment of topical wounds (Thomas[6–8]), as an antireflux remedy (Hagstam,[9] Mandel et al.[10]), and as a tablet excipient (Onsøyen[11]). The purity level and the current means of manufacture make it difficult to believe, however, that commodity alginates will find a use in implantable devices and drug formulations for parenteral administration.

Ultrapure alginates, made in accordance with GMP/ISO 9000 guidelines, have been successfully employed for applications inside the human body,[12,13] and several products containing ultrapure alginate are in the process of being clinically evaluated. TABLE 1 lists potential applications where ultrapure alginate could play a role.

## THE ASTM

The American Society for Testing and Materials was organized in 1898 as a not-for-profit organization to develop standards and technical information for materials, products, systems, and services. Originally the engineers who formed the ASTM recognized a need for standards for the steel used in railroad rails, which often was of inferior quality. The ASTM standards may be test methods, specifications, practices, guides, classifications, or terminology. To date there are over 10,000 standards published in virtually all areas of material technology. A further description can be found at the ASTM web site.[32]

ASTM Committee F04 on Medical and Surgical Materials and Devices established a separate division, Division IV, on Tissue-Engineered Medical Products (TEMPS) in 1997. The purpose of Division IV is to develop standards for tissue-engineered medical products focusing on components of combination medical products, intended to repair, replace, or regenerate human tissue.[33,34] These comprise biological components, such as cells, tissue, cellular products and/or biomolecules, and biomaterials used in combination, including biologic, biomimetic, and/or synthetic materials. That there is a need for biomaterial standardization has been discussed elsewhere.[35–37]

Division IV includes about 10 subcommittees and more than 37 task groups working to develop TEMPS standards. The subcommittee F04.43, for example, is working within the field of biomaterials. The task groups for alginate and chitosan (F04.43.4 and F04.43.10, respectively) are a part of this subcommittee.

## THE ASTM GUIDE FOR ALGINATE

In February of 2001 the guide entitled *Standard Guide for Characterization and Testing of Alginates as Starting Materials Intended for Use in Biomedical and Tissue-Engineered Medical Products Application* was published in the ASTM Book of Standards under the designation F 2064. The aim of the guide is to identify key parameters relevant for the functionality and characterization of alginates for the development of new commercial applications of alginates for the biomedical and pharmaceutical industries.

Alginate has found uses in a variety of products ranging from simple technical applications, such as viscosifiers, to advanced biomedical matrices providing controlled drug delivery from immobilized living cells.[38] Alginates are a family of non-branched binary copolymers of 1–4 glycosidically linked β-D-mannuronic acid (M) and α-L-guluronic acid (G) residues (see FIGURE 1). The relative amount of the two uronic acid monomers and their sequential arrangement along the polymer chain vary widely, depending on the origin of the alginate. The distribution of the uronic acid residues can be considered as patterns of homopolymeric blocks of G and M, respectively, and blocks with an alternating sequence, all in coexistence. Alginates isolated from different algae can vary both in monomer composition and block arrangement, and these variations are also reflected in the properties of the alginate (see TABLE 2). Although viscosity depends mainly on molecular size, the affinity for cations and the gel-forming properties are mostly related to the block structure of

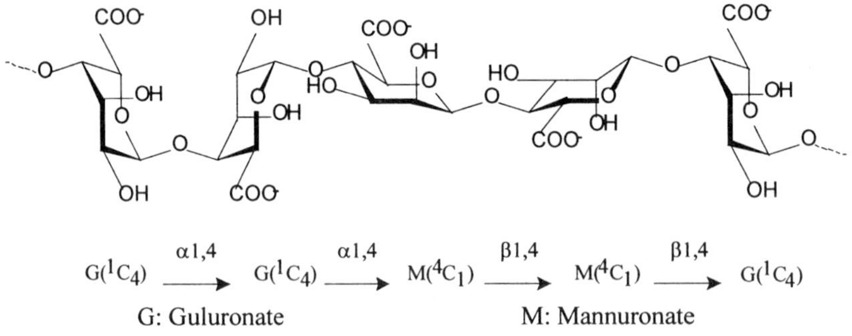

$$G(^1C_4) \xrightarrow{\alpha 1,4} G(^1C_4) \xrightarrow{\alpha 1,4} M(^4C_1) \xrightarrow{\beta 1,4} M(^4C_1) \xrightarrow{\beta 1,4} G(^1C_4)$$

G: Guluronate          M: Mannuronate

**FIGURE 1.** Chemical block structures of alginate.

TABLE 2. Typical values for M and G content in seaweed used for alginate production

| Seaweed | M/G | %M | %G | %MM | %GG |
|---|---|---|---|---|---|
| *Laminaria hyperborea* (stem) | 0.45 | 30 | 70 | 18 | 58 |
| *Laminaria hyperborea* (leaf) | 1.22 | 55 | 45 | 36 | 26 |
| *Laminaria digitata* | 1.22 | 55 | 45 | 39 | 29 |
| *Macrocystis pyrifera* | 1.50 | 60 | 40 | 40 | 20 |
| *Lessonia nigrescens* | 1.50 | 60 | 40 | 43 | 23 |
| *Ascophyllum nodosum* | 1.86 | 65 | 35 | 56 | 26 |
| *Laminaria japonica* | 1.86 | 65 | 35 | 48 | 18 |
| *Durvillea antarctica* | 2.45 | 71 | 29 | 58 | 16 |
| *Durvillea potarum* | 3.33 | 77 | 23 | 69 | 13 |

repeating guluronic acid residues. When two guluronic acid residues are adjacent in the polymer, they form a binding site for polyvalent cations. The content of G blocks is the main structural feature contributing to gel strength and stability of the gel. Reactivity with calcium, causing gel formation, is a direct function of the average length of the G blocks occurring in the polymer chain[39,40] (see FIGURE 2). The greater the length of G blocks, the more calcium crosslinking can occur. This results in a gel with a higher gel strength than one formed from a mannuronate-rich alginate. Thus, knowledge of the M/G relationship of an alginate will have direct relevance to the functionality of a gel and, possibly, also to how cells respond to encapsulation.

Composition and sequential structure, together with molecular weight and molecular conformation, are the key characteristics of alginate in determining its properties and functionality. The composition and sequential structure can be determined by high-resolution $^1$H- and $^{13}$C-nuclear magnetic resonance spectroscopy (NMR) (see FIGURE 3). Techniques have been developed to determine the monad frequencies, as

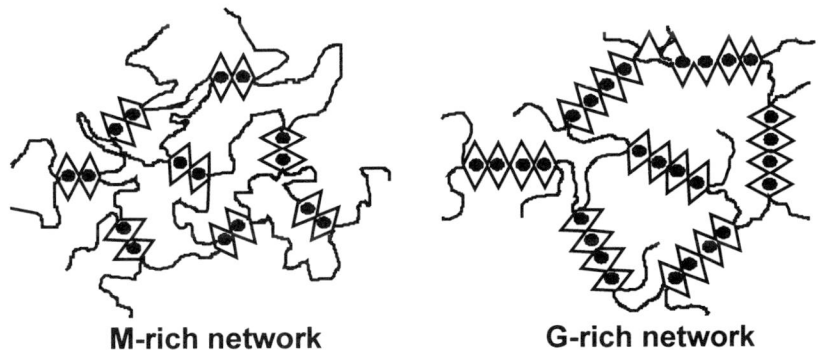

**FIGURE 2.** Schematic of the internal structure of calcium alginate gels. ◯ represents M-fractions; ◈◈ represents crosslinked G-fractions.

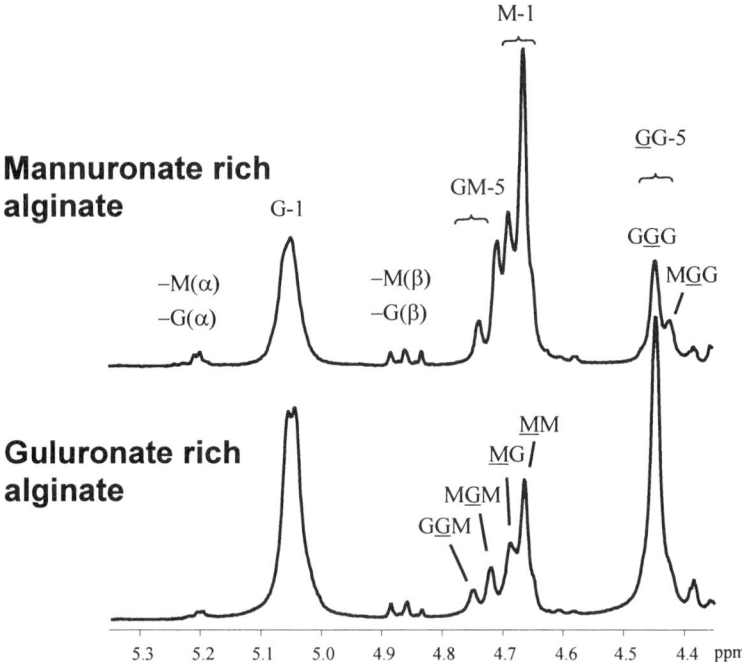

**FIGURE 3.** $^1$H-NMR spectra of mannuronate- and guluronate-rich alginate.

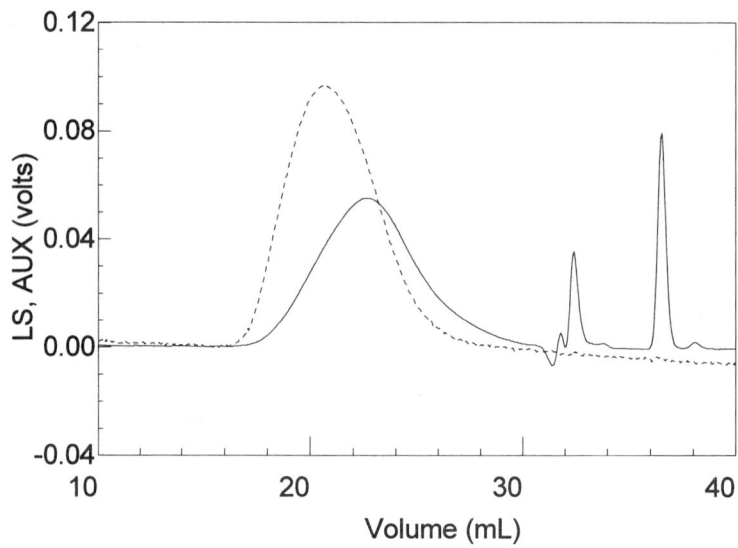

**FIGURE 4.** Size exclusion chromatography of sodium alginate.

well as diads and triads. Based upon such measurements, parameters like M/G ratio, G-content with consecutive G > 1 blocks, M-content with consecutive M > 1 blocks, and average length of blocks of G and M, respectively, can be calculated and are useful parameters in the characterization of the polymer.

Molecular weight can be determined by several methods. The most common methods in general use are calculations based upon intrinsic viscosity (Mark-Houwink-Sakurada equation), and size-exclusion chromatography with light-scattering measurement (see FIGURE 4). In addition to average molecular weight, expressed as number average and weight average, the ratio between the two, referred to as the polydispersity index, is often used to describe the molecular weight distribution within a population.

## THE ASTM GUIDE FOR CHITOSAN

The ASTM guide entitled *Standard Guide for Characterization and Testing of Chitosan Salts as Starting Materials Intended for Use in Biomedical and Tissue-Engineered Medical Product Applications* was published in the ASTM Book of Standards in May 2001 under the designation F 2103.

Chitosan is a high molecular weight cationic polysaccharide derived from crustacean shells by deacetylation of naturally occurring chitin. Chitosan is also a linear polymer that is composed of glucosamine and *N*-acetyl glucosamine units linked in a β(1–4) manner (see FIGURE 5). The glucosamine and *N*-acetyl glucosamine can theoretically be arranged by a similar sequential structure as M and G in alginate. Most often, commercial products have a random distribution of the remaining *N*-acetyl glucosamine units after deacetylation. The ratio between glucosamine and *N*-acetyl glucosamine is referred to as the degree of deacetylation. In solution, chitosan salts carry a positive charge through protonization of the free amino group on glucosamine. Reactivity with negatively charged surfaces is a direct function of the

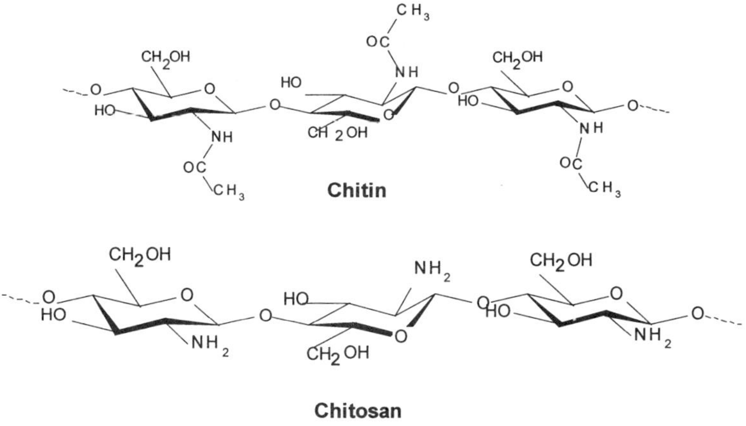

**FIGURE 5.** Chemical structure of chitin and chitosan.

positive charge density of chitosan. The cationic nature of chitosan gives this polymer a mucoadhesive property.[41–43]

## REGULATORY ISSUES

When alginate or chitosan are to be used for applications inside the body, as an implantable device or for parenteral administration of drugs, strict requirements of manufacture, characterization, and purity need to be met for the biomaterial. Common to both ASTM guides is the following.

### *Documentation*

Alginate and chitosan for use in biomedical and pharmaceutical applications and in tissue-engineered medical products (TEMPS) should ideally be documented in drug master files (DMF) to which end users may obtain a letter of cross reference from suppliers. Such DMF should be submitted to the US FDA and to other regulatory authorities, both national and international.

### *Impurity Levels*

The term *impurity* relates to the presence of extraneous substances and materials in the biopolymer sample. Impurities can also arise from the presence of other biopolymer salts (for example, calcium alginate or alginic acid in the sodium alginate material). Additionally, and depending on the end use, a high molecular weight material present in a sample of low molecular weight could constitute an impurity. The major impurities of concern include, but are not limited to, the following:

*Endotoxin Content*

The endotoxin level in alginate is ultimately critical to its use in biomedical applications, where there are regulatory limits to the amount of endotoxin that can be implanted into humans. For example, for implantable devices the endotoxin level must be below 5 EU/kg of body weight.

*Protein Content*

Residual protein in alginate and chitosan could cause allergic reactions such as hypersensitivity. The biopolymer supplier should demonstrate protein removal and protein quantitative methods of satisfactory sensitivity.

*Heavy Metals*

The marine source of both alginate and chitosan indicates that possible heavy metal contaminates such as lead and mercury should be analyzed.

*Microbiological Burden*

Bacteria, yeast and mold are also impurities that can arise in processed material. The presence of bacteria may also contribute to the presence of endotoxins.

## Safety and Toxicology

The safety of alginate and chitosan in biomedical and pharmaceutical applications and in TEMPS should be established according to current guidelines, such as ISO 10993 and ASTM F748. Preclinical safety studies specific to the clinical application under consideration must also be done in accordance with 21CFR312.

## GMP/ISO

Reproducibility in the manufacture of the compound is very important, and this is ensured under a series of good manufacturing practice (GMP) guidelines (21CFR211).

## Regulatory Standards

Sodium alginate is listed on the list of materials affirmed generally recognized as safe (GRAS) by the US Food and Drug Administration (FDA) (21CFR184.1724). This permits sodium alginate (but not other salts such as magnesium) to be used in foods as a thickener or gelling agent. That sodium alginate is listed on the GRAS list does not indicate approval for the use of alginate in pharmaceutical and/or biomedical applications.

In the US Pharmacopeia alginate is still described as poly mannuronate, even though guluronate and the block forming structure of alginate are now well known. Therefore, there is a need for revision of regulatory monographs and for establishing new guidance standards. Chitosan chloride has just recently been approved for inclusion into the European Pharmacopoeia.[44]

## CONCLUSIONS

The use of naturally occurring biopolymers for biomedical and pharmaceutical applications, and in TEMPS, is increasing. Knowledge of the physical and chemical properties of alginate and chitosan will assist users in choosing the correct biomaterials for their particular applications. Establishing parameters, such as M/G ratio and G-block size for alginate, degree of deacetylation for chitosan, and common parameters, such as molecular weight, viscosity, and the endotoxin content, will ensure uniformity and repeatability for those using such materials. Characterization of these biopolymers in accordance with a guidance document will also assist in documentation of formulations and devices. Finally, standardization of test methods and characterization parameters will allow the functionality of alginate or chitosan to fit the requirement of the application or end product.

## REFERENCES

1. KIM, B.S., C.E. BACZ & A. ATALA. 2000. Biomaterials for tissue engineering. World J. Urol. **18:** 2–9.
2. ROWLEY, J.A., G. MADLAMBAYAN & D.J. MOONEY. 1999. Alginate hydrogels as synthetic extracellular matrix materials. Biomaterials **20:** 45–53.

3. MIYAZAKI, S., W. KUBO & D. ATTWOOD. 2000. Oral sustained delivery of theophylline using *in situ* gelation of sodium alginate. J. Control. Rel. **67:** 275-280.
4. RAMDAS, M., *et al.* 1999. Alginate encapsulated bioadhesive chitosan microspheres for intestinal drug delivery. J. Biomater. Appl. **13:** 290–296.
5. ULUDAG, H., P. DEVOS & P.A. TRESCO. 2000. Technology of mammalian cell encapsulation. Adv. Drug Deliv. Rev. **42:** 29–64.
6. THOMAS, S. 2000. Alginate dressings in surgery and wound management—part 1. J. Wound Care **9:** 56–60.
7. THOMAS, S. 2000. Alginate dressings in surgery and wound management: part 2. J. Wound Care **9:** 115–119.
8. THOMAS, S. 2000. Alginate dressings in surgery and wound management: part 3. J. Wound Care **9:** 163–166.
9. HAGSTAM, H. 1986. Alginates and heartburn—evaluation of a medicine with a mechanical mode of action. *In* Gums and Stabilizers in the Food Industry. G.O. Phillips, Ed.: 363–370. Elsevier, Amsterdam.
10. MANDEL, K.G., B.G. DAGGY, D.A. BRODIE, & H.I. JACOBY. 2000. Review article: alginate-raft formulations in the treatment of heartburn and acid reflux. Aliment. Pharmacol. Ther. **14:** 669–690.
11. ONSØYEN, E. 1995. Hydration induced swelling of alginate based matrix tablets at GI-tract pH conditions. *In* Excipients and Delivery Systems for Pharmaceutical Formulations. D.R. Karse & R.A. Stephenson, Eds.: 108–122. The Royal Society of Chemistry, Cambridge, UK.
12. SOON-SHIONG, P., *et al.* 1994. Insulin independence in a type I diabetic patient after encapsulated islet transplantation. Lancet **343:** 950–951.
13. DIAMOND, D.A. & A.A. CALDAMONE. 1999. Endoscopic correction of vesicoureteral reflux in children using autologous chondrocytes: preliminary results. J. Urol. **162:** 1185–1188.
14. MARUYAMA, M. *et al.* 1995. Hydroxyapatite clay for gap filling and adequate bone ingrowth. J. Biomed. Mater. Res. **29:** 329–336.
15. KENLEY, R., *et al.* 1994. Osseous regeneration in the rat calvarium using novel delivery systems for recombinant human bone morphogenetic protein-2 (rhBMP-2). J. Biomed. Mater. Res. **28:** 1139–1147.
16. SUZUKI, K., *et al.* 1999. Regeneration of transected spinal cord in young adult rats using freeze-dried alginate gel. Neuroreport **10:** 2891–2894.
17. ATALA, A., *et al.* 1994. Endoscopic treatment of vesicoureteral reflux with a chondrocyte-alginate suspension. J. Urol. **152:** 641–644.
18. GENTILE, F.T. 1999. Vesicoureteral Reflux. Sci. Med. Nov/Dec: 6–7.
19. BRUNSTEDT, M., B. PURKAIT, A. BHATE & Y.R. WOO, inventors; Mentor Corporation, assignee. 1996. Filling material for soft tissue implant prostheses and implants made therewith. Eur. Patent Application 0 727 232 A2. February 5.
20. REED, T-A., *et al.* 2001. Local endostatin treatment of gliomas administered by microencapsulated producer cells. Nature Biotech. **19:** 29–34.
21. JOKI, T., *et al.* 2001. Continuous release of endostatin from micro-encapsulated engineered cells for tumor therapy. Nature Biotech. **19:** 35–39.
22. EMERICH, D.F., *et al.* 1992. A novel approach to neural transplantation in Parkinson's disease: use of polymer-encapsulated cell therapy. Neurosci. Biobehav. Rev. **16:** 437–447.
23. CHANG, P.L., *et al.* 1994. Growth of recombinant fibroblasts in alginate microcapsules. Biotechnol. Bioeng. **43:** 925–933.
24. PEIRONE, M.A., *et al.* 1998. Delivery of recombinant gene product to canines with nonautologous microencapsulated cells. Hum. Gene Ther. **9:** 195–206.
25. STOCKLEY, T.L., *et al.* 2000. Delivery of recombinant product from subcutaneous implants of encapsulated recombinant cells in canines. J. Lab. Clin. Med. **135:** 484–492.
26. CHEN, Z.P. & G. MOHR. 1996. Microencapsulation for cell implants into the central nervous system: the importance of alginate viscosity and related factors. Stereotact. Funct. Neurosurg. **66:** 141–146.

27. LIM, F. & A.M. SUN. 1980. Microencapsulated islets as bioartificial endocrine pancreas. Science **210:** 908–910.
28. SUN, A.M., G.M. O'SHEA & M.F. GOOSEN. 1984. Injectable microencapsulated islet cells as a bioartificial pancreas. Appl. Biochem. Biotech. **10:** 87–99.
29. WONG, H. & T.M. CHANG. 1986. Bioartificial liver: implanted artificial cells microencapsulated living hepatocytes increases survival of liver failure rats. Int. J. Artif. Organs **9:** 335–336.
30. SUN, A.M., et al. 1987. Microencapsulated hepatocytes: an *in vitro* and *in vivo* study. Biomater. Artif. Cells Artif. Organs **15:** 483–496.
31. CHANG, T.M. & N. MALAVE. 2000. The development and first clinical use of semipermeable microcapsules (artificial cells) as a compact artificial kidney. 1970 [classical article]. Ther. Apher. **4:** 108–116.
32. ASTM web site: <www.astm.org>
33. PICCIOLO, G.L. 2000. Regenerative medicine: tissue engineering standards come to ASTM. ASTM Standardization News **28:** 7–8.
34. PICCIOLO, G.L. & D.L. STOCUM. 2001. ASTM lights the way for tissue engineered medical products standards. ASTM Standardization News **29:** 30–35.
35. HELLMAN, K.B. 1997. Bioartificial organs as outcomes of tissue engineering. Scientific and regulatory issues. Ann. N.Y. Acad. Sci. **831:** 1–9.
36. BRUCK, S.D. & E.P. MUELLER. 1989. Reference standards for implantable materials: problems and needs. Med. Prog. Technol. **15:** 5–20.
37. HELLMAN, K.B., G.L. PICCIOLO & E.P. MUELLER. 1993. Biomaterials and biotechnology. The union of these technologies promises solutions to recalcitrant problems. Biotechnology **11:** 1179–1180.
38. SKAUGRUD, Ø., et al. 1999. Biomedical and pharmaceutical applications of alginate and chitosan. Biotechnol. Genet. Eng. Rev. **16:** 23–40.
39. SMIDSRØD, O. & K.I. DRAGET. 1996. Chemistry and physical properties of alginates. Carbohydrates in Europe **14:** 6–13.
40. SMIDSRØD, O. & G. SKJÅK-BRÆK. 1990. Alginate as immobilization matrix for cells. TIBTECH **8:** 71–78.
41. SKAUGRUD, Ø. 1995. Drug delivery systems with alginate and chitosan. *In* Excipients and Delivery Systems for Pharmaceutical Formulations. D.R. Karse & R.A. Stephenson, Eds.: 96–107. Spec. Publ. Roy. Soc. Chem. No. 161. Cambridge, UK.
42. ALLAN, G.G., et al. 1984. Biomedical applications of chitin and chitosan. *In* Chitin, Chitosan and Related Enzymes. J.P. Zikakis, Ed.: 119–133. Academic Press, Inc., New York.
43. LI, Q., E.T. DUNN, E.W. GRANDMAISON & M.F.A. GOOSEN. 1992. Applications and properties of chitosan. J. Bioact. Compat. Polymers **7:** 370–397.
44. Chitosan Chloride. 1999. Pharmaeuropa **11:** 515.

# Hepatic Progenitors and Strategies for Liver Cell Therapies

R. SUSICK,[a] N. MOSS,[b] H. KUBOTA,[b] E. LECLUYSE,[c] G. HAMILTON,[c] T. LUNTZ,[b] J. LUDLOW,[a] J. FAIR,[d] D. GERBER,[d] K. BERGSTRAND,[a] J. WHITE,[a] A. BRUCE,[a] O. DRURY,[a] S. GUPTA,[e] AND L.M. REID[b,f]

[a]*Incara Cell Technologies, 79 TW Alexander Drive, Building 4401, Suite 200, Research Triangle Park, North Carolina, USA*

[b]*Department of Cell and Molecular Physiology, UNC School of Medicine, Chapel Hill, North Carolina, USA*

[c]*Division of Pharmaceutics, UNC School of Pharmacy, Chapel Hill, North Carolina, USA*

[d]*Department of Surgery, UNC School of Medicine, Chapel Hill, North Carolina, USA*

[e]*Department of Medicine, Liver Center, Albert Einstein College of Medicine, 1300 Morris Park Avenue, Bronx, New York, USA*

[f]*Program in Molecular Biology and Biotechnology, UNC School of Medicine, Chapel Hill, North Carolina, USA*

ABSTRACT: Liver cell therapies, including liver cell transplantation and bioartificial livers, are being developed as alternatives to whole liver transplantation for some patients with severe liver dysfunction. Hepatic progenitors are proposed as ideal cells for use in these liver cell therapies given their ability to expand extensively, differentiate into all mature liver cells, have minimal immunogenicity, be cryopreservable, and reconstitute liver tissue when transplanted. We summarize our ongoing efforts to develop clinical programs of hepatic progenitor cell therapies with a focus on hepatic stem cell biology and strategies that have emerged in analyzing that biology.

KEYWORDS: stem cells; hepatic progenitors; liver cell therapies; liver; liver transplantation

## INTRODUCTION

Severe liver dysfunction or terminal liver failure can be reversed by orthotopic liver transplantation, but with the necessity for chronic immunosuppression of the recipient and with the need to wait for a donor liver, sometimes for years, due to the paucity of liver donors available <www.unos.org>.[1–7] Given the problem of the small number of liver donors, an average of 4,500 per year, rules have been promulgated by organ procurement and liver transplant programs to prioritize the potential recipients. The net result is that there are many patients who do not qualify for liver transplantation despite a desperate need for one. We propose to alleviate or over-

Address for correspondence: L.M. Reid, 116 Glaxo Building, Campus Box 7038, UNC School of Medicine, Chapel Hill, NC 27599, USA. Voice: 919-966-0347; fax: 919-966-6112.
stemcell@med.unc.edu

come this problem by developing liver cell therapies using hepatic progenitors and methods analogous to bone marrow transplantations provided to patients with hemopoietic dysfunctions. We discuss here an overview of progenitor cell biology and its potential influence on cell therapies using liver as a model.

## STEM CELLS AND COMMITTED PROGENITORS

Stem cells are immature cells that are pluripotent in that they give rise to daughter cells maturing into multiple possible cell types and have extensive growth potential.[8,9] Several broad classes of stem cells have been defined:

- *Totipotent stem cells* have the capacity to produce adult cell types derived from all three embryonic germ layers (ectoderm, endoderm, and mesoderm), can enter into the germ line, and have proven ability to self-replicate, that is, produce daughter cells that are identical to the parent.[10,11] The known and well characterized totipotent stem cells are found in embryonic tissues. Recent, controversial evidence suggests that there may be either a small population of totipotent stem cells that persist into adulthood in the bone marrow *or* a collection of determined stem cells in the bone marrow that give rise to fates such as liver or brain, fates not realized heretofore as derived from a subpopulation of bone marrow cells.[12–15]

- *Embryonic stem cells (ES cells)* are also totipotent in that they can give rise to all adult cell types. However, a criteria for non-human embryonic stem cells is that they can enter the germ line, a criterion that cannot be tested for human embryonic stem cell cultures. Therefore, we accept the definition for human ES cells provided by Thomson and associates that they are "(i) derived from pre-implantation or peri-implantation embryos; (ii) have prolonged undifferentiated proliferation; and (iii) have stable developmental potential to form derivatives of all three embryonic germ layers even after culture."[16]

- *Determined stem cells,* pluripotent cells that give rise to some, but not all, possible adult cell types, have extensive growth potential and questionable ability to self-replicate.[17] Committed progenitors, derived from the stem cells, have lost their pluripotency, and are precursors for a single cell type.

Whereas all forms of progenitors (see TABLE 1) are found in embryonic tissues, most adult tissues contain only determined stem cells and/or committed progenitors.[17] The exceptions are the adult heart, which is thought to have either no progenitors or perhaps only committed progenitors,[18,19] resulting in the heart's limited regenerative capacity, and the bone marrow, now being studied as a possible adult reservoir of totipotent stem cells or a novel location for various types of determined stem cells.[12–15]

The known properties of the different classes of progenitors help to define their potential in academic, clinical, or industrial programs. Of the types of progenitors studied (e.g., mesenchymal, neuronal, muscle, and epidermal), all have been found to be readily cryopreserved[20–22] and expanded *ex vivo*.[23,24] However, the embryonic stem cells are especially renowned for their ability to survive freezing and to expand without differentiating if maintained under precise culture conditions.[16,18,20,21,25] By

TABLE 1. Classes and properties of progenitors

| Properties | Totipotent Stem Cells or ES Cells | Determined Stem Cells | Committed Progenitors |
|---|---|---|---|
| Representatives of the class | embryonic stem cells (ES cells); cells from preimplantation or peri-implantation embryos such as morula cells | hemopoietic, neuronal, mesenchymal, hepatic stem cells | hepatocytic, biliary |
| Potency | pluripotent | pluripotent | not pluripotent |
| Fate(s) | all possible fates | restricted fates | single fate |
| Growth potential | extensive | extensive | extensive |
| Self-replicative ability | yes | debatable | no |
| Tumorigenicity | tumorigenic if injected at ectopic site and with tumorigenicity reduced but not eliminated by lineage-restriction | non-tumorigenic | non-tumorigenic |
| Advantages in clinical or industrial programs | ease in *ex vivo* expansion and cryopreservation; ability to form all cell types | safe for cell transplantation in humans; possible to control differentiation to specific cell types *ex vivo* or *in vivo*. | |
| Disadvantages with respect to clinical or industrial programs | tumorigenicity issues preclude use in cell transplantation; inability to control strictly the differentiation to specific fates | difficulties in obtaining high quality human tissue reproducibly (especially true for organ tissue); need for enrichment or purification procedures and cryopreservation methodology; need to use distinct determined stem cell that can give rise to specific mature cell types | |

contrast, cryopreservation of adult cells, such as hepatocytes, has met with limited success and even that limited success is achieved only by embedding the cells in alginate or a form of extracellular matrix.[26-29] Significant *ex vivo* expansion of and the ability to subculture adult liver cells have been found to occur only with the so-called "small hepatocytes", assumed to be a diploid subpopulation of the liver.[30,31] Typically, the mature cells undergo one or two rounds of division and then survive for a matter of days in culture, or with appropriate extracellular matrix and medium conditions will survive for a few weeks.[32-36]

The ability of totipotent cells and embryonic stem cells to give rise to all or almost all possible adult fates makes them appealing as a "one serves all" approach for cell therapies and makes them the most exploitable of the classes of stem or progenitor cells. However, their use in cell transplantation for patients is precluded by their tumorigenic potential.[16,20,37,38] The tumorigenicity of ES cells when injected at ectopic sites is being investigated extensively, especially by biotechnology companies, in hopes that it can be controlled to enable ES cells to reach their full potential both industrially and clinically.[37]

Although determined stem cells are more restricted in their adult cell fates, they have not been found to be tumorigenic, enabling them to be the first choice for clinical programs in cell transplantation or for bioartificial organs. Bone marrow and cord blood transplants, qualifying as the first forms of progenitor cell therapies, have been performed for years.[39-41] More recently, other forms of progenitor cell therapies are being tested in clinical trials; these include mesenchymal progenitor cells,[15,24] neuronal progenitor cells,[23,42,43] and fetal pancreatic islet cell tranplants,[44,45] and the early data from these trials are very encouraging for the future for progenitor cell therapies as a class. The problems with determined stem cells include (1) identification of tissue sources, an especial problem for organs that until now have derived only from brain-dead, but beating-heart donors; (2) the need for the development of purification schemes for isolation of the cells; (3) identification of optimal cryopreservation conditions; and (4) defining the *ex vivo* expansion and differentiation conditions.

## THE MODEL OF THE LIVER AS A STEM CELL AND LINEAGE SYSTEM

Reid and associates have hypothesized that hepatic progenitor cells should optimize the reconstitution of livers in patients with inadequate liver functions by reducing or eliminating the difficulties observed in liver cell therapies using unfractionated adult liver cells.[46,47] This assumption is based on the model of the liver as a stem cell and maturational lineage system.[46,48-52] The essential feature of liver histology is the acinus, demarcated by a peripheral vasculature, consisting of six sets of portal triads, and a central vasculature consisting of the central vein; the two vascular structures are connected by plates of liver cells, like spokes in a wheel, and that are flanked by sinusoidal endothelia. The blood flow originates in the portal triads, flows across the plates of liver cells and endothelia, and then into the central vein that drains into the vena cava. Historically, the liver acinus has been described as having three zones with liver functions differing depending on the zone: zone 1 is the periportal region and contains the liver's progenitors and adult diploid cells;

zone 2, the midacinar region, and zone 3, the pericentral zone, contain only or predominantly polyploid cells, mostly tetraploid cells, and express many of the highly differentiated functions of the liver. The extent of polyploidy varies with the species: young adult rodent livers are approximately 90% polyploid,[53-55] whereas young adult humans have livers estimated to be approximately 50% polyploid.[56] However, rigorous studies of polyploidy in livers of humans of varying age have not yet been done. Old studies on human liver that considered cells with a single nucleus to be diploid have been discredited with the recognition of mononucleated tetraploid cells, and the more recent studies using reliable technologies for evaluating ploidy have focused on a relatively small number of samples due to the difficulties in obtaining human liver tissue.[56-58]

The liver's progenitors have been found associated with the canals of Hering near each of the portal triads.[9,59-61] The canals of Hering extend like bottle-brush fibers throughout zone 1 of the liver.[61] The hepatic progenitors produce daughter cells that lead either to biliary or hepatocytic differentiation and undergo a stepwise, unidirectional maturation to yield cells with all the known parenchymal cell phenotypes of the liver ending in terminally differentiated cells near the central vein.[51] In parallel, the cells produce an extracellular matrix in the space of Disse between the parenchymal cells and the endothelia, and with a chemistry that forms a gradient. That associated with the progenitors consists of fetal forms of cell adhesion molecules (CAMs), type IV collagen, laminin, and multiple forms of heparan sulfate proteoglycans; that associated with the mature cells consists of distinct and adult-specific forms of CAMs, fibrillar collagens, fibronectin, and heparin proteoglycan. For various reviews of the liver matrix chemistry, see References 62–66.

Liver-specific gene expression has long been known to have discrete patterns associated with the zones of the liver acinus. For lengthy reviews by several investigators, see References 46, 67–69. Based on the maturational lineage model, the heterogeneity can be interpreted as a *combination* of distinct microenvironments and maturational changes within the cells, the net sum of the two resulting in lineage-position dependence of gene expression resulting in *early, intermediate,* and *late* gene expression. Representative early genes include alpha-fetoprotein (AFP), albumin, insulin-like growth factor II (IGF II), and specific extracellular matrix components (type IV collagen, fetal laminin, and fetal heparan sulfate proteoglycans); intermediate genes include PEPCK, insulin-like growth factor I (IGF I), and connexin 26; late genes include connexin 32, P450 isoforms 3A4 and 2E, glutathione–S-transferase, and late forms of extracellular matrix molecules (fibrillar collagens, fibronectins, and heparin proteoglycan). The kinetics of the lineage is quite slow in the quiescent liver with preliminary (and unconfirmed) evidence suggesting it to exceed one year in rodents.[70,71] No studies have been done yet in humans. In TABLE 2 are given representative properties of cells in each of the three zones and part of the data supporting the model of the liver as a maturational lineage system. It should be noted that the maturational lineage model is not accepted universally. It has been proposed that the renowned heterogeneity of the liver is due only to variations in the local microenvironment; representative reviews of this alternate point of view are given by Gebhardt and by Gumucio.[67,69]

TABLE 2. Major liver lineage stages: adult rat parenchymal cells

| Periportal zone 1 | Midacinar zone 2 | Pericentral zone 3 |
|---|---|---|
| diploid | tetraploid | 4N and 8N |
| less than 25 μ in size | about 25–35 μ in size | greater than 35 μ in size |
| zone 1 genes PepCK, CX 26, glutathione peroxidase | zone 2 genes transferrin, tyrosine aminotransferase, CX 32 | zone 3 genes glutathione-S-transferase, CX 32, CYP3A4, MUP |
| can undergo 8–10 rounds of complete cell division | can undergo 1–2 rounds of nuclear division with variable occurrence of cytokinesis | little to no cell division; often multinucleated many apoptotic cells (Tunel assay) |

## PURIFICATION OF RODENT HEPATIC PROGENITORS INCLUDING HEPATIC STEM CELLS

Methods for identification and purification of the hepatic progenitors including hepatic stem cells were developed in rodent systems using procedures that have been published[48,50,72–75] and aspects of the technologies and procedures patented.[75–79] In general, the approach has been to use multiparametric flow cytometry in combination with multiple fluoroprobe-labeled monoclonal antibodies to purify cells of a defined antigenic profile. Antigenic profiles and particular properties identified for clonogenic hepatic cells, including hepatic stem cells, are given in TABLE 3. However, even when no antigens are known to define the cells of interest, one can enrich significantly for these cells by doing a "negative sort". This is carried out by using fluoroprobe-labeled antibodies to markers on cells not of interest and then separating the population into

TABLE 3. Antigenic profiles and phenotype of clonogenic parenchymal cells

|  | Clonogenic Adult Cells | Hepatic Stem Cells |
|---|---|---|
| Antigenic profile | RT1A$^+$, OX18$^+$, ICAM-1$^+$ | RT1A$^-$, OX18$^{dull}$, ICAM-1$^+$ |
| Ploidy | diploid[a] | diploid |
| Number of cells from one cell in 20 days | 120 | 3,000–4,000 |
| Pluripotent | no | yes |
| Gene expression[b] | AFP, albumin | AFP, albumin |
| Strict mitogens | EGF, insulin | insulin, transferrin |

[a]The cells seeded are a mixture of diploid and polyploid cells; those that emerge in the colonies in culture are diploid. It is unknown if only the diploid cells were able to survive and grow under the conditions, or whether the tetraploid cells under these conditions can undergo cytokinesis to become diploid.

[b]Although colonies from both the stem cells and the adult cells express both AFP and albumin, the AFP expression in the cells from the stem cells is markedly stronger as detected by immunohistochemistry assays.

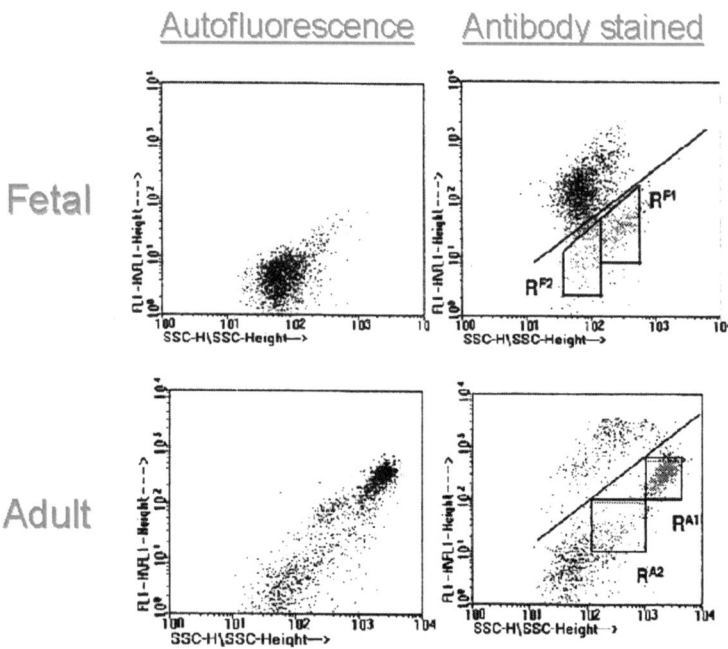

**FIGURE 1.** Sorting progenitor and mature liver cells. Mature parenchyma, $R^{F1}$, $R^{A1}$; hepatic progenitors, $R^{F2}$, $R^{A2}$.

those expressing those markers and those not. Secondarily, one can use side scattering, a flow cytometric parameter, in which the intensity of scattered light is related to the number of cytoplasmic particles (e.g., mitochondria and ribosomes). The less mature cells are agranular or lower in granularity, whereas the more mature cells are more granular, enabling one to enrich for cell populations of given granularity. A representative flow cytometric sort for enrichment of parenchymal cells using a negative sort and side scatter is shown in FIGURE 1. The agranular cells isolated by this approach are shown in FIGURE 2. Some unique properties of the hepatic stem cells are given in TABLE 3; general properties are summarized in TABLE 4.

**TABLE 4. Hepatoblasts (hepatic stem cells)**

| |
| --- |
| Bipotent precursors for hepatocytes and biliary cells |
| Most, if not all, hepatic cells in early fetus (e.g., E13 in rats) are hepatoblasts |
| Express α-fetoprotein and albumin |
| Found in fetal to young adult liver |
| These cells or related cells are present in all endodermal tissues (e.g., liver, lung, pancreas) and bone marrow |

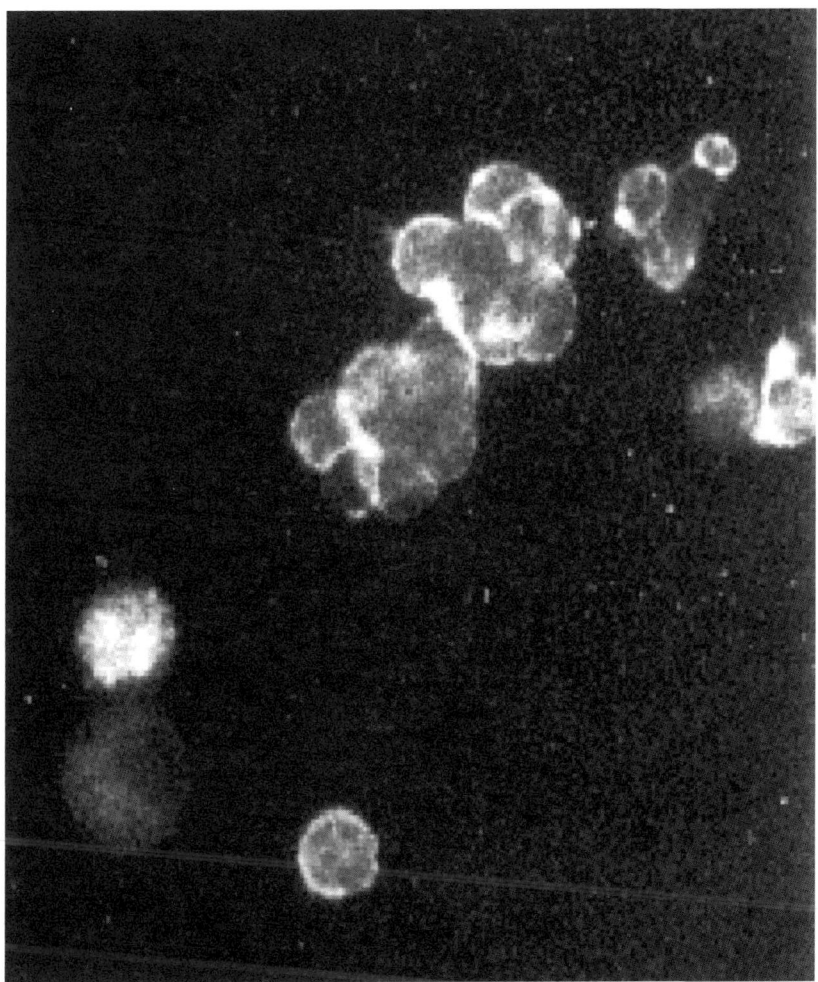

**FIGURE 2.** Sorted rodent hepatic progenitor cells. MARKERS: α-fetoprotein, albumin (weak), connexin 43, connexin 26, IGF II receptors, diploid, less than 15 μ in diameter, agranular by side scatter.

## PURIFICATION OF HUMAN LIVER PROGENITORS

Methodologies have been developed for purification of liver progenitors from human livers derived from fetal (abortuses) to adult livers (rejects or "cut-downs") from liver transplant programs).[80] In brief, the donor livers are enzymatically dissociated and then cryopreserved. The freshly isolated cells or the cryopreserved cells are flow-cytometrically sorted by:

1. Debulking of the cell suspension to reduce or eliminate non-progenitor cell populations (polyploid cells with adult specific markers such as connexin 32 and/or non-parenchymal cells bearing markers such as CD45 or glycophorin A) to yield enriched liver progenitor cell populations comprising hepatic, hemopoietic, and mesenchymal progenitor cells.
2. Staining of the enriched progenitor cell population with several fluroprobe-labeled antibodies to specific cell surface markers that are shared with all of the progenitor cell populations as well as those that define unique lineages.
3. Use of multiparametric flow cytometric (fluorescence, forward scatter, and side scatter) to purify the progenitors into the subpopulations of hepatic, hemopoietic, and mesenchymal progenitors. The sorting strategies needed to provide the liver progenitors have an antigenic profile that results in cells that are negative for hemopoietic markers (e.g., CD45-), positive for hepatic-specific markers (e.g., alpha-fetoprotein and albumin), agranular by side scatter, less than 15 µ in diameter, and diploid.

Although this approach works on small samples (approximately 100 grams), it is being modified to scaled-up protocols to work successfully for whole human livers. These protocols are now under development.

## SOURCING OF HUMAN LIVERS

All human liver tissue derives from donors who have undergone brain death but not cardiac arrest, accounting for 1–2% of the deaths in the United States, and resulting in approximately 4,500 donor livers/year <www.unos.org>. The starting material for all research and for candidate novel clinical programs, such as liver cell therapies, in the United States has been the rejected livers from the organ transplantation programs, constituting only approximately 1–5% of the donor livers (45–225 livers/year). Therefore, in preparation for efforts to establish a clinical program of liver cell therapies, it has been essential to identify alternate sources of human liver. We have just established the first cadaveric liver procurement program, that is, livers from donors who have undergone heart arrest, constituting 98% of the deaths in the United States, and to include neonatal, pediatric, and adult livers.[81] The issues currently under investigation are to define the restrictions, in terms of length of warm and/or cold ischemic time and conditions associated with the dying process, that dictate the quality and the number of viable cells that can be obtained from the donor livers. Yet even though this program is in its infancy, the initial findings are encouraging that cadaveric livers may become a viable alternative as a source of liver cells.

## CRYOPRESERVATION

An advantage of using the progenitor cell populations is that they can be cryopreserved successfully.[80] The cells can be suspended in a cryopreservative buffer, aliquoted into 3-ml cryovials or cryocyte bags at appropriate cell densities, and frozen to liquid nitrogen temperatures ($-160°C$) using a computerized control rate freezer. The samples are stored in the vapor phase of liquid nitrogen ($-160°C$) to minimize cross contamination. The ability to cryopreserve the cells enables the establishment of a cell bank greatly facilitating the logistics for rigorous screening of samples for disease or genetic defects, for genotyping, tissue typing, for clinical cell therapy programs, and for distribution to academic and industrial investigators.

## *EX VIVO* EXPANSION OF PROGENITORS

*Ex vivo* expansion and differentiation of cells will be critical both for research purposes, for bioartificial organs, and for eventual use of progenitors in clinical forms of autologous cell therapies. Facets of the development of novel bioreactors and of biodegradable scaffolding for cells are presented elsewhere.[82–85] Here are summarized the matrix and hormonal conditions for *ex vivo* expansion and differentiation of liver cells. These have been identified and can be summarized as those required by cells at all stages of the maturational lineage and those that differ depending on the stage of the lineage[32,74,76,78,86–90] and reviewed by Brill and others.[47,49] A summary of the

TABLE 5. Common requirements for all stages of the lineage

|  | Growth | Differentiation |
|---|---|---|
| Substratum | type IV collagen and laminin | fibrillar collagens and fibronectin |
| Calcium | less than 0.5 mM | more than 0.5 mM |
| Proteoglycans/GAGs | heparan sulfate proteoglycans or heparan sulfates | heparin proteoglycans or heparins |
| Basal Medium | rich basal medium supplemented with selenium, copper, zinc, nicotinamide | |

TABLE 6. Requirements differing with maturational stage

|  | Stem Cells | Committed Progenitors | Mature Cells |
|---|---|---|---|
| Substratum | strict requirement for porosity and flexibility | | tolerate impervious, rigid surfaces |
| Lipid Requirements | strict requirement for complex lipids comprising mixture of free fatty acids and appropriate carrier proteins (e.g., HDL) | | tolerate single lipid source, i.e., linoleic acid |
| Strict Mitogens | insulin, transferrin | insulin, transferrin, EGF | insulin, EGF |
| Feeder Layers | strict requirement of embryonic stroma, ideally from embryonic liver | tolerate stromal feeders from diverse sources | not required |

NOTE: For the details, see some of the noted refereed articles[50,73,74,92] and reviews.[47,49,66,76]

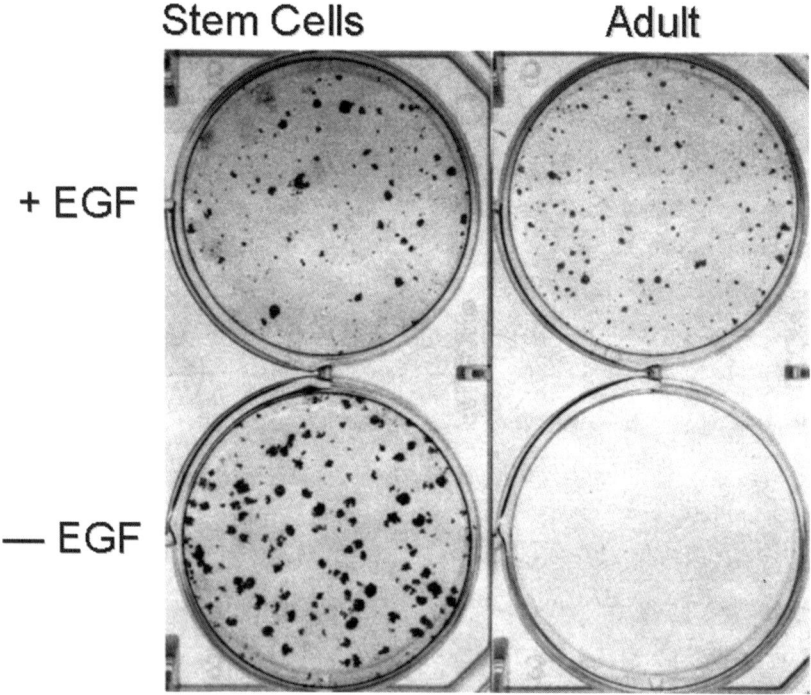

**FIGURE 3.** Colony formation of adult cells versus stem cells (both diploid).

highlights of these requirements is provided in TABLES 5 and 6. Under the defined conditions, one can seed a single cell into the dish and observe it to form a colony of cells, demonstrating conclusively its clonogenic properties.[74] Whereas others have shown colony formation after seeding at relatively high densities,[31,91] the conditions indicated below and described in detail elsewhere are the only ones known to permit clonogenic growth.[74] A subpopulation of adult liver cells will grow at low densities under these conditions but cannot be verified as clonogenic given their propensity for aggregation. Representative colonies of the adult cells versus stem cells are shown in FIGURES 3 and 4. In FIGURE 3 is shown evidence that the stem cells do not require epidermal growth factor, EGF, whereas it is a strict requirement for the adult cells, and in FIGURE 4 is noted the distinct morphology of the colonies of stem cells versus adult cells.

## THE ROLE OF PROGENITORS IN LIVER REGENERATION

Two distinct forms of liver regeneration have been known by investigators since the 1930s.[93] There is a form of liver regeneration involving predominantly hypertrophic responses and occurring after partial hepatectomy,[52,69,94] and a form of liver regeneration involving predominantly a hyperplastic response and occurring after

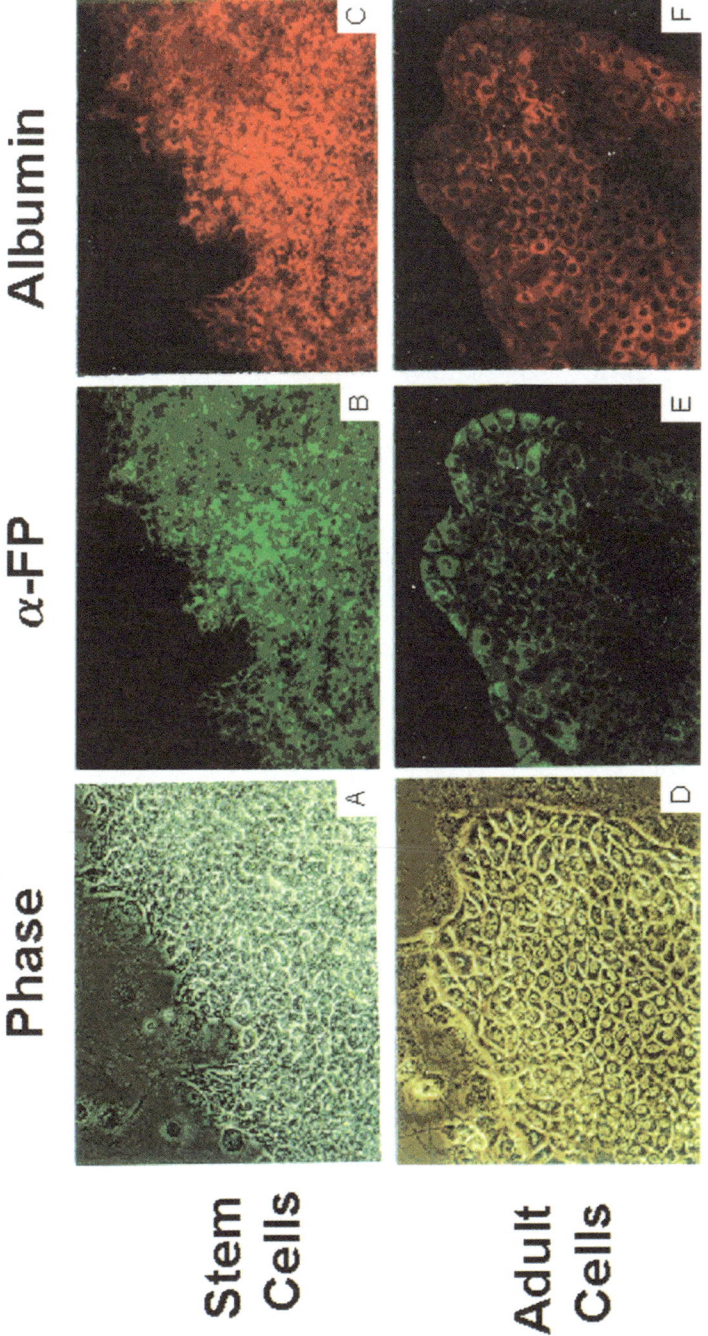

**FIGURE 4.** Colonies grown from hepatic stem cells versus adult cells.

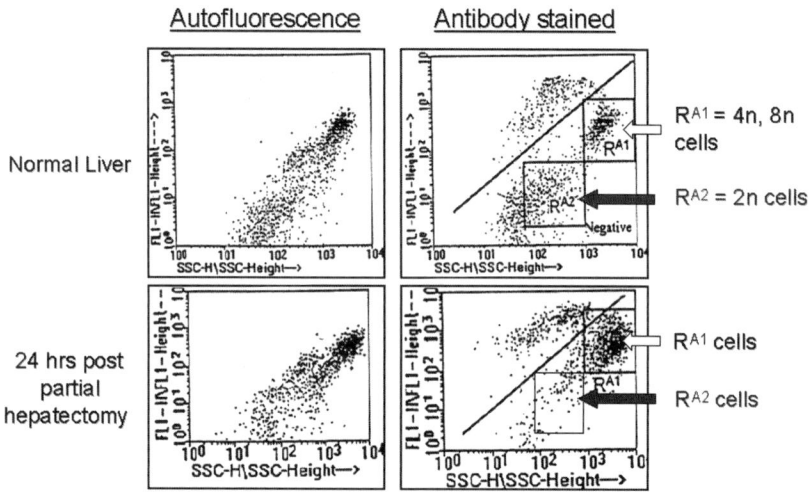

**Hepatectomy leads to DNA synthesis with minimal cytokinesis.**

**FIGURE 5.** *In vivo* growth control.

various forms of toxic injury or oncogenic insults. These are summarized in numerous reviews.[9,69,95] In brief, the cells behave as follows:

1. After partial hepatectomy, the adult cells undergo nuclear division with incomplete cytoplasmic division resulting in a dramatic increase in tetraploid and octaploid cells and with a slow (2–3 week) restoration of the diploid cell population. A representative flow cytometric analysis of this process is shown in FIGURE 5; versus
2. After chemical, viral or radiation injuries that most often results in preferential loss of cells in zones 2 and 3 (predominantly if not entirely the polyploid cells of the liver), the diploid cells, including the progenitor cells, expand rapidly and then mature to reconstitute the rest of the liver.

## RECONSTITUTION OF LIVER BY CELL TRANSPLANTATION

An important consideration in the development of different liver cell therapies is the relative ability of each class of cells to reconstitute damaged livers. Various preparations of cells have been used in experimental trials of liver cell therapies:
1. unfractionated adult liver cells,[96–100]
2. adult liver cells fractionated by size,[101]
3. progenitor cells,[102,103]
4. bone marrow cells[12,13] and purified hemopoietic progenitors.[14]

For all these preparations of cells, *in vivo* expansion of donor cells *in vivo* has been found to depend on a "cellular vacuum" in the recipient, in which a significant percentage of the liver cells from zones 2 and/or 3 are lost due to (a) drugs such as retrorsine[104] or carbon tetrachloride[105]; (b) viral infections such as hepatitis[106,107]; (c) oncogenic insults[9,108]; or (d) aberrant genetics (whether occurring naturally or artificially induced) that result in liver cell loss.[109,110] Thus, inoculation of progenitor cells into quiescent livers is associated with integration and rapid maturation into adult liver cells;[102] a representative *in vivo* fate assay following inoculation of progenitor cells into quiescent liver is shown in FIGURE 6. By contrast, inoculation of cells into livers associated with a cellular vacuum results in extensive expansion followed by maturation.[14,97,110,111] The implications for liver cell strategies are that recipients with liver failure associated with massive cell loss would be predicted to require fewer donor cells, since the donor cells should expand under those *in vivo* conditions. By contrast, recipients with inborn errors of metabolism, consisting of livers with normal cell numbers but with an aberrant liver-specific function, should require high numbers of donor cells that should demonstrate limited growth and rapid differentiation.

Bone marrow is a well established tissue source and with the dramatic, recent realization that some bone marrow cells can mature into liver cells, leading to an exciting new type of liver cell therapy.[12] Yet, in studies to date, bone-marrow-derived cells have proven to have poor efficiency in reconstituting liver, perhaps due either to a small number of cells in the bone marrow capable of differentiating into liver cells or to the need for a factor(s) to facilitate their ability to grow when in the liver.[13,14] Therefore, more research is needed to assess the requirements or limitations of bone marrow as a source of cells capable of reconstituting damaged liver tissue.

The relative ability of hepatic progenitors versus mature liver cells to reconstitute damaged livers is not known for certain. Contradictory evidence has been published. Grompe and associates have isolated liver cells of varying sizes by centrifugal elutriation and have found that the liver cells in the intermediate sizes, about 25 µ, proved best able to restore host livers damaged by tyrosinemia.[101] However, the experimental design may have skewed the data:[101] they co-injected unfractionated adult liver cells with preparations of each size of donor cells; adult liver cells produce a conditioned medium, therefore a secreted factor(s), that inhibits the growth of hepatic progenitors (Reid *et al.*, unpublished data). Other investigators have tested the relative efficacy of progenitors versus adult liver cells to grow in retrosine-treated rats and have demonstrated that the progenitors have far greater regenerative capacity than the adult cells.[103,108] These findings complement *in vitro* studies in which only small hepatocytes, those under 17 µ in size, are able to grow readily in culture or to be able to survive subculturing.[30,31,112] Therefore, more studies are needed to draw firm conclusions.

The optimal methods for introduction of the cells *in vivo*, methods that will be critical for liver cell therapies, are the focus of investigations by Dr. Sanjeev Gupta and associates.[113] Although most of the studies have been done in rodents, the presumed best route for reintroduction of the cells into patients is likely to be directly into the liver or, in cases of cirrhosis, intrasplenic.[102,114] With intrasplenic injection, any emboli that form during the injection are likely to become lodged within the spleen, where they cause little harm. Furthermore, the intrasplenic injections are

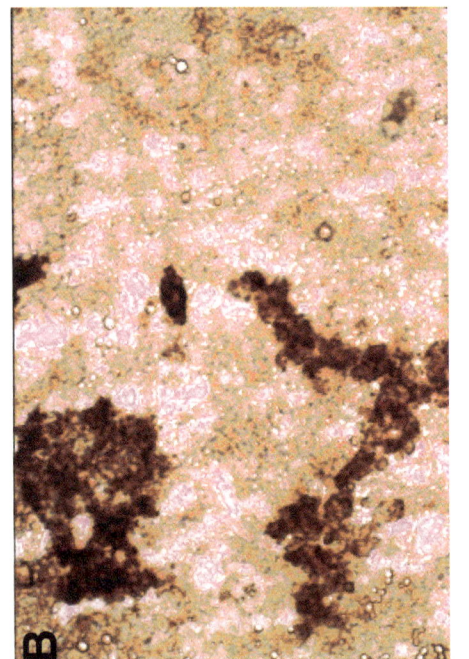
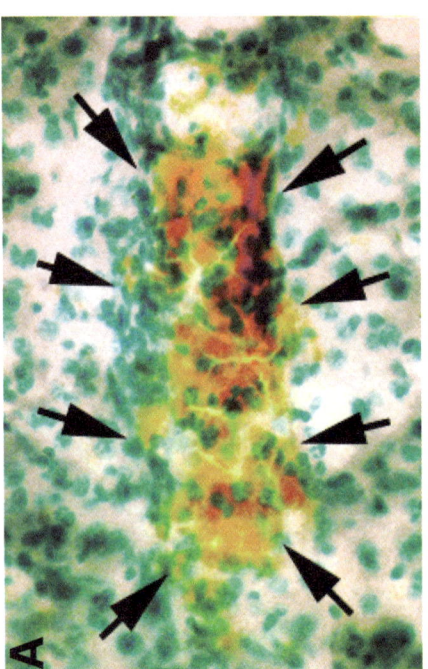

**FIGURE 6.** *In vivo* fate assays. **A.** Liver (several weeks after transplantation): donor DPPIV$^+$, fetal liver cells (*orange*, indicated by *arrows*) adjacent to portal area of DPPIV$^-$ host liver. Methyl green counterstain. DPPIV, dipeptidyl peptidase IV. **B.** Spleen: glucose-6-phosphatase staining in fetal liver cells transplanted into the spleen. No counterstain.

TABLE 7. Advantages of progeitor cells versus mature liver cells

| |
|---|
| Full lineage potential |
| Superior lifespan |
| Maximum proliferative capacity |
| Resistance to ischemia |
| Can be obtained from cadaveric livers |
| Ability to be cryopreserved with high viability and function |
| Small cell volume for transplant |

likely to minimize the number of cells that escape into the capillary beds of lungs or other sites. The cells that remain as single cell suspensions can flow from the spleen into the liver, where they attach via adhesion mechanisms that are tissue specific.

The few studies on cell transplantation of unfractionated adult liver cells into humans have indicated that they can indeed offer an alternative to liver transplantation.[115–119] However, their success has been limited for multiple reasons[116,118–120] and include:

1. the propensity for adult cells (that in general are large, 30–50 μ) to form aggregates that can cause portal hypertension, lung emboli, or other severe clinical problems;
2. rejection phenomena due to allogenic immunological issues that require chronic immunosuppression of the recipient;
3. difficulties in cryopreserving adult liver cells;
4. the limited growth observed for injected cells; and
5. the need to obtain cells from the limited number of rejected livers from the organ transplantation program, severely constraining the availability of source tissue.

Most of these difficulties, even that of immunological rejection, are likely to be alleviated or eliminated by using progenitor cell populations given that progenitors are small (5–15 μ) resulting in smaller aggregates, are readily cryopreserved, have extensive growth properties both *in vitro* and *in vivo,* and tolerate ischemia more than mature cells enabling them to be isolated from cadaveric livers and resulting in a dramatic expansion of source material.[81] Even the need for immunosuppression may be alleviated or eliminated. The hepatic stem cells have minimal immunogencity.[74] Although the stem cell's descendants should certainly become immunogenic, their extraordinary expansion potential and cryopreservability enables the samples to be tissue typed, facilitating matching of donor to recipients. A summary of these advantages is given in TABLE 7.

## CONCLUSIONS

A program for procurement of cadaveric neonatal and adult livers has been established recently that offers an alternate source of liver tissue from that currently available. Methods for purification and cryopreservation of hepatic progenitors have been developed using fetal livers and portions of adult human liver tissue.[80] At present, efforts are under way to develop scale-up protocols for the purification of progenitors from whole cadaveric livers. The scale-up protocols, in combination with cryopreservation methods, are laying the foundation for the establishment of a cell bank of liver cells of varying maturational stages. These cells may be used in the future for clinical trials as well as for academic, pharmaceutical, and biotechnological investigations. We propose that liver cell therapies, bioartificial human livers, and gene therapies will be done most efficiently when performed with enriched populations of liver progenitors that have the greatest capacity for growth and differentiation and the best ability to be cryopreserved. In the near future, we propose to assess the efficacy of the liver progenitors to correct liver dysfunctions in children or adults with inborn errors of metabolism or in patients with acute or chronic liver failure and who do not qualify for liver transplantation.

## ACKNOWLEDGMENTS

Funding for the studies on rodent livers derives from an NIH Grant (R01-DK52851); that for human livers from a sponsored research grant to UNC from Incara Cell Technologies (formerly Renaissance Cell Technologies), and from Incara Pharmaceuticals, Inc. We thank Cynthia Lodestro for laboratory management, Lucendia English for technical assistance, and Donna Rogers for assistance with the database and computers.

### REFERENCES

1. SHAW, B.W. 1994. Transplantation in the elderly patient. Surgical Clinics of North America **74:** 389–400.
2. SAITO, S., A.N. LANGNAS, R.J. STRATTON, *et al.* 1992. Hepatic re-transplantation: University of Nebraska Medical Center Experience. Clin. Transplant. **46:** 430–435.
3. STARZL, T.E., C.G. GROTH, L. BRETSCHNEIDER, *et al.* 1968. Orthotopic homotransplantation of the human liver. Ann. Surg. **168:** 392–415.
4. STARZL, T.E., T.L. MARCHIORO, K.A. PORTER & L. BRETTSCHNEIDER. 1967. Homotransplantation of the liver. Transplantation **5:** 790–803.
5. GORDON, R.D., J. FUNG, A.G. TZAKIS, *et al.* 1991. Liver transplantation at the University of Pittsburgh from 1984 to 1990. Clin. Transplant. **177:** 105–117.
6. KHANNA, A., A. JAIN, B. EGHTESAD & J. RAKELA. 1999. Liver transplantation for metabolic liver diseases. Surgical Clinics of North America **79:** 153–162.
7. DODSON, S.F., S. ISSA & A. BONHAM. 1999. Liver transplantation for chronic hepatitis. Surgical Clinics of North America **79:** 131–145.
8. MORRISON, S.J., N.M. SHAH & D.J. ANDERSON. 1997. Regulatory mechanisms in stem cell biology. Cell **88:** 287–298.
9. GRISHAM, J.W. & S.S. THORGEIRSSON. 1997. Liver stem cells. *In* Stem Cells. C.S. Potter, Ed.: 233–282. Academic Press, London.
10. BRINSTER, R.L. 1974. The effect of cells transferred into the mouse blastocyst on subsequent development. J. Exp. Med. **140:** 1049–1056.
11. MINTZ, B. & K. ILLMENSEE. 1975. Normal genetically mosaic mice produced from malignant teratocarcinoma cells. Proc. Natl. Acad. Sci. USA **72:** 3585–3589.
12. PETERSEN, B.E., W.C. BOWEN, K.D. PATRENE, *et al.* 1999. Bone marrow as a potential source of hepatic oval cells. Science **284:** 1168–1170.
13. THEISE, N.D., M. NIMMAKAYALU, R. GARDNER, *et al.* 2000. Liver from bone marrow in humans. Hepatology **32:** 11–16.
14. LEGASSE, E., H. CONNORS, M. AL-DHALIMYM, *et al.* 2000. Purified hemopoietic stem cells can differentiate into hepatocytes *in vivo*. Nat. Med. **11:** 1229–1234.

15. PITTENGER, M.E., A.M. MACKAY, S.C. BECK, et al. 1999. Multilineage potential of adult human mesenchymal stem cells. Science **284:** 143–147.
16. THOMSON, J.A., J. ITSKOVITZ-ELDOR, S.S. SHAPIRO, et al. 1998. Embryonic stem cell lines derived from human blastocysts. Science **282:** 1145–1146.
17. POTTEN, C.S., Ed. 1997. Stem Cells. Academic Press, London.
18. MALTSEV, V.A., J. ROHWEDEL, J. HESCHELER & A.M. WOBUS. 1993. Embryonic stem cells differentiate *in vitro* into cardiomyocytes representing sinusnodal, atrial and ventricular cell types. Mech. Devel. **44:** 41–50.
19. LINTZ, T.J., L.M. PARSONS, L. HARTLEY, et al. 1993. Nkx-2.5: a novel murine homeobox gene expressed in early heart progenitor cells and their myogenic descendants. Development **119:** 419–431.
20. CHEN, U. 1992. Careful maintenance of undifferentiated mouse embryonic stem cells is necessary for their capacity to differentiate to hematopoietic lineages *in vitro*. Current Topic. Microbiol. Immunol. **177:** 3–12.
21. RESNICK, J.L., L.S. BIXLER, L. CHENG & P.J. DONOVAN. 1992. Long-term proliferation of mouse primordial germ cells in culture [see comments]. Nature **359:** 550–551.
22. EK, S., O. RINGDEN, L. MARKLING, et al. 1993. Effects of cryopreservation on subsets of fetal liver cells. Bone Marrow Transplant. **11:** 395–398.
23. GAGE, F.H. 1994. Neuronal stem cells: their characterization and utilization. Neurobiol. Aging **15**(Supple. 2): S191.
24. DEANS, R.J. & A.B. MOSELEY. 2000. Mesenchymal stem cells: biology and potential uses. Exp. Hematol. **28:** 875–884.
25. SCHULDINER, M., O. YANUKA, J. ITSKOVITZ-ELDOR, et al. 2000. Effects of eight growth factors on the differentiation of cells derived from human embryonic stem cells. Proc. Natl. Acad. Sci. USA **97:** 11307–11312.
26. KOEBE, H.G., J.C. DUNN, M. TONER, et al. 1990. A new approach to the cryopreservation of hepatocytes in a sandwich culture configuration. Cryobiology **27:** 576–584.
27. GUYOMARD, C., L. RIALLAND, B. FREMOND, et al. 1996. Influence of alginate gel entrapment and cryopreservation on survival and xenobiotic metabolism capacity of rat hepatocytes. Toxicol. Appl. Pharmacol. **141:** 349–356.
28. LIN, C., K.Y. HOU & W.X. ZHANG. 1994. Studies of long-term cryopreservation of hepatocytes and their transplantation treating acute hepatic failure in Wistar rats. Chinese J. Surg. **32:** 633–635.
29. SWALES, N.J., C. LUONG & J. CALDWELL. 1996. Cryopreservation of rat and mouse hepatocytes. I. Comparative viability studies. Drug Metab. Dispos. **24:** 1218–1223.
30. TATENO, C. & K. YOSHIZATO. 1999. Growth potential and differentiation capacity of adult rat hepatocytes *in vitro*. Wound Repair Regen. **7:** 36–44.
31. MITAKA, T., T. KOJIMA, T. MIZUGUCHI & Y. MOCHIZUKI. 1995. Growth and maturation of small hepatocytes isolated from adult rat liver. Biochem. Biophys. Res. Commun. **214:** 310–317.
32. ENAT, R., D.M. JEFFERSON, N. RUIZ-OPAZO, et al. 1984. Hepatocyte proliferation in vitro: its dependence on the use of serum-free hormonally defined medium and substrata of extracellular matrix. Proc. Natl. Acad. Sci. USA **81:** 1411–1415.
33. REID, L.M. & T.L. LUNTZ. 1997. *Ex vivo* maintenance of differentiated mammalian cells. Meth. Molec. Biol. **75:** 31–57.
34. REID, L.M. & D.M. JEFFERSON. 1984. Culturing hepatocytes and other differentiated cells. Hepatology **4:** 548–559.
35. LECLUYSE, E.L., P.L. BULLOCK, A. MADAN, et al. 1999. Influence of extracellular matrix composition and medium formulation on the induction of cytochrome P450 2B enzymes in primary cultures of rat hepatocytes. Drug Metab. Dispos. **27:** 909–915.
36. LECLUYSE, E.L., A. MADAN, J. FORSTER, et al. 2001. Induction of cytochrome P450 enzymes in primary cultures of human hepatocytes. J. Biochem. Molec. Toxicol. In press.
37. MENDIOLA, M.M., T. PETERS, E.W. YOUNG & L. ZOLOTH-DORFMAN. 1999. Research with human embryonic stem cells: ethical considerations. Hastings Center Report **29:** 31–36.

38. MARTIN, G.R. 1981. Isolation of a pluripotent cell line from early mouse embryos cultured in medium conditioned by teratocarcinoma stem cells. Proc. Natl. Acad. Sci. USA **78:** 7634–7638.
39. GLUCKMAN, E., H.A. BROXMEYER, A.D. AUERBACH, et al. 1989. Hematopoietic reconstitution in a patient with Fanconi's anemia by means of umbilical cord blood from an HLA-identical sibling. N. Engl. J. Med. **321:** 1174–1178.
40. LIAN, Z.X., B. FENG, K. SUGIURA, et al. 1999. c-kit(< low) pluripotent hemopoietic stem cells form CFU-S on day 16. Stem Cells **17:** 39–44.
41. MAYANI, H., L.J. GUILBERT & A. JANOWSKA-WIECZOREK. 1992. Biology of the hemopoietic microenvironment. Eur. J. Hæmatol. **49:** 225–233.
42. CATTANEO, E. & R. MCKAY. 1991. Identifying and manipulating neuronal stem cells. Trend. Neurosci. **14:** 338–340.
43. ALVAREZ-BUYLLA, A. & C. LOIS. 1995. Neuronal stem cells in the brain of adult vertebrates. Stem Cells **13:** 263–272.
44. SHUMAKOV, V.I., V.N. BLIUMKIN, S.N. IGNATENKO, et al. 1983. Transplantation of cultures of human fetal pancreatic islet cells to diabetes mellitus patients. Klinicheskaia Meditsina **61:** 46–51.
45. REINHOLT, F.P., K. HULTENBY, A. TIBELL, et al. 1998. Survival of fetal porcine pancreatic islet tissue transplanted to a diabetic patient. Xenotransplantation **5:** 222–225.
46. SIGAL, S.H., S. BRILL, A.S. FIORINO & L.M. REID. 1992. The liver as a stem cell and lineage system. Am. J. Physiol. 263: G139–G148.
47. XU, A., T. LUNTZ, J. MACDONALD, et al. 2000. Liver stem cells and lineage biology. In Principles of Tissue Engineering, 2nd edit. R. Lanza, R. Langer & J. Vacanti, Eds. Academic Press, San Diego.
48. BRILL, S., P. HOLST, S. SIGAL, et al. 1993. Hepatic progenitor populations in embryonic, neonatal, and adult liver. Proc. Soc. Exp. Biol. Med. **204:** 261–269.
49. BRILL, S., P.A. HOLST, I. ZVIBEL, et al. 1994. Extracellular matrix regulation of growth and gene expression in liver cell lineages and hepatomas. In Liver Biology and Pathobiology, 3rd edit. I.M. Arias, J.L. Boyer, N. Fausto, et al., Eds.: 869–897. Raven Press, New York.
50. BRILL, S., I. ZVIBEL & L.M. REID. 1999. Expansion conditions for early hepatic progenitor cells from embryonal and neonatal rat livers. Digest. Dis. Sci. **44:** 364–371.
51. SIGAL, S.H., S. GUPTA, D.F. GEBHARD, JR., et al. 1995. Evidence for a terminal differentiation process in the rat liver. Differentiation **59:** 35–42.
52. SIGAL, S.H., P. RAJVANSHI, G.R. GORLA, et al. 1999. Partial hepatectomy-induced polyploidy attenuates hepatocyte replication and activates cell aging events. Am. J. Physiol. **276:** G1260–G1272.
53. ANATSKAYA, O.V., A.E. VINOGRADOV & B.N. KUDRYAVTSEV. 1994. Hepatocyte polyploidy and metabolism/life-history traits: hypotheses testing. J. Theor. Biol. **168:** 191–199.
54. GERLYNG, P., A. ABYHOLM, T. GROTMOL, et al. 1993. Binucleation and polyploidization patterns in developmental and regenerative rat liver growth. Cell Prolif. **26:** 557–565.
55. MOSSIN, L., H. BLANKSON, H. HUITFELDT & P.O. SEGLEN. 1994. Ploidy-dependent growth and binucleation in cultured rat hepatocytes. Exp. Cell Res. **214:** 551–60.
56. SAETER, G., C.Z. LEE, P.E. SCHWARZE, et al. 1988. Changes in ploidy distributions in human liver carcinogenesis. J. Natl. Cancer Inst. **80:** 1480–1485.
57. KUDRIAVTSEV, B.N., M.V. KUDRIAVTSEVA, G.A. SAKUTA, et al. 1993. Hepatocyte polyploidization in chronic liver diseases in man. Tsitologiia **35:** 70–83.
58. KUDRYAVTSEV, B.N., M.V. KUDRYAVTSEVA, G.A. SAKUTA & G.I. STEIN. 1993. Human hepatocyte polyploidization kinetics in the course of life cycle. Virchows Archiv. B. Cell Pathol. Including Molec. Pathol. **64:** 387–393.
59. WILSON, J.W. & E.H. LEDUC. 1958. Role of cholangioles in restoration of the liver of the mouse after dietary injury. J. Pathol. Bacteriol. **76:** 441–449.
60. SELL, S. 1994. Liver stem cells. Mod. Pathol. **7:** 105–112.
61. THEISE, N.D., R. SAXENA, B.C. PORTMANN, et al. 1999. The canals of Hering and hepatic stem cells in humans. Hepatology **30:** 1425–1433.

62. MARTINEZ-HERNANDEZ, A., F.M. DELGADO & P.S. AMENTA. 1991. The extracellular matrix in hepatic regeneration. Localization of collagen types I, III, IV, laminin, and fibronectin [published erratum appears in Lab. Invest. 1991, **65**(2): 257]. Lab. Invest. **64:** 157–166.
63. MARTINEZ-HERNANDEZ, A. & P.S. AMENTA. 1993. Morphology, localization, and origin of the hepatic extracellular matrix. *In* Extracellular Matrix: Chemistry, Biology, and Pathobiology with Emphasis on the Liver. M. Zern & L.M. Reid, Eds.: 255–330. Marcel Dekker, New York.
64. PIERCE, A., M. LYON, I.N. HAMPSON, *et al.* 1992. Molecular cloning of the major cell surface heparan sulfate proteoglycan from rat liver. J. Biol. Chem. **267:** 3894–3900.
65. STAMATOGLOU, S.C. & R.C. HUGHES. 1994. Cell adhesion molecules in liver function and pattern formation. FASEB J. **8:** 420–427.
66. REID, L.M., A.S. FIORINO, S.H. SIGAL, *et al.* 1992. Extracellular matrix gradients in the space of Disse: relevance to liver biology [editorial]. Hepatology **15:** 1198–1203.
67. GUMUCIO, J.J., Ed. 1989. Hepatocyte Heterogeneity and Liver Function, Vol. 19. Springer International, Madrid.
68. TRABER, P.G., J. CHIANALE & J.J. GUMUCIO. 1988. Physiologic significance and regulation of hepatocellular heterogeneity [see comments]. Gastroenterology **95:** 1130–1143.
69. GEBHARDT, R. 1992. Metabolic zonation of the liver: regulation and implications for liver function. Pharmacol. Therapeut. **53:** 275–354.
70. ARBER, N., G. ZAJICEK & I. ARIEL. 1988. The streaming liver. II. Hepatocyte life history. Liver **8:** 80–87.
71. ZAJICEK, G., N. ARBER & D. SCHWARTZ-ARAD. 1991. Streaming liver. VIII: Cell production rates following partial hepatectomy. Liver **11:** 347–351.
72. SIGAL, S.H., S. BRILL, L.M. REID, *et al.* 1994. Characterization and enrichment of fetal rat hepatoblasts by immunoadsorption ("panning") and fluorescence-activated cell sorting. Hepatology **19:** 999–1006.
73. BRILL, S., I. ZVIBEL & L.M. REID. 1995. Maturation-dependent changes in the regulation of liver-specific gene expression in embryonal versus adult primary liver cultures [published erratum appears in Differentiation 1995, **59**(5): 331]. Differentiation **59:** 95–102.
74. KUBOTA, H. & L.M. REID. 2000. Clonogenic hepatoblasts, common precursors for hepatocytic and biliary lineages, are lacking classical major histocompatiblity complex class I antigen. Proc. Natl. Acad. Sci. USA **97:** 12132–12137.
75. REID, L.M. & M. AGELLI. 1996. Compositions comprising hepatocyte precursors. U.S. Patent # 5,789,246. Date of application: August 7, 1991.
76. REID, L.M., M. AGELLI & A. OCHS. 1994. Method of expanding hepatic precursor cells. U.S. Patent # 5,576,207. Date of application: August 7, 1991.
77. REID, L.M. & M. AGELLI. 1991. Hepatic precursors. U.S. Patent. Date of application: August 7, 1991.
78. KUBOTA, H. & L.M. REID. 1999. Processes for clonal growth of hepatic progenitor cells. U.S. Patent Application # 113918.500.
79. KUBOTA, H. & L.M. REID. 1999. Methods of isolating bipotent hepatic progenitor cells. U.S. Patent Application # 113918.400.
80. MOSS, N., H. KUBOTA, T. LUNTZ, *et al.* 2001. Antigenic profile of hepatic progenitors from human livers. In preparation.
81. REID, L.M., E. LECLUYSE & H. KUBOTA. 2000. Liver tissue source. U.S. Patent Application # 113918. Date of application: January 23, 2000.
82. MACDONALD, J.M. & S.P. WOLFE. 1999. Bioreactor design and process for engineering tissue from cells. U.S. Patent # 113918.200. Filed June 3, 1999.
83. MACDONALD, J.M., S.P. WOLFE, I. CHOWDHURY, *et al.* 2001. Effect of flow configuration and membrane characteristics on membrane fouling in a novel multi-coaxial hollow fiber bioartificial liver. Ann. N.Y. Acad. Sci. **944:** this volume.
84. WOLFE, S.P., E. HSU, L.M. REID & J.M. MACDONALD. 2001. A novel multi-coaxial tubular bioreactor for adherent cell types. Part 1: Hydrodynamic studies. Biotechnol. Bioengin. **944**: in press.

85. XU, A. & L.M. REID. 2001. Biodegradable microcarriers for use with progenitor cells. Ann. N.Y. Acad. Sci. **944:** this volume.
86. ROJKIND, M., Z. GATMAITAN, S. MACKENSEN, *et al.* 1980. Connective tissue biomatrix: its isolation and utilization for long-term cultures of normal rat hepatocytes. J. Cell Biol. **87:** 255–263.
87. JEFFERSON, D.M., D.F. CLAYTON, J.E. DARNELL, JR. & L.M. REID. 1984. Posttranscriptional modulation of gene expression in cultured rat hepatocytes. Molec. Cell. Biol. **4:** 1929–1934.
88. SPRAY, D.C., M. FUJITA, J.C. SAEZ, *et al.* 1987. Proteoglycans and glycosaminoglycans induce gap junction synthesis and function in primary liver cultures. J. Cell Biol. **105:** 541–551.
89. ROSENBERG, E., D.C. SPRAY & L.M. REID. 1992. Transcriptional and posttranscriptional control of connexin mRNAs in periportal and pericentral rat hepatocytes. Eur. J. Cell Biol. **59:** 21–26.
90. ZVIBEL, I., A.S. FIORINO, S. BRILL & L.M. REID. 1998. Phenotypic characterization of rat hepatoma cell lines and lineage-specific regulation of gene expression by differentiation agents. Differentiation **63:** 215–223.
91. TATENO, C.T.-K.K., C. YAMASAKI, H. SATO & K. YOSHIZATO. 2000. Heterogeneity of growth potential of adult rat hepatocytes *in vitro*. Hepatology **31:** 65–74.
92. CHESSEBEUF, M. & P. PADIEU. 1984. Rat liver epithelial cultures in a serum-free medium: primary cultures and derived cell lines expressing differentiated functions. In Vitro **20:** 780–795.
93. HIGGINS, G.M. & R.M. ANDERSON. 1931. Arch. Pathol. **12:** 186–202.
94. CARRIERE, R. 1969. The growth of liver parenchymal nuclei and its endocrine regulation. Int. Rev. Cytol. **25:** 201–277.
95. FAUSTO, N., J.M. LEMIRE & N. SHIOJIRI. 1993. Cell lineages in hepatic development and the identification of progenitor cells in normal and injured liver. Proc. Soc. Exp. Biol. Med. **204:** 237–241.
96. OVERTURF, K., M. AL-DHALIMY, C.N. OU, *et al.* 1997. Serial transplantation reveals the stem-cell-like regenerative potential of adult mouse hepatocytes. Am. J. Pathol. **151:** 1273–1280.
97. GUPTA, S., P. RAJVANSHI, E. ARAGONA, *et al.* 1999. Transplanted hepatocytes proliferate differently after CCl4 treatment and hepatocyte growth factor infusion. Am. J. Physiol. **276:** G629–G638.
98. GUPTA, S., P. RAJVANSHI, A.N. IRANI, *et al.* 2000. Integration and proliferation of transplanted cells in hepatic parenchyma following D-galactosamine-induced acute injury in F344 rats. J. Pathol. **190:** 203–210.
99. RHIM, J.A., E.P. SANDGREN, R.D. PALMITER & R.L. BRINSTER. 1995. Complete reconstitution of mouse liver with xenogeneic hepatocytes. Proc. Natl. Acad. Sci. USA **92:** 4942–4946.
100. RHIM, J.A., E.P. SANDGREN, J.L. DEGEN, *et al.* 1994. Replacement of diseased mouse liver by hepatic cell transplantation. Science **263:** 1149–1152.
101. OVERTURF, K.A.-D.M., M. FINEGOLD & M. GROMPE. 1999. The repopulation potential of hepatocyte populations differing in size and prior mitotic expansion. Am. J. Pathol. **155:** 2135–2143.
102. SIGAL, S.H., P. RAJVANSHI, L.M. REID & S. GUPTA. 1995. Demonstration of differentiation in hepatocyte progenitor cells using dipeptidyl peptidase IV deficient mutant rats. Cell Mol. Biol. Res. **41:** 39–47.
103. DABEVA, M.D., P.M. PETKOV, J. SANDHU, *et al.* 2000. Proliferation and differentiation of fetal liver epithelial progenitor cells after transplantation in adult rat liver. Am. J. Pathol. **156:** 2017–2031.
104. LACONI, E., R. OREN, D.K. MUKHOPADHYAY, *et al.* 1998. Long-term, near total liver replacement by transplantation of isolated hepatocytes in rats treated with retrorsine. Am. J. Pathol. **153:** 319–329.
105. GAGANDEEP, S., P. RAJVANSHI, R.P. SOKHI, *et al.* 2000. Transplanted hepatocytes engraft, survive, and proliferate in the liver of rats with carbon tetrachloride-induced cirrhosis. J. Pathol. **191:** 78–85.

106. BILIR, B., D. KUMPE, J. KRYSL, *et al.* 1998. Hepatocyte transplantation in patients with liver cirrhosis. Digestive Diseases (published conference abstracts) AASLD Meetings, May 16th–22nd, 1998: Abstract #LOO56.
107. BILIR, B.M., D. GUINETTE, F. KARRER, *et al.* 2000. Hepatocyte transplantation in acute liver failure. Liver Transplant. **6:** 41–43.
108. SHAFRITZ, D.A. 2000. Rat liver stem cells: prospects for the future. Hepatology **32:** 1399–1400.
109. OVERTURF, K., M. AL-DHALIMY, R. TANGUAY, *et al.* 1996. Hepatocytes corrected by gene therapy are selected *in vivo* in a murine model of hereditary tyrosinaemia type I [see comments] [published erratum appears in Nat. Genet. 1996, 12(4): 458]. Nat. Genet. **12:** 266–273.
110. SANDGREN, E.P., R.D. PALMITER, J.L. HECKEL, *et al.* 1991. Complete hepatic regeneration after somatic deletion of an albumin-plasminogen activator transgene. Cell **66:** 245–256.
111. BRAUN, K.M., J.L. DEGEN & E.P. SANDGREN. 2000. Hepatocyte transplantation in a model of toxin-induced liver disease: variable therapeutic effect during replacement of damaged parenchyma by donor adult liver cells. Nat. Med. **6:** 320–326.
112. MITAKA, T., M. MIKAMI, G.L. SATTLER, *et al.* 1992. Small cell colonies appear in the primary culture of adult rat hepatocytes in the presence of nicotinamide and epidermal growth factor. Hepatology **16:** 440–447.
113. GUPTA, S., P. RAJVANSHI, R. SOKHI, *et al.* 1999. Entry and integration of transplanted hepatocytes in rat liver plates occur by disruption of hepatic sinusoidal endothelium. Hepatology **29:** 509–519.
114. GUPTA, S., H. MALHI, S. GAGANDEEP & P. NOVIKOFF. 1999. Liver repopulation with hepatocyte transplantation: new avenues for gene and cell therapy [review]. J. Gene Med. **1:** 386–392.
115. STROM, S., R. FISHER, W. RUBINSTEIN, *et al.* 1997. Transplantation of human hepatocytes. Transplant. Proc. **29:** 2103–2106.
116. STROM, S.C., J.R. CHOWDHURY & I.J. FOX. 1999. Hepatocyte transplantation for the treatment of human disease (Review). Semin. Liver Dis. **19:** 39–48.
117. RUNGE, D., W. FLEIG, G. MICHALOPOULOS, *et al.* 2000. Hepatocyte transplantation. Possibilities for use and examples of practical clinical application. Deutsche Meedizinische Wochenschrift **125:** 397–400.
118. CHOWDHURY, J.R., N.R. CHOWDHURY, S.C. STROM, *et al.* 1998. Human hepatocyte transplantation: gene therapy and more? Pediatrics **102:** 647–648.
119. FOX, I.J., J.R. CHOWDHURY, S.S. KAUFMAN, *et al.* 1998. Treatment of the Crigler-Najjar Syndrome Type I with hepatocyte transplantation. N. Engl. J. Med. **338:** 1422–1426.
120. STROM, S., R. FISHER, M. THOMPSON, *et al.* 1997. Hepatocyte transplantation as a bridge to orthotopic liver transplantation in terminal liver failure. Transplantation **63:** 559–569.

# Formation of Sertoli Cell–Enriched Tissue Constructs Utilizing Simulated Microgravity Technology

DON F. CAMERON,[a,b,c] JOELLE J. HUSHEN,[a,c] STANLEY J. NAZIAN,[d] ALISON WILLING,[c] SAM SAPORTA,[a,c] AND PAUL R. SANBERG[d]

[a]*Department of Anatomy, University of South Florida College of Medicine, Tampa, Florida, USA*

[b]*Department of Surgery, University of South Florida College of Medicine, Tampa, Florida, USA*

[c]*Department of Neurosurgery, University of South Florida College of Medicine, Tampa, Florida, USA*

[d]*Department of Physiology and Biophysics, University of South Florida College of Medicine, Tampa, Florida, USA*

ABSTRACT: Cell transplantation therapy for diabetes and Parkinson's disease offers hope for long-term alleviation of symptoms. However, successful protocols remain elusive due to obstacles, including rejection and lack of tropic support for the graft. To enhance engraftment, testis-derived postmitotic Sertoli cells have been cotransplanted with islets in the diabetic rat (Db) and neurons in the Parkinsonian rat (PD). Sertoli cell tropic, regulatory, and nutritive factors that nourish and stimulate germ cells also support isolated neurons and islets *in vitro*. Likewise, immunosuppressive properties of Sertoli cells, extant in the testis, are expressed by extratesticular Sertoli cells evidenced by allo- and xenograft immunoprotection of grafts in both the CNS (in the PD model) and the periphery (in the Db model). On this basis, we have created Sertoli islet cell aggregates (SICA) and Sertoli neuron aggregated cells (SNAC) using simulated microgravity culture technology developed by NASA. Isolated rat and pig Sertoli cells were cocultured with neonatal pig islets (SICA) and with immortalized *N*-Terra-2 (NT2) neurons (SNAC) in the HARV biochamber. Formed aggregates were assayed for desirable functional and structural characteristics. Cell viability in SICA and SNAC exceeded 90% and FasL immunopositive Sertoli cells were present in both. Sertoli cells did not interfere with insulin secretion by SICA and promoted differentiation of NT2 cells to the dopaminergic hNT cell type in SNAC. Addition of Matrigel resulted in structural reorganization of the aggregates and enhanced insulin secretion. We conclude that SICA, SNAC, and Matrigel-induced islet- and neuron-filled "Sertoli cell biochambers" are suitable for long-term transplantation treatment of Db and PD.

KEYWORDS: Sertoli cells; microgravity; HARV; coculture

Address for correspondence: Don F. Cameron, Ph.D., Department of Anatomy, MDC-6, University of South Florida College of Medicine, 12901 Bruce B. Downs Blvd., Tampa, FL 33612, USA. Voice: 813-974-9434; fax: 813-974-2058.
dcameron@HSC.usf.edu

## INTRODUCTION

### Testicular Sertoli Cells

The testicular nurse cell, known as the Sertoli cell, resides in the testis, where it provides a nutrient-rich environment for germ cell expansion and differentiation. Among these proteins are insulin-like growth factor I, basic fibroblast growth factor, transforming growth factors α and β, platelet-derived growth factor, neurturin, interleukin 1α and interleukin 6, and the transport proteins, transferrin and ceruloplasmin.[1] Sertoli cells also protect spermatids from immune detection and destruction, principally by formation of the so-called "blood–testis" barrier, which is, in fact, the collective population of Sertol–Sertoli junctional complexes. Clearly, immunoprotection by testicular Sertoli cells is imparted to the highly antigenic germ cell population. However, it is imparted by mechanisms that are not yet clearly defined, possibly facilitated by the fact that Sertoli cells do not express major histocompatibility complex class I or II antigens and, therefore, may not be detected by the immune system. One suggested mechanism by which Sertoli cells provide immune protection is the constitutive expression of FasL (CD95 ligand). Bellgrau and coworkers[2] showed that the *gld* mouse survived indefinitely when Sertoli cells were transplanted under the kidney capsule. They concluded that the expression of functional FasL by Sertoli cells accounts for the immune-privileged nature of the testis.

### Extratesticular Sertoli Cells

Bellgrau and coworkers went further and suggested that FasL expression was the mechanism by which isolated Sertoli cells induce localized immune privilege to cotransplanted cells and tissues,[2] which is appealing in that this is similar to the already well defined mechanism of downregulation of the immune response naturally occurring in the mammalian system. The role of FasL in promoting immunosuppression by extratesticular Sertoli cells in transplantation has received much attention since it was first suggested that Sertoli cells impart their immunoprotective function by this pathway. An alternative or additional mechanism of extratesticular Sertoli cell immunoprotective activity is by way of suppression of activated lymphocytic proliferation. Sertoli cell–conditioned media has been shown to inhibit Con A-stimulated spleen lymphocyte proliferation in a dose-dependent manner. This appears to occur through a dose-dependent inhibition of interleukin 2 (IL-2) production, since the addition of exogenous IL-2 was not able to reverse this effection.[3]

Characteristics of Sertoli cells that make them ideal transplantation facilitators are that (1) they are terminally differentiated and mitotically quiescent when isolated, (2) they live for the life of the donor and may, therefore, live for the life of the host, (3) they do not express MHC I or II antigens, (4) they express and secrete numerous tropic, growth and immunosuppressive factors, and (5) they are easily isolated and cryopreserved.

### Transplantation Facilitation by Sertoli Cells

In the course of finding a suitable organ or tissue site for islet transplantation, it was discovered that the relocated abdominal testis (at 37°C) provided an extraordinarily safe environment for extended survival of islet grafts and some relief of the diabetic complications.[4–7] It is now clear that immunosuppressive and supportive properties exhibited by the abdominal testis were generated by the organ's Sertoli cell population[8,9] and, thus, have been used in cotransplantation protocols to "facilitate" the success of islet engraftment.[8,9] The first direct evidence that SCs could, in fact, provide for immunosuppression by a mechanism not involving the B–T barrier was realized when Selawry and Cameron[9] created an abdominal testis-like immunoprivileged site outside of the testis by cotransplanting isolated islets with isolated Sertoli cells beneath to the kidney capsule in the diabetic rat. This protocol, when accompanied with a short two-day course of cyclosporin A, extended the viability of both islet allo- and xenografts, prevented the rejection of the graft in the otherwise immunologically hostile site, and rendered the once hyperglycemic diabetic rat normoglycemic for the life of the animal.[9] Additionally, SCs may facilitate islet graft success by providing for a supportive tropic environment illustrated, in part, by their ability to significantly enhance islet cellular viability following cryopreservation[10] if the islets are thawed in established SC cultures.

On the basis that Sertoli cells might serve as useful "transplantation facilitators" in other cell transplantation protocols, for example Parkinson's disease, isolated SCs were transplanted with rat ventral mesencephalic cells (VM) into the DA-depleted rat striatum, resulting in an increase of graft survival, an increase of surviving TH-positive neurons and an increase of TH-neuron soma size when compared to VM-only grafts.[11] Additionally, Sanberg and coworkers[12] showed that SCs enhanced the survival of bovine adrenal chromaffin cells when cotransplanted in the rat striatum, whereas no chromaffin cells survived in the absence of SCs. Additionally, we have shown that all hNT neuron grafts will survive in the striatum when cotransplanted with SCs without systemic immunosuppression as compared to only 50% survival in hNT-only grafts.[13] This latter observation was accompanied with a 60% reduction of gliosis, indicating a significant suppression of the CNS immune response at the graft site. When transplanted alone, both rat (allografts) and porcine (xenografts) SCs survive in the brain without systemic immunosuppression for ten months post transplantation.[14]

As with islets, SCs provide a supportive tropic environment for neurons illustrated, in part, by their ability to significantly enhance cellular viability following cryopreservation if the VM cells are thawed in established SC cultures.[15] Furthermore, we have shown a significant increase in the numbers of TH-positive neurons in coculture with SCs when compared with neuron-only monocultures.[16] As with the islets studies, Sertoli cells needed to be present to effect these supportive tropic results.

Although extratesticular Sertoli cells support isolated cells and immunoprotect grafts as well as might be expected when using systemic immunoprotection, there are inherent problems limiting the usefulness of this protocol, including the difficulty of insuring the obligatory close proximity of the two cell types following transplantation. To overcome these limitations, it would be beneficial to have a transplantable, viable, tissue-like aggregate composed of Sertoli cells and the transplantable cell type in which the cells types retain their differentiated functions—that is, for example, normal insulin secretion by β-cells of the islets and dopamine production by the neurons and immunoprotection and tropic support by the Sertoli cells.

In this report, we describe the tissue engineering, morphology and functional assay of a Sertoli islet cell aggregate (SICA) and Sertoli neuron aggregated cells (SNAC) created by simulated microgravity coculture using the NASA-developed rotating cell culture system (RCCS).

## Simulated Microgravity

The RCCS is a relatively new development in bioreactor technology that enables the cultivation of highly differentiated three-dimensional cell aggregates mimicking the structure and function of parental tissue.[18] The RCCS was originally designed to protect delicate tissue cultures during space flight. However, it quickly became apparent that the unique environment provided by the RCCS of low shear force, high mass transfer, and microgravity, enables three-dimensional cell growth to take place in a conventional tissue culture incubator. The RCCS has a wide range of cell and clinical research applications, including cancer research, *in vitro* toxicology testing, and tissue engineering.

## Principle of Rotary Cell Culture

Most culture systems address one specific parameter, shear force, at the expense of others such as mass transfer of nutrients and metabolic wastes, three-dimensionality, and/or cocultivation of dissimilar cell types. The RCCS is the first bioreactor designed to simultaneously integrate cocultivation, low shear, high mass transfer, and three-dimensional growth without sacrificing any other parameter. The RCCS is a zero head space, aqueous medium-filled bioreactor that suspends particles or cell aggregates by rotating the vessel wall and integral gas diffusion membrane around the horizontal axis. The rotation vessel can hold particles/aggregates of up to 1 cm in diameter in orbital suspension, since the sedimentation forces induced by gravity are balanced by the centrifugal force generated by the rotation of the vessel. As the aggregates expand, the rotational speed is increased. Over 40 different cell types have been successfully grown in the RCCS and, to date, no tissue type tested (either suspension or anchorage dependent cells) has failed to grow in the RCCS. For example, hepatocytes have been expanded in RCCS into high fidelity models of liver tissue.[21] Human cancer cells grown include those of melanoma, prostate cancer, breast cancer, ovarian cancer, and osteosarcoma. As an example, normal human fibroblasts have been cocultured with human colon cancer cells and, in less than a month, the coculture producing hundreds of differentiated colon cancer polyps, each exceeding one centimeter in diameter.

To our knowledge, our work is the first attempt to develop Sertoli cell–enriched tissue constructs with highly differentiated cell types suitable for transplantation. This report summarizes our results relating to the creation and definition of SICA and SNAC intended to be used in cell transplantation therapies of experimental diabetes and Parkinson's disease, respectively. The type of RCCS used to create SICA and SNAC was the high aspect ratio vessel (HARV). It is a 10-ml cylindrical RCCS bioreactor with a variable speed power supply. Cocultures were placed in the HARV and then the HARV was placed in a convention incubator at 37°C and 5% $CO_2$–95% air. The methods for isolating cells and the use of HARV coculture reported herein are described in detail elsewhere.[17]

## RESULTS

The detailed morphology and selective assay of SICA and SNAC are reported elsewhere.[17] Presented herein is a summary of those results.

### SICA

SICA were formed in the HARV following five days coincubation of isolated neonatal pig Sertoli cells and pancreatic islets. They ranged in size between 1–6 mm in diameter, depending on whether or not 1% Matrigel was added to the coculture medium. Consistently, SICA formed in the presence of Matrigel (i.e., $SICA_{MG}$) were larger than those formed in the absence of Matrigel.

Islets were incorporated within the SICA, as verified by sectional morphology (see FIGURE 1) and illustrated with scanning electron microscopy (see FIGURE 2). All islet endocrine cell types were present, as determined by the unique ultrastructure of secretion granules. Only in the presence of Matrigel did Sertoli cells segregate to the periphery of the aggregate, leaving the islet cells more centrally located and closely associated with lumen-like spaces. In the latter, Sertoli cells were highly polarized and gave the appearance of a simple columnar epithelium, similar to their morphological and histological appearance *in situ*. This phenomenon of Sertoli cell epithelialization *in vitro* has been observed in conventional culture when Sertoli cells are plated on a Martigel substratum,[19,20] but this is the first time that Sertoli cells have been reported to undergo such a dramatic cytoskeletal reorganization when not in direct contact with the substratum.

Cryosections of fixed SICA showed the expression of FasL on Sertoli cells and insulin in β cells by positive immunostaining. In $SICA_{MG}$ there appeared to be an

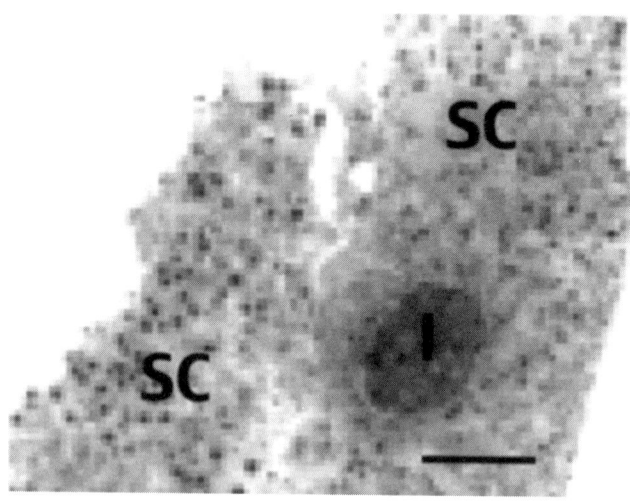

**FIGURE 1.** When sectioned (0.5 μm), SICA reveal Sertoli cells (*SC*) surrounding intact islets (*I*). Toluidine blue stain. *Bar*, 100 μm.

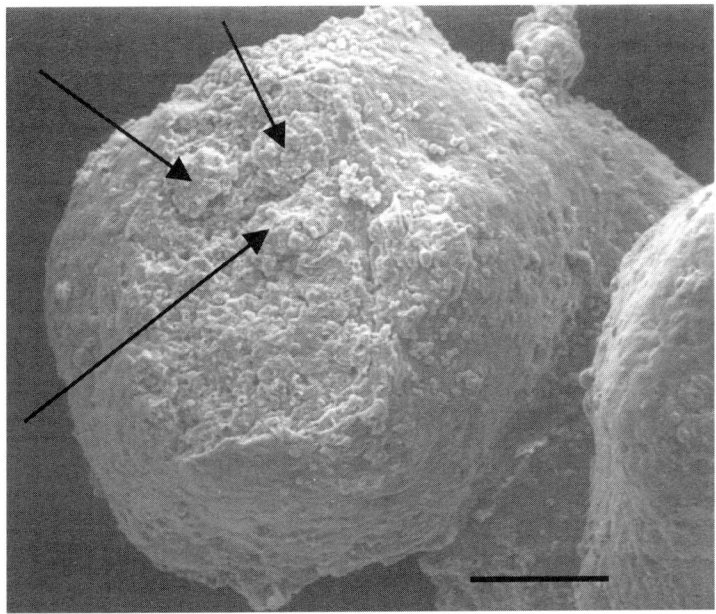

**FIGURE 2.** This scanning electron micrograph shows a SICA partially fractured. Islets (*arrows*) are present within a matrix of Sertoli cells. Bar, 100 μm.

increased density of β cells, although this was not quantified. When exposed to elevated glucose (180 mg%), SICA were capable of secreting insulin as determined by elevated RIA detectable insulin in the medium (see FIGURE 3). Additionally, isolated SICA were capable of suppressing Con-A–stimulated lymphocytic proliferation *in vitro* when compared to islet cell–only coincubation with the mixed lymphocytes.

## *SNAC*

SNAC measuring 1–3 mm in diameter were formed in the HARV following one-week coincubation of isolated rat prepubertal Sertoli cells and the NTerra2 (Nt2) neuron precursor cell line generously supplied by Layton Bioscience, Inc. The NT2 cell acquires a dopaminergic phenotype, illustrated by positive tyrosine hydroxylase (TH) immunostaining, following five weeks of exposure to retinoic acid *in vitro*. As with SICA, Sertoli cell segregation and lumen formation could be induced by adding 1% Matigel to the coculture medium, as demonstrated, in this case, by the peripheral distribution of FasL and centralization of NuMa-positive NT2 cells. The most striking observation of these aggregates was the appearance of TH-positive cells in cryosectioned SNAC, since *in vitro* formation required only one-week incubation, and in the absence of retinoic acid. It would appear that the bioreactor environment of simulated microgravity and/or Sertoli cells accelerated the conditions necessary for dopaminergic differentiation by a mechanism not requiring the retinoic acid.

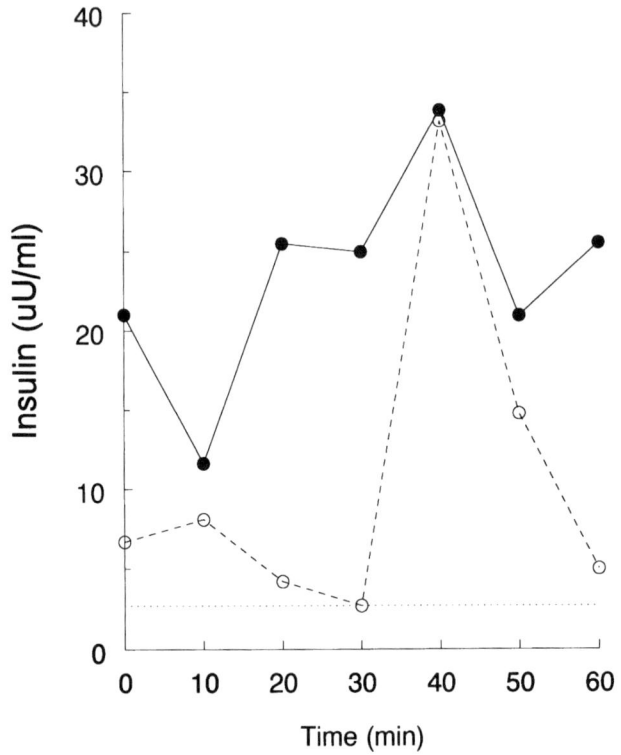

**FIGURE 3.** This graph illustrates insulin production against time as measured by RIA following exposure to elevated glucose (180 mg%) by isolated SICA (*solid line*), islets alone (*dashed line*), and in medium alone (*dotted line*).

## DISCUSSION

Results from this study showed that when cocultured in simulated microgravity utilizing the HARV biochamber, organized three-dimensional aggregates form, following coculture of Sertoli cells with neonatal pig islets (SICA) and NT2 cells (SNAC). In both cases, the transplantable cells exhibited desirable characteristics such as insulin production by β cells in the SICA and TH expression in SNAC neurons. Both prepubertal rat Sertoli cells and neonatal pig Sertoli cells were used in the formation of aggregates, but it is not clear whether one cell type was better than the other in inducing desirable characteristics in SICA or SNAC since the observations were not quantified. Whether or not these novel tissue constructs will enhance the long-term success of cell transplantation therapies for the therapeutic treatment of experimental diabetes and Parkinson's disease also is yet to be determined. However, they do provide a new and promising approach to the ever-growing armamentaria of methods applied to the amelioration of devastating symptoms of these two serious diseases, in particular, and to a number of conditions and diseases involving the replacement of dysfunctional cells, in general.

## ACKNOWLEDGMENT

This study was supported, in part, by NASA (NAG8-1381).

## REFERENCES

1. SKINNER, M.K. 1993. Secretion of growth factors and other regulatory factors. *In* The Sertoli Cell. L.D. Russell & M.D. Griswold, Eds.: 493–508. Cache River Press, Clearwater, FL.
2. BELLGRAU, D., D. GOLD, H.P. SELAWRY, *et al.* 1995. A role for CD95 ligand in preventing graft rejection. Nature **377:** 630–632.
3. SELAWRY, H., M. KOTB, H. HERROED & Z.-N. LU. 1991. Production of a factor, or factors, suppressing IL-2 production and T cell proliferation by Sertoli cell-enriched preparations. Transplantation **52:** 846–850.
4. SELAWRY, H., R. FOJACO & K. WHITTINGTON. 1985. Intratesticular islet allografts in the spontaneously diabetic B/W Rat. Diabetes **34:** 1019–1023.
5. CAMERON, D.F., K. WHITTINGTON, R.E. SCHULTZ & H. SELAWRY. 1990. Successful islet/abdominal testis transplantation does not require Leydig cells. Transplantation **50:** 649–653.
6. SELAWRY, H. & D.F. CAMERON. 1993. Sertoli cell-enriched fractions in successful islet cell transplantation. Cell Transplant. **2:** 123–129.
7. WHITMORE, W.F. & F.R. GITTLES. 1978. Intratesticular grafts: the testis as an exceptionally immunologically privileged site. Trans. Am. Assoc. Gen. Urinary Surg. **70:** 76–80.
8. SELAWRY, H., R. FOJACO & K. WHITTINGTON. 1987. Extended survival of the MHC-compatible islet isografts in the spontaneously diabetic BB/W rat. Diabetes **36:** 1061–1070.
9. SELAWRY, H., K. WHITTINGTON & R. FOJACO. 1986. Effect of cyclosporine on islet xenograft survival in the BB/W rat. Transplantation **42:** 568–575.
10. SELAWRY, H.P., X. WANG & L. ALLOUSH. 1996. Sertoli cell-induced effects on functional and structural characteristics of isolated neonatal porcine islets. Cell Transplant. **5:** 517–524.
11. WILLING, A.E., A.I. OTHBERG, S. SAPORTA, *et al.* 1999. Sertoli cells enhance the survival of co-transplanted dopamine neurons. Brain Res. **822:** 246–250.
12. SANBERG, P.R., C.V. BORLONGAN, S. SAPORTA & D.F. CAMERON. 1996. Testis-derived Sertoli cells survive and provide localized immunoprotection for xenogragfts in rat brain. Nat. Biotech. **14:** 1692–1695.
13. WILLING, A.E., J.J. SUDBURY, A.I. OTHBERG, *et al.* 1999. Sertoli cells decrease microglia response and increase engraftment of human hNT neurons in the hemiparkinson rat striatum. Brain Res. Bul. **48:** 441–444.
14. SAPORTA, S.S., D.F. CAMERON, C. BORLONGAN & P.R. SANBERG. 1997. Survival of rat and porcine Sertoli cell transplants into rat striatum with or without short-term cyclosporine immunosuppression. Exp. Neurol. **146:** 299–304.
15. CAMERON, D.F., A.I. OTHBERG, C.V. BORLONGAN, *et al.* 1997. Post-thaw viability and functionality of cryopreserved rat fetal brain. Cell Transplant. **6:** 185–189.
16. OTHBERG, A.I., D.F. CAMERON, A. ANTON, *et al.* 1997. Evidence for a direct trophic effect of porcine Sertoli cells on rat fetal dopaminergic neurons *in vitro*. Proc. 4th Am. So. Neural. Transplantation.
17. CAMERON, D.F., J.J. HUSHEN & S.J. NAZIAN. 2001. Formation of insulin-secreting, Sertoli-enriched tissue constructs by microgravity coculture of isolated pig islets and Sertoli cells. In Vitro. In press.
18. SCHWARZ, R.P., T.J. GOODWIN & D.A. WOLF. 1992. Cell culture for three-dimensional modeling in rotating-wall vessels: an application of simulated microgravity. J. Tiss. Cult. Meth. **14:** 51–58.
19. HADLEY, M., C. BYERS, C. SUAREZ-QUIAN & M. DYM. 1985. Extracellular matrix regulates Sertoli cell differentiation *in vitro*. J. Cell. Biol. **101:** 1511–1522.

20. CAMERON, D.F., K.E. MUFFLY & S.J. NAZIAN. 1993. Testosterone stimulates spermatid binding to competent Sertoli cells *in vitro*. Endocrinol. J. **1:** 61–65.
21. KHAOUSTOV, V.I., G.J. DARLINGTON, H.E. SORIANO, *et al.* 1999. Induction of three-dimensional assembly of human liver cells by simulated microgravity. In Vitro Cell Dev. Biol. Animal **35:** 501–509.

# The Influence of Extracellular Matrix on the Generation of Vascularized, Engineered, Transplantable Tissue

OLIVER C.S. CASSELL,[a] WAYNE A. MORRISON,[a] AURORA MESSINA,[a] ANTHONY J. PENINGTON,[a] ERIK W. THOMPSON,[b] GEOFFREY W. STEVENS,[c] JILSKA M. PERERA,[c] HYNDA K. KLEINMAN,[d] JOHN V. HURLEY,[a] ROSALIND ROMEO,[a] AND KENNETH R. KNIGHT[a]

[a]*Bernard O'Brien Institute of Microsurgery, University of Melbourne, St. Vincent's Hospital, Fitzroy, Victoria 3065, Australia*

[b]*Department of Surgery, University of Melbourne, St. Vincent's Hospital, Fitzroy, Victoria 3065, Australia*

[c]*Department of Chemical Engineering, University of Melbourne, Victoria 3010, Australia*

[d]*Cell Biology Section, National Institute of Dental and Craniofacial Research, National Institutes of Health, Bethesda, Maryland, USA*

ABSTRACT: In a recently described model for tissue engineering, an arteriovenous loop comprising the femoral artery and vein with interposed vein graft is fabricated in the groin of an adult male rat, placed inside a polycarbonate chamber, and incubated subcutaneously. New vascularized granulation tissue will generate on this loop for up to 12 weeks. In the study described in this paper three different extracellular matrices were investigated for their ability to accelerate the amount of tissue generated compared with a no-matrix control. Poly-D,L-lactic-co-glycolic acid (PLGA) produced the maximal weight of new tissue and vascularization and this peaked at two weeks, but regressed by four weeks. Matrigel was next best. It peaked at four weeks but by eight weeks it also had regressed. Fibrin (20 and 80 mg/ml), by contrast, did not integrate with the generating vascularized tissue and produced less weight and volume of tissue than controls without matrix. The limiting factors to growth appear to be the chamber size and the capacity of the neotissue to integrate with the matrix. Once the sides of the chamber are reached or tissue fails to integrate, encapsulation and regression follow. The intrinsic position of the blood supply within the neotissue has many advantages for tissue and organ engineering, such as ability to seed the construct with stem cells and microsurgically transfer new tissue to another site within the individual. In conclusion, this study has found that PLGA and Matrigel are the best matrices for the rapid growth of new vascularized tissue suitable for replantation or transplantation.

KEYWORDS: tissue engineering; extracellular matrix; angiogenesis; chamber model; fibrin; Matrigel; poly-D,L-lactic-co-glycolic acid (PLGA)

Address for correspondence: Dr. Kenneth R. Knight, Bernard O'Brien Institute of Microsurgery, St. Vincent's Hospital, 42 Fitzroy Street, Fitzroy, Victoria 3065, Australia. Voice: + 613 9288 4020; fax: + 613 9416 0926.
knightkr@svhm.org.au

## BACKGROUND

Tissue engineering offers the prospect of replacing missing or non-functioning body parts with newly created, living tissue. It has the potential to minimize the donor site morbidity of conventional reconstructive surgery, and to create specialized tissue for which there is no donor site. It combines the techniques of cell and tissue culture with the use of biocompatible materials and the manipulation of angiogenesis to generate new tissue.[1]

We have developed an *in vivo* model that meets many of these needs. It is based on the insertion of an arteriovenous (AV) loop and an extracellular matrix scaffold into a polycarbonate chamber.[2] This model allows *de novo* generation of vascularized tissues that can be moved to the desired recipient site with no donor site morbidity. The model expands the finding of Erol and Spira,[3] who showed that the creation of an AV loop beneath the skin leads to spontaneous angiogenesis capable of vascularizing an overlying skin graft, thus creating a neo "skin flap". It extends the findings of Khouri *et al.*[4] and Tanaka *et al.*,[5] who demonstrated that an AV shunt can intrinsically generate new, vascularized tissue when it is sandwiched between sheets of collagenous matrix and separated from the surrounding tissue within a plastic chamber. In our model, new tissue can be generated from an AV loop enclosed in a chamber in the absence of added matrix.[6,7] Under these circumstances a fibrin-rich plasma exudate fills the chamber in the first 24 hours and acts as the scaffold.

To further develop this model we tested three matrices—fibrin, Matrigel, and poly-D,L-lactic-co-glycolic (PLGA)—for their ability to accelerate the process of vascularized tissue formation in the chamber. The ideal extracellular matrix (ECM) should be biodegradable, nontoxic, enhance cellular colonization and vascularization, and offer structural support.

Fibrin clots have been used in cartilage tissue engineering to prepare an injectable form of chondrocytes for joint cartilage repair.[8]

The properties of Matrigel, a recombined form of basement membrane derived from the mouse EHS sarcoma,[9] have been mainly gleaned from *in vitro* cell biology and angiogenesis studies.[10] In tissue engineering experiments to date, Matrigel has proven to be beneficial for the formation of new neural tissue[11] and adipose tissue.[12]

PLGA, a widely used scaffold in tissue engineering, comprises polylactic acid and polyglycolic acid.[13] The relative amounts can be varied to produce the desired scaffold properties, where polylactic acid imparts rigidity and polyglycolic acid imparts biodegradability. Commonly, 75% polylactic acid/25% polyglycolic acid provides a rigid but biodegradable scaffold.[13] PLGA prolongs the activity of exogenously added growth factors,[12,14] and the pore size can be varied to accommodate cellular and vascular infiltration.[13] The much heralded success of the human ear, built on a PLGA scaffold, on the nude mouse was a significant advance in cartilage tissue engineering.[15] PLGA has also been applied to the formation of adipose tissue,[16] blood vessels,[17] and liver tissue.[18]

## MATERIALS AND METHODS

Full ethical approval was received from the Animal Ethics Committee of St. Vincent's Hospital, Melbourne, Australia, for these experiments.

### Animals

All the rats used were male inbred Sprague Dawley, weighing between 220–280 g. They were housed individually and were fed standard rat chow and water ad libitum.

### The Chamber

The polycarbonate chamber was manufactured by the Department of Chemical Engineering, University of Melbourne, Australia. It comprises a base and lid that clip together to form a 0.5 ml semi-sealed chamber with an internal diameter of 14 mm and height of 5 mm. An opening, comprising 20% of the circumference, allows for entry and exit of the artery and vein of the arteriovenous loop. The base of the chamber has four small holes that allow it to be anchored to surrounding tissues with sutures.

### The Arteriovenous (AV) Loop Chamber Model

This model has been described elsewhere[2,6] (see FIGURE 1). Briefly, an arteriovenous loop using the femoral artery and vein with interposed vein graft were created in the groin. This loop was laid inside the base of a polycarbonate chamber, an appropriate matrix was inserted around it, and the lid placed over the top to close it. At the specified exploration time the chamber was exposed, the vessels examined for patency, and the tissue generated harvested for analysis.

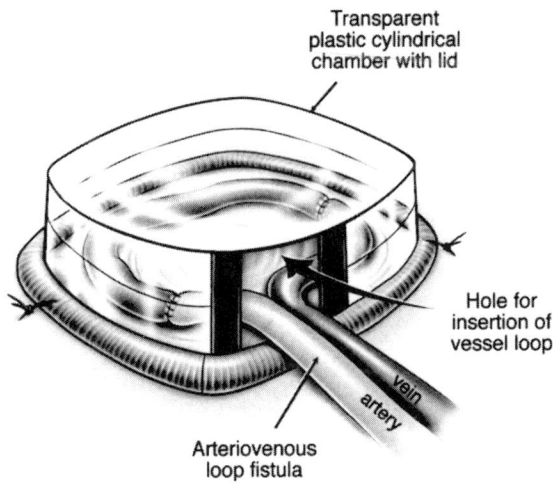

**FIGURE 1.** Schematic diagram of the arteriovenous shunt loop model used to generate new vascularized tissues. (From Mian et al.[6] Reproduced by permission of Mary Ann Liebert Inc.)

## Volume and Weight

The volume of the tissue generated was determined using a standard water displacement technique. A beaker of isotonic saline was placed on a balance and the balance zeroed. The tissue was suspended from a wooden strut placed across the beaker and totally submerged in the saline without touching the sides of the beaker. The weight of the displaced fluid was recorded ($W$) and the volume equivalent calculated by dividing $W$ by 1.0048 (the specific gravity for normal saline).

## Microfil Technique

In two of the six rats in each group Microfil® (Canton Bio-medical, Boulder, CO) was injected intraarterially to perfuse the flap for qualitative determination of flap vascularization. The artery of the tissue flap was cannulated with a catheter connected to a 24 gauge needle. The tissue was pulse infused with 5 ml of heparinized saline, followed by 5 ml of phosphate buffered saline (PBS) and finally 5 ml of Microfil. Intermittent clamping of the vein was carried out to ensure good perfusion of peripheral flap tissues. The tissue was refrigerated at 4°C for 24 hours to allow the Microfil to set, subsequently dehydrated by immersion in 70% ethanol for two hours, 90% ethanol for two hours, and 100% ethanol overnight, and was cleared by two days immersion in Cedar wood oil. Note that this technique was used for qualitative not quantitative analysis.

## Histology and Immunohistochemistry

The remaining four specimens were immersion fixed in buffered 10% formol saline (BFS), processed, and embedded in paraffin. Sections were cut at 5 μm and stained with hematoxylin and eosin (H&E), Masson's Trichrome, or immunohistochemically with an antibody to α-smooth muscle actin (Dako, Denmark), the latter used to detect myofibroblasts. An avidin-biotin method was used to label the antibody–horseradish peroxidase complex.[19]

## Preparation of Matrices

### Fibrin

Bovine plasma fibrinogen, Fraction 1, type I/S (Sigma, St. Louis, Missouri) was dissolved in DMEM (Gibco-BRL, Life Technologies, Melbourne, Australia) containing 1% penicillin G/streptomycin (CSL, Melbourne, Australia) and 1% L-glutamine (Sigma) at concentrations between 20 and 160 mg/ml. Bovine plasma thrombin (Sigma) was diluted to 5 units/ml in 44 mM calcium chloride. Equal volumes (250 μl) of the solutions were mixed and allowed to clot (this starts to form after 15 sec) at room temperature in a chamber.

For experiments using fibrinolytic agents, aprotinin (Bayer, Melbourne) and tranexamic acid (St. Vincent's Hospital Pharmacy, Melbourne) were added to the fibrinogen solution, to give final concentrations of 3,500 units/ml and 8.5 mg/ml, respectively. Preliminary studies were performed to determine the minimum concentration of fibrin required to form a stable clot in the chamber. Fibrinogen solutions from 10 to 80 mg/ml, with and without antifibrinolytic agents, were placed with a loop in a chamber for 20 min. The chamber was weighed before and after this procedure to determine the fibrin loss.

*Matrigel*

Matrigel (Collaborative Research Inc., Bedford, MA), 10–12 mg protein/ml of DMEM containing 10 μg/ml of Gentamycin, was stored at −20°C, thawed overnight at 4°C, and manipulated using precooled pipettes prior to use.[9] Growth factor reduced (GFR) Matrigel was prepared from the original Matrigel according to the method of Vukicevic *et al.*[20] The protein concentration of GFR Matrigel was found to be approximately 7 mg/ml.

*PLGA*

PLGA (Birmingham Polymers, Alabama, USA) was prepared using a particulate leaching method.[13,17] In essence the PLGA was dissolved in chloroform and NaCl crystals were added. After evaporation of the chloroform the salt was leached from the scaffold leaving non-communicating pores the size of the salt crystals. The PLGA used in this experiment had a pore size of 300–420 μm and a mean porosity of 84%. PLGA was machined in two parts to fit inside the chamber—a base plate containing a groove for the AV loop and a flat disc to cover the loop and base plate. The dimensions of the PLGA discs were 1.4 mm in diameter by 2.5 mm thick. The PLGA was sterilized and pre-wet by the technique of Patrick.[17] They were soaked in 100% alcohol for 30 minutes on a mechanical stirrer before being washed three times for 30 minutes in sterile saline immediately prior to use.

## *Experimental Groups*

Using groups of six rats, unless otherwise specified, the following groups were adopted:

1. controls, comprising chambers with an AV loop but no ECM;
2. fibrin (20 mg/ml), with and without fibrinolytics, and fibrin (80 mg/ml);
3. Matrigel and growth-factor reduced (GFR) Matrigel; and
4. PLGA.

All groups were assessed at four weeks. Additional Matrigel groups were assessed at two and eight weeks, a second PLGA group at two weeks, and a loop-only control ($n = 3$) at time zero.

## *Statistics*

Data are reported as mean ± standard error of the mean (SEM) for the total number of observations, where $n$ denotes the number of rats. Statistical comparisons between groups using analysis of variance and a *post hoc* Dunnett's test were considered significant when $p < 0.05$.

## RESULTS

### Macroscopic Appearance, Weights, and Volumes of New Tissue

The weights and volumes of tissue in the chambers are shown in TABLE 1 and FIGURE 2.

#### Controls

At day 0, AV loops alone weighed 0.045 g and occupied a volume of 0.030 ml. After four weeks a soft tissue mass of pulsating, encapsulated, vascularized tissue of 0.23 g weight and 0.21 ml volume had grown in the chamber.

#### Fibrin

Fibrinolysis commenced immediately upon contact of the AV loop with the fibrin matrix in the chamber. The amount of dissolved fibrin after 20 minutes contact with the loop decreased progressively as the fibrin concentration was increased. At 10, 20, 25, and 80 mg/ml fibrin, 67%, 44%, 42%, and 10% of the total fibrin dissolved, respectively. The presence of antifibrinolytics, aprotinin (7,000 units/ml), and tranexamic acid (17 mg/ml) did not alter these results.

After four weeks incubation, there was no difference in the amount of tissue generated between fibrin groups. The weights of new tissue, excluding residual unincorporated fibrin, were 0.17, 0.16, and 0.15 g, and volumes 0.15, 0.13, and 0.12 ml, for the 80 mg/ml, 20 mg/ml, and 20 mg/ml plus antifibrinolytics groups, respectively. The latter two groups were significantly smaller than control flaps generated with AV loop alone ($p < 0.05$).

TABLE 1. Tissue generation in chamber with arteriovenous loop and selected extracellular matrices after two, four, or eight weeks incubation[a]

| Treatment | Number | Exploration Time (weeks) | Weight (g) | Volume (ml) |
|---|---|---|---|---|
| AV loop at time of insertion into chamber | 3 | 0 | 0.045 | 0.030 |
| Control (AV loop without matrix) | 6 | 4 | 0.23 (0.03) | 0.21 (0.03) |
| Fibrin (80 mg/ml) | 6 | 4 | 0.17 (0.02) | 0.15 (0.02) |
| Fibrin (20 mg/ml) | 6 | 4 | 0.16 (0.02) | 0.13 (0.02) |
| Fibrin (20 mg/ml) plus antifibrinolytics | 6 | 4 | 0.15 (0.02) | 0.12 (0.02) |
| Matrigel | 6 | 2 | 0.32 (0.03) | 0.30 (0.03) |
|  | 6 | 4 | 35 (0.03) | 33 (0.03) |
|  | 8 | 8 | 0.18 (0.02) | 0.16 (0.02) |
| Growth factor reduced matrigel | 5 | 4 | 0.27 (0.02) | 0.24 (0.01) |
| PGLA | 5 | 2 | 43 (0.05) | 38 (0.04) |
|  | 5 | 4 | 0.33 (0.04) | 0.29 (0.04) |

[a]Results are presented as means with standard errors of the mean (SEM) in parentheses.

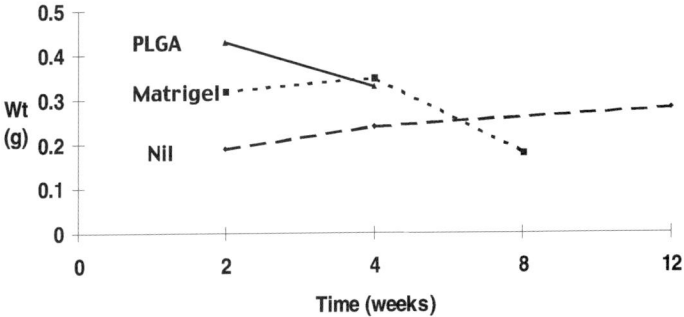

**FIGURE 2.** A comparison of the weight of new tissue generated after 2, 4, 8, or 12 weeks in a chamber containing an arteriovenous loop and the extracellular matrices indicated. Note that historical data were used for the control values at 2 and 12 weeks (see Mian et al.[6]).

*Matrigel*

Addition of Matrigel to the chamber resulted in significantly more tissue, excluding unincorporated Matrigel, after two weeks (0.32 g and 0.30 ml) compared with the flap generated after four weeks with loop alone (0.23 g and 0.21 ml, $p < 0.05$). The amount of tissue generated remained constant up to four weeks (0.35 g and 0.33 ml, $p < 0.01$ compared with control) but decreased to control levels by eight weeks (0.18 g and 0.16 ml, not significant, NS; see FIGURE 3). A small amount of unabsorbed, partly incorporated Matrigel, observed by microscopy to be present within the newly generated tissue, was included in these weight/volume measurements. GFR Matrigel had only a minor effect on the amount of tissue generated after

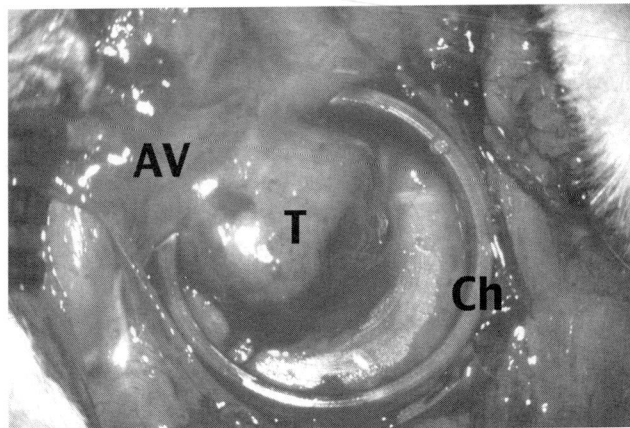

**FIGURE 3.** Macroscopic view of new vascularized tissue formed after eight weeks in Matrigel, showing the tissue (*T*) retracted from the edges of the chamber (*Ch*). The position of the arteriovenous pedicle (*AV*) supplying nutrition to the new tissue is indicated.

four weeks compared with controls (0.27 g and 0.24 ml, NS for weight, $p < 0.05$ compared with normal Matrigel for volume).

*PLGA*

The contents of the chamber after two weeks incubation weighed 0.43 g and occupied 0.38 ml. This was considerably larger than Matrigel at two weeks and the control loop at four weeks. However, since these measurements included a variable and undefined amount of undissolved PLGA, statistical comparison with other groups was not considered appropriate. There was a small decrease in flap size to 0.33 g and 0.29 ml between two and four weeks (NS).

## Histological Appearance

*Controls*

After four weeks incubation alone the AV loop was surrounded by an inner core of mature blood vessels in a collagen-based matrix, with more active tissue on the periphery containing some hemorrhage and immature sprouts (see FIGURE 4). Some inflammatory cells were present. Microfil injection demonstrated good interconnection between loop vessels and new flap vasculature.

*Fibrin*

In all three groups there was a small but well formed flap similar to that developed with the AV loop alone. However, at the periphery there was an intense inflammatory reaction and no capsule formation. Microfil injection demonstrated continuity between the AV loop and the vasculature of the flap, including new vessels at the flap edge. There was negligible penetration of cells or vessels in the residual fibrin adjacent to the new flap.

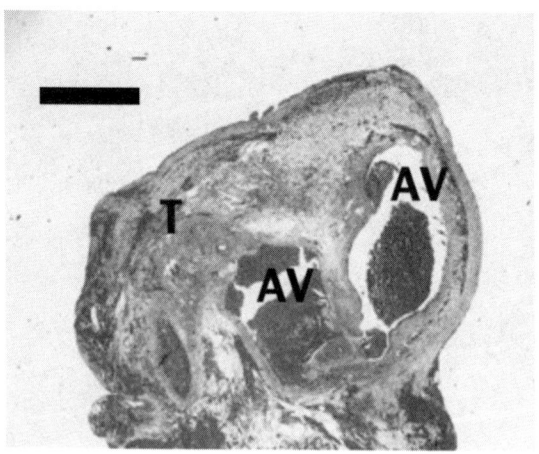

**FIGURE 4.** Controls tissue (*T*) generated with no added matrix at four weeks. Portions of the arteriovenous loop (*AV*) are shown on this section. Stained with Masson's Trichrome; *scale bar*, 320 µm.

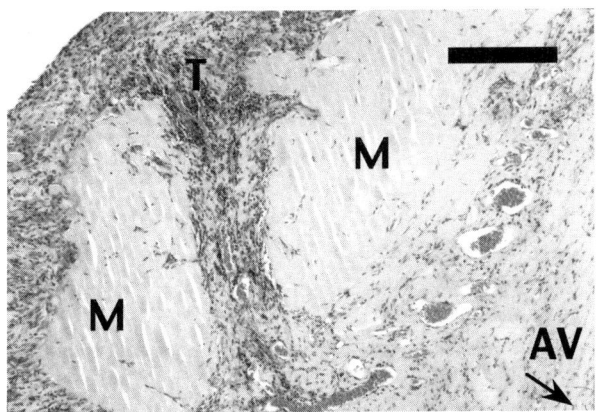

**FIGURE 5.** New tissue formed at four weeks in the presence of Matrigel. There is an extensive cellular infiltration (*T*) between zones of acellular, unincorporated Matrigel (*M*). H & E stained; *scale bar*, 40 μm.

*Matrigel*

At two weeks there were many mature vessels extending to the flap edge, numerous vascular sprouts, and extravasated red blood cells. These vessels were supported in a loose connective tissue matrix and surrounded by areas of unincorporated Matrigel within the flap. By four weeks the density and size of vessels throughout the flap increased; there were fewer extravasated blood cells and small amounts of unincorporated Matrigel

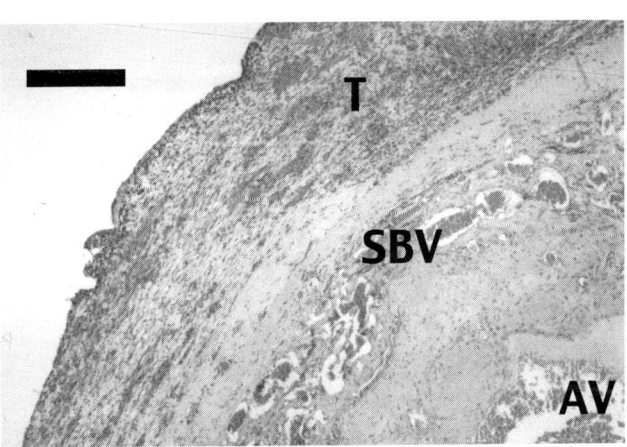

**FIGURE 6.** New tissue formed at eight weeks in the presence of Matrigel. There is a more extensive connective tissue (*T*) compared to the four week specimen. Many small blood vessels (*SBV*) have branched from the AV loop (*AV*). H & E stained; *scale bar*, 120 μm.

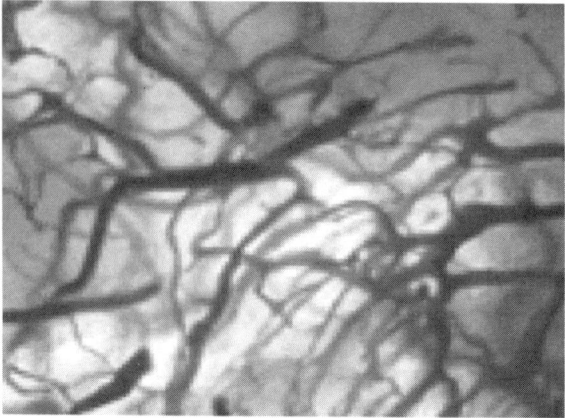

**FIGURE 7.** Microfil injected, cedar wood oil cleared specimen of tissue generated using a Matrigel scaffold at four weeks, showing extensive network of blood vessels. *Scale bar*, 40 µm.

containing leukocytes, fibroblasts, and the occasional vascular sprout (see FIGURE 5). In the eight-week group, tissue appeared more mature with fewer cells, denser collagen, and larger vessels nearer the loop. A capsule had formed around the generated tissue and there was no residual Matrigel remaining (see FIGURE 6). At all times Microfil injection demonstrated good vascular connectivity between the loop and the flap vessels (see FIGURE 7).

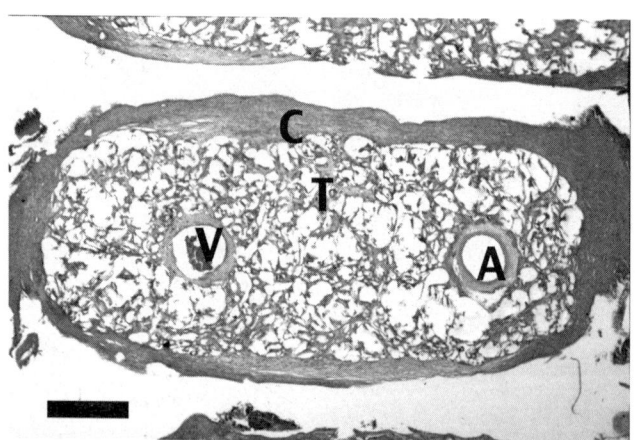

**FIGURE 8.** New tissue (*T*) forming in pores of the unstained PLGA after four weeks incubation. The artery (*A*) and vein (*V*) of the AV loop are clearly visible. Note also the well formed, vascularized capsule (*C*) surrounding the new tissue. H & E stained; *scale bar*, 160 µm.

The GFR Matrigel flap tissue was similar in appearance to larger vessels in the center and less active angiogenesis at the periphery. There was evidence of early capsule formation and leukocytes were present.

*PLGA*

At two and four weeks there was excellent vascular outgrowth to the edge of the PLGA. Residual PLGA was lined by a mononuclear cell infiltrate and the pores in between were filled with a loose connective tissue matrix heavily seeded with myofibroblasts. From two to four weeks the density of the vasculature increased, the amount of residual PLGA decreased, and a thick connective tissue capsule formed at the periphery (see FIGURE 8).

## DISCUSSION

Tissue engineering aspires to the creation of large quantities of vascularized, differentiated tissue. The challenge in this field is to bring together specialized cells, extracellular matrix, and a blood supply in circumstances that promote formation of a functional three-dimensional construct. We have previously reported spontaneous angiogenesis in a chamber model.[2,6] In this study we explored the capacity of various extracellular matrices to modulate this neovascularization. We have shown that new tissue spontaneously generated by placing an arteriovenous loop inside a chamber can be accelerated when PLGA or, to a lesser extent Matrigel, is used as an additional matrix, but inhibited when high concentrations of fibrin are used.

Fibrin has many potential advantages as a tissue engineering matrix. It can support vascular growth *in vitro*[21,22] and is cheap and non toxic. It is the main component of the scaffold on which new tissue grows in a wound or when the loop alone is placed in the chamber.[6,7] Fibrin has been used successfully as a matrix in several models of tissue engineering.[8,23,24] In our *in vivo* model fibrin is unstable because it is subject to degradation by fibrinolytic enzymes as part of the wound healing process and is, therefore, impractical as a tissue engineering matrix. Although this lysis is reduced by increasing concentrations of fibrin and by adding antifibrinolytics,[8] these measures drastically reduce neovascularization. At 20 mg/ml fibrin there was an acceptable degree of fibrinolysis but no augmentation of tissue growth. At 80 mg/ml fibrin there was negligible fibrinolysis, but the fibrin formed an inert mass within the chamber, occupying space and, thereby, preventing further growth of new tissue. Fibrin may be useful at lower concentrations, approximating normal plasma levels (3 mg/ml) and the conditions in the loop alone controls, if fibrinolysis can be prevented. In other *in vivo* models, fibrin was "stabilized" after the addition of cells.[24,25]

Matrigel, a reconstituted basement membrane purified from the mouse tumor, Engelbrecht Swarm Holm sarcoma,[9] has also been shown to support angiogenesis *in vitro*.[10] Its greatest attraction for tissue engineering is that it provides a supportive medium for cultured cells[26] and is likely to be useful for transferring differentiated cells or stem cells into the chamber. Matrigel demonstrates an ability to enhance and accelerate vascular growth *in vivo*. Unrefined Matrigel contains a number of growth factors, including PDGF and TGFβ, that have proangiogenic properties, and this may be partly responsible for the increased vascular growth observed.[20,27] Support for this hypothesis is found in the reduced amount of growth into growth factor reduced Matrigel.[20] From a tissue engineering perspective the greatest disadvantage of Matrigel is that as a mouse tumor product it may not be acceptable for human use. It is, however, useful for development of the concept until a human equivalent, such as "Humatrix"[28] or "Amgel",[29] becomes widely available.

PLGA proved to be the most successful of the three matrices studied, particularly with respect to vascular outgrowth reaching the edge of the chamber within two weeks of implantation. This occurred without the addition of exogenous angiogenic factors. The rate of absorption of PLGA can be modified by varying the proportions of polyglycolic and polylactic acid. PLGA has previously been shown to provide as supportive an environment for cultured cells, notably chondrocytes[15] and preadipocytes.[16] However, the optimal scaffold for our application may involve a combination of PLGA and Matrigel, or new configurations of PLGA.[30] PLGA is already approved by the FDA for human use, for example as suture material (e.g., Dexon®) and for other applications.

In all groups the size of the construct decreased after reaching its maximum size. The exception was the loop only chambers, in which the maximum size of the construct was not reached within the time frame of the experiment. This contracture was associated with the development histologically of a *capsule* surrounding the tissue and the presence of myofibroblasts. In parallel with processes commonly observed in wound healing, myofibroblast-mediated contracture, together with apoptosis of these cells 3–4 weeks postinjury,[31] may be features of this new tissue formed in the presence of PLGA and Matrigel. This capsular tissue may be forming in response to contact with the walls of the hydrophobic polycarbonate chamber.

## CONCLUSION

The presence of Matrigel or PLGA accelerates vascularization and enhances the amount of tissue generated from an AV loop in a chamber. However, this effect is short lived since the amount of tissue eventually decreases, possibly due to exhaustion of the ECM, encapsulation and contraction, or lack of a functional application of the tissue generated. Experiments to increase the size of the chamber, surface coating of the chamber walls, and cellular seeding of these constructs may overcome these limitations. Fibrin has limited use in this tissue engineering model. The AV loop chamber model has proven to be a useful and dynamic means of testing matrices previously tested *in vitro* or in immune compromised animals. Importantly, the vascularized tissue or organoid produced by this method is potentially suitable for replantation or transplantation using microsurgical connection of the attached pedicle blood vessels to blood vessels at the recipient or repair site.

## ACKNOWLEDGMENTS

Thanks to the staff of the Experimental Medical and Surgical Unit, St. Vincent's Hospital Melbourne, for their expert surgical assistance. This study was supported by grants from Transport Accident Commission, National Health and Medical

Research Council (Australia), Particulate Fluid Processing Special Research Center of the Australian Research Council, the Jack Brockhoff Foundation, and the L.E.W. Carty Charitable Fund, Melbourne.

## REFERENCES

1. VACANTI, J.P. & R. LANGER. 1999. Tissue engineering: the design and fabrication of living replacement devices for surgical reconstruction and transplantation. Lancet **354**(Suppl. 1): 32–34.
2. TANAKA, Y., A. TSUTSUMI, D.M. CROWE, et al. 2000. Generation of autologous tissue (matrix) flap by combining an arteriovenous shunt loop with artificial skin in rats: preliminary report. Br. J. Plast. Surg. **53:** 51–57.
3. EROL, O. & M. SPIRA. 1980. New capillary bed formation with a surgically constructed arteriovenous fistula. Plast. Reconstr. Surg. **66:** 109–115.
4. KHOURI, R.K., S.P. HONG, E.G. DEUNE, et al. 1994. De novo generation of permanent neovascularized soft tissue appendages by platelet-derived growth factor. J. Clin. Invest. **94:** 1757–1763.
5. TANAKA, Y., S. TAJIMA, A.TSUTSUMI, et al. 1996. New matrix flap prefabricated by arteriovenous shunting and artificial skin dermis in rats. II. Effect of interpositional vein and artery grafts and bFGF on new tissue generation. J. Jpn. Plast. Reconstr. Surg. **16:** 679–686.
6. MIAN, R., W.A. MORRISON, J.V. HURLEY, et al. 2000. Formation of new tissue from an arteriovenous loop in the absence of added extracellular matrix. Tissue Eng. **6:** 595–603.
7. MIAN, R., K.R. KNIGHT, A.J. PENINGTON, et al. 2001. Stimulating effect of an arteriovenous shunt on the in vivo growth of isografted fibroblasts: a preliminary report. Tissue Eng. **7:** 73–80.
8. SILVERMAN, R.P., D. PASSARETTI, W. HUANG, et al. 1999. Injectable tissue-engineered cartilage using a fibrin glue polymer. Plast. Reconstr. Surg. **103:** 1809–1818.
9. KLEINMAN, H.K., M.L. MCGARVEY, J.R. HASSELL, et al. 1986. Basement membrane complexes with biological activity. Biochemistry **25:** 312–318.
10. NICOSIA, R.F. & A. OTTINELLI. 1991. Modulation of microvascular growth and morphogenesis by reconstituted basement membrane gel in three-dimensional cultures of rat aorta: a comparative study of angiogenesis in Matrigel, collagen, fibrin and plasma clot. In Vitro Cell Devel. Biol. **26:** 119–128.
11. MADISON, R., C.F. DA SILVA, P. DIKKES, et al. 1985. Increased rate of peripheral nerve regeneration using bioresorbable nerve guides and a laminin-containing gel. Exp. Neurol. **88:** 767–772.
12. KAWAGUCHI, N., K. TORIYAMA, E. NICODEMOU-LENA, et al. 1998. De novo adipogenesis in mice at the site of injection of basement membrane and basic fibroblast growth factor. Proc. Nat. Acad. Sci. USA **95:** 1062–1066.
13. MIKOS, A.G., A.J. THORSEN, L.A. CZERWONKA, et al. 1994. Preparation and characterisation of poly(L-lactic acid) foams. Polymer **35:** 1068–1077.
14. ISHAUG-RILEY, S.L., G.M. CRANE-KRUGER, M.J. YASZEMSKI, et al. 1998. Three-dimensional culture of rat calvarial osteoblasts in porous biodegradable polymers. Biomaterials **19:** 1405–1412.
15. CAO, Y., J.P. VACANTI, K.T. PAIGE, et al. 1997. Transplantation of chondrocytes utilizing a polymer-cell construct to produce tissue-engineered cartilage in the shape of a human ear. Plast. Reconstr. Surg. **100:** 297–304.
16. PATRICK, C.W. JR., P.B. CHAUVIN, J. HOBLEY, et al. 1999. Preadipocyte seeded PLGA scaffolds for adipose tissue engineering. Tissue Eng. **5:** 139–151.
17. SHINOKA, T., D. SHUM-TIM, P.X. MA, et al. 1998. Creation of viable pulmonary artery autografts through tissue engineering. J. Thorac. Cardiovasc. Surg. **115:** 536–546.
18. DAVIS, M.W. & J.P. VACANTI. 1996. Toward development of an implantable tissue engineered liver. Biomaterials **17:** 365–372.

19. MESSINA, A., K.R. KNIGHT, B.J. DOWSING, et al. 2000. Localisation of inducible nitric oxide synthase to mast cells during ischemia/reperfusion injury of skeletal muscle. Lab. Invest. **80:** 423–431.
20. VUKICEVIC, S., H.K. KLEINMAN, F.P. LUYTEN, et al. 1992. Identification of multiple active growth factors in basement membrane Matrigel suggests caution in interpretation of cellular activity related to extracellular matrix components. Exp. Cell Res. **202:** 1–8.
21. SALTZ, R., D. SIERRA, D. FELDMAN, et al. 1991. Experimental and clinical application of fibrin glue. Plast. Reconstr. Surg. **88:** 1005–1015.
22. DVORAK, H.F., V.S. HARVEY, P. ESTRELLA, et al. 1987. Fibrin containing gels induce angiogenesis. Lab. Invest. **57:** 673–686.
23. DVORAK, H.F., M. DETMAR, K.P. CLAFFEY, et al. 1995. Vascular permeability factor/vascular endothelial growth factor: an important mediator of angiogenesis in malignancy and inflammation. Int. Arch. Allergy Immunol. **107:** 233–235.
24. WECHSELBERGER, G., T. SCHOELLER, A. STENZL, et al. 1998. Fibrin glue as a delivery vehicle for autologous urothelial cell transplantation onto a prefabricated pouch. J. Urol. **160:** 583–586.
25. MEINHART, J., M. DEUTSCH & P. ZILLA. 1997. Eight years of clinical endothelial transplantation. Closing the gap between prosthetic grafts and vein grafts. ASAIO Journal **43:** M515–M521.
26. EMONARD, H., A. CALLE, J.-A. GRIMAUD, et al. 1987. Interactions between fibroblasts and a reconstituted basement membrane matrix. J. Invest. Dermatol. **89:** 156–163.
27. BROWN, K.J., S.F. MAYNES, A. BEZOS, et al. 1996. A novel *in vitro* assay for human angiogenesis. Lab. Invest. **75:** 539–555.
28. STERNLICH, M.D., P. KEDESHIAN, Z.M. SHAO, et al. 1997. The human myoepithelial cell is a natural tumor suppressor. Clin. Cancer Res. **3:** 1949–1958.
29. XIE, H., T. TURNER, M.H. WANG, et al. 1995. In vitro invasiveness of DU-145 human protate carcinoma cells is modulated by EGF receptor-mediated signals. Clin. Exp. Metastas. **13:** 407–419.
30. WAKE, M.C., C.W. PATRICK, JR. & A.G. MIKOS. 1994. Pore morphology effects on the fibrovascular tissue growth in porous polymer substrates. Cell Transplant. **3:** 339–343.
31. DARBY, I., O. SKALLI, & G. GABBIANI. 1990. Alpha-smooth muscle actin is transiently expressed by myofibroblasts during experimental wound healing. Lab. Invest. **63:** 21–29.

# An Approach to Constructing Three-Dimensional Tissue

IN KAP KO AND HIROO IWATA

*Institute for Frontier Medical Sciences, Kyoto University,
53 Kawara-cho, Shogoin, Sakyo-ku, Kyoto, Japan*

ABSTRACT: The authors propose an approach to constructing three-dimensional tissue with capillaries using cellulose hollow fibers. Fibronectin (FN) was immobilized on hollow fibers to assure cell attachment. Bovine coronary artery smooth muscle cells (BCASMC) and L cells were seeded on FN-immobilized fibers and cultured for an extended period of time. The cells proliferated and formed multicellular layers on the fibers. The hollow fibers were removed by enzymatic digestion using cellulase. The cellulase treatment did not damage L cells, although some cells fell off from the fibers. On the other hand, no deterioration was observed in the BCASMC aggregate structure. The BCASMC aggregates maintained several lumens after removal of the hollow fibers by cellulase digestion. The authors believe that their approach offers a useful method to tissue engineering in preparation of three-dimensional tissue structure.

KEYWORDS: cellulose hollow fiber; FN immobilization; BCASMC; cellulase; three-dimensional capillary structure

## INTRODUCTION

Tissue engineering has attracted significant research attention as a means to yield new biomedical engineering products and applications.[1] Tissue engineering is growing, based on advances in molecular biology, cell biology, biomedical material sciences, and medical engineering. Some of the tissue-engineered products, such as bioartificial skin[2,3] and articular cartilage,[4,5] have been commercialized. Promising results have also been reported in the development of the external ear,[6] esophagus,[7] urethra,[8] and bladder.[9] The common features of these products are thin tissue composed of single or few kinds of cells and poorly organized blood capillaries. Oxygen and nutrients are supplied to cells through the diffusion process from surroundings. We claim that the first approach to tissue engineering has been developed and completed.

Most of natural tissue and organs have a three-dimensional structure, into which blood capillaries intensively penetrate to supply a sufficient amount of oxygen and nutrients to cells in the tissue. A new departure should be made from the conventional approaches to reconstruct such tissues and organs. Although some approaches

---

Address for correspondence: Hiroo Iwata, Institute for Frontier Medical Sciences, Kyoto University, 53 Kawara-cho, Shogoin, Sakyo-ku, Kyoto, 606-8507, Japan. Voice: +81-75-751-4119; fax: +81-75-751-4144.
iwata@frontier.kyoto-u.ac.jp

have been attempted to reconstruct three-dimensional tissue,[10–12] a method to prepare three-dimensional tissue with blood capillaries has not yet been established.

In this paper, the authors present one approach to reconstructing three-dimensional tissue with capillaries using hollow fibers. Cellulose hollow fibers were employed as a substrate for the cell culture. During *in vitro* cell culture, cells proliferated and formed multicellular layers on the hollow fibers. The hollow fibers were removed by digestion using cellulase without damaging living tissue. Tissue with capillaries was obtained.

## MATERIALS AND METHODS

### Materials

Regenerated cellulose hollow fibers (inner radius, 200 μm, outer radius, 230 μm) and cellulase were kindly donated from Japan Medical Supply Ltd. (Hiroshima, Japan) and from Meiji Seika Kaisha Ltd. (Tokyo, Japan), respectively. Sources of other chemicals, culture media and cells are listed here: Regenerated cellulose dialysis membrane from Sanko Pharmaceutical Co., Ltd., (Tokyo, Japan), 2,2,2-trifluoroethanesulfonyl chloride (tresyl chloride) and lyophilized bovine serum fibronectin (FN) from Nacalai Tesque Inc. (Kyoto, Japan), Eagle's MEM culture medium and Dulbecco's PBS(-) from Nissui Pharmaceutical Co., Ltd., (Tokyo, Japan), D-MEM/F12 culture medium from Gibco, BRL, Life Technologies, Inc. (Tokyo, Japan), fetal bovine serum (FBS) from Bio Whittaker (Walkersville, Maryland), sodium L-ascorbate and cell counting kit from Wako Pure Chemical Industries, Ltd., (Osaka, Japan), Trypsin250 from Difco LAB. (Detroit MI), and bovine coronary artery smooth muscle cell (BCASMC) from Cell Application Toyobo (Osaka, Japan).

Fibronectin was immobilized onto regenerated cellulose fibers and membrane discs by the tresyl chloride-activated method.[13] Regenerated cellulose fibers and membrane discs were boiled in water for 30 min to remove impurities. The water was exchanged twice and the fibers dried under reduced pressure. The dried fibers and membrane discs were sterilized by the ethylene oxide (E.O.) gas method. A total of 0.2 g of the dried fibers or membranes were activated in 40 ml of 0.14 M tresyl chloride solution in dry acetone containing 0.5 M dried pyridine at room temperature for one hour while shaking. The reaction products were thoroughly washed with dried acetone to remove free tresyl chloride. The activated products were immersed in 0.1 mg/ml FN aqueous solution under shaking at 4°C for 24 h. After FN immobilization, the FN-immobilized fibers and membranes were washed with phosphate buffered saline (PBS) and Milli-Q water. The membranes were dried under reduced pressure and stored in a drier until used.

Surfaces of regenerated cellulose fibers, tresyl-activated fibers, and FN-immobilized fibers were characterized by X-ray photoelectron spectroscopy (ESCA) using an ESCA 750 spectrometer (Shimadzu Corp., Kyoto, Japan). MgKα X-ray from a magnesium anode source at 8 kV and 30 mA was used and the pressure in the instrument was maintained at $5 \times 10^{-5}$ Pa throughout the analysis. The angle of the electron detector to the film surface was fixed at 90°.

The amount of immobilized FN on the hollow fibers was determined after hydrolysis by amino acid analysis, using a high performance liquid chromatograph

(OPA-NaClO, HPLC) (Tosho Corp., Osaka, Japan).[14] In brief, FN immobilized on the hollow fibers was hydrolyzed to amino acids in a 6 M HCl solution at 110°C for 24 h. Concentrations of amino acids from FN in the resulting solution were quantitatively analyzed by HPLC. Known amounts of FN in PBS were processed by the same procedure to obtain standard chromatograms. The amount of FN immobilized onto the hollow fiber was calculated by comparing peak heights of aspartic acid (Asp), threonine (Thr), valine (Val), isoleucine (Ile), and arginine (Arg) of sample chromatograms with those of standard chromatograms.

To examine the effect of FN immobilization on cell attachment, cellulose film discs of 1.5 cm diameter were used. Fibronectin was immobilized on cellulose films by the procedure mentioned above. A disc was placed in a well of a 24-well culture plate. L cells or BCASMC that were grown to subconfluence on polystyrene tissue culture flask were collected by the trypsin digestion method using a 0.05% trypsin–EDTA solution. 0.3 ml of cell suspension ($4 \times 10^5$ cells/ml) in serum free culture medium was loaded into each well and incubated under 5% $CO_2$ at 37°C for two hours. After a two-hour incubation, the cell-adhered films were rinsed with the serum free culture medium to remove weakly bounded cells and then incubated in culture medium supplemented with serum under 5% $CO_2$ at 37°C. After a certain time culture, the number of cells on the surfaces were determined to examine cell proliferation on the surfaces. The culture media were Eagle's MEM supplemented with 10% FBS for L cells and D-MEM/F-12 supplemented with 10% FBS and 0.05 mg/ml ascorbate for BCASMC, respectively. The number of cells adhered on the films was determined using a cell counting kit (a colorimetric method).[15]

Plain, tresyl-activated, and FN-immobilized hollow fibers were digested with cellulase in 0.1 M acetate buffer solution (pH 4.1), PBS (pH 7.0), MEM with 10% serum (pH 7.0), MEM without serum (pH 7.0), and MEM without glucose or serum (pH 7.0). Cellulose hollow fibers were placed in each well of the 24-well culture plate and 0.4 ml of cellulase solution (8 mg/ml) was loaded. The cellulase solution was exchanged every 24 h. At predetermined periods, the morphology of hollow fiber was observed using a phase contrast optical microscope.

Bundles of 10 hollow fibers were used for the preparation of cell aggregates. Prior to cell adhesion, FN-immobilized hollow-fiber bundles were incubated in PBS in 24-well culture plates for one hour. Phosphate buffered saline was removed before the seeding of cells. One ml of cell suspension ($8 \times 10^5$ cells/ml) in serum free medium was applied to each well. The plates were incubated under 5% $CO_2$ at 37°C for two hours. After that period, the hollow-fiber bundles with cells were rinsed with the serum free culture medium to remove weakly bounded cells, and then moved into a well containing 2 ml of medium with serum and incubated under 5% $CO_2$ at 37°C for predetermined periods. Hollow-fiber bundles carrying cell aggregates, formed after nine days' culture for L cells and 30 days' culture for BCASMC, were placed in new wells. One ml of cellulase solution in serum free medium (8 mg/ml, pH 7.0) was added and incubated under 5% $CO_2$ at 37°C. The cellulase solution was exchanged every 24 h. After two days, the cellulase solution was removed and culture medium with 10% serum was added in each well. The cell aggregates were then cultured for an additional three days. During these processes, morphologies of the cell aggregates were observed using a phase contrast microscope.

Cell aggregates before and after cellulase digestion were fixed with 10% neutral formalin solution, dehydrated with ethanol, and embedded in paraffin. Tissue thin sections with 5 μm were prepared for optical microscopic observation. The sections were stained with Mayer's hematoxylin-eosin solution and Masson trichrome to identify the morphology of cells and the distribution of an extracellular matrix (ECM) inside the cell constructs.

## RESULTS

Procedures to immobilize FN on cellulose hollow fibers are represented in SCHEME 1. Hydroxyl groups on a surface of cellulose fibers were activated by tresyl chloride in acetone for FN immobilization on the surface by immersing the activated fibers in a FN solution. TABLE 1 shows the results of the ESCA analyses of the fiber surfaces in each step. The atomic ratio, F/C, of the tresylated fiber indicates that approximately one tresyl group was introduced per three pyranose groups existing on the surface of the cellulose fiber. By immobilizing FN onto the fibers, although the N/C atomic ratio was expected to increase to 0.2, a clear increase was not observed. A large signal noise might hide the nitrogen signal due to the low signal sensitivity of the nitrogen atom in the ESCA analysis. After the FN immobilization, the F/C ratio decreased to 0.04 indicating co-occurrence of hydrolysis of the tresyl

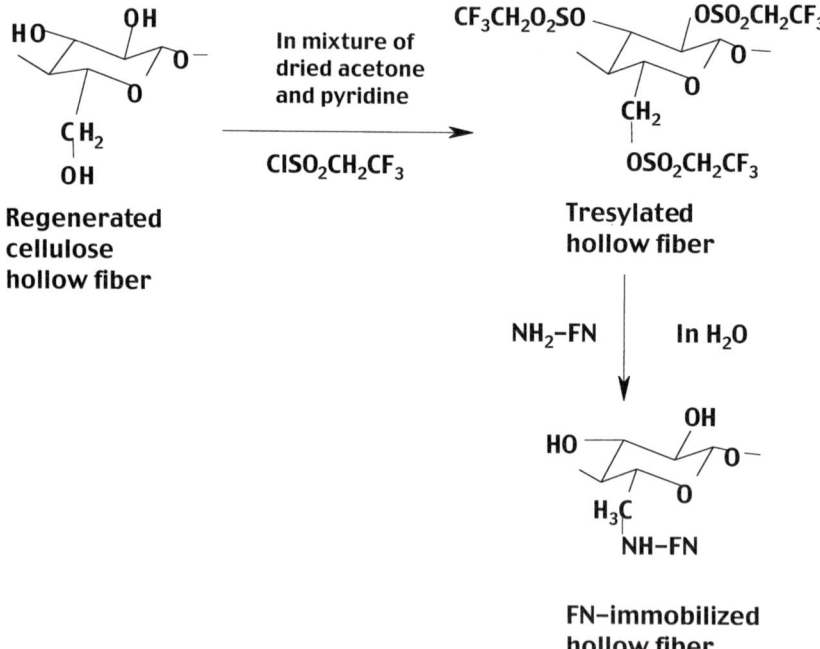

**SCHEME 1.** Immobilization of fibronectin on hollow fiber.

TABLE 1. ESCA analysis

| Sample | Atomic Ratio | | |
| --- | --- | --- | --- |
| | O/C | F/C | N/C |
| Regenerated fiber | 0.65 | 0.02 | 0.03 |
| Tresylated fiber | 0.58 | 0.15 | 0.03 |
| FN-immobilized fiber | 0.68 | 0.04 | 0.04 |

groups during the FN immobilization. The amounts of FN immobilized onto the hollow fibers were determined by amino acid analyses using HPLC. FIGURE 1 reveals the dependence of the immobilized amount on the immersion time of the tresylated fibers in the FN solution. An increase in immobilization is observed with a plateau of 0.15 µg/cm$^2$ reached after 24 hours.

L cells and BCASMC were cultured on unmodified and FN-immobilized cellulose membrane discs to examine the effects of FN immobilization on cell adhesion and cell proliferation. FIGURE 2 shows densities of cells attached on the films. After two hours' incubation in the culture medium without serum, the cell density of BCASMC adhered onto the FN-immobilized film was four times higher than that on untreated cellulose film. L cells and BCASMC proliferated from $6 \times 10^4$ and $5 \times 10^4$ cells/cm$^2$ to $1.6 \times 10^5$ and $1.6 \times 10^5$ cells/cm$^2$, respectively, on the FN-immobilized surfaces during a seven-day culture in media with serum. However, no cell proliferation was observed on the native cellulose films for either kind of cells. Fibronectin immobilization rendered the cellulose membrane suitable for cell culture.

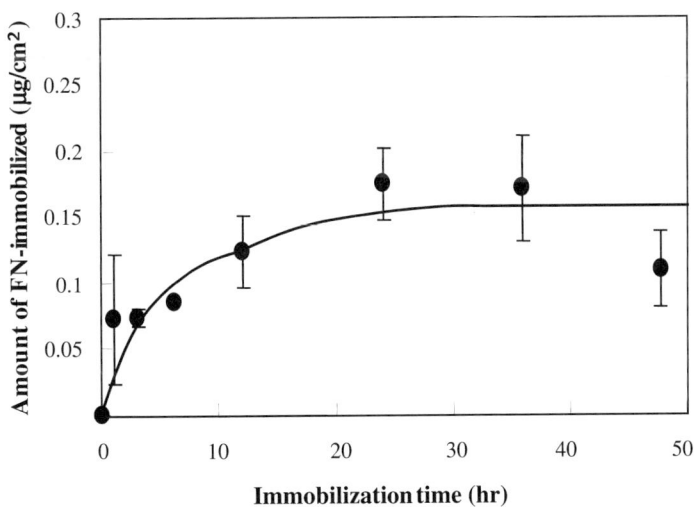

FIGURE 1. Effect of reaction time on the amount of FN immobilized onto hollow fiber.

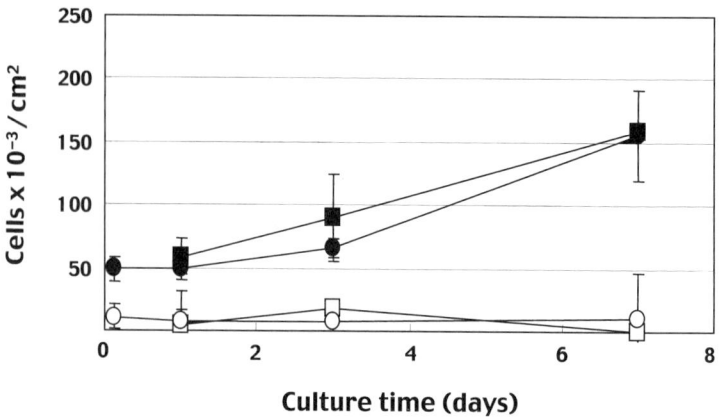

**FIGURE 2.** Growth of L cells and BCASMC on untreated cellulose film and FN-immobilized cellulose film. □, untreated film (L cells); ■, FN-immobilized film (L cells); ○, untreated film (BCASMC); ●, FN-immobilized film (BCASMC).

Morphologies of L cells and BCASMC adhered on hollow fibers were observed using a phase contrast optical microscope. As shown in FIGURE 3(a), L cells did not adhere well to untreated fiber, as indicated by round-shaped morphologies. During a three-day culture in the medium with serum, some cells adhered to the fiber surface, as indicated by flattened shapes. However, most cells took a round shape again and fell off of the fibers during additional days of culture. On the FN-immobilized fibers, L cells adhered well and rapidly proliferated. After nine days' culture, L cells formed 3–4 cell layers on the fibers. During this period, some cells fell from the fibers onto the tissue culture plate and grew on it. FIGURE 3(b) shows the morphologies of BCASMC on FN-immobilized fibers. BCASMC also adhered and grew well on FN-immobilized fibers. After 40 days' culture, BCASMC proliferated and formed multicellular layers in spaces between the fibers. During observation, no cell was dislodged from the fibers onto the culture plate in the case of BCASMC.

TABLE 2. Digestion of hollow cellulose fibers by cellulase in various buffered solutions

| Sample | Buffer Solution | | Culture Medium | | |
|---|---|---|---|---|---|
| | pH 4.1 | pH 7.0 | MEM(−)[a] | MEM(−) | MEM(+) |
| Plain regenerated cellulose fiber | +++ | +++ | ++ | + | ± |
| Tresylated fiber | +++ | ++ | + | + | ± |
| FN-immobilized fiber | +++ | ++ | + | + | ± |

NOTES: +++, completely degraded; ++, virtually degraded; +, small number of fragments observed; ±, partially degraded.

pH 4.1, acetate buffer; pH 7.0, PBS(−) buffer; MEM(−)[a], medium without glucose or serum (pH 7.0); MEM(−), medium without serum (pH 7.0); MEM(+), medium with 10% serum (pH 7.0).

Cellulase solution (8 mg/ml) was exchanged daily.

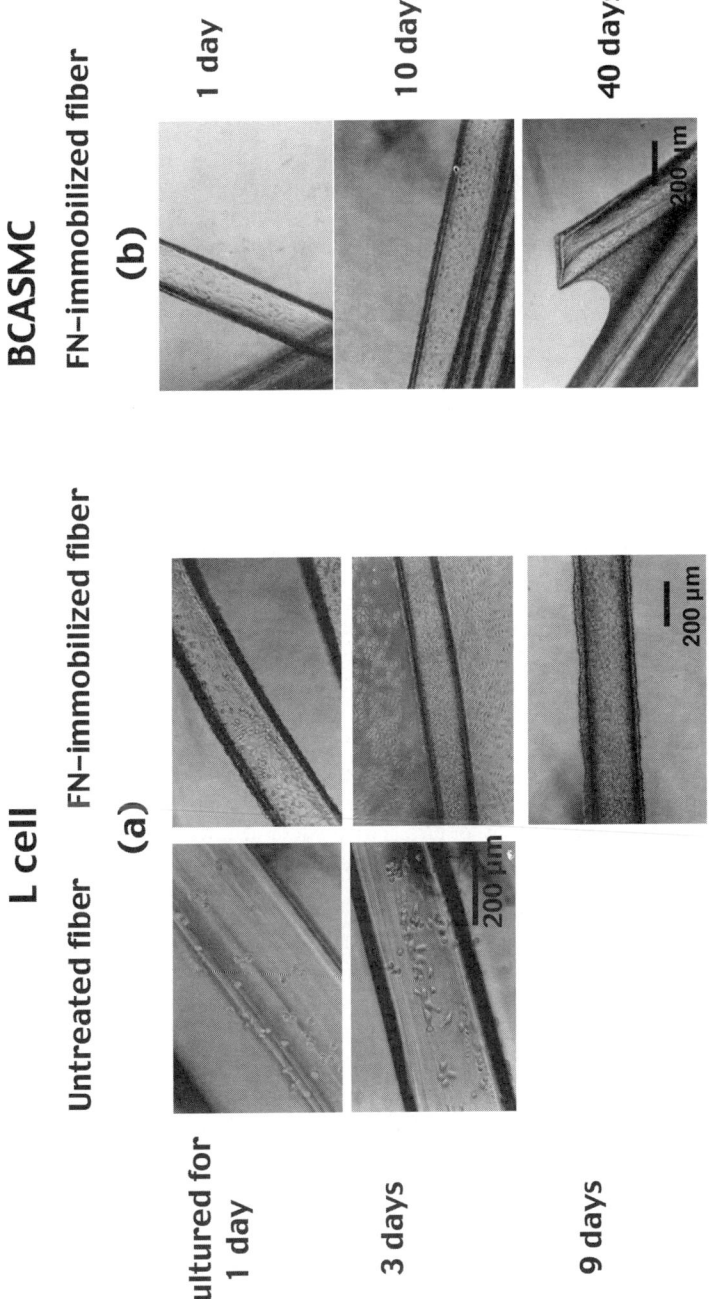

**FIGURE 3.** Optical microphotographs of L cells and BCASMC cultured on untreated fiber and FN-immobilized fiber.

Cellulose fibers should be decomposed and removed to obtain a three-dimensional cell aggregate without a foreign material. Therefore, degradation of cellulose hollow fibers by cellulase was examined in various solutions. The results are summarized in TABLE 2. The cellulase demonstrates the maximum enzymatic activity at pH 4–5. Cellulose hollow fibers were effectively decomposed in acetate buffer solution at pH 4.1 within one day, regardless of chemical modifications of the fibers. In phosphate buffered saline at pH 7.0, more than two days were required to completely decompose unmodified fibers. When chemically modified fibers were exposed to the enzyme solution, tiny particles were still remaining after two days of degradation. In the culture medium supplemented with 10% serum, hollow fibers were partially decomposed during the initial three days, although no apparent further degradation was observed during seven additional days. In culture medium without glucose and serum, the shape of the fibers deteriorated during the initial period (several days) and the degradation continued, although a small number of fragments was found in the reaction mixture, even after seven days.

A BCASMC cell aggregate on a hollow fiber bundle was treated by a cellulase solution and its morphological change was observed using a phase contrast microscope. As shown in FIGURE 4, the aggregate did not change drastically in morphology during two days of treatment. After the cellulase solution was replaced with a new culture medium supplemented with 10% serum, the aggregate was incubated for an additional three days. The BCASMC aggregate slightly contracted during this period. On the other hand, an L cell aggregate on the fibers became unstable and many cells fell from fibers onto the surface of a culture plate during cellulase treatment for one day. These began to proliferate on the plate after the cellulose solution was replaced with new medium with 10% serum. FIGURE 5 presents microphotographs of thin sections of the BCASMC aggregate stained with hematoxylin-eosin and Masson trichrome before and after cellulase treatment, respectively. As seen in FIGURE 5(a), BCASMC formed multi-cellular layers between the fibers. Even after the BCASMC aggregate was exposed to the cellulase solution, no deterioration was observed in its structure. After an additional culture in culture medium supplemented with 10% serum, the aggregate shrunk, although it still maintained several lumens. FIGURE 5(b) shows its thin section stained with Masson trichrome. In the aggregate, BCASMC adhered well to each other and ECM spread over the cell aggregate. It was also observed that most of cells exist on the periphery of the aggregate.

## DISCUSSION

Natural tissue composed of cells having high metabolic rates is well vascularized for sufficient supply of oxygen and nutrient to cells in the tissue. Tissue-engineered constructs from these cells require an adequate supply of nutrient and oxygen, of which the latter is thought to be critical. The tissue construct without blood capillaries leads rapidly to death of most of the cells. Several approaches are being investigated to promote vascularization of engineered tissue. Angiogenic factors such as VEGF and bFGF were locally delivered to promote vascularization of engineered tissue.[16] Endothelial cells were cotransplanted with functional cells to enhance angiogenesis.[17] However, these methods have not been as successful in thick, complex tissues, particularly those comprising the large vital tissue. All of these

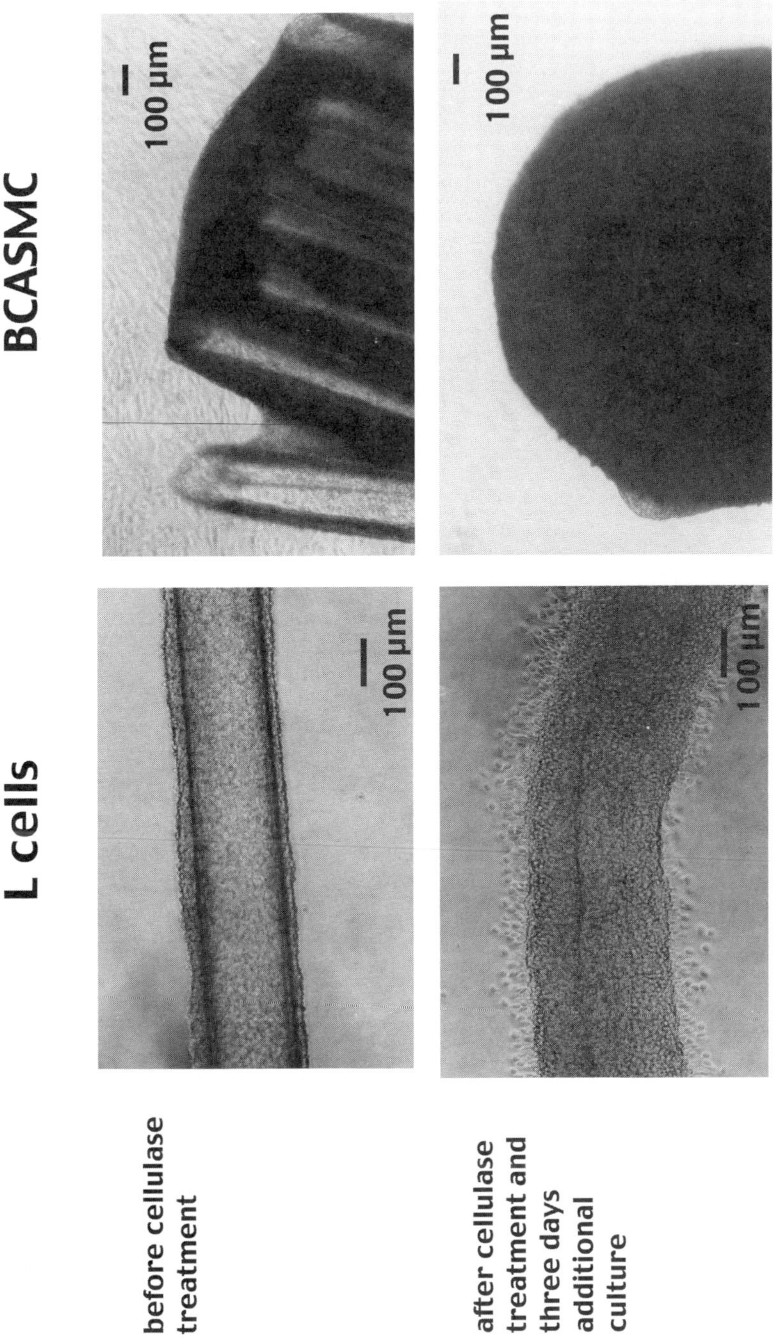

FIGURE 4. Optical microscopic observation of morphology of L cells and BCASMC aggregate on hollow fibers before and after cellulase treatment.

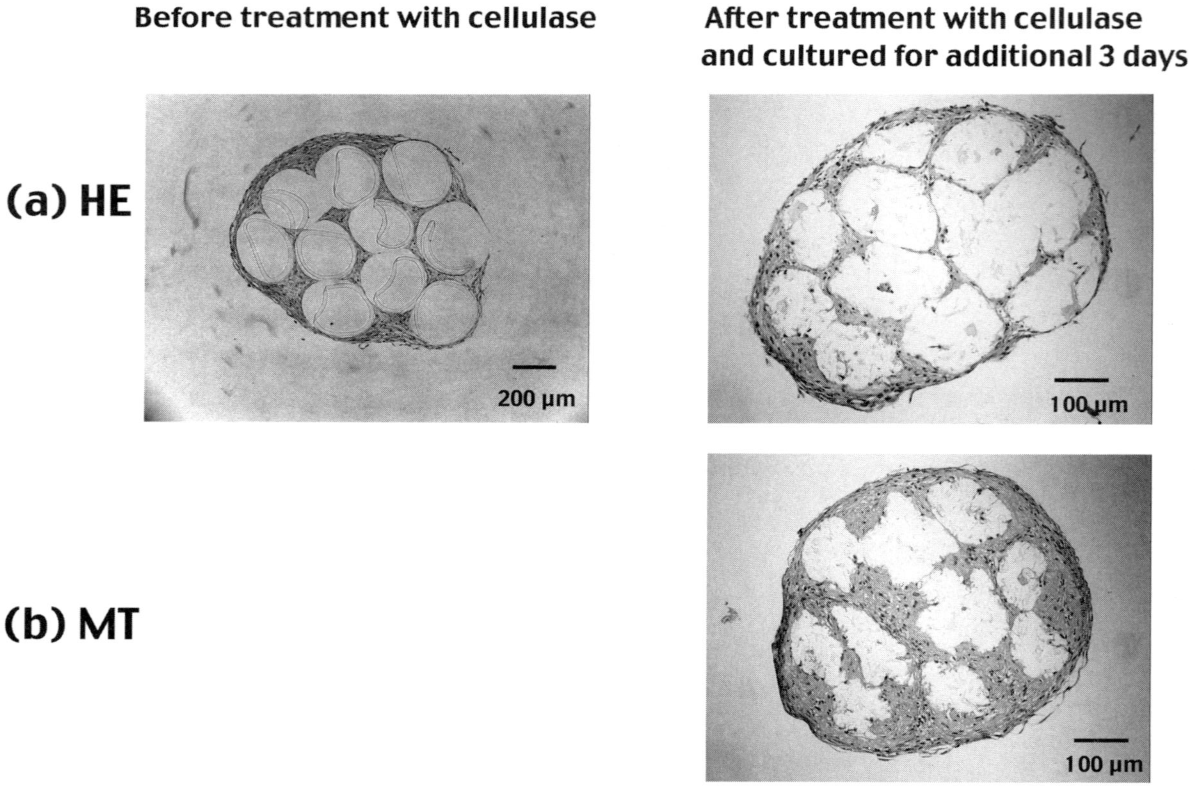

**FIGURE 5.** Various stainings of BCASMC aggregate before and after cellulase treatment.

approaches rely on the in-growth of blood vessels into tissue-engineered constructs to achieve permanent vascularization. Vacanti et al.[18] reported a method to integrate a vascular system into engineered tissue before implantation. Using photolithography techniques, trench patterns reminiscent of branched architecture of vascular and capillary networks were etched onto silicon and Pyrex surfaces to serve as template. Cell monolayers formed on the surfaces were folded into compact three-dimensional tissues. However, they could not generate complex, vascularized, thick tissue. Their method is quite interesting, but it remains preliminary. Scaffolds made of degradable hollow fibers for tissue-engineered constructs seem to offer another promising approach to develop engineering tissue with capillaries without foreign materials.

Biodegradable materials that are used to construct three-dimensional tissues *in vitro* should fulfill several requirements. There should be an appropriate scaffold for cell adhesion and proliferation, and one that can be degraded and removed from tissue. Aliphatic polyesters such as poly(lactic acid) and poly(glycolic acid),[9,11,17,19] alginate-$Ca^{2+}$ hydrogel, and cellulose are candidates for this purpose. Each has merits and disadvantages. Polyesters have been used to prepare scaffolds for tissue-engineered constructs and are approved for medical uses in many countries, but they cannot be removed immediately when the scaffold is no longer needed. Alginate is also approved for medical uses and is easily handled for preparation of hydrogel scaffolds with various shapes by reacting with polyvalent cations, although cells cannot adhere well on these hydrogels.

In this study, the authors examined cellulose hollow fibers to prepare three-dimensional cell aggregates with capillaries. Cellulose has a high density of reactive hydroxyl groups in its structure that can be used for immobilization cell adhesive proteins, such as fibronectin[20] and laminin.[21] Hollow cellulose fibers have sufficient mechanical strength to support a cell aggregate structure. Since mammalian cells do not metabolize cellulose and its related polysaccharides, enzymes that can hydrolyze cellulose are expected not to damage mammalian cells. Such enzymes can be used to remove a cellulose scaffold from a tissue-engineered construct when no longer needed.

Both L cells and BCASMC adhered and proliferated on FN-immobilized fibers. Quasi three-dimensional tissue constructs with capillaries could be prepared from BCASMC using FN-immobilized cellulose hollow fibers and cellulase. In case of L cells, some cells fell from the fiber bundle either during cell growth on the fibers or on cellulase treatment of the cell aggregate formed on the fiber bundle. This might be due to the fact that L cells do not express cadherins.[22] Thus, L cells do not adhere well to each other.

Hollow cellulose fibers used as a scaffold should be degraded and removed to construct three-dimensional tissue without foreign materials. The cellulase used in this study is a mixture of various enzymes. Avlcelase, carboxymethyl cellulase, and endo-1,4-glucosidase in the cellulase used in this study demonstrate maximum activities between pH 4 and pH 5. As expected from these facts, hollow cellulose fibers were effectively degraded in an acetate buffer solution at pH 4.1.[23] However, exposure of a cell aggregate to such a low pH damages cells. Matrices should be treated with cellulase in culture medium at between pH 7 and pH 7.4. As indicated in the caption of TABLE 2, the hollow fibers could be decomposed at pH 7.0, although small fragments remained, even after prolonged treatment. Small fragments of the hollow fibers were also detected in the thin sections of the cell aggregates treated by cellulase, as shown in FIGURE 5.

Various cellulases are commercially available. We are examining these and will select a more suitable cellulase for our purpose. Most cellulases contain endoglucanases and exoglucanases. The former enzyme hydrolyzes the middle of the disordered regions of cellulose and the latter attacks the chain ends of cellulose in the crystalline area. However, the crystalline part is expected to be minimally hydrolyzed. Hollow cellulose fibers with low crystallinity are expected to be easily removed from cell aggregates. They are suitable for our purpose.

Hollow cellulose fibers were used to construct three-dimensional tissue constructs with capillaries. Fibronectin was immobilized on hollow fibers to give cell attachment ability to them. After multicellular layers (BCASMC) were formed on the fiber bundle, the hollow fibers were removed by enzymatic digestion using cellulase. No deterioration was observed in the BCASMC aggregate structure with quasi three-dimensional tissue with capillaries. Although this is a preliminary trial to prepare three-dimensional tissue with capillaries *in vitro*, we believe that our approach will stimulate other research to commence trials.

## REFERENCES

1. R. LANGER & J.P. VACANTI. 1993. Tissue engineering. Science **260**: 920–926.
2. J.F. HANSBURG, J. MORGAN, G. GREENLEAF & J. UNDERWOOD. 1994. Development of a temporary living skin replacement composed of human neonatal fibroblasts cultured in biobrane, a synthetic dressing material. Surgery **115**(5): 633–644.
3. G.D. GENTZKOW, S.D. IWASAKI, K.S. HERSHON, *et al.* 1996. Use of dermagraft, a cultured human dermis, to treat diabetic foot ulcers. Diabetes Care **19**(4): 350–354.
4. M. BRITTBERG, A. LINDAHL, A. NILSSON, *et al.* 1994. Treatment of deep cartilage defects in the knee with autologous chondrocyte transplantation. N. Eng. J. Med. **331**(14): 889–895.
5. T. MINAS & S. NEHRER. 1997. Current concepts in the treatment of articular cartilage defects. Orthopedics **20**(6): 525–538.
6. Y. CAO, J.P. VACANTI, K.T. PAIGE, *et al.* 1997. Transplantation of chondrocytes utilizing a polymer-cell construct to produce tissue-engineered cartilage in the shape of a human ear. Plast. Reconstr. Surg. **100**(2): 297–302; discussion 303–304.
7. Y. TAKIMOTO, T. NAKAMURA, Y. YAMAMOTO, *et al.* 1998. The experimental replacement of a cervical esophageal segment with an artificial prosthesis with the use of collagen matrix and a silicone stent. J. Thor. Cardiovasc. Surg. **116**(1): 98–106.
8. K.D. SIEVERT, M.E. BAKIRCIOGLU, L. NUNES, *et al.* 2000. Homologous acellular matrix graft for urethral reconstruction in the rabbit: histological and functional evaluation. J. Urol. **163**(6): 1958–1965.
9. F. OBERPENNING, J. MENG. J.J. YOO & A. ATALA. 1999. De novo reconstitution of a functional mammalian urinary bladder by tissue engineering. Nat. Biotech. **17**: 149–155.
10. N. L'HEUREUX, S. PAQUET, R. LABBE, *et al.* 1998. A completely biological tissue-engineered human blood vessel. FASEB J. **12**: 47–56.
11. L.E. NIKLASON, J. GAO, W.M. ABBOTT, *et al.* 1999. Functional arteries grown *in vitro*. Science **284**(5413): 489–493.
12. C.A. SUNDBACK & J.P. VACANTI. Alternatives to liver transplantation: from hepatocyte transplatation to tissue-engineered organs. Gastroenterology **118**(2): 438–442.
13. K. NILSON & K. MOSBACH. 1981. Immobilization of enzyme and affinity ligands to various hydroxyl group carrying supports using reactive sulfonyl cholorides. Biochem. Biophys. Res. Commun. **102**: 449–457.

14. Y. HIRANO, Y. KANDO, T. HAYASI, et al. 1991. Synthesis and cell attachment activity of bioactive oligopeptides: RGD, RGDS, RGDV, and RGDT. J. Biomed. Mater. Res. **25**(12): 1523–1534.
15. T. MOSMANN. 1983. Rapid colorimetric assay for cellular growth and survival: application to proliferation and cytotoxicity assay. J. Immunol. Meth. **65**(1–2): 55–63
16. M.H. SHERIDAN, L.D. SHEA, M.C. PETERS & D.J. MOONEY. 2000. Bioabsorbable polymer scaffolds for tissue engineering capable of sustained growth factor delivery. J. Control. Rel. **64**(1–3): 91–102.
17. J.E. NOR, J. CHRISTENSEN, D.J. MOONEY & P.J. POLVERINI. 1999. Vascular endothelial growth factor (VEGF)-mediated angiogenesis is associated with enhanced endothelial cell survival and induction of Bcl-2 expression. Am. J. Pathol. **154**(2): 375–384.
18. S. KAIHARA, J. BORENSTEIN, R. KOKA, et al. 2000. Silicon micromachining to tissue engineer branched vascular channels for liver fabrication. Tissue Engineering **6**(2): 105–117.
19. J. GAO, L. NIKLASON & R. LANGER. 1998. Surface hydrolysis of poly (glycolic acid) meshes increases the seeding density of vascular smooth muscle cells. J. Biomed. Mater. Res. **42**: 417–424.
20. O. NOISET, Y.-J. SCHNEIDER & J. MARCHAND-BRYNAERT. 1999. Fibronectin adsorption or/and covalent grafting on chemically modified PEEK film surfaces. J. Biomater. Sci. Polymer Edn. **10**(6): 657–677.
21. X. YU, G.P. DILLON & R.V. BELLAMKONDA. 1999. A laminin and nerve growth factor-laden three dimensional scaffold for enhanced neurite extension. Tissue Engin. **5**(4): 291–304.
22. M. TAKEICHI. 1988. The cadherin: cell–cell adhesion molecules controlling animal morphogenesis. Development **102**(4): 639–655.
23. P.L. HURST, J. NIELSEN, P.A. SULLIVAN & M.G. SHEPHERD. 1977. Purification and properties of a cellulase from *Aspergillus niger*. Biochem. J. **165**: 33–41.

# Objectively Assessing Bioartificial Organs

D. HUNKELER, A. REHOR, I. CEAUSOGLU, U. SCHULDT, L. CANAPLE,
P. BERNARD, A. RENKEN, L. RINDISBACHER, AND N. ANGELOVA

*Laboratory of Polyelectrolytes and BioMacromolecules,*
*Swiss Federal Institute of Technology, CH-1015 Lausanne, Switzerland*

ABSTRACT: The metrics used, thus far, to assess bioartificial organ function are shown to be subjective and requiring validation. Therefore, four categories of correlations are proposed based on, respectively, device, *in vitro* and *in vivo* evaluations, and clinical function. Examples are presented whereby the correlations among individual indicators are used as a means to expedite the development of immunoisolated cells. Specifically, a case study illustrating the validation of *in vitro* indicators of *in vivo* graft function for the bioartificial pancreas (microencapsulated islets) is summarized. This has revealed thresholds with respect to given metrics relating to *in vivo* device function, the necessity to couple bioartificial organ design with transplant site selection, as well as the lack of objectivity involved in the evaluation and establishment of hypotheses. Specific quantitative indicators illustrate the need for quality-controlled measures, for example, relating to the tolerance of microcapsule diameter and membrane thickness distributions. Qualitative indices representing fibrosis and device properties (e.g., sphericity) are also used to describe the need for *in vitro* experiments in the development of bioartificial organs.

KEYWORDS: bioartificial pancreas; bioindicators; biostatistics; FDA; immunoisolation; microencapsulation; tissue engineering

## INTRODUCTION

The development of bioartificial organs, transplantable devices in which tissue is immunoisolated by non-physiological material barriers, offers the possibility for relatively burdenless therapies for patients suffering from hormone-deficient and neurodegenerative disorders. This includes individuals suffering from Parkinson's and Alzheimer's diseases as well as Huntington's chorea.[1] The *in vitro*, and ultimately *in vivo*, evaluation of the efficacy of such "devices" requires the validation of *indicators*, or *metrics*, that correlate material properties and process conditions to bioartifical organ function. Specifically, given that the large animal and clinical evaluation of bioartificial organs involve lengthy *in vivo* protocols, the experimental design must be parsimonious. Furthermore, the need for enzymatic tissue digestion, based on scarce resources if auto- or allografts are employed, also places cost constraints on the development program. Therefore, the optimization of a transplantable bioartificial organ, including the definition of transplant mass and site,[2] as well as immunobarrier permeability, durability, and size, requires validated metrics.

Address for correspondence: David Hunkeler, Laboratory of Polyelectrolytes and BioMacromolecules, Swiss Federal Institute of Technology, CH-1015 Lausanne, Switzerland. Voice: + 41-21-693-3114; fax: + 41-21-693 5690.
david.hunkeler@epfl.ch

Furthermore, *in vitro* indicators that can be correlated with the *in vivo* metrics that ultimately judge the efficiency of the device will be needed if the field is to advance towards its forecasted potential.

TABLE 1 summarizes the metrics proposed to date for bioartificial organs including the extracorporeal bioartificial liver,[3] somatic gene therapy,[4] and the delivery of dopamine for the treatment of Parkinson's disease.[5] TABLE 1 includes *in vitro* material and microcapsule indicators as well as explant-related measures and semiquantitative parameters characterizing histological analyses. It is evident that a variety of means have been proposed to judge microcapsule mechanical stability in media and buffer (Sections 1–3 of TABLE 1) as well as following explantation (Section 4). Indicators of capsule morphology and permeability complement biological markers of fibrosis, and cellular and humoral immunoreactions with the immunoisolation barriers.

## *Bioartificial Pancreas*

Given the socioeconomic importance of diabetes as the third leading cause of death in developed countries, the bioartificial pancreas, a therapy aimed at providing minute to minute regulation of blood glucose levels via the transplantation of immunoisolated islets of Langerhans, will be employed herein as a case study. Specifically, the means by which *in vitro* metrics can be validated, by using *in vivo* experimentation, will be demonstrated. TABLE 2 summarizes the indicators employed for the immobilization of islets, with sub-categorizations related to the effect of encapsulation material on the tissue, as well as those indicators related to *in vitro* and *in vivo* graft function. There are a set of indicators that are valid only for specific organs. For example, islet stimulation, insulin storage, and glucose tolerance can be applied for the bioartificial pancreas. Alternatively, if one were assessing a different device, such as the extracorporeal bioartificial liver, presently in Phase I/II clinical testing,[6] the *in vitro* analyses of urea and protein synthesis, as well as *in vivo* monitoring of conjugated bilirubin and alanine aminotransferase, mean arterial pressure, survival time, and the grade of hepatic coma, would be essential.[7]

## *Bioindicator Subjectivity*

The metrics to assess bioartificial organ function, listed in TABLES 1 and 2, are widely representative of the indicators currently used in the literature, as well as those applied to justified prior clinical studies. Neither table is intended to be an exhaustive summary. Rather, this paper will demonstrate that the definition of a metric to preassess graft function and the hypotheses for which the metric is used, are subjective unless systematically validated and independently verified. Although the latter may be the norm for scientific results, and FDA evaluations, a call for metric validation in the preregulatory stage is novel.

## RESULTS

There is a maximum of ten interindicator correlations:

Category I: (a) *Device* properties versus *raw material/process* characteristics.

**TABLE 1. Metrics proposed to characterize immunoisolation devices and bioartificial organs**

| No. | Metric | Description of Metric | Ref. |
|---|---|---|---|
| | | 1. Transport and interfacial properties of immunoisolation devices *in vitro* | |
| 1.1 | Permeability | Ingress or egress of standard molecules (e.g., dextran). Quantification of the external concentration of standard proteins. | Brissova[8] |
| 1.2 | Antibody exclusion | Encapsulation protein-A-sepharose (PAS); incubation of capsules with radio-labeled antibody (ab) and measurement of entrapped radioactivity. Non-radioactive labeling (fluoro-chrome) would allow localization of ab. | Wang[9] |
| 1.3 | Molecular exclusion | Encapsulation of PAS pre-incubated with ab specific for test molecule (mol x); incubate with labeled mol x (see Metric 1.2) | Wang[9] |
| 1.4 | Immunoglobulin binding | Rapid screening of immunoisolation material chemistry. | Calafiore[10] |
| | | 2. Mechanical properties of empty capsules *in vitro* | |
| 2.1 | Dry bursting | Measure the force applied to burst the capsule. | Dautzenberg[11] |
| 2.2 | Hypotonic bursting | Idem 2.1 in hypotonic solution; measure corresponding strain (more physiological than Metric 2.1). | Renken[12] |
| 2.3 | Stress-strain hysteresis | Measure loading-unloading curves and the difference between the areas below the curves without capsule rupture. | Renken[12] |
| 2.4 | Force until 60% compression | Measure force-strain until given compression without capsule rupture. | Renken[12] |
| 2.5 | Fatigue at compression | Multiple compression; measure force-strain and compare cycles (loading/unloading) on sequential tests of a capsule. | proposed herein |
| 2.6 | Centrifugation | Measure the gravity force applied by centrifugation for a given time at which a certain amount of capsules break (individual capsule characteristics unattainable). | Dautzenberg[11] |
| 2.7 | Percentage broken capsules | Mix capsules for a given time with glass beads; measure liberated dye indicating burst capsule concentration. | Leblond[13] |
| 2.8 | Load at 50% break | Measure force required to break 50% of the capsules contained between two parallel plates. | Ohtsubo[14] |
| 2.9 | Relaxation time | Measure the time required to recover original shape after a given compression. | proposed herein |
| 2.10 | Osmotic stress | Measurement of capsule size after storage in solution over a range of saline concentrations; determination of salt concentration at which capsules burst due to osmotic pressure. | Van Raamsdonk[15] |

TABLE 1/continued.

| No. | Metric | Description of Metric | Ref. |
|---|---|---|---|
| 2.11 | Stress–strain modeling | Positive aspects: Comprehensive description, universal physical parameters such as Young's modulus. Negative aspects: very complicated, requires assumption on material kind (e.g. Mooney-Rivlin). | Liu[16] |
| 2.12 | Temporal stability | Time-dependent stability in buffer. | Pathak[17] |
| 2.13 | Swelling | Swelling/shrinking in media or saline. | Long[18] |
| 3. Mechanical properties of empty capsules *in vivo* | | | |
| 3.1 | Leakage | Measuring the concentration of an encapsulated test molecule (e.g., ab) in the bloodstream over time post-transplantation. | proposed herein |
| 3.2 | *In vivo* mechanical resistance | Deformation at break and the force-strain curve are measured for explanted capsules. | proposed herein |
| 3.3 | Fibrotic overgrowth | Fibrosis is correlated with microcapsule integrity. | De Vos[19] |
| 4. Post-explantation graft characteristics | | | |
| 4.1 | Fibrosis | Histological observation of the thickness of the fibrotic layer. This can also be measured in terms of the number of cell layers. | Lanza[20] |
| 4.2 | Cellular immunoreactions | Immunohistochemical observation of immune cell infiltration. | Horcher[21] |
| 4.3 | Humoral immunoreactions | Detection of anti-xenograft ab in serum. | adapted standard medical protocol |
| 4.4 | Capsule retrieval | Percentage of retrieved capsules relative to the implanted number. | Lanza[20] |
| 4.5 | Complement | Complement activation. | Berger[22] |
| 4.6 | Explant function | Demonstration of reoccurrence of symptoms following bioartificial organ explant. | Juang[23] |
| 4.7 | Device starvation | Permeability reduction due to fibrotic tissue adsorption. | Burczak[24] |
| 4.8 | Explant permeability | Permeability of generally polymeric explanted immune barriers assessing the influence of implantation on ingress or egress. | Sharkawy[25] |
| 4.9 | Giant cells | The presence of giant cells (fused macrophages) at the tissue/implant interface. | Khuow[26] |

TABLE 2. Metrics proposed to characterize the bioartificial pancreas

| No. | Metric | Description of Metric | Ref. |
|---|---|---|---|
| | | 5. Effect of the encapsulation materials on the pancreatic islets | |
| 5.1 | Cytotoxicity | Incubation of islets in presence of polymer solution and polyelectrolyte complex; measure the release of an internal marker molecule. Cytotoxicity distinguishes necrosis from apoptosis by the choice of markers (e.g., LDH marks cell membrane integrity). | Hunkeler[27] |
| 5.2 | Polymer effect on islet insulin release (static) | Culture islets in presence of polymer solution and polyelectrolyte complex; change glucose concentration in the culture medium; measure insulin concentration in the culture supernatant over time. | Prokop[28] |
| 5.3 | Polymer effect on islet insulin release (perifusion) | Culture islets in presence of polymer solution and polyelectrolyte complex for a defined period of time, followed by perifusion. | proposed herein |
| | | 6. *In vitro* graft function | |
| 6.1 | Tissue pre-selection | Ranking with respect to: lack of histological lesions, lack of lymphocyte infiltration, lack of intraislet capillary congestion, lack of extreme exocrine tissue degradation. | Basta[29] |
| 6.2 | Islet morphology/ ultrastructure | Microscopic observation of islet size, shape. | Warnock[30] |
| 6.3 | Islet number | Count number of islets within ranges of defined diameters; calculate islet equivalents (IEQ). | Warnock[30] |
| 6.4 | Islet purity | Microscopic detection of contaminating tissue. | Warnock[30] |
| 6.5 | Fluorometric assay | Test islet viability using inclusion and exclusion dyes. | Warnock[30] |
| 6.6 | Insulin storage | Immunohistochemical staining of insulin in islets. Quantitative measurements are possible with a CCD camera [32]. | Maki[31] |
| 6.7 | Static insulin release | Change glucose concentration in culture medium; measure insulin concentration in the culture supernatant over time. | Warnock[30] |

TABLE 2/continued.

| No. | Metric | Description of Metric | Ref. |
|---|---|---|---|
| 6.8 | Perifusion | Incubation under continuous flow of perfusate containing variable glucose concentrations; measure insulin concentration in perfusate over time. An assessment of the biphasic nature of the response curve is also often included. | Warnock[30] |
| 6.9 | C-Peptide | Concentration of C-Peptide released into culture medium. | Neerman-Arbez[33] |
| | | 7. *In vivo* graft function | |
| 7.1 | Glycemia | Measurement of blood glucose levels after transplantation into diabetic rats. Diabetes: $\geq 20$ mmol/l; normoglycemia: $\leq 11$ mmol/l. | Lim[34] |
| 7.2 | Glycosylated hemoglobin | Measure glycosylated hemoglobin (HbA1c) levels after transplantation into diabetic mice. | adapted standard medical protocol |
| 7.3 | Glucose tolerance | Measure blood glucose and insulin levels upon injection of glucose (i.v., oral). | Maki[31] |
| 7.4 | Glucose variance | Day-to-day variance in blood glucose level versus the baseline level. | Soon-Shiong[35] |
| 7.5 | Body weight | Monitor body weight of the animal post-implantation. | Lanza[36] |
| 7.6 | Polydypsia | Monitor daily fluid consumption of single mice or groups. | De Vos[37] |
| 7.7 | Polyurea | Measure daily urine volume. | De Vos[37] |
| 7.8 | C-peptide | Plasma based measure representative of integrated glucose level over a period generally spanning approximately one month. | Soon-Shiong[35] |
| 7.9 | Glycosylated albumin | Similar to the measurement of glycosylated hemoglobin, the level of protein glycosylation reflects, in part, the glucose level. In diabetic patients, albumin and hemoglobin, as well as other proteins, are overglycosylated. Following transplantation, the level of glycosylation should return to normal levels. | Soon-Shiong[35] |

Category II: (a) *In vitro* performance versus *raw material/process* characteristics.
(b) *In vitro* performance versus *device* properties.
Category III:(a) *In vivo* function versus *raw material/process* characteristics.
(b) *In vivo* function versus device properties.
(c) *In vivo* function versus *in vitro* performance.
Category IV:(a) *Clinical* followup data versus *raw material/process* characteristics.
(b) *Clinical* followup data versus *device* properties.
(c) *Clinical* followup data versus *in vitro* performance.
(d) *Clinical* followup data versus *in vivo* function.

### *Category I Indicators: Bioartificial Organ Specificity*

An example of a Category I indicator is shown in FIGURE 1, where microcapsule mechanical resistance and permeability are related to the membrane chemical composition. The dependent variables, mechanical resistance and permeability, are fundamental properties of the bioartificial organ that relate to a specific process characteristic (in this case, the polyelectrolyte complex network density) that is itself

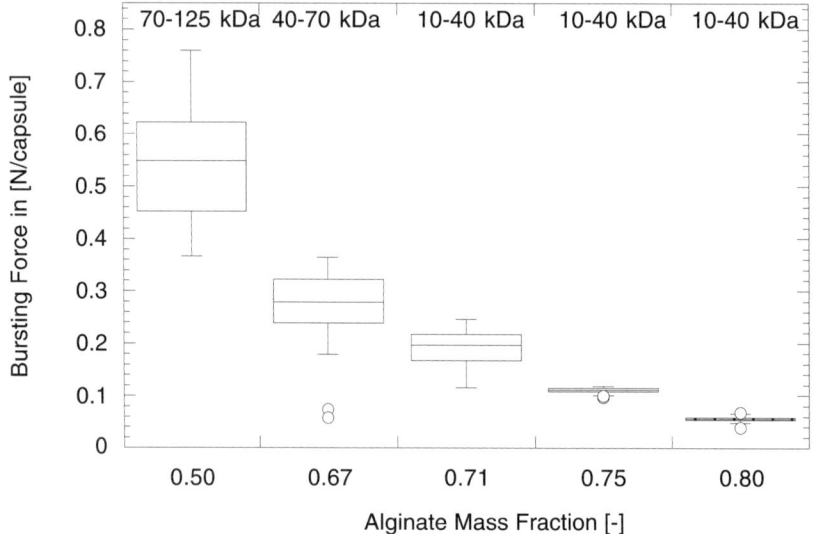

**FIGURE 1.** An example of a Category I indicator correlation showing the relationship between microcapsule mechanical properties and permeability as a function of the composition of the polyanion blend given by its alginate content in the solution used to produce the microcapsule. The microcapsule was produced from a 1.2 wt% sodium alginate/cellulose sulfate solution in sodium chloride, gelled with calcium chloride and reacted with poly(methylene-co-guanidine) hydrochloride in a second reactive step. Data are represented in a box plot where the *rectangle* defines the middle half of the data, with the mean indicated as a *horizontal line* within the box. *Vertical lines* represent the upper and lower quartiles of the data, with discrete data indicating outliers that are not considered in the statistics. For further information, see Reference 12.

governed by the reaction time, solution pH, polymer chemical composition, as well as polymer molar masses and concentrations.[12] Such correlations are the easiest to establish, among the aforementioned seven categories, since they do not require particular caution related to tissue handling, nor do they involve animal experimentation. With such degrees of liberty, an extensive set of rapid and economical experiments can be envisioned to produce Category I correlations. For example, Ma *et al.* have shown that membrane thickness increases with sodium alginate, poly-L-lysine, and calcium chloride concentration, and is reciprocally related to the solution pH and polycation molar mass.[38] Various authors have also demonstrated that capsules based on polyelectrolyte complexes have time-dependent stabilities, under physiological conditions. Category I correlations are clearly non-risky from an ultimate clinical perspective since they are not based on human, or even animal, testing.

## *Semiquantitative Indicators and Quality-Control Issues*

The ultimate clinical use of Category I–III correlations to assess bioartificial organ potential, or functioning, requires the incorporation of elements of statistical process control. Therefore, quality plots such as that shown in FIGURE 2, which illustrates the interbatch microcapsule reproducibility in capsule and membrane diameters, are necessary. Furthermore, the tolerance range, such as the ±10% used for microcapsule diameter control in FIGURE 2A, can be established based on medical criteria and need not be arbitrary. In the case of a bioartificial pancreas intended for intrahepatic transplant, 400-µm microcapsules permit oxygen diffusion to the tissue (maximum distance is 200 µm) and ensure a lack of capillary blockage, while providing 100% islet coverage by the membranes (immunoprotection). In addition, the 10% tolerance corresponds to the maximum volume (20 ml) which can be transplanted into one lobe of the liver. That is, 440 µm (400 µm + 10%) is an upper limit for transplants into the portal vein. Statistical plots such as that shown in FIGURES 2A and B are required as bioartificial organs move through the FDA's clinical testing stages and, in particular, are required to verify the effectiveness of good manufacturing practice (GMP) programs.

Metrics used to assess device properties can also be semiquantitative. For example, a sphericity index has been proposed to quantify the quality of a potential bioartificial organ (see FIGURE 3). Additionally, traditionally qualitative assessments, such as fibrotic reactions to transplanted materials, can be assessed using indices (see FIGURE 4). Both of these metrics will be employed within this paper. Other semiquantitative Category IVa correlations include Calafiore's use of islet purification criteria as metrics of islet morphogenic integrity, as well as *in vitro* and *in vivo* viability.[29]

## *Category IIb and IIIb Indicators:*
## *Correlating Biological Behavior and Device Properties*

A more elaborate means to examine a potential bioartificial organ involves tissue immobilization experiments. For example, FIGURE 5 illustrates the *in vivo* stimulation indices of free islets, 400-µm or 1-mm islet-containing capsules, in response to a glucose stimulation (Category IIb correlation). Category IIa and IIIa correlations are abundant in the literature and include comparison of *in vitro* or *in vivo* data as a function of material chemistry. Clearly, there is a trend in the stimulation index

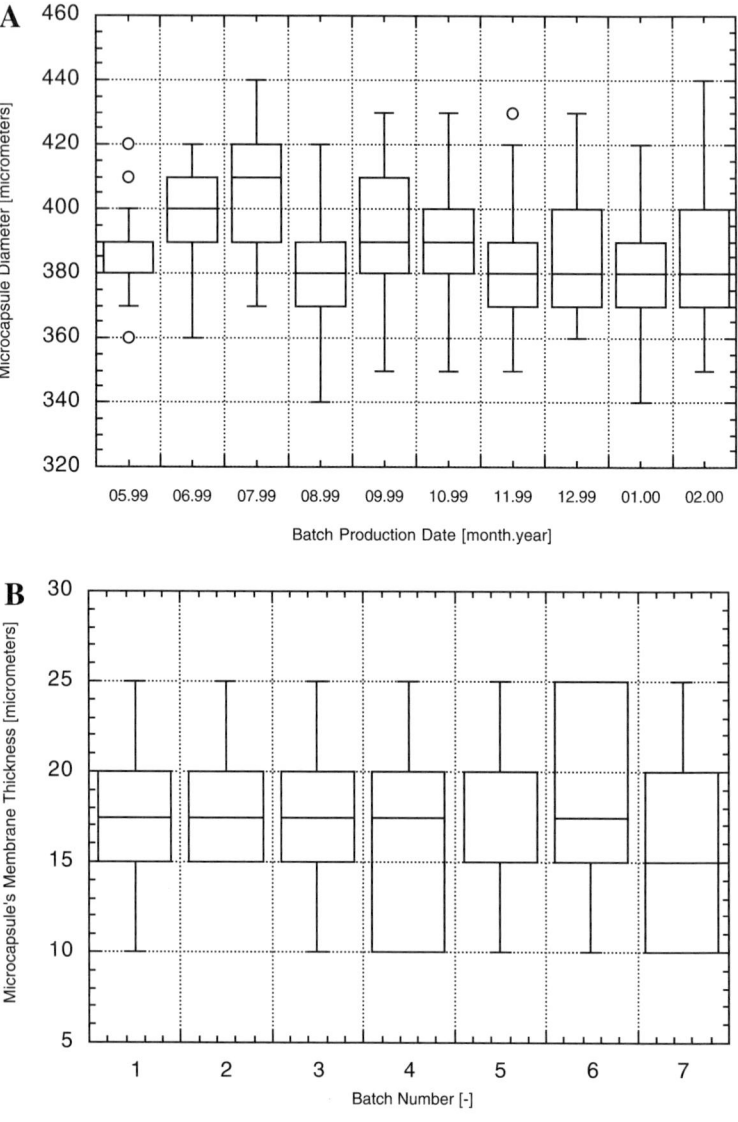

**FIGURE 2.** Quality plots illustrating the interbatch reproducibility of microcapsule diameter (**A**) and membrane thickness (**B**) as a function of batch number. Batches were prepared on subsequent weeks with the dates noted in (**A**) and the batch numbers noted in (**B**). In all cases batches were based on new solutions and a completely recalibrated encapsulation apparatus. The microcapsules were produced, in a two-step process, from 1.2 wt% sodium alginate/cellulose sulfate solution in sodium chloride, gelled with calcium chloride and reacted with poly(methylene-co-guanidine) hydrochloride.

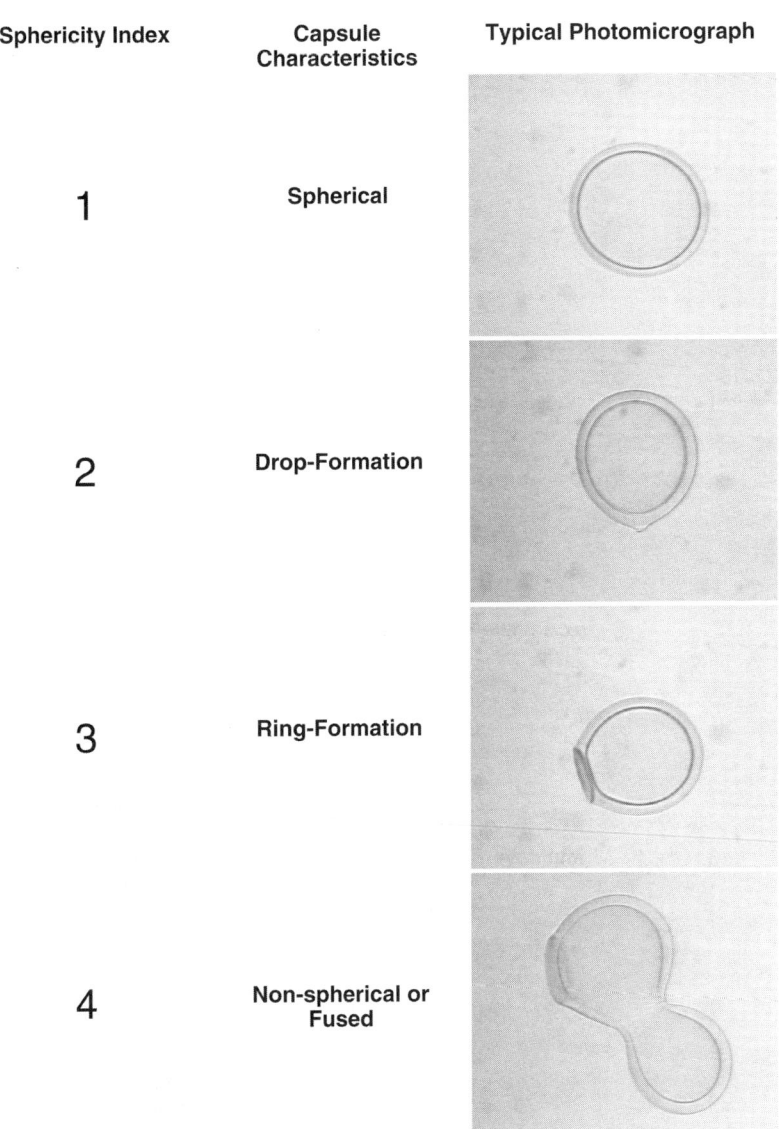

**FIGURE 3.** Photomicrographs illustrating the evaluation of a semiquantitative sphericity index. Drop formation indicates an elongation of one extreme of the microcapsule, whereas a ring designates a flattened surface, usually due to a prolonged reaction at an interface (e.g., air/buffer).

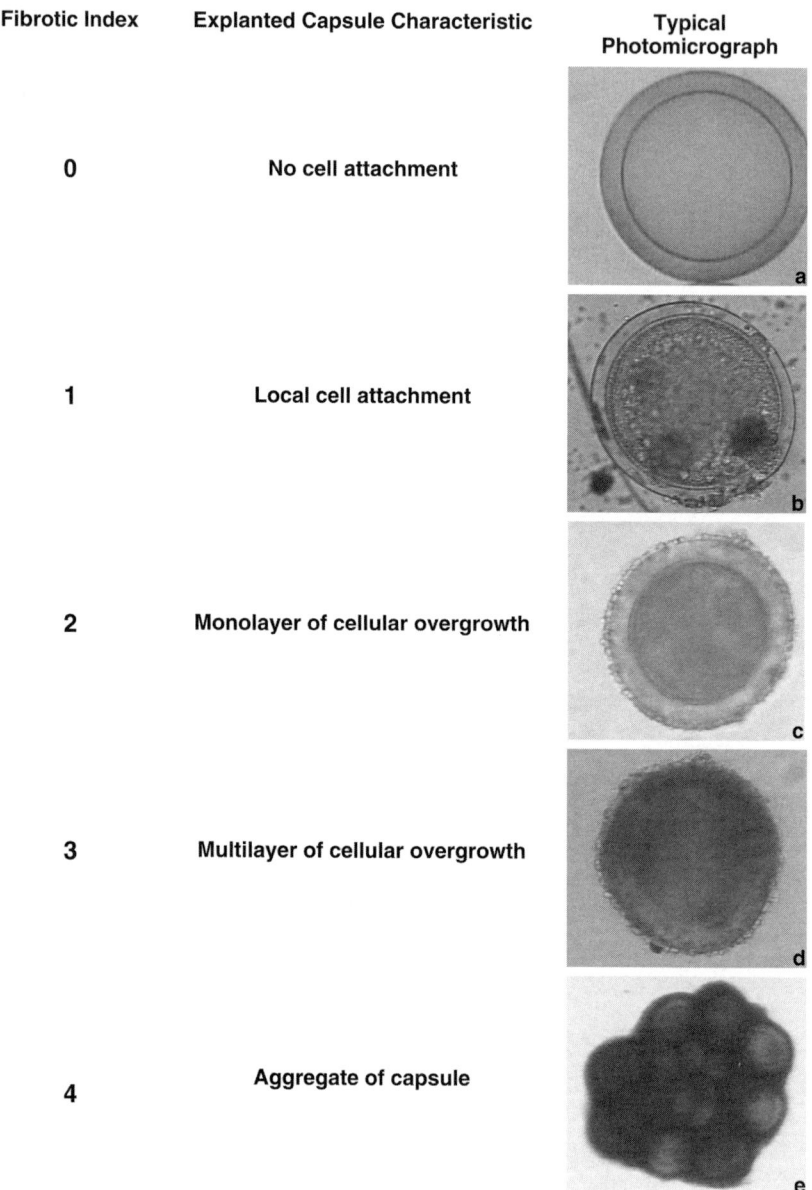

**FIGURE 4.** Photomicrographs illustrating the determination of a semiquantitative fibrotic index.

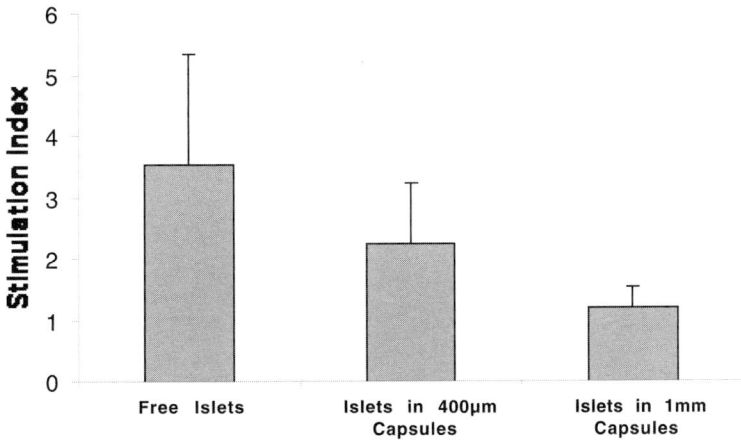

**FIGURE 5.** An example of a category IIb indicator correlation showing the relationship between *in vitro* glucose stimulation index and capsule diameter. Isolated rat islets were encapsulated within multicomponent capsules of 400 μm or 1 mm diameter. The microcapsules were produced from a 1.2 wt% sodium alginate/cellulose sulfate solution in sodium chloride, gelled with calcium chloride and reacted with poly(methylene-co-guanidine) hydrochloride. Two days after encapsulation, glucose stimulation was performed and the released insulin quantified by radioimmunoassay. Stimulation indices were calculated by dividing the amount of insulin released at high glucose (20 mmol/l) by that released at low glucose (5 mmol/l). Islets were considered functional if they had a stimulation index greater than 2.

reported as a function of the capsule size, with larger capsules providing reduced insulin responses. The low stimulation index of islets in 1-mm capsules (1.2 ± 0.35) is probably due to the long diffusion distance for oxygen and nutrients inside the capsule, leading to a poor cellular state.

FIGURE 6 extends the aforementioned experimentation on the effect of microcapsule size to *in vivo* studies. A correlation between the fibrotic index of capsules transplanted intraperitoneally (IP) and the microcapsule diameter is observed (Category IIIb). FIGURES 6B and C are photomicrographs of microencapsulated islets and the corresponding 400-μm microcapsules that were their *in vitro* precursors. The latter were also well tolerated intraportally in large animal models (25-kg mini-pigs),[39,40] indicating that a Category III indicator can be used to identify the optimal transplant site. Specifically, 400 μm appears to be the ideal diameter for internal organ transplantation since there is no serious increase in portal pressure,[39] the oxygen diffusion distance corresponds to the radius of the device and the 400-μm microcapsules are less fibrotic when transplanted intraportally.[41] Fortunately, 400 μm also corresponds to a total transplant volume of 14 ml, which is below the maximum tolerated in one lobe of the liver. Conversely, in the peritoneum, larger microcapsules, with a much smaller surface to volume ratio, are less fibrinogenic, and have even been demonstrated to regulate glucose for extended periods in xenografted rodents[9] whereas the smaller devices, of the same chemistry, are rapidly rejected intraperitoneally (FIG. 6C). FIGURE 6D also validates a Category I indicator, the dependence of microcapsule sphericity on the

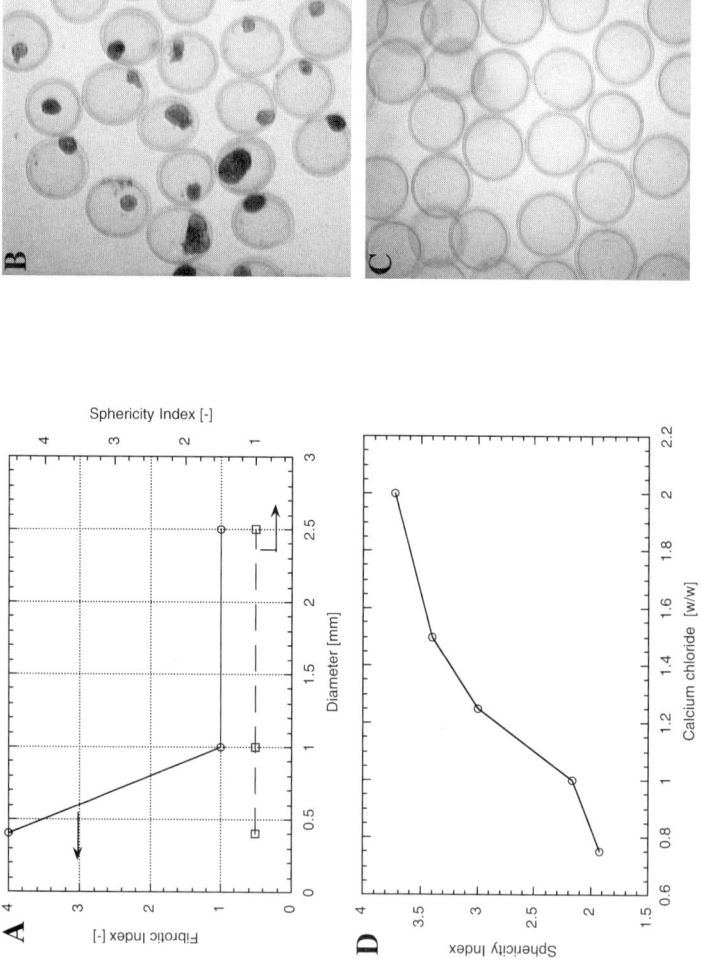

**FIGURE 6.** (**A**) An example of a Category IIIb indicator correlation showing the relationship between the sphericity index (defined in FIGURE 3) and the fibrotic index (defined in FIGURE 4) of an intraperitoneally implanted microcapsule as a function of a device property (capsule diameter). The capsules were produced from a 1.2 wt% alginate/cellulose sulfate solution in sodium chloride, gelled with calcium chloride and reacted with poly(methylene-co-guanidine) hydrochloride. (**B**) and (**C**) represent 400-μm microcapsules, respectively, with and without human islets. (**D**) Illustrates the effect of sodium chloride concentration, in the reaction media, on capsule sphericity. **A** and **D** represent Category IIIb correlations.

sodium chloride level of the reaction medium. Therefore, the use of Category I, II, and III correlations has permitted the authors to determine that the characteristics of a bioartificial pancreas will be transplantation site–dependent. This implies that, from the outset, a bioartifical pancreas will need to be designed with a given transplantation site in mind. Furthermore, a chemistry, or morphology, that works in the intraperitoneum of small animals cannot be applied in internal organs clinically. In this sense, the use of metrics and correlations, such as advocated herein, has strong implications in early stage experimental design.

### *Category IIIc Indicators:* in Vitro–in Vivo *Correlations*

Given that the number of animals available, particularly as tissue donors but also as recipients, limits the number of possible experiments, the use of *in vivo* data for optimization of bioartificial organs remains a tedious, although necessary, task. Therefore, the aim of several research groups is to validate *in vitro* tests with *in vivo* data since *in vivo* graft function is, in the end, the only metric that can be used to justify transplant success. Unfortunately, Category IIIc indicators, although necessary, are absent, to the authors' knowledge, from any of the bioartificial organ studies presented to date in the literature.

One could anticipate a Category IIIc correlation showing the relationship between diabetes reversal and the implant stimulation index. Preliminary data published by various groups indicate that, despite the scatter in the measurements and the lack of statistically significant sample numbers, a threshold in stimulation index below which graft function is not observed may exist. Therefore, the *in vitro* metric (stimulation index) may eventually be validated as an advanced predictor of *in vivo* response. Without such a Category IIIc correlation, the *in vitro* stimulation index is an arbitrary invalidated metric upon which experimental designs and conclusions should not be based. Clearly, a single Category IIIc correlation is not sufficient to replace animal experimentation. However, by prevalidating metrics, the process of bioartificial organ testing and optimization could be expedited.

## DISCUSSION

Should the metrics employed to evaluate bioartificial organs be standardized? The indicators used to assess graft function are clearly tissue- and site-specific. However, prior to the demonstration of concept of a given bioartificial organ, product development costs prohibit extensive experimental design. Therefore, the information that agencies such as the FDA require should be based on statistically validated metrics. The authors of this paper propose the development of Category I–III correlations, such as those described herein, as mandatory means to demonstrate, and validate, graft function. During clinical trials the traditional Category IV correlations[a] used in medical research centers, which relate patient follow-up data to device characteris-

---

[a]Those non-governmental organizations, who are against animal testing, usually base their arguments on the lack of correlation between clinical outcomes and animal model data. Without Category IV correlations the justification for extensive *in vivo* experimentation, which are necessary in bioartificial organ research, becomes questionable.

tics, would serve as the basis for conclusions. Therefore, the present paper *states the case for the need for the standardization of pre-FDA Stage I hypothesis, experimentation, and conclusions. This information should be a required part of the data to be supplied to the accrediting or regulatory organization.*

Metrics to evaluate bioartificial organs are device- and application-specific, implying the need for an evolving list as new therapies are created. The necessity for the definition of biomarkers as diagnostics for graft rejection and acceptance has also been announced. However, with the exception of Waldmann's statements,[b] the question as to which type of committee should regulate metric use has not been debated. Clearly the FDA, in its existing capacity, can deal with the issue of metric subjectivity, and data quality issues. However, the discussions concerning xenotransplantation,[43,44] and genetically modified tissue[45] set a precedence for the creation of international advisory committees. Their composition, and the relation of such committees to regulating bodies poses, if nothing else, a set of legal issues related to the verification and implementation of bioartificial organs.

## CONCLUSIONS

Bioartificial organs promise to provide multibillion dollar health care cost reductions, while improving the quality, and duration, of life. Clearly, the ultimate metrics in assessing either type of product are graft survival and its influence on the reduction in the severity of the associated disease's symptoms. The authors of this paper recommend *the use of validated correlations between* in vivo *and* in vitro *indicators as a means to improve bioartificial organ quality in the pre-FDA phase,* and concomitantly reducing subjectivity and time required for development.[c]

### REFERENCES

1. ROBERTS, T., U. DEBONI & M.V. SEFTON. 1996. Biomaterials **17:** 267.
2. DE VOS, P., D. VEGLER, B.J. DEHAAN, *et al.* 1996. Diabetologia **45:** 1102.
3. NOSÉ, Y., J. MIKAMI, Y. KASAI, *et al.* 1963. ASAIO Trans. **IX:** 358.
4. CHANG, P.L. 1996. Transfus. Sci. **17:** 35.
5. SANBERG, P.R., C.V. BORLONGAN, A.I. OTHBERG, *et al.* 1997. Nat. Med. **3:** 1129.
6. CHEN, S.C., E. KAKAHU, F. WATANABE, *et al.* 1997. *In* Bioartificial Organs. A. Prokop, D. Hunkeler & A. Cherrington, Eds. Ann. N.Y. Acad. Sci. **350:** 1–350.
7. DIXIT, V. & G. GITNICK. 1996. Scand. J. Gastroent. **31:** 101.
8. BRISSOVA, M., I. LACIK, A.C. POWERS, *et al.* 1998. J. Biomed. Mater. Res. **39:** 61.
9. WANG, T., I. LACIK, M. BRISSOVA, *et al.* 1997. Nat. Biotech. **15:** 258.
10. CALAFIORE, R., G. BASTA, P. SARCHIELLI, *et al.* 1996. Acta Diabetologica **33:** 150.
11. DAUTZENBERG, H., B. LUKANOFF, U. ECKERT, *et al.* 1996. Ber. Bunsenges. Phys. Chem. **100:** 1045.
12. RENKEN, A. 2000. Ph.D. Thesis. Swiss Federal Institute of Technology, Lausanne, Switzerland.

---

[b]Establishing tolerance induction as a viable alternative for immunosuppression after organ transplant is, however, a reasonable goal that can be achieved through the cooperation between basic and clinical researchers, regulatory authorities and industry."[42]

[c]The conclusions from this paper were published as a Letter to the Editor in *Nature Biotechnology* **18:** 1021 [2000].

13. LEBLOND, F.A., J. TESSIER & J.P. HALL. 1996. Biomaterials **17:** 2097.
14. OHTSUBO, T., S. TSUDA & K. TSUJI. 1991. Polymer **32:** 2395.
15. VAN RAAMSDONK, J.M. & P.L. CHANG. 2001. J. Biomed. Mater. Res. **54:** 264.
16. LIU, G.G., D.R. WILLIAMS & B.B. BRISCOE. 1996. Phys. Rev. **E54:** 6673.
17. PATHAK, C.P., A.S. SAWHREY & J.A. HUBBELL. 1992. J. Am. Chem. Soc. **114:** 8311.
18. LONG, D. & D. VAN LUYEN. 1996. J. Makromol. Sci. Pure. Appl. Chem. **A33:** 1875.
19. DE VOS, P., G.D.H. WOLTERS & R. VAN SCHIFGAARDE. 1994. Transplant. Proc. **26:** 782.
20. LANZA, R.P., W.M. KUHTREIBER, D. ECKER, *et al.* 1995. Transplantation **59:** 1377.
21. HORCHER, A., T. ZEKORN, U. SIEBERS, *et al.* 1994. Transplant. Proc. **26:** 784.
22. BERGER, M., B. BIOXUP & M.V. SEFTON. 1994. J. Mat. Sci. Mat. in Med. **5:** 622.
23. JUANG, J.H., S. BONNER-WEIR, Y.J. WU & C.G. WEIR. 1994. Diabetes **43:** 1334.
24. BURCZAK, K., E. GAMION & A. KOCKMAN. 1996. Biomaterials **17:** 2351.
25. SHARKAWY, A.A., B. KLIZMAN, G.A. TRUSKEY & W.M. REICHERT. 1997, 1998, 2000. J. Biomed. Mater. Res. **37:** 401 (1997); **40:** 586 (1998); **40:** 598 (2000).
26. KHOUW, I.M.S., P.B. VAN WACHEM, G. MOLEMA, *et al.* 2000. J. Biomed. Mater. Res, **52:** 439.
27. HUNKELER, D., A. PROKOP, A. POWERS, *et al.* 1997. Polymer News **7:** 232.
28. PROKOP, A., D. HUNKELER, M. HARALSON, *et al.* 1998. Adv. Polym. Sci. **136:** 55.
29. BASTA, G., A. FALOUNI, L. OSTICIOLI, *et al.* 1995. J. Inv. Med. **43:** 555.
30. WARNOCK, G.L. 1995. *In* Cell Transplantation. C. Riccordi, Ed. Springer, Berlin.
31. MAKI, T., I. OTSU, J.J. O'NEIL, *et al.* 1996. Diabetes **45:** 342.
32. RULLI, M., A. KUUSISTO, J. SALO, *et al.* 1997. J. Immunol. Meth. **208:** 169.
33. NEERMAN-ARBEZ, M. & P.A. HALBAN. 1993. J. Biol. Chem. **268:** 16248.
34. LIM, F. & A.M. SUN. 1980. Science **210:** 908.
35. SOON-SHIONG, P. 1994. *In* Pancreatic Islet Transplantation III: Immunoprotection of Pancreatic Islets. R.P. Lanza, Ed. R.G. Landes Co., Austin, TX.
36. LANZA, R.P., A.M. BEYER, J.E. STARUK & W.L. CHICK. 1993. Transplantation **56:** 1067.
37. DE VOS, P., B.J. DEHAAN, G.H. WOLTERS, *et al.* 1997. Diabetologia **46:** 262.
38. MA, X.Y., I. VACEK & A. SUN. 1994. Art. Cells, Blood Subst. and Immobiliz. Biotech. **22:** 43.
39. OBERHOLZER, J., C. TOSO & PH. MOREL. 2001. Implantation of microcapsules via the portal vein of pigs. Transplantation. Submitted.
40. OBERHOLZER, J., C. TOSO & PH. MOREL. 2000. Intraportal injection of microcapsules in a large animal model. Personal communication.
41. LEBLOND, F.A., G. SIMARD, N. HENLEY, *et al.* 1999. Cell Transplant. **8:** 327.
42. WALDMANN, H. 1999. Nat. Med. **5:** 1245.
43. BACH, F.H. & H.V. FINEBERG. 1998. Nature **391:** 326.
44. HUNKELER, D., A. SUN, G. KORBUTT, *et al.* 1999. Nat. Biotech. **17:** 1045.
45. BRAMSTEDT, K.A. 1999. TIBTECH **17:** 428.

# Bioartificial Organs in the Twenty-first Century Nanobiological Devices

ALEŠ PROKOP

*Vanderbilt University, Department of Chemical Engineering, Nashville, Tennessee, USA*

ABSTRACT: Bioartificial organs involve the design, modification, growth and maintenance of living tissues embedded in natural or synthetic scaffolds to enable them to perform complex biochemical functions, including adaptive control and the replacement of normal living tissues. Future directions in this area will lead to an abandonment of the trial-and-error implant optimization approach and a switch to the rational production of precisely formulated nanobiological devices. This will be accomplished with the help of three major thrusts: (1) use of molecularly manipulated *nanostructured biomimetic materials*; (2) application of microelectronic and *nanoelectronic interfacing* for sensing and control; and (3) application of *drug delivery and medical nanosystems* to induce, maintain, and replace a missing function that cannot be readily substituted with a living cell and to accelerate tissue regeneration. Biomimetics involves employment of microstructures and functional domains of organismal tissue function, correlation of processes and structures with physical and chemical processes, and use of this knowledge base to design and synthesize new materials for health applications. Nanostructured materials should involve biological materials (rather then synthetic ones) because their prefabricated structure is suitable for modular control of devices from existing materials. Nanostructured tools should encompass surface patterned molecular arrays, nanoscale synthetic scaffolding mimicking the cell–extracellular matrix microenvironment, precise positioning of molecules with specific signals to provide microheterogeneity, composites of bioinorganic and organic molecules, molecular layering (coating), and molecular and supramolecular self-assembly and self-organization (template-directed) assembly. The nanoelectronic interface includes electronic or optoelectronic biointerfaced devices based on individual cells, their aggregates and tissues, organelles, and molecules, such as enzyme-based devices, transport and ion-channel membrane proteins, and receptor–ligand structures, including nanostructured semiconductor chips and microfluidic components. Delivery nanosystems encompass both water and lipid core vehicles (for hydrophilic and lipophilic components) of various geometries: liposomes, micelles, nanoparticles, lipid shells (as imaging and contrasting agents), solid nanosuspensions, lipid nanospheres, and coated film surfaces (molecular layering), all for use in delivering drugs, proteins, cell modifiers, and genes. Nanoelectronic interface and delivery nanosystems will be used for sensing, feedback, control, and analysis of function of bioartificial organs.

KEYWORDS: bioartificial organs; nanobiological devices; outlook

Address for correspondence: Aleš Prokop, Vanderbilt University, Department of Chemical Engineering, Nashville, TN 37235, USA. Voice: 651-343-3515; fax: 615-343-7951.
ales.prokop@mcmail.vanderbilt.edu

## INTRODUCTION

An excerpt from a 1993 lecture on the future of biomaterials states: "Our existing biomaterials, although demonstrating generally satisfactory clinical performance, were developed upon a trial-and-error optimization approach rather than being engineered to produce the desired interfacial reaction."[1] Buddy Ratner proceeds to emphasize the need to develop material science nanotechnology and molecular biology to permit the synthesis of precisely engineered surfaces.

In the author's opinion, the aforementioned evaluation of biomaterials can be translated into future directions of bioartificial organs. The production of rationally formulated prosthetic devices will be accomplished with help of three major thrusts: (1) employment of molecularly manipulated nanostructured biomimetic materials; (2) application of microelectronic and nanoelectronic interfacing technologies for sensing and control; and (3) application of drug delivery nanosystems within existing macro-, micro-, and future nanomedical systems to induce, maintain and replace a missing function that cannot be readily substituted by a living cell. The problems associated with the use of cells and tissues, the main components of bioartificial organs, are not addressed in this review. From this list it can be concluded that a nanoapproach within these three areas is a common denominator, resulting in *nanobiological devices*.

The literature reviewed herein points towards *nanotechnology*, that is, miniaturization, as a major thrust in the coming years (with the exception of extracorporeal devices). There are several reasons for miniaturization in bioartificial organs:

- Some complex specific tissue functions cannot be easily mimicked with presently employed macromaterials and devices.

- To provide implantable biointerface sensing and feedback in mimetic organs, based, for example on secretagogue-triggered hormone release, for cell/tissue implants with impaired sensing capability. Miniaturization of sensors to nano-dimensions decreases typical time constants down to the milliseconds time scale.

- To speed-up functional tissue/organ development by providing localized drug delivery systems, unless a suitable gene is introduced.

- To eliminate effects of often-deleterious physical phenomena by matching the physical relaxation times (time constants) to the reaction constants of cellular phenomena.

The scaling laws that govern the miniaturization of mechanical devices have been studied extensively, although little is known about how miniaturization of cell culture might affect the chemical and physical parameters required for maintaining them *in vitro*. There has been, however, substantial work on scaling bioreactors to larger volumes. Commercial bioreactors have volumes typically from $10^4$ to $10^5$ liters. It is well known that in scaling-up an industrial bioreactor, many physical similarities break down, because certain properties become dominant, such as viscosity or diffusion. For example, when one physical parameter, such as the power input of a mixer in an aerated bioreactor, is fixed, other relationships are considerably disturbed, such as the level of turbulent liquid motion, liquid circulation time, impeller tip speed, and heat transfer.[2] As a result, scaling up a bioreactor can lead to damage to shear-sensitive organisms, such as mammalian cells. Hence, mixing and liquid homogenization times are increased.

A scaled down cell/tissue reactor would benefit from the scaling, or lack thereof, of a number of key physical and biological parameters and phenomena. In particular, there are a number of biological phenomena that occur quite rapidly ($10^{-3}$–$10^{-5}$ sec) at cellular dimensions of 10 μm, such as quiescent mass and heat transfer within the interior of a living cell, but are much slower at the spatial scale of a typical cell culture environment. The dynamic hierarchy of biological systems and subsystems, including physical and biological phenomena, is listed in TABLE 1 in terms of relaxation times or time constants. Those biological processes with very long time constants, such as DNA replication and messenger RNA synthesis ($10^2$–$10^4$ sec) will not benefit from scale-down. However, many cellular processes occur in sub-second, millisecond, and even microsecond intervals, and it is for these processes, that scaling down the size of the physical environment and its concomitant variables to more closely match those of the biological process offers the greatest potential. The real-time dynamics include the faster relaxation times of enzymatic systems, enzyme–substrate–inhibitor interactions, and receptor–ligand interactions, all of which are

TABLE 1. Dynamic hierarchy of physical (reactor) and biological systems (Prokop[2])

| System (subsystem) | Relaxation time, sec |
|---|---|
| Mixing time to homogenize liquid in a large-scale bioreactor (10–100 m$^3$) | $10^4$–$10^8$ |
| Time to exchange liquid volume to 90% level (depending on growth rate) in a continuous reactor | $10^5$–$10^6$ |
| Oxygen transfer (forced, not free diffusion) | $10^2$–$10^3$ |
| Heat transfer (forced convection) | $10^3$–$10^4$ |
| Cell proliferation, DNA replication | $10^2$–$10^4$ |
| Response to environmental changes (temperature, oxygen) | $10^3$–$10^4$ |
| Messenger RNA synthesis | $10^3$–$10^4$ |
| Translocation of substances into cells (active transport) | $10^1$–$10^3$ |
| Intracellular quiescent mass and heat transfer (dimension $10^{-5}$ m) | $10^{-5}$–$10^{-3}$ |
| Protein synthesis | $10^2$–$10^1$ |
| Allosteric control of enzyme action | 1 |
| Glycolysis | $10^{-1}$–$10^1$ |
| Oxydative phosphorylation in mitochondria | $10^{-2}$ |
| Enzymatic reaction and turnover | $10^{-6}$–$10^{-3}$ |
| Bonding between enzyme and substrate, inhibitor | $10^{-6}$ |
| Receptor–ligand interaction | $10^{-6}$ |

TABLE 2. Time constants at scale-down for a stagnant sphere[a]

| Subsystem | Relaxation Time | |
|---|---|---|
| | 2,000 μm | 200 μm |
| Oxygen quiescent (free) diffusion in/from the liquid phase within a sphere[3] | 0.5 sec | 5 msec |
| Heat transfer by convection into/out of sphere[4] | 7.0 sec | 70 msec |

[a] In practice, gradients at the interface facilitate higher transfer rates and shorter relaxation times.

involved in the immediate response of the cell to an external physical or chemical stimuli.

In TABLE 2, results of our calculations on the scale dependence of chemical and thermal diffusion time constants for two reactor sizes are listed: a spherical reaction phase (droplet) with 2-mm and 200-μm diameters (with volumes 24 ml and 24 nl, respectively). As seen from this table, the time constants for oxygen diffusion from these spheres (to achieve about 50% depletion or saturation) and heat transfer time constants (to heat up these spheres from ambient to 50% of the targeted 37°C temperature; no heat source is considered within the sphere) have a strong dependence upon sphere size. This is due to a squared dependency on the droplet size in both cases (e.g., for the oxygen transfer time constant $t = 4R^2 E/D$, where $R$ is the sphere radius, $E$ is a fractional oxygen depletion, and $D$ is oxygen diffusivity in water; for the heat transfer the relationship is similar). The reduction of the linear scale by a factor of ten from 2,000 mm to 200 mm results in a one 100-fold decrease in both relaxation times and provides the ultimate rationale for microminiaturization of the cell culture system: by scaling down, the cell/tissue reactor chemical and thermal time constants are matched to those of the cells. Within such a small-scale reactor, it would be possible to monitor and employ intracellular processes (usually exhibiting much larger time constants) to the benefit of bioartificial organs, and not experience common physical process limitations of a macrodevice. One relevant example involves the reduction in the size of the implant design, whereby one can avoid necrotic zones, due to oxygen and nutrient limitation, within the mass of cells. This is typically encountered with hepatocytes and pancreatic islets, and is a major concern for long term function.

## NANOSTRUCTURED BIOMIMETIC MATERIALS FOR TISSUE CONSTRUCTS

Biomimetics employs microstructures and functional domains of organismal design principles, a correlation of processes and structures with physical and chemical processes, and the use of this knowledge to assemble or synthesize new materials for health applications. The most common method to achieve this goal is by molecular self-assembly. Specifically, biomimetics attempts to simulate:

- Surface topology (polymeric patterning, positional assembly) germane to micro- and nanoenvironment of tissues having significant effects on cell adhesion, migration, function and tissue integration.

- *In vivo* chemical micro-environment (protein and other macromolecular patterning) via surface functionalization of biomaterials.

- Micro- and nanoscale mechanical stresses (mechanophysical patterning) generated by cell–biomaterial interactions, since they may have significant effects on phenotypic behavior (e.g., by using elastomeric materials as substrates to maintain skeletal and heart myocytes, and chondrocytes).

- *In vivo* biological microenvironment (cell patterning) via precise positioning of cells on biomaterials to enable controlled homotypic and heterotypic interactions.

## *Assembly, Self Assembly*

It is unlikely that any process can be developed in the near future to mimic the ability of specific cells to synthesize and organize hierarchical materials with very fine features. However, a hybrid approach of using synthetic matrices, provided that the required mechanical properties and functional characteristics are available and that such matrices are capable of being populated by specific cells for tissue constructs, has been taken by many researchers. Highly functionalized biomaterials with an inherent capability of some natural polymers (such as proteins, polysaccharides, and lipids) and also of some synthetic analogs can be allowed to assemble into structures of a given size and shape to mediate the end-use function. Most often, this formation of systems from individual parts (positional assembly) is driven by local geometry and molecular forces and it does not require any additional external forces. The development of such "smart" materials that, in addition to shape (position), integrate sensing, actuation (secretion), and control, can benefit from lessons learned from biological systems. This knowledge can be useful for design of future generation of bioartificial organs.

Nature uses macromolecular assemblies for the key processes of life, including nucleic acid synthesis, protein (and other biopolymers) synthesis, energy transduction, and control of cell growth and division. Biomimetics then employs biological macromolecules as the building blocks for composite molecular structures and devices. Self-organizing synthesis refers to an assembly of units (parts) in which the units themselves are single molecules, biomolecules, or complex molecular clusters in a predesigned pattern with control over molecular placement (position), orientation, spacing, and interaction, and in which this control is manifested over supermolecular length scales. In self-assembly, the parts move randomly and explore the space of possible molecular orientations. If some particular arrangement is more stable, then it will be preferred and adapted.[5] Molecular assembly is the spontaneous assortment of molecules under equilibrium conditions into stable, structurally well defined aggregates joined by noncovalent bonds.[6] Such assembly relies on weak bonds, such as ionic bonds, hydrogen bonds, hydrophobic interactions, and van der Waals interactions, occurring at the length scales of biological systems. Shape complementarity, determined by size and positioning of functional groups, in addition to the above, plays a dominant role in the stoichiometry and final shape of the assembled architecture.[7] Multiple bonding interactions are often needed to stabilize complex nanostructures. Spontaneous association of a large number of components often results in specific microscopic and nanoscopic structures (films, layers, membranes, vesicles, capsules, micelles, tubes, mesophases, rods, coils, nanoparticles, etc.).[8,9]

On a practical level, relevant to bioartificial organs, a hybrid nanocomposite material compound of inorganic, organic, and bioorganic (biological) bear typically nanometer scale crystals of hydroxyapatite, suitable as a bone substitute,[10,11] are suspended to produce a hybrid composition. Another example involves assembly of diblock or triblock synthetic polymers, generating microphase separation of coiled blocks into regular domains, while macrophase separation is precluded.[12,13] Such structures are suitable for controlled delivery in conjunction with bioartificial organs. The molecular layering (surface coating), resulting from repeated and alternate processing of the surface by an excess of appropriate reagent (often polyelectrolyte or another charged molecule), belongs to a special mode of assembly, template-directed assembly,[14] where a solid template of some particular chemistry is used to create a more complex initial pattern for subsequent self-assembly. Molecular imprinting of synthetic polymers is another example. This method is a process in which functional and polymerizing monomers are copolymerized in the presence of the target molecule, which acts as a molecular template. The functional groups of the monomers are held in position by the highly crosslinked polymeric structure. Subsequent removal of the template by solvent extraction or chemical cleavage reveals binding sites that are complementary in size and shape to the target molecule.[15] The self-assembled monolayers (SAMs) will be mentioned later.

## *Polymer Patterning*

This biomimetic route uses traditional processing methods for preparing polymeric matrices, as well as several more advanced techniques. First, the generation of nanoscale scaffolding (nanofibrous extracellular matrix) is described. It is based on polymer phase separation from a solvent, followed by porogen leaching in water. By using different geometrical porogen elements, made from salt or sugar, very high surface-to-volume ratio matrices are produced with various architectures.[16] A similar method uses thermally induced gelation, followed by solvent exchange and freeze-drying.[17] Another technique involves mechanical or chemical surface treatments to obtain surface roughness 10 to 100 micrometer in size from initially smooth material.[18]

Recently, progress has been made to employ polymers in electronic device manufacturing. The widespread use of polymeric materials arises from their film-forming properties, ease of fabrication, and the ability to synthesize and modify such materials for specific functionalities. Patterning of such polymeric materials at micro- and nanoscale is a key in electronic device manufacturing.[19] This technology also finds use in other areas such as biology and medicine.[20] Of particular interest are functional polymeric micro- and nanostructures that can be prepared via self assembly. Among standard techniques are microlithographic chemical processing, film deposition, etching, bonding, and microinjection molding. The driving force that is behind this development is a demand for precise and improved resolution of chemical patterns.[19]

Microfabrication can sometimes enable devices with novel capabilities. Geometrical control can be very important, for example. The present microfabrication technologies make it possible to pattern varying geometries on the same matrix with a micrometer positional accuracy. As a consequence, a microisland of culture space of defined size (say 50 to 250 µm), each containing different number of cells, can be generated.[21,22] Precise control over the degree of homotypic and heterotypic interactions between hepatocytes and fibroblasts in a coculture was achieved via spatial control[23] (see FIGURES 1 and 2). The author found that liver-specific functions (albumin and urea synthesis) depend on the amount of the heterotypic interface. An *optimal* coculture pattern size (with an appropriate ratio of hepatocytes to fibroblasts) is in the vicinity of 500 micrometers and is amenable to scale-up to a new liver extracorporeal device. Micropatterned substrates (as above) prevent cells from migrating (and from proliferating) and, hence, can keep adherent cells in well defined and stable positions. The lower limit for cell culture pattern size, in general, may be due to their need for proximity to the same or other cell types, sharing diffusive substances and cell–cell contact. This notion is supported by the next example. Progressive restrictions of area where bovine and human endothelial cells are cultured on smaller and smaller micropatterned adhesive islands regulate transition from growth to apoptosis. This observation can also be explained on the basis of the control role of cell shape in cell function.[24] A *contact guidance* of fibroblasts has been studied using grooves 1 µm deep and 1–10 µm wide,[25] or of neural cells on micrometer-sized pillars.[26] For fibroblasts, the dynamics of cytoskeleton polymerization due to mechanical stress was put forward as an explanation.

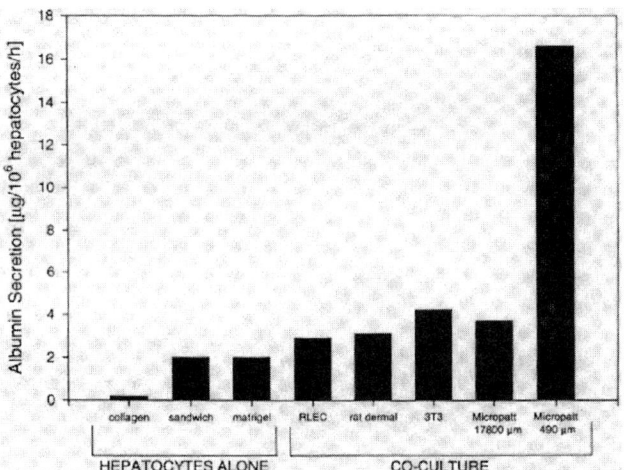

**FIGURE 1.** A comparison of albumin synthesis in hepatocyte culture. The albumin secretion (*last two columns*) is contrasted to other literature data.[23] Collagen, collagen support; sandwich, collagen I support; Matrigel, Matrigel support; RLEC, coculture with rate liver epithelial cells; rat dermal, coculture with rat dermal fibroblasts; 3T3, coculture with 3T3 fibroblast subclones; Micropatt 1,780 µm, coculture islet of 1,780 µm size; Micropatt 490 µm, coculture islet of 490 µm size. (From Bhatia.[23] Reproduced by permission.)

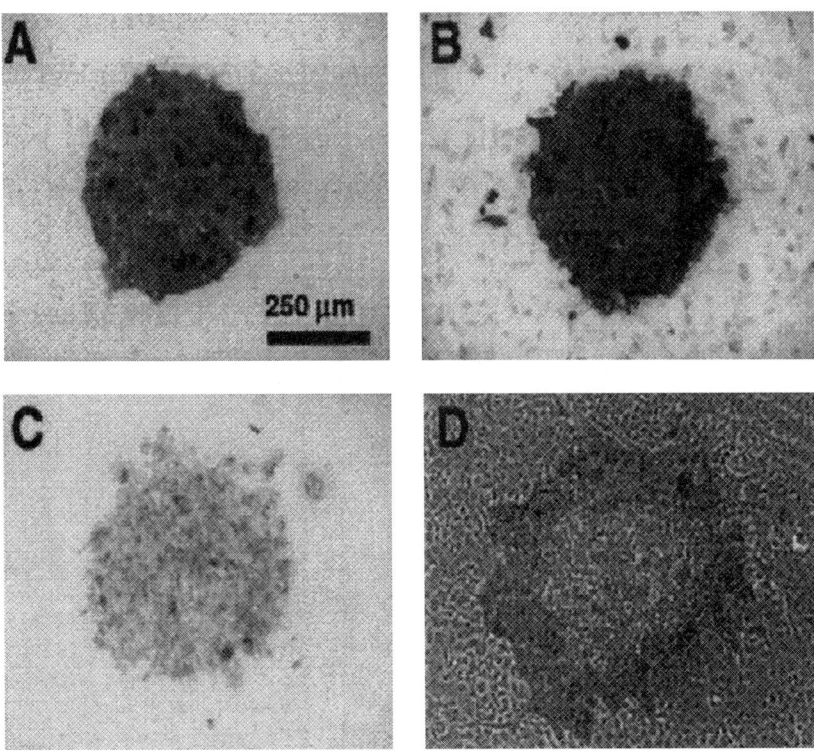

**FIGURE 2.** Immunochemical staining of intracellular albumin in micropatterned hepatocytes and fibroblasts for 490 μm pattern (Bhatia, 1999). Bright-field microscopy of micropatterned hepatocytes (no fibroblasts) on days 1 and 6 (**A** and **C**). Phase contrast micrograph of micropatterned coculture (hepatocytes/fibroblasts) on day 1 and 6 (**B** and **D**) do not display a uniform decline in albumin content on day 6. Fibroblasts in **D** are located on the pattern periphery. (From Bhatia.[23] Reproduced by permission.)

## *Protein Patterning*

This route provides for three-dimensional molecular chemical imprinting resulting in nanometer scale features representing the specific surface molecules, providing highly stable and biospecific surfaces for maintenance of tissue equivalents. Two methods are worth mentioning. One creates an inverse replica of the subcellular (in the specific case subendothelial) extracellular cell matrix (ECM) surface generated by a gentle removal of adhered cells. The lumenal space is then coated with a biocompatible polymeric resin. The resulting replica provides a complex submicrometer topology at the cellular to macromolecular level.[27] This fabrication technology does not preclude the incorporation of materials of biological origin, such as signaling molecules (to be expanded below) and allows the examination of the influence of matrix on cell adhesion and differentiation. Likewise, protein imprinting in polymers was reported.[28] Radio-frequency glow-discharge plasma deposition was used to form polymeric thin films around proteins coated with disaccharide molecules. Following a covalent attachment of disaccharides to polymer film, polysaccharide-like cavities exhibit highly selective recognition site for specific proteins.

Direct two-dimensional protein patterning (in contrast to indirect patterning described above) at a microscale is reviewed in.[29] In this review, examples of patterning using conventional photolithographic methods, photochemistry and self-assembled monolayers (SAMs) are given. S-layer nanopatterning[30] and three-dimensional patterning are discussed as possible future directions. S-layers are crystalline outermost bacterial envelope layers composed of a single protein or glycoprotein species that exhibit a self-assembling property. Protein-patterned materials for cellular systems are considered vehicles for engineering of tissues and organ grafts.[31]

A special case of protein patterning is that providing for proper biological signals. Micropatterning with cell adhesion molecules and growth factors are reviewed in Reference 32. Biomaterials with immobilized signal molecules have a potential to regulate cellular functions and their precise behavior. In some instances, the immobilized signal molecules are more active, as compared to diffusible ones.[33] The immobilization of a growth factor is considered to inhibit the downregulation induced by the cellular internalization of the receptor–signal molecule complex.

### *Mechanochemical Patterning*

Micropatterning of regions of a cell substrate with stimuli-responsive polymers is reviewed in Reference 32. Thermo-responsive polymers can be uniquely used to provide selective cell detachment by temperature and have been exploited in spheroids composed of hepatocytes and fibroblasts as well as keratinocytes and fibroblasts.[34,35] A three-dimensional polymeric elastomeric scaffold, featuring micrometer heterogeneity, was recently described for terminal differentiation of skeletal myoblast culture.[36] The scaffold was fabricated by means of a spin-casting method. Practical utilization of mechanochemical signaling at a micro- and nanometer scales remains open for bioartificial organ applications.

### *Cell Positioning*

The ultimate goal of the bioartificial organ effort should be a control over the spatial assignment of cells to effectively mimic the natural ordering of tissues. Two-dimensional patterns of single cells have been explored (see FIGURE 3) and patterning of two cell types to provide heterotypic interactions has also been suggested.[37] Recently, two- and three-dimensional positioning of multiple cells has been demonstrated with neurite cells[38] (see FIGURE 4). This method, called "laser-guided direct writing", allows parallel processing of a large growth support and may help to identify key cellular and molecular interactions that define organ-specific functions. Such technology, still in its infancy, may form a platform for future hybrid bioartificial organs.

### *Significance of Nanopatterning for Bioartificial Organs*

The previous discussion on nanopatterning of macromolecules demonstrated the importance of intimate substrate (polymer) architecture in the vicinity of cells and

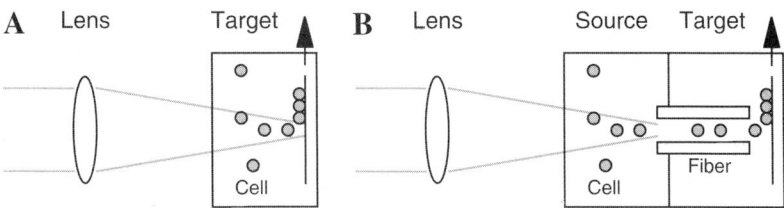

**FIGURE 3.** Laser-guided direct-writing system. (**A**) Laser light is focused weakly into a suspension of cells. The cells are propelled by light through the fluid and deposited on a target surface. (**B**) Light is coupled into a hollow optical fiber and cells are carried through the fiber and deposited. (From Odde and Renn.[38] Reprinted by permission.)

tissues. The presence of any foreign object is always traumatic. It is clear that there are marked differences between implants with smooth and those with coarse surfaces, with the coarse surfaces displaying less necrosis (apoptosis) and reactive capsule formation. The coarse or micropillared surfaces induce less capsule formation, as compared to smooth ones, perhaps, due to differences in the effect of the surface texture on cell phenotype, or differences in mechanical shear.[39] Similar observations were noted for single-polymer filament implants of varying diameters.[40] Stresses on the tissue are higher for large fibers because they are relatively inflexible. Small diameter fibers (a few micrometers) induce a lower activity of surrounding cells (smaller capsule thickness) and smaller inflammatory response (lower macrophage density) compared to thicker filaments of 10–30 μm (see FIGURES 5 and 6). A concept has been proposed to explain these findings which suggest that, below a certain threshold of cell–material contact surface area, there is an insufficient signal from the cytoskeleton and membrane to nucleus to induce an unfavorable cell response. Thin-fiber meshes could, thus, offer an appropriate material for implants, avoiding

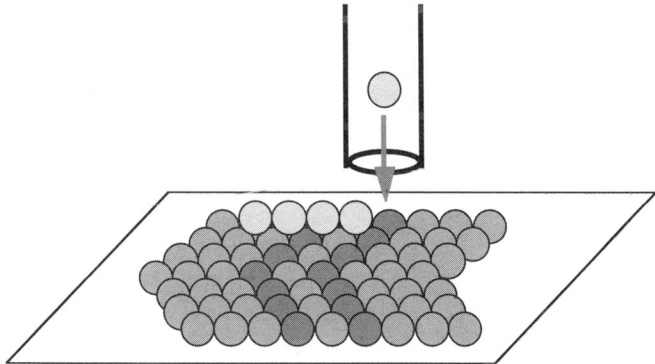

**FIGURE 4.** Schematic illustration of three-dimensional patterning of multiple cell types. ◉, cell type 1; ●, cell type 2; ○, cell type 1. (From Odde and Renn.[38] Reprinted by permission.)

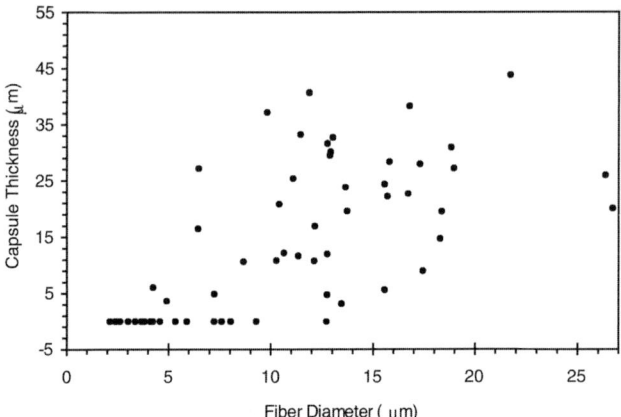

**FIGURE 5.** Capsule thickness in rats for polypropylene fibers of different fiber diameter. Fibers with diameters smaller than 6 μm demonstrate minimal or no fibrous capsule compared with those larger than 6 μm in diameter. (From Sanders et al.[40] Reprinted by permission.)

avascular thick encapsulation. Based on the above discussion, one can conclude that the miniaturization of bioartificial organs would be very desirable. Micro- and nano-patterning technologies may serve as a suitable tool to arrive at acceptable long term therapeutic applications.

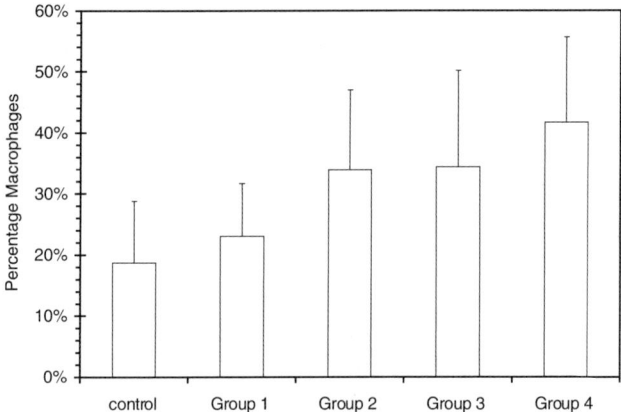

**FIGURE 6.** Macrophage densities for polypropylene fibers of different fiber diameter. Densities expressed as percentage of tissue volume are comparable for control and Group 1, whereas densities for groups 2, 3, and 4 are much larger than the control values. Group 1 (2.1–5.9 μm), Group 2 (6.5–10.6 μm), Group 3 (11.1–15.8 μm), Group 4 (16.7–26.7 μm). Control, no fiber. (From Sanders et al.[40] Reprinted by permission.)

## NANOELECTRONIC INTERFACE TOOLS FOR TISSUE CONSTRUCTS

Nanoelectronic interface tools include optoelectronic biointerfaced devices based on individual cells, their aggregates and tissues, organelles, and molecules, such as enzyme-based devices, transport and ion-channel membrane proteins, and receptor-ligand structures. The sensing elements are typically integrated into nanostructured semiconductor chips and microfluidic components (nanopipetters for fluid dispensing and withdrawal, micropumps, microchannels for fluid flow and splitting, microseparators, and microvalves). Several categories of such sensing tools are visualized:

- Tissue- (cell-) based biosensors on nanoporous silicon.
- Ion-channel-based sensing using reconstituted mimetic or synthetic receptors.
- Cell-based combined sensing and secretion, utilizing a process of secretagogue-induced exocytosis (e.g., immunoprotected allograft or xenograft implant as a sensing and secretory cell).

The need for sensing in bioartificial organs can be addressed by identifying the present status of the regulation of processes that maintain homeostatic balance. Islets appear to be a very good example of an ideal sensor. They respond to several secretagogues (e.g., glucose) and secrete insulin. However, islet cells can partially loose their differentiation characteristics, due to their isolation from the pancreas (damage) or their expansion *in vitro*. Pancreatic endocrine cell lines are characterized by aberrant regulation of hormone production and secretion. It should be stated that only porcine islets respond in a similar way as human islets in terms of response threshold and its dynamics. They may be also imperfect depending on the ontogeny status of the source. Even gene transfer has not yet helped to reconstitute physiological glucose-responsive insulin secretion in these cell lines or islets. If such cells are not responsive to alternations of physiological state or global metabolism, clinical consequences can be devastating. Similar arguments about the responsiveness to special secretagogues can be made for other tissues to be used for bioartificial organ constructs. In the following section, the status of sensing at a micro- and nanoscale is summarized.

### *Tissue-Based Sensing*

This type of biorecognition is based on entire cell/tissue being capable of specific binding to certain chemical species. It should be pointed out that by using this approach the detection limits can be very low because of signal amplification by the intracellular cascading system and that the recognition abilities of cells for substances is unparalleled. As an indicator for measurement of specific substances, several non-specific cellular phenomena can be used: cell growth, substrate uptake, and metabolic product formation (e.g., acidification of media), oxygen uptake (respiration), and heat flux (release). The output signal can be optical, electrical (pH, redox potential, or dissolved oxygen) or via heat release (calorimetry). Similar results can be obtained by means of isolated organelles used as bioreceptors (sensors). Without going into details of their design, a few examples are listed below: a tissue-based biosensor has been proposed using an acidification rate (pH measurement);[41] another uses a heat flux[42] or a combination of heat flux and oxygen uptake;[43] the last employs a microwell array combined with a distal tip of an optical imaging fiber.[44]

### Biomimetic Receptor–Based Sensing

Functionalized biomolecular interfaces that incorporate membrane-associated proteins (MAP) can form the basis for advanced materials that serve as biological sensors.[45] MAP are used as active components to facilitate important cellular processes, such as nerve conduction, energy transduction, active-ion and molecular transport, and cell–cell adhesion (interaction). These proteins are intercalated and firmly tethered within the lipid membrane, in which they are free to laterally diffuse. The employment of biomimetic receptors for sensing involves artificial membrane fabrication. Phospholipids can be allowed to self-assemble into Langmuir-Blodgett layers on a SAM attached to gold or silicon support.[46] MAP can be then integrated into such lipid structures to perform a very specific analysis.[47] Another way of integrating MAP is based on their natural tendency to self-assemble into two-dimensional lattices. Gap junction and S-layer proteins can readily do that.[30] Practical applications already exist.

Cornell et al.[47] have applied, besides MAP, other sensing molecules, such as antibodies, enzymes, DNA, and even synthetic ligands for blood typing, detection of bacteria, virus particles, drugs, and electrolytes. For example, by incorporating $K^+$ ionophore valinomycin into a tethered lipid membrane, potassium release at physiologically relevant concentrations can be measured. Cytion SA (Switzerland) is marketing a multichannel instrument for parallel measurements using lipid-vesicle integrated ion-channels, electrophoretically attached to a silicon chip (see FIGURE 7).[48] This is the first time that a fully automated and miniaturized patch clamp technique has been introduced into commercial use (for drug screening). Rapid progress in this field will also allow direct applications in bioartificial organs. Extracellular calcium sensing G-protein, coupled to calcium-sensing receptor

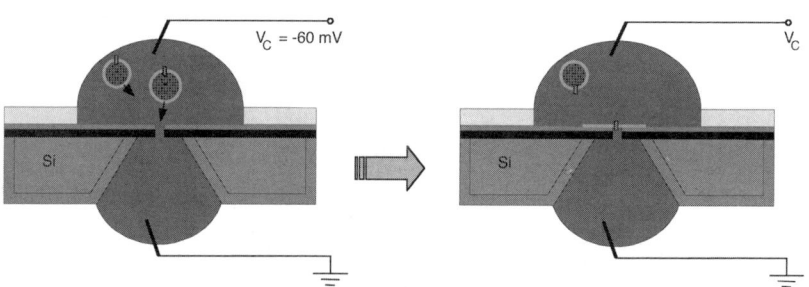

**FIGURE 7.** Schematic diagram of ion-channel based sensor. A fluid compartment is etched into a 400-μm thick silicon chip. The $Si_3N_4$ diaphragm has an aperture between 0.6 to 7 μm in diameter. Ag/AgCl redox electrode is used for voltage application for electrophoretic positioning of lipidic vesicles containing ion-channel protein (left). Once a GΩ seal is formed from the vesicle-derived planar bilayer, an activation of ion-channel via a proper ligand can be detected by means of transmembrane ion current measurement (right). (Reprinted by permission of Cytion SA.)

(CaSR), described in thyroid, has been shown to be functional in pancreatic islet cells.[49] Because the calcium sensing is a part of a complex secretagogue-induced insulin release mechanism, this receptor could be used as a sensing element in conjunction with ion-channel chip design.[50] The applications could involve other tissues where calcium is of importance. The interfacing of such chips into a living implant would pose another problem.

### Cell-Based Sensing/Secretion

The best biosensor/release system is that of transplanted living cells/tissues[51] ("sensor/secretor" cells). It provides substances in a regulated manner. It may not be always optimal due to the possible damage associated with cell isolation prior to implantation and cross-species differences in the threshold levels of sensing. The intricacies of the sensory/secretory systems in transplants have been a quite neglected area.

### Drug Delivery Nanosystems and Accelerated Tissue Regeneration

In many situations, implanted cells do not regenerate into a functional organ or integrate into the existing niche. The environment may not contain the signaling molecules that stimulate regeneration and/or there may be inhibitory signal that directs the cells from a repair pathway. In the absence of knowledge of the inhibitory substances and ways of eliminating these inhibitory signals, the attention is focused on stimulatory substances. The present understanding of factors and mechanisms involved in the cell proliferation and patterning of regenerating tissues is neither complete. The objective of stimulation therapy for regeneration, where it does not occur naturally, is the promotion of full implant integration, involving processes to promote the migration, proliferation, and differentiation of the local regeneration-competent cells. The coupling of a bioartificial organ construct with a delivery system may appear to be beneficial for shortening of the integration period. This is of a great significance for systems where stem cells (progenitor cells) are used as a cellular implant, requiring an environment rich in plethora stimulatory factors for implant mass expansion.

Some examples of accelerated tissue regeneration are known in the bone area (e.g., use of BMP and FGF) to facilitate osteoblast induction and bone regeneration process.[52] Partial functional axon regeneration across spinal cord lesions has been demonstrated with help of FGFa,[53] supplied as an impregnated fibrin matrix. Other example includes vascularization of implants by exogenous supply of VEGF, released from poly(D,L-lactide-co-glycolide) microspheres[54] or gel matrix embedded with FGFb.[55] Carriers have been shown to enhance therapeutic potential of many drugs reducing systemic toxicity, stabilizing the drug, protecting its degradation, decreasing its clearance, and providing effective delivery to a target site.

A brief review of delivery options available at micro- and nanoscale levels is provided below. The substances that can augment the implant integration, in addition to growth factors, include cell modifiers (cytokines), antigens, genes, and other pharmaceuticals (biologics). Delivery vehicles can be broadly classified into three groups: (1) vehicles for water-soluble substances (water-core vehicles); (2) vehicles for water-insoluble substances (lipophilic-core vehicles); and (3) special case of film-coated (tethered) surfaces. Among several technical parameters, the entrapment efficiency, drug loading capacity and release profile are the most important.

The vehicles for water-soluble substances include nanoparticles, micelles, and microspheres made from various polymers.[56,57] Such vehicles can be formulated with the help of:

- diblock or triblock copolymer assembly and drug loading;
- complexing synthetic or natural macromolecules;
- protein emulsification/thermal denaturation; and
- protein emulsification and glutaradehyde crosslinking.

One biocompatible nanoparticulate delivery system was suggested by Prokop et al.[57] This is based on the complexing of multicomponent polymeric systems in absence of drastic chemical reactions or solvents. It is suitable for protein entrapment, with very high loading and bioavailability. These nanoparticles have been tested for administration by various routes, including oral antigen delivery, with very good results. A special mention should be given to another gentle method, based on self-induced gelling of protein mimics (e.g., of silk or elastin).[59–61] Its utility for delivery remains, however, to be demonstrated.

Hydrophobic drug delivery vehicles employ various processing methods:[62–64]

- interfacial polymerization in presence of a solvent or water;
- emulsion polymerization in presence of a solvent;
- emulsification and solvent evaporation;
- emulsification/solvent or non-solvent precipitation (solvent or water);
- self-assembly of hydrophobized polyelectrolytes; and
- high-pressure homogenization for nanosuspension preparation.

Depending on the processing method, the lipophilic-core vehicles assume various geometries: liposomes, micelles, core-corona (core-shell) nanoparticles, lipid nanospheres, and solid nanosuspensions. The process to generate such a system typically involves sonication as well as exposure to organic solvents, high temperature and high concentrations of surfactants. These conditions may promote a therapeutic protein degradation. The main drawback could be the presence of residual solvents in the implanted material and possible toxic breakdown products for some synthetic polymer-based nanoparticles.[65]

The film delivery systems are convenient since they may be used in conjunction with the bioartificial organ constructs. Prokop et al.[58] applied a nonabsorbable polymeric mesh to provide a retrievable support for microencapsulated islets. The mesh material was coated with a polymeric gel, incorporating an angiogenic growth factor. The resulting vascularized bed could be used for a support of implants that require an efficient access to blood supply. The micro- and macrovasculature lasted for several months because of sustained factor delivery. FGF-loaded nanoparticulate vehicle can also be used as an injectable form to encourage angiogenesis.

Problems of gene delivery by means of polymeric systems are reviewed in Reference 66. Formulation may include sponges, gel particles, paste and coating, all providing a sustained-release. Future bioartificial organ products involve regulated therapeutic gene expression, with a low baseline, high induction ratio, and positive control by a small molecule drug, perhaps orally or intravenously delivered.[66] However, gene silencing is considered a threat to the success of gene therapy. Transplantation of modified cells lines (i.e., with a gene transfer) often leads to a rapid diminution of gene expression, following a brief period of a transient (and rather low) expression.[67] Silencing-resistant gene expression constructs remain to be developed.

## CONCLUSIONS

The following conclusions are drawn from the presented literature review:
1. NANO/MICRO-miniaturization at all levels (cellular, sensor, delivery vehicle) will be needed.
2. The provision of a NANO-structured polymeric support environment for cells and tissues is required to better control their phenotype.
3. The provision of cellular mimic detection systems (artificial membranes with receptors and nanoelectric interface capable of full integration into tissues) should be developed.
4. Cell transplantation of "sensor/secretor" cells with a homeostatic mechanism is an optimal means to replace a missing sensory function.
5. The combination of tissue constructs with miniature chemical delivery systems to accelerate tissue development and integration will be common in the near future.

## REFERENCES

1. RATNER, B.D. 1993. Society for Biomaterials 1992 Presidential Address. New ideas in biomaterials science—a path to engineered biomaterials. J. Biomed. Mat. Res. **27:** 837–850.
2. OLDSHUE, J.Y. 1983. Fluid Mixing Technology. McGraw Hill, New York.
3. NEWMAN, A.B. 1931. Trans. Amer. Inst. Chem. Eng. **27:** 203–310.
4. CROSBY, E.J. 1961. Experiments in Transport Phenomena. Wiley, New York.
5. MERKLE, R.C. 1999. Biotechnology as a route to nanotechnology. Trends Biotechnol. **17:** 271–274.
6. WHITESIDES, G.M., J.P. MATHIAS & C.T. SETO. 1991. Molecular self-assembly and nanochemistry: A chemical strategy for the synthesis of nanosystems. Science **254:** 1312–1319.
7. MCGRATH, K.P. & M.M. BUTLER. 1997. Self-assembling protein systems: a model for materials science. *In* Protein-Based Materials, K. McGrath & D. Kaplan, Eds.: 251–279. Birkhauser, Boston.
8. STRUPP, S.I., V. LEBOUHEUR, K. WALKER, *et al.* 1997. Supramolecular materials: self-organized nanostructures. Science **276:** 384–389.
9. DECHER, D. 1997. Fuzzy nanoassemblies: towards layered polymeric multicomposites. Science **277:** 384–389.
10. DU, C., F.Z. CUI, X.D. ZHU & K. DEGROOT. 1999. Three-dimensional nano-HAp/collagen matrix loading with osteogenic cells in organ culture. J. Biomed. Mat. Res. **44:** 407–415.

11. LIU, J., A.Y. KIM, L.Q. WANG, et al. 1996. Self-assembly in the synthesis of ceramic materials and composites. Advan. Coll. Interface Sci. **69:** 131–180.
12. MUTHUKUMAR, M. C.K. OBER & E.L. THOMAS. 1997. Competing interactions and levels of ordering in self-organizing polymeric materials. Science **277:** 1225–1232.
13. CHEN, J.T., E.L. THOMAS, C.K. OBER & G.-P. MOO. 1996. Self-assembled smectic phases in rod-coil block copolymers. Science **273:** 343–346.
14. LAVAL, J.-M., J. CHOPINEAU & D. THOMAS. 1995. Nanotechnology: R&D challenges and opportunities for application in biotechnology. Trends Biotechnol. **13:** 474–481.
15. HAUPT, K. & K. MOSBACH. 1999. Molecularly imprinted polymers in chemical and biological sensing. Biochem. Soc. Trans. **27:** 344–350.
16. WIDMER, M.S., P.K. GUPTA, L. LU, et al. 1998. Manufacture of porous biodegradable polymer conduits. Biomaterials **19:** 1945–1955.
17. ZHANG, R. & P.X. MA. 2000. Synthetic nano-fibrilar extracellular matrices with predesigned macroporous architectures. J. Biomed. Mat. Res. **52:** 430–438.
18. LEITAO, E.R.D.S.F., Inventor. 1997. Nanotechnology forms for treatment of implant surface, Eur. Pat. Appl. EP 97-201424.
19. ITO, H., E. REICHMANIS, O. NALAMASU & T. UENO, Eds. 1998. Micro- and Nanopatterning Polymers. ACS Symp. Ser. 706.
20. VOLDMAN, J., M.L. GRAY & M.A. SCHMIDT. 1999. Microfabrication in biology and medicine. Ann. Rev. Biomed. Eng. **1:** 401–525.
21. FOLCH, A., N.-H. JO, O. HURTADO, et al. 2000: Microfabricated elastomeric stencils for micropatterning cell cultures. J. Biomed. Mat. Res. **52:** 346–353.
22. VAIDYA, R., L.M. TENDER, G. BRADLEY, et al. 1998. Computer-controlled laser ablation: a convenient and versatile tool for micropatterning bifuntional synthetic surfaces for applications in biosensing and tissue engineering. Biotechno. Progr. **14:** 371–377.
23. BHATIA, S. 1999. Microfabrication in Tissue Engineering and Bioartificial Organs. Kluwer Academic, Boston.
24. CHEN, C.S., M. MRKSICH, S. HUANG, et al. 1998. Micropatterned surfaces for control of cell shape, position, and function. Biotechnol. Progr. **14:** 356–363.
25. WALBOOMERS, X.F., H.J.E. CROES, L.A. GINSEL & J.A. JANSEN. 1998. Growth behavior of fibroblasts on microgrooved polystyrene. Biomaterials **19:** 1861–1868.
26. TURNER, A.M.P., N. DOWELL, S.W.P. TURNER, et al. 2000. Attachment of astroglial cells to microfabricated pillar arrays of different geometries. J. Biomed. Mat. Res. **51:** 430–441.
27. GOODMAN, S.L., P.A. SIMS & R.M. ALBRECHT. 1996. Three-dimensional extracellular matrix textured biomaterials. Biomaterials **17:** 2087–2095.
28. SHI, H., W.-B. TSAI, M.D. GARRISON, et al. 1999. Template-imprinted nanostructured surfaces for protein recognition. Nature **398:** 593–507.
29. BLAWAS, A.S. & W.M. REICHERT. 1998. Protein patterning. Biomaterials **19:** 595–609.
30. PUM, D. & U.B. SLEYTR. 1999. The application of bacterial S-layers in molecular nanotechnology. Trends Biotechnol. **17:** 8–12.
31. TAN, J., H. SHEN, K.L. CARTER & W.M. SALTZMAN. 2000. Controlling human polymorphonuclear leukocytes motility using microfabrication technology. J. Biomed. Mat. Res. **51:** 694–702.
32. ITO, Y. 1999. Surface micropatterning to regulate cell functions. Biomaterials **20:** 2333–2342.
33. ITO, Y., L.-S. LI, T. TAKAHASHI, et al. 1997. Enhancement of the mitogen effect by artificial juxtacrine stimulation using immobilized EGF. J. Biochem. **121:** 514–520.
34. TAKEZAWA, T., M. YAMAZAKI, Y. MORI, et al. 1992. Morphological and immunocytochemical characterization of a heterospheroid composed of fibroblasts and hepatocytes. J. Cell Sci. **101:** 495–501.
35. TAKEZAWA, T., A. ITO & Y. MORI. 1994. Histological observations of heterospheroid consisting of human dermal fibroblasts and human epidermal keratinocytes. Connect. Tissue **26:** 1110–1115.
36. MULDER, M.M., R.W. HITCHOCK & P.A. TRESCO. 1998. Skeletal myogenesis on elastomeric substrates: Implications for tissue engineering. J. Biomat. Sci. Polymer Edn. **9:** 731–748.

37. ODDE, D.J. & M.J. RENN. 2000. Laser-guided direct writing of living cells. Biotechnol. Bioeng. **67:** 312–318.
38. ODDE, D.J. & M.J. RENN. 1999. Laser-guided direct writing for applications in biotechnology. Trends Biotechnol. **17:** 385–389.
39. ROSENGREN, A., N. DANIELSEN & L.M. BJURSTEN. 1999. Reactive capsule formation and soft-tissue implants is related to cell necrosis. J. Biomed. Mat. Res. **46:** 458–464.
40. SANDERS, J.E., C.E. STILES & C.L. HAYES. 2000. Tissue response to single-polymer fibers of varying diameters: evaluation of fibrous encapsulation and macrophage density. J. Biomed. Mat. Res. **52:** 231–237.
41. OWICKI, J.C. & J.W. PARCE. 1992. Biosensors based on the energy metabolism of living cells: the physical chemistry and cell biology of extracellular acidification. Biosens. Biolectr. **7:** 255–272.
42. PIZZICONI, V.B. & D.L. PAGE. 1997. A cell-based immunosensor with engineered molecular recognition—Part I: Design feasibility. Biosens. Bioelectr. **12:** 287–299.
43. KEMP, R.B. & Y. GUAN. 1997. Heat flux and the calorimetric-respirometric ratio as measures of catabolic flux in mammalian cells. Themochim. Acta **300:** 199–211.
44. TAYLOR, L.C. & D.R. WALT. 2000. Application of high-density optical microwell arrays in a live-cell biosensing system. Anal. Biochem. **178:** 132–142.
45. ANONYMOUS. 1996. Biomolecular Self-Assembling Materials. Scientific and Technological Frontiers. National Academy Press. Washington, DC.
46. LAVAL, J.-M., P.-E. MAZERAN & D. THOMAS. 2000. Nanobiotechnology and its role in the development of new analytical devices. Analyst **125:** 29–33.
47. CORNELL, B.A., V.L.B. BRAACH-MAKSVYTLS, L.G. KING, et al. 1997. A biosensor that uses ion-channel switches. Nature **387:** 580–583.
48. SCHMIDT, C., M. MAYER & H. VOGEL. 2000. A chip-based biosensor for the functional analysis of single ion channels. Angew. Chem. Int. Ed. **39:** 3137–3140.
49. RASSCHAERT, J. & W.J. MALAISSE. 1999. Expression of the calcium-sensing receptor in pancreatic islet B-cells. Biochem. Biphys. Res. Commun. **264:** 615–618.
50. MORISHIGE, K., A. INANOBE, Y. YOSHIMOTO, et al. 1999. Secretagogue-induced exocytosis recruits G protein-gated $K^+$ channels to plasma membrane in endocrine cells. J. Biol. Chem. **274:** 7969–7974.
51. TRESCO, P.A., R. BIRAN & M.D. NOBLE. 2000. Cellular transplants as sources for therapeutic agents. Advan. Drug. Del. Revs. **42:** 3–27.
52. REDDI, A.H. 1998. Role of morphogenetic proteins in skeletal tissue engineering and regeneration. Nature Biotechnol. **16:** 247–252.
53. CHENG, H., Y. CAO & L. OLSON. 1996. Spinal cord repair in adult paraplegic rats: Partial restoration of hind limb function. Science **273:** 510–513.
54. KING, T.W. & C.W. PATRICK, JR. 2000. Development and in vitro characterization of vascular endothelial growth factor (VEGF)-loaded poly(DL-lactic-co-glycolic acid)/poly(ethylene glycol) microspheres using a solid encapsulation/single emulsion/solvent extraction technique. J. Biomed. Mat. Sci. **51:** 383–390.
55. PROKOP, A., E. KOZLOV, S.N. NON, et al. 2001. Towards retrievable vascularized bioartificial pancreas (VBAP): induction and long-lasting stability of polymeric mesh implant vascularized with help of fibroblast growth factors a and b and hydrogel coating. J. Biomed. Mat. Res. **3:** 245–261.
56. ALLEN, C., A. EISENBERG & D. MAYSINGER. 1999. Copolymer drug carriers: conjugates, micelles and microspheres. STP Pharma Sci. **9:** 139–151.
57. NAKACHE, E., N. POULAIN, F. CANDAU, et al. 2000. Biopolymer and polymer nanoparticles and their biomedical applications. In Handbook of Nanostructured Materials and Nanotechnology. H.S. Nalwa, Ed.: 577–634. Academic Press, New York.
58. PROKOP, A., C.A. HOLLAND, E. KOZLOV & R.D. TANNER. 2001. Water-based nanoparticulate polymeric system for protein delivery: physical and chemical characterization. Biotechnol. Bioeng. In press.
59. CAPPELLO, J., J.W. CRISSMAN, M. SRISSMAN, et al.1998. In situ self-assembling protein polymer gel systems for administration, delivery, and release of drugs. J. Control. Rel. **53:** 105–117.

60. PETKA, W.A., J.L. HARDEN, K.P. MCGRATH, et al. 1998. Reversible hydrogels from self-assembling artificial proteins. Science **281:** 389–392.
61. LEON, E.J., N. VERMA, S. ZHANG, et al. 1998. Mechanical properties of a self-assembling oligopeptide matrix. J. Biomat. Sci. Polymer Edn. **9:** 297–312.
62. VAUTHIER-HOLZSCHERER, C., S. BENABBOU, G. SPENLEHAUR, et al. 1991. Methodology for the preparation of ultra-dispersed polymer systems. STP Pharma Sci. **1:** 109–116.
63. ALLEN, C., D. MAYSINGER & A. EISENBERG. 1999. Nano-engineering block copolymer aggregates for drug delivery. Coll. Surf. Biointerfaces **16B:** 3–27.
64. MULLER, R.H. & K. PETERS. 1998. Nanosuspensions for the formulation of poorly soluble drugs. I. Preparation by size-reduction technique. Int. J. Pharm. **160:** 229–237.
65. CRUZ, T., R. GASPAR, A. DONATO & C. LOPES. 1997. Interaction between polyalkylcyanoacrylate nanoparticles and peritoneal macrophages: MTT metabolism, NBT reduction, and NO production. Pharm. Res. **14:** 73–79.
66. BONADIO, J. 2000. Tissue engineering via local gene delivery: Update and future prospects for enhancing the technology. Advan. Drug Del. Revs. **44:** 185–194.
67. BESTER, T.H. 2000. Gene silencing as a threat to the success of gene therapy. J. Clin. Invest. **105:** 409–441.

# Index of Contributors

**A**ksenova, N., 180–186
Ammon, H.P.T., 271–276
Angelova, N., 350–361, 456–471

**B**artkowiak, A., 120–134
Basta, G., 240–251
Becchetti, E., 240–251
Becker, H.D., 271–276
Bergstrand, K., 398–419
Bernard, P., 456–471
Binette, T.M., 47–61
Bonner-Weir, S., 96–119
Bruce, A., 398–419
Brunetti, P., 240–251
Brunnenmeier, F., 199–215
Bucher, P., 373–387

**C**alafiore, R., 240–251
Calvitti, M., 240–251
Cameron, D.F., 420–428
Canaple, L., 350–361, 456–471
Capitani, S., 240–251
Cassell, O.C.S., 429–442
Ceausoglu, I., 456–471
Cheng, L.L., 96–119
Cline, G.W., 96–119
Colton, C.K., 96–119
Cortesi, R., 160–179
Cottet, S., 267–270

**D**emirag, A., 373–387
Desvergne, B., 350–361
Dorian, R., 252–266
Dornish, M., 388–397
Doser, M., 271–276
Drury, O., 398–419
Dufour, J.M., 47–61
Dupraz, P., 267–270

**E**hler, E., 135–143
Enderle, A., 271–276
Eppenberger, H.M., 135–143
Espevik, T., 216–225
Esposito, E., 160–179

**F**air, J., 398–419
Fissell, W.H., 284–295
Fuhr, G., 199–215
Funatsu, K., 344–349
Funke, A., 284–295

**G**erber, D., 398–419
Gerlach, J.C., 308–319
Gill, R.G., 35–46
Gounarides, J.S., 96–119
Gray, D.W.R., 226–239
Gupta, S., 398–419

**H**aase, A., 199–215
Hamilton, G., 398–419
Hendrich, C., 199–215
Hillgärtner, M., 199–215
Hoffman, A.S., 62–73
Humes, H.D., 284–295
Hunkeler, D., i, 1–6, 7–17, 350–361, 456–471
Hurley, J.V., 429–442
Hushen, J.J., 420–428

**I**jima, H., 277–283, 344–349
Ikada, Y., 296–307
Ioannis Constantinidis, 83–95
Isidorov, R., 180–186
Iwata, H., 296–307, 443–455

**J**arema, M.A.C, 96–119
Jork, A., 199–215

Kaplan, D., 388–397
Kardassis, D., 308–319
Katsuno, T., 344–349
Kawakami, K., 277–283, 344–349
Kimball, J., 284–295
King, S.R., 252–266
Kleinman, H.K., 429–442
Knight, K.R., 429–442
Ko, I.K., 443–455
Kolokoltsova, T., 180–186
Korbutt, G.S., 47–61
Kubota, H., 334–343, 398–419
Kulseng, B., 216–225

Lakey, J., 252–266
LeCluyse, E., 398–419
Lembert, N., 271–276
Long, Jr., R., 83–95
Lou, J., 373–387
Luca, G., 160–179, 240–251
Ludlow, J., 398–419
Luntz, T., 398–419

MacDonald, J.M., 334–343
MacKay, S., 284–295
Magyar, J.P., 135–143
Messina, A., 429–442
Mimietz, S., 199–215
Ming Swi Chang, T., 362–372
Morel, P., 373–387
Morrison, W.A., 429–442
Moss, N., 398–419

Nakazawa, K., 344–349
Nastruzzi, C., 160–179
Nazian, S.J., 420–428
Nechaeva, E.A., 180–186
Nemir, M., 135–143
Neri, L.M., 240–251
Noguchi, A., 344–349
Nosé, Y., 18–34
Nöth, U., 199–215
Nurdin, N., 350–361

Oberholzer, J., 373–387
Obermeyer, N., 308–319
Ono, T., 277–283
Ono, T., 344–349

Papas, K.K., 96–119
Park, Y.-G., 296–307
Patzer II, J.F., 320–333
Penington, A.J., 429–442
Perera, J.M., 429–442
Perriard, J.-C., 135–143
Petersen, P., 271–276
Planck, H., 271–276
Poncelet, D., 74–82
Prokop, A., 472–490

Rehor, A., 456–471
Reid, L.M., 144–159, 334–343, 398–419
Renken, A., 456–471
Rilo, H., 252–266
Rindisbacher, L., 456–471
Ris, F., 373–387
Rokstad, A.M., 216–225
Romeo, R., 429–442
Roos, E.S., 96–119
Roy-Chowdhury, I., 334–343
Ryabicheva, T., 180–186

Safley, S., 83–95
Sainz Vidal, D., 187–198
Sakai, S., 277–283
Sambanis, A., 83–95
Sanberg, P.R., 420–428
Saporta, S., 420–428
Sauer, I.M., 308–319
Schuldt, U., 456–471
Shapiro, M.J., 96–119
Shulman, G.I., 96–119
Skaugrud, Ø., 388–397
Skjåk-Bræk, G., 216–225
Smolina, M., 180–186
Stankevich, R., 180–186
Steinert, A., 199–215

# INDEX OF CONTRIBUTORS

Stevens, G.W., 429–442
Storrs, R., 252–266
Strand, B.L., 216–225
Susick, R., 398–419
Suter, N., 135–143

**T**heruvath, T., 308–319
Thompson, E.W., 429–442
Thorens, B., 267–270
Thürmer, F., 199–215
Toso, C., 373–387
Triponez, F., 373–387

**V**araksin, N., 180–186
Vilesov, A., 180–186

**W**andrey, C., 187
Weber, C., 83–95
Weber, M., 199–215
Weir, G.C., 96–119
Wesche, J., 271–276
Westphal, I., 199–215
White, J., 398–419
Willing, A., 420–428
Wolfe, S.P., 334–343
Wu, H., 96–119

**X**u, A.S.I., 144–159

**Z**immermann, H., 199–215
Zimmermann, U., 199
Zschocke, P., 271–276